The Burdens of Mental Disorders

Global Perspectives from the WHO World Mental Health Surveys

Edited by

Jordi Alonso
IMIM – Institut Hospital del Mar d'Investigacions Mèdiques, Barcelona, Spain

Somnath Chatterji
World Health Organization, Geneva, Switzerland

Yanling He
Shanghai Mental Health Center, Shanghai, People's Republic of China

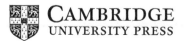

CAMBRIDGE UNIVERSITY PRESS
Cambridge, New York, Melbourne, Madrid, Cape Town,
Singapore, São Paulo, Delhi, Mexico City

Cambridge University Press
The Edinburgh Building, Cambridge CB2 8RU, UK

Published in the United States of America by Cambridge University Press, New York

www.cambridge.org
Information on this title: www.cambridge.org/9781107019287

© World Health Organization 2013

First published 2013

Printed and bound in the United Kingdom by the MPG Books Group

A catalog record for this publication is available from the British Library

Library of Congress Cataloging in Publication data
The burdens of mental disorders : Global Perspectives from the WHO world mental health surveys / edited by Jordi Alonso,
Somnath Chatterji, Yanling He.
   p. ; cm.
Includes bibliographical references and index.
ISBN 978-1-107-01928-7 (Hardback)
I. Alonso, J. (Jordi)   II. Chatterji, Somnath.   III. He, Yanling, 1962–   IV. World Health Organization.
[DNLM: 1. Health Surveys.   2. Mental Disorders.   3. Cost of Illness.   4. World Health. WM 140]
362.19689–dc33

                                                                                          2012045050

ISBN 978-1-107-01928-7 Hardback

Contents

Acknowledgments

The editors would like to acknowledge the amazing efforts of all the investigators, staff members, and others who help with all aspects of the WHO World Mental Health (WMH) surveys. Only a fraction of those involved in this work are listed as authors of the chapters included in this volume, and we are merely representatives of the many people who made this important project a reality. We would like to express our gratitude also to those who helped with the preparation of this volume. In particular, we thank Gemma Vilagut and Masha Petukhova for their invaluable collaboration, particularly their crucial analyses and checks which assured data accuracy and reliability. Also Colleen Bouzan and Alison Hoffnagle for the myriad of institutional, professional, and administrative activities and information supplied. Additional thanks for their contribution to the collaborators at IMIM – Hospital del Mar Medical Research Institute in Barcelona, Núria Duran, Gabi Barbaglia, Oleguer Pares, Raquel Gómez, Carme Gasull, and Puri Barbas. Also, to collaborators at the Harvard Health Care Program in Boston, Jerry Garcia, Nancy Sampson, and Eric A. Bourke. At Cambridge University Press in the UK, thanks to Joanna Chamberlin.

This project was carried out in conjunction with the World Health Organization World Mental Health (WMH) Survey Initiative. We thank the WMH staff for assistance with instrumentation, fieldwork, and data analysis. These activities were supported by the National Institute of Mental Health (NIMH R01MH070884, R01MH077883), the John D. and Catherine T. MacArthur Foundation, the Pfizer Foundation, the US Public Health Service (R13-MH066849, R01-MH069864, R01-DA016558), the Fogarty International Center (FIRCA R03-TW006481), the Pan American Health Organization, the Eli Lilly and Company Foundation, Ortho-McNeil Pharmaceutical, GlaxoSmithKline, and Bristol-Myers Squibb. A complete list of all within-country and cross-national WMH publications can be found at www.hcp.med.harvard.edu/wmh.

The São Paulo Megacity Mental Health Survey is supported by the State of São Paulo Research Foundation (FAPESP) Thematic Project Grant 03/00204-3. The Bulgarian Epidemiological Study of common mental disorders (EPIBUL) is supported by the Ministry of Health and the National Center for Public Health Protection. The Chinese World Mental Health Survey Initiative is supported by the Pfizer Foundation. The Shenzhen Mental Health Survey is supported by the Shenzhen Bureau of Health and the Shenzhen Bureau of Science, Technology, and Information. The Colombian National Study of Mental Health (NSMH) is supported by the Ministry of Social Protection. The ESEMeD project is funded by the European Commission (Contracts QLG5-1999-01042, SANCO 2004123, EAPH 20081308), the Piedmont Region (Italy), Fondo de Investigación Sanitaria, Instituto de Salud Carlos III, Spain (FIS 00/0028), Ministerio de Ciencia y Tecnología, Spain (SAF 2000-158-CE), Departament de Salut, Generalitat de Catalunya, Spain, Instituto de Salud Carlos III (CIBER CB06/02/0046, RETICS RD06/0011 REM-TAP), and other local agencies, and by an unrestricted educational grant from GlaxoSmithKline. The Epidemiological Study on Mental Disorders in India was funded jointly by the Government of India and WHO. Implementation of the Iraq Mental Health Survey (IMHS) and data entry were carried out by the staff of the Iraqi MOH and MOP with direct support from the Iraqi IMHS team, with funding from both the Japanese and European Funds through United Nations Development Group Iraq Trust Fund (UNDG ITF). The Israel National Health Survey is funded by the Ministry of Health with support from the Israel National Institute for Health Policy and Health Services Research and the National Insurance Institute of Israel. The World Mental Health Japan (WMHJ) Survey is supported by the Grant for

Research on Psychiatric and Neurological Diseases and Mental Health (H13-SHOGAI-023, H14-TOKUBETSU-026, H16-KOKORO-013) from the Japan Ministry of Health, Labor, and Welfare. The Lebanese National Mental Health Survey (LEBANON) is supported by the Lebanese Ministry of Public Health, the WHO (Lebanon), the Fogarty International Center (FIRCA R01-TW006481), anonymous private donations to IDRAAC, Lebanon, and unrestricted grants from Janssen Cilag, Eli Lilly, GlaxoSmithKline, Roche, and Novartis. The Mexican National Comorbidity Survey (MNCS) is supported by the National Institute of Psychiatry Ramon de la Fuente (INPRFMDIES 4280) and by the National Council on Science and Technology (CONACyT-G30544-H), with supplemental support from the Pan American Health Organization (PAHO). The New Zealand Mental Health Survey (NZMHS) is supported by the New Zealand Ministry of Health, the Alcohol Advisory Council, and the Health Research Council. The Nigerian Survey of Mental Health and Wellbeing (NSMHW) is supported by the WHO (Geneva), the WHO (Nigeria), and the Federal Ministry of Health, Abuja, Nigeria. The Northern Ireland Study of Mental Health was funded by the Health & Social Care Research & Development Division of the Public Health Agency. The Portuguese Mental Health Study was carried out by the Department of Mental Health, Faculty of Medical Sciences, Universidade Nova de Lisboa, with the collaboration of the Portuguese Catholic University, and was funded by the Champalimaud Foundation, the Gulbenkian Foundation, the Foundation for Science and Technology (FCT), and the Ministry of Health. The Romanian WMH study projects "Policies in Mental Health Area" and "National Study regarding Mental Health and Services Use" were carried out by the National School of Public Health & Health Services Management (former National Institute for Research & Development in Health, present National School of Public Health Management & Professional Development), Bucharest, with technical support from Metro Media Transylvania, the National Institute of Statistics – National Center for Training in Statistics, SC Cheyenne Services SRL, Statistics Netherlands, and were funded by the Ministry of Public Health (former Ministry of Health) with supplemental support of Eli Lilly Romania SRL. The South Africa Stress and Health Study (SASH) is supported by the US National Institute of Mental Health (R01-MH059575) and the National Institute of Drug Abuse, with supplemental funding from the South African Department of Health and the University of Michigan. The Ukraine Comorbid Mental Disorders during Periods of Social Disruption (CMDPSD) study is funded by the US National Institute of Mental Health (R01-MH61905). The US National Comorbidity Survey Replication (NCS-R) is supported by the National Institute of Mental Health (NIMH; U01-MH60220), with supplemental support from the National Institute of Drug Abuse (NIDA), the Substance Abuse and Mental Health Services Administration (SAMHSA), the Robert Wood Johnson Foundation (RWJF; Grant 044780), and the John W. Alden Trust.

Contributors

Núria Duran Adroher
CIBER en Epidemiología y Salud
Pública (CIBERESP), IMIM – Institut
Hospital del Mar d'Investigacions Mèdiques,
Barcelona, Spain

Sergio Aguilar-Gaxiola, MD, PhD
Center for Reducing Health Disparities,
University of California Davis School of Medicine,
Davis, CA, USA

Jordi Alonso, MD, PhD
Epidemiology and Public Health Program, IMIM –
Institut Hospital del Mar d'Investigacions Mèdiques;
Pompeu Fabra University (UPF); CIBER en
Epidemiología y Salud Pública (CIBERESP),
Barcelona, Spain

Ali Obaid Al-Hamzawi, MD
World Health Organization, Al-Qadisia University/
College of Medicine, Diwania Teaching Hospital,
Diwania, Iraq

Laura Helena Andrade, MD, PhD
Department and Institute of Psychiatry,
University of São Paulo Medical School, São
Paulo, Brazil

Matthias C. Angermeyer, MD, PhD
Center for Public Mental Health, Gösing am Wagram,
Austria

James Anthony, PhD
Department of Epidemiology, Michigan State
University, East Lansing, MI, USA

Corina Benjet, PhD
National Institute of Psychiatry Ramón de la Fuente
Muñiz, Mexico City, Mexico

Guilherme Borges, ScD
National Institute of Psychiatry Ramón de la
Fuente Muñiz, Mexico City, Mexico

Joshua Breslau, PhD, ScD
RAND Corporation, Pittsburgh, PA, USA

Evelyn J. Bromet, PhD
Department of Psychiatry and Behavioral
Science, Stony Brook University, Stony Brook,
NY, USA

Ronny Bruffaerts, PhD
Research Group Psychiatry, Katholieke Universiteit
Leuven, Leuven, Belgium

Brendan Bunting, PhD
Psychology Research Institute, University of Ulster,
Londonderry, Northern Ireland, UK

Huibert Burger, MD, PhD
University Medical Center Groningen, Groningen,
the Netherlands

José Miguel Caldas de Almeida, MD
Departamento de Saúde Mental, Faculdade de
Ciências Médicas, Universidade Nova de Lisboa,
Lisboa, Portugal

Graça Cardoso, MD, PhD
Departamento de Saúde Mental, Faculdade de
Ciências Médicas, Universidade Nova de Lisboa,
Lisboa, Portugal

Somnath Chatterji, MD
Multi-Country Studies, Health Statistics and
Information Systems (HSI), World Health
Organization, Geneva, Switzerland

Wai Tat Chiu, MA
Department of Health Care Policy, Harvard Medical
School, Boston, MA, USA

Giovanni de Girolamo, MD
IRCCS Fatebenefratelli, Brescia, Lombardy, Italy

Ron de Graaf, MSc, PhD
Netherlands Institute of Mental Health and Addiction,
Utrecht, the Netherlands

Peter de Jonge, PhD
University Medical Center Groningen, Groningen, the Netherlands

Koen Demyttenaere, MD, PhD
Research Group Psychiatry, Katholieke Universiteit Leuven, Leuven, Belgium

John Fayyad, MD
Child and Adolescent Psychiatry, Institute for Development, Research, Advocacy, and Applied Care (IDRAAC); Department of Psychiatry and Clinical Psychology, St. George Hospital University Medical Center, Beirut, Lebanon

Alize J. Ferrari
Queensland Centre for Mental Health Research, Wacol, Queensland, Australia

Silvia Florescu, MD, PhD
Public Health Research and Evidence Based Medicine Department, National School of Public Health and Health Services Management, Bucharest, Romania

Anne M. Gadermann, PhD
The Human Early Learning Partnership, University of British Columbia, Vancouver, BC, Canada

Meyer Glantz, PhD
Division of Epidemiology Statistics and Prevention Research (DESPR), National Institutes on Drug Abuse, Bethesda, MD, USA

Jen Green, PhD
School of Education, Boston University, Boston, MA, USA

Michael J. Gruber, MS
Department of Health Care Policy, Harvard Medical School, Boston, MA, USA

Oye Gureje, MSc
Department of Psychiatry, University of Ibadan, College of Medicine, Ibadan, Nigeria

Josep Maria Haro, MD, MPH, PhD
Parc Sanitari Sant Joan de Déu, Sant Boi de Llobregat, Barcelona, Spain

Yanling He, MD
Department of Epidemiology, Shanghai Mental Health Center, Wan Ping Nan Lu, Shanghai, People's Republic of China

Steven G. Heeringa, PhD
Institute for Social Research, University of Michigan, Ann Arbor, MI, USA

Hristo Hinkov, MD
National Center for Public Health and Analysis, Sofia, Bulgaria

Chiyi Hu, MD, PhD
Shenzhen Institute of Mental Health & Shenzhen Kangning Hospital, Shenzhen, People's Republic of China

Yueqin Huang, MD, MPH, PhD
Institute of Mental Health, Peking University, Beijing, People's Republic of China

Irving Hwang, MA
Department of Health Care Policy, Harvard Medical School, Boston, MA, USA

Robert Jin, MD, PhD
Department of Health Care Policy, Harvard Medical School, Boston, MA, USA

Elie G. Karam, MD
Department of Psychiatry & Clinical Psychology, Balamand University, Faculty of Medicine, St. George Hospital University Medical Center; Institute for Development, Research, Advocacy and Applied Care (IDRAAC), Beirut, Lebanon

Norito Kawakami, MD, PhD
School of Public Health, University of Tokyo, Tokyo, Japan

Ronald C. Kessler, PhD
Department of Health Care Policy, Harvard Medical School, Boston, MA, USA

Lola Kola, MSc
Department of Psychiatry, University of Ibadan College of Medicine, Ibadan, Nigeria

Viviane Kovess-Masféty, MD, PhD
Department of Epidemiology and Paris Descartes University Research Unit, EHESP – School of Public Health, Rennes, France

Michael C. Lane, PhD
Department of Health Care Policy, Harvard Medical School, Boston, MA, USA

Carmen Lara, MD, PhD
Autonomous University of Puebla, Puebla, Mexico

William LeBlanc, PhD
Department of Health Care Policy, Harvard Medical School, Boston, MA, USA

Sing Lee, MBBS, FRCPsych
Department of Psychiatry, The Chinese University of Hong Kong, Prince of Wales Hospital, Hong Kong, People's Republic of China

Jean-Pierre Lépine, MD, HDR
Hôpital Lariboisière Fernand Widal, Assistance Publique Hôpitaux de Paris; INSERM U 705, University Paris Diderot and Paris Descartes, Paris, France

Daphna Levinson, PhD
Research and Planning, Mental Health Services, Ministry of Health, Jerusalem, Israel

Zhaorui Liu, MD, MPH
Institute of Mental Health, Peking University, Beijing, People's Republic of China

Gustavo Loera, EdD
Center for Reducing Health Disparities, University of California Davis School of Medicine, Davis, CA, USA

Herbert Marschinger, PhD
Institute of Social Medicine, Occupational Health and Public Health, Public Health Research Unit, University of Leipzig, Leipzig, Germany

Katie A. McLaughlin, PhD
Children's Hospital Boston, Boston, MA, USA

Maria Elena Medina-Mora, PhD
National Institute of Psychiatry Ramón de la Fuente Muñiz, Mexico City, Mexico

Elizabeth Miller, MD, PhD
Division of Adolescent Medicine, Children's Hospital of Pittsburgh, University of Pittsburgh Medical Center, Pittsburgh, PA, USA

Samuel D. Murphy, DrPH
Psychology Research Unit, University of Ulster, Londonderry, Northern Ireland, UK

Aimee Nasser Karam, PhD
Department of Psychiatry & Clinical Psychology, Balamand University, Faculty of Medicine, St. George Hospital University Medical Center; Institute for Development, Research, Advocacy and Applied Care (IDRAAC), Beirut, Lebanon

Matthew K. Nock, PhD
Department of Psychology, Harvard University, Cambridge, MA, USA

Mark A. Oakley Browne, MBChB, PhD, FRANZCP
Statewide and Mental Health Services, Department of Health and Human Services; Division of Psychiatry, School of Medicine, The University of Tasmania, Australia

Siobhan O'Neill, PhD
Psychology Research Unit, University of Ulster, Londonderry, Northern Ireland, UK

Johan Ormel, PhD
Department of Psychiatric Epidemiology, University Medical Center Groningen, Groningen, the Netherlands

Beth-Ellen Pennell, MA
Institute for Social Research, University of Michigan, Ann Arbor, MI, USA

Maria V. Petukhova, PhD
Department of Health Care Policy, Harvard Medical School, Boston, MA, USA

José Posada-Villa, MD
Instituto Colombiano del Sistema Nervioso, Bogotá, Colombia

Rajesh Sagar, MD
Department of Psychiatry, All India Institute of Medical Sciences, New Delhi, India

Mohammad Salih Khalaf, MD
Day Care and Rehabilitation Center, Ibn Seena Teaching Hospital, Mosul, Iraq

Nancy A. Sampson, BA
Department of Health Care Policy, Harvard Medical School, Boston, MA, USA

Kathleen Saunders, JD
Goup Health Research Institute, Seattle, WA, USA

Michael Schoenbaum, PhD
RAND Corporation, Santa Monica, CA, USA

Kate M. Scott, PhD
Department of Psychological Medicine, Dunedin
School of Medicine, Otago University, Dunedin,
New Zealand

Soraya Seedat, MD
Department of Psychiatry, Stellenbosch University,
and MRC Research Unit on Anxiety and Stress
Disorders, Cape Town, South Africa

Victoria Shahly, PhD
Department of Health Care Policy, Harvard Medical
School, Boston, MA, USA

Dan J. Stein, MD, PhD
Department of Psychiatry, University of Cape Town,
Cape Town, South Africa

Hisateru Tachimori, PhD
National Center of Neurology and Psychiatry,
Kodaira, Tokyo, Japan

Nezar Ismet Taib, MD
Mental Health Center-Duhok, Duhok, Kurdistan
Region, Iraq

Adley Tsang, BSoSc
Hong Kong Mood Disorders Center, The
Chinese University of Hong Kong; Prince of
Wales Hospital, Hong Kong, People's Republic
of China

T. Bedirhan Üstün, MD, PhD
World Health Organization, Geneva, Switzerland

Maria Carmen Viana, MD, PhD
Universidad Federal de Espirito Santo, Departamento
de Medicina Social, Vitoria, Brazil

Gemma Vilagut, MSc
Health Services Research Group, IMIM – Institut
Hospital del Mar d'Investigacions Mèdiques; CIBER
en Epidemiología y Salud Pública (CIBERESP),
Barcelona, Spain

Michael R. Von Korff, ScD
Group Health Cooperative, Center for Health Studies,
Seattle, WA, USA

J. Elisabeth Wells, PhD
Department of Public Health and General Practice,
University of Otago, Christchurch, New Zealand

Harvey A. Whiteford, MD
School of Population Health, University of
Queensland, Herston, Queensland, Australia

David R. Williams, PhD, MPH
Department of Society, Human Development, and
Health, Harvard University, Boston, MA, USA

Ben Wu, MS
Department of Health Care Policy, Harvard Medical
School, Boston, MA, USA

Miguel Xavier, MD, PhD
Faculdade de Ciências Médicas, Universidade Nova de
Lisboa, Lisboa, Portugal

Alan M. Zaslavsky, PhD
Department of Health Care Policy, Harvard Medical
School, Boston, MA, USA

Chapter

1

Burdens of mental disorders: the approach of the World Mental Health (WMH) surveys

Jordi Alonso, Somnath Chatterji, Yanling He, and Ronald C. Kessler

Introduction

The concept of global burden of disease was first publicized in a landmark report commissioned by the World Bank (1993). The measure developed in that report to operationalize the definition of disease burden was designed to assess the gap in the health of a population, taking into account not only mortality but also the non-fatal consequences of injury and disease. This was accomplished by creating a single summary measure that combined the number of years lost due to premature mortality with the number of years "lost" due to living with disabling non-fatal conditions. As a continuation of that work, the World Health Organization (WHO) and Harvard University published the Global Burden of Disease (GBD) study (Murray & López 1996) in an effort to provide systematic estimates of the leading causes of death globally and to combine these estimates with the leading causes of disability. The GBD study took exhaustive measurements of the disability-adjusted life years (DALYs) lost due to more than 100 diseases and 19 risk factors. The first publication of the GBD study estimated that in 1990 unipolar major depression was the fourth leading cause of the loss of DALYs worldwide (3.7%), exceeded only by respiratory infections (8.2%), diarrheal diseases (7.2%), and perinatal conditions (6.7%). Projections estimate that unipolar major depression will be the number one leading cause of total disability worldwide by the year 2030 (World Health Organization 2008). The GBD made it very clear, almost for the first time, that mental disorders are a major challenge to global health. A totally renewed set of GBD estimates for the year 2010, with more conditions and risk factors, was released at the end of 2012 (Murray et al. 2012).

A subsequent systematic review of epidemiological studies on mental disorders examined estimates of frequency (one-year prevalence), risk of mortality, and disability associated with 10 mental disorders (Eaton et al. 2007). In that review, the one-year prevalence of major depressive disorders (median of 42 studies) was 5.3% of the adult population, with a median excess risk of mortality of 70% (OR = 1.7) and a disability weighting between 0.35 (0 [worst] to 1 [best]) and a Sheehan Disability Score of 58 (0 [worst] to 100 [best]). Because of their high prevalence and associated significant disability, the review estimated that the cost of mental disorders in Western countries were huge. In Europe, the total cost of mental disorders in 2011 was estimated to be €461 billion (nearly €1,000 per inhabitant) (Gustavsson et al. 2011). Of those, 39% corresponded to direct medical costs (due to the use of professional services, medical interventions, and medication), 13% to other direct non-medical services, and almost half (48%) to indirect costs (those incurred due to sick leave, early retirement, and premature death) (Gustavsson et al. 2011). Affective disorders, and especially unipolar depression, alone accounted for more than half of the indirect costs, indicating the considerable toll such disorders place on European social productivity.

The World Mental Health surveys approach to the burden of mental disorders

Initiated a decade after the GBD study, the WHO World Mental Health (WMH) surveys, with over 121,000 respondents surveyed across 24 different countries, is the largest ongoing cross-national series of community epidemiological surveys of mental disorders ever carried out (Kessler & Üstün 2008). The WMH surveys represent an important contribution to

The Burdens of Mental Disorders, ed. Jordi Alonso, Somnath Chatterji, and Yanling He. Published by Cambridge University Press. © World Health Organization 2013.

the body of knowledge on the global burden of mental disorders, as they assess the prevalence of these disorders using the most comprehensive and sophisticated instrument available, the WHO Composite International Diagnostic Interview (CIDI) version 3.0 (Kessler & Üstün 2004) and thoroughly and comparably evaluate disabilities across many countries. (At the time of the publishing of this volume, additional WMH surveys have been completed and others are under way or planned in other countries, but the data are not yet ready for presentation.)

The WMH surveys have some particular strengths in terms of their contribution to the body of knowledge on the burdens of mental disorders, including the large size and geographical representativeness of their samples, the exhaustive and well-standardized evaluation of disorders and health outcomes, and the use of sophisticated analytical approaches capable of accurately estimating the population distribution of the consequences of disease. As detailed in Chapter 2 of the present volume, respondents from 24 countries covering all six WHO world regions have been studied. Using common well-established measures and strictly standardized data collection procedures, the community-based epidemiological surveys carried out within the WMH project can be used to estimate diminished functioning and negative long-term consequences attributable to a wider range of mental disorders than considered in the GBD study. In addition, while the GBD study focuses on decrements in current health and mortality associated with the health conditions, the WMH data allow for the consideration of a much wider range of adverse outcomes. For example, the WMH examines the long-term effects of early-onset mental disorders on educational attainment and earnings as well as on marital timing, stability, and quality.

A particular innovation of the WMH analyses reported in this volume is the assessment of the consequences of mental disorders at both the individual and societal levels. While the first level allows inferences to be made about those who suffer from a particular disorder, the second level, which also takes into account the prevalence of the disorder, provides information more closely related to public health. The inclusion of both levels in the analysis should make this volume an important empirical contribution to public health decision-making. A final significant feature of this volume is that for a good part of the health consequences assessed, a broad range of both

mental disorders and chronic physical conditions were analyzed. The inclusion of both types of health problems represents quite a unique opportunity to identify the disorders that are most closely linked to impairments at the community level, as well as the domains of functioning and long-term consequences.

Three compilations of the results of the WMH surveys have already been published. The first described epidemiologic information on mental disorders, including prevalence and use of services (Kessler & Üstün 2008). The second focused on the epidemiology of coexisting mental and physical disorders, covering risk factors, consequences, and implications for research (Von Korff *et al.* 2009). The third presented and discussed a wealth of data on the prevalence, onset, persistence, risk, protective factors, and treatment of suicidal behaviors (Nock *et al.* 2012).

In this volume we describe and discuss a wide range of consequences associated with mental disorders across the life course of the individuals who have participated in the WMH surveys. Many relevant outcomes that are affected by mental disorders are considered in the domains of *personal disadvantages*, *productivity losses*, *disability*, and *worsened perceived health* (Figure 1.1). Each end of the figure depicts the main variables of interest in our analyses (i.e., mental disorders and the relevant outcomes). The figure also includes some of the possible intermediate variables that the vast body of literature suggests may play a role in the association between the two.

In Section 2 of this volume, we assess the extent to which early-onset mental disorders impact the individual and give rise to long-lasting *personal disadvantages*. To do so we considered only mental disorders with onset prior to the outcome of interest and apply a survival analysis approach to the data. Chapter 3 provides new information concerning how parental psychopathology is related to mental disorders in offspring: most of the parental disorders examined are indeed associated with an increased risk for every class of offspring mental disorder. This pattern is evident even after controlling for the presence of comorbid parental disorders, as well as for number of parent disorders. Chapter 4 shows that early-onset mental disorders are associated with a decreased likelihood of satisfactory educational attainment at each of the educational periods (primary, secondary, and college entry and termination). These results suggest that some of the later-life effects attributed to lower educational attainment should be considered, at

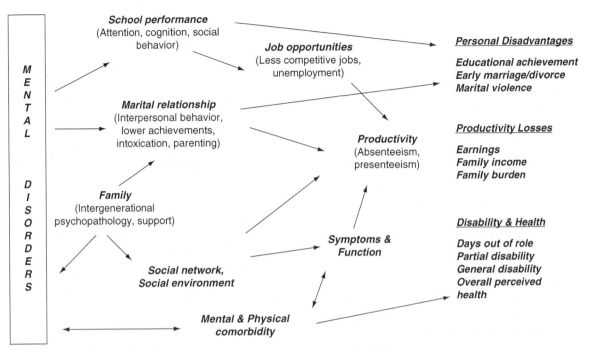

Figure 1.1 Intermediate and final outcomes of the impact of mental disorders in the WMH surveys.

least in part, consequences of early-onset mental disorders. Chapters 5 and 6 describe how early-onset mental disorders affect marital status and quality. Our results suggest that mental disorders reduce the amount of time people spend in marital relationships both by reducing the likelihood that they will marry and, more importantly, by increasing the likelihood that they will divorce or separate after marrying. No single disorder or group of disorders accounts for the majority of this pattern of associations, but many different disorders are involved. The second of these two chapters also reveals that mental disorders developed prior to marriage are associated with a significantly elevated risk of marital violence in most of the countries studied. The final chapter in Section 2, Chapter 7, expands the analysis of life-course consequences of early mental disorders by showing that these are associated with a significantly elevated risk of a wide range of adult-onset chronic physical conditions, such as heart disease, asthma, arthritis, chronic back pain, and severe headache. Taken together, the results shown in Section 2 provide compelling evidence for the widespread existence of diverse personal disadvantages associated with early-onset mental disorders across the full range of countries considered in the WMH surveys.

The next section of the volume, Section 3, is devoted to another important set of consequences of mental disorders: *productivity loss*. Frequently under-evaluated, productivity loss is a major disease burden, which, from a purely economic point of view, might justify intense investments in health restoration (Suhrcke *et al.* 2008). Chapter 8 focuses on the reduction of individual earnings among those with serious mental disorders. Our data show that individuals with serious mental illness earn, on average, almost one-third less than others in the population (29% in high-income countries to 31% in low/lower-middle-income countries). Chapter 9 presents data documenting a strong association of common early-onset mental disorders (in this particular case defined as disorders present before completion of educational attainment) with current household income, after adjusting for education. This association is considerably stronger in high-income than in upper-middle-income countries, and not significant at all in low/lower-middle-income countries. Chapter 10 estimates the population-level contribution of both serious mental and serious physical conditions to the family burden associated with the full range of health problems affecting first-degree relatives. We consider both the psychological burden (e.g., worry, embarrassment) and the objective burden. The latter is defined in terms of time and finances devoted to informal caregiving activities. As the chapter shows, these objective burdens are substantial and mental disorders greatly contribute to them. As a whole, the results in Section 3 provide compelling evidence of the considerable decreases in productivity associated with mental disorders.

The largest section in this volume, Section 4, compares the relative importance of mental disorders and selected chronic physical conditions for disability and perceived health. *Disability* is comprehensively assessed and analyzed in this section, with the objective of evaluating the contribution of mental and physical disorders as thoroughly as possible at both the individual and the societal level. Comorbidity (i.e., the co-occurrence of disorders) is carefully taken into account in each of the chapters in this section. In an attempt to capture significant disability, Chapter 11 considers only the number of days that respondents reported that they were totally unable to perform their primary activities. Neurological disorders and several mental disorders (e.g., bipolar and post-traumatic stress) are responsible for a high number of days out of role at the individual level, while at the societal level pain conditions are the main contributors. In Chapter 12 we consider "partial" disability (that is, days performing normal activities in lesser amounts, or performing them worse and/or with extreme effort), where we found similar results. In all, the mental disorders considered in the WMH surveys can be considered responsible for about 15–17% of disability at the societal level. Next, Chapter 13 describes the interference with daily functioning of each particular disorder using the Sheehan Disability Scale (SDS) (Leon *et al.* 1997). The SDS assesses activities in four role domains (home management, ability to work, social life, and ability to manage personal relationships) and our results show that interference ratings are generally higher for mental disorders than for physical disorders, due to a higher degree of social interference. Importantly, the same chapter describes how the use of health services among sufferers from mental and physical disorders is considerably lower among those with mental disorders, even when their disability is more severe; these trends are common in both high- and low-income countries. Chapter 14 presents data suggesting that when disabilities are measured with a comprehensive instrument, such as the World Health Organization's Disability Assessment Schedule 2.0

(WHODAS 2) (Üstün *et al.* 2010), mental disorders are found to contribute to more than 25% of disability at the societal level, in particular in middle- and higher-income countries. The final two chapters of the section deal with the impact of mental disorders and chronic physical conditions on *perceived health*. Chapter 15 shows that, in general, physical conditions are more strongly associated with perceived health than mental disorders, especially when societal distribution is considered. Chapter 16 attempts to establish the mediating role of disability in the association between disease and perceived health. More than a third of the effect of disease on perceived health is mediated by the WHODAS disabilities. Importantly, mediating subdomains are different for the health effects of mental disorders (mediated by role function but also by social influences and stigmas) than for the health effects of chronic physical conditions (mediated by role functioning and mobility).

The final section of this volume, Section 5, is devoted to considering several of the implications of our results. Chapter 17 looks at the similarities, differences, and complementarity of our data with the burden information from the GBD study, in particular the 2010 edition. It underlines the respective strengths and limitations of each study in terms of their contributions to the field of public health. While the WMH study is more comprehensive at the population level and more methodologically homogeneous, the GBD study is more comprehensive at the disorder level and yields data on epidemiological estimates other than prevalence, such as incidence, remission, duration, and excess mortality. In Chapter 18 we identify the most relevant implications of the results presented in this volume for mental health policy and service practice. These implications include the need to invest in mental health services worldwide and to apply a more thorough understanding of the burdens of mental disorders to improving the planning, organization, provision, and evaluation of health services devoted to mental health problems.

Strengths and limitations of the WMH surveys

As mentioned above, the WMH surveys have several strengths that make them a unique source of information on the epidemiology of mental disorders across the globe. Some general strengths include the large size of the overall sample, which results in greater precision when analyzing relatively rare phenomena such as some of the less prevalent disorders studied in this volume, and the geographical amplitude and representativity of the samples surveyed, which allow for international comparisons to be made. In this volume, data are shown not only for the overall participating sample, but also for three broad categories of countries according to their income level, in keeping with the classification of the World Bank (2008): low/lower-middle-, upper-middle-, and high-income countries. International comparisons are of particular value since the epidemiological evidence about common mental disorders is mostly based on studies conducted in Western countries. Finally, the WMH surveys use exhaustive and well-standardized evaluations of disorders and health outcomes, as discussed in detail in Chapter 2. This standardization process, which encompasses everything from survey design to data collection methods, database implementation, and data analysis, represents an unprecedented contribution to the validity and interpretability of the epidemiology of mental disorders across the globe.

A second set of strengths is related to the use of sophisticated analytical approaches which result in an accurate estimate of the population distribution of the consequences of disease. The analysis of the effects of lifetime mental disorders on role transitions has shown that lifetime disorders are *time-varying*; that is, a given disorder may have started at different ages for different respondents. As a result, in order to maintain the temporal sequence between predictors and outcomes, timing must be taken into consideration in estimating risk-factor models. This is done in the discrete-time survival analysis by coding each year of each respondent's life separately for each lifetime disorder. Another innovative approach of the WMH surveys is the inclusion of comorbidity (both mental and physical) in the analysis of the association between disorders and the various outcomes addressed in this volume. In particular, whether comorbid conditions have an additive or a *sub-additive effect* (i.e., that the level of association between a specific disorder and an outcome increases with each additional coexisting disorder, but it does so at a decreasing rate) has been tested in a number of analyses. Chapters 11–16 use this type of approach. These analytic methods are described in more detail in Chapter 2.

Along with these strengths, a number of limitations call for necessary caution in the interpretation of the results of the WMH surveys presented in this volume.

While limitations specific to particular topics are addressed in each chapter concerned, an overall review of the major general limitations is presented below.

WMH data were collected retrospectively, relying on respondent recall, rather than prospectively. Recall bias of the occurrence of mental disorders would generally tend towards under-reporting, as some respondents cannot remember well enough to respond accurately and in full (Wells & Horwood 2004). Recall bias also affects the age-of-onset of mental disorders parameter (Simon & Von Korff 1995), which is relevant for several of the chapters in Section 2 of this volume, dealing with individual disadvantages associated with mental disorders starting early in life (early-onset mental disorders). The task of recalling symptoms over the course of a lifetime is more difficult for older respondents than for younger respondents, simply because they have to remember across longer periods of time. In addition, respondents whose current mental health is poor may be more likely to report having had poor mental health in the past than respondents whose current mental health is good. Due to this recall bias, the respondents who report disorders are more likely to have more severe and persistent disorders compared to the actual group of people with a lifetime disorder in the general population. These biases may result in overestimating the impact of mental disorders on the outcomes of interest, such as educational attainment or chronic physical conditions. Also, reporting accuracy may differ across countries, because of differences in the extent to which mental disorders are stigmatized.

A source of bias that limits the analyses which include both mental and physical disorders is that they were differently assessed. While mental disorders were thoroughly evaluated with the CIDI 3.0, chronic physical conditions were assessed using self-report condition checklists. Although there is generally good agreement between self-reporting of medical diagnoses and physician or medical-record confirmation of those diagnoses (Kriegsman *et al.* 1996), bias assessment cannot be ignored. The direction of such bias is unclear, and there may also be variations across countries.

It is important to note that only a restricted set of the most common mental and physical conditions was included. In particular, some burdensome conditions, such as dementia and psychosis, were not included. Some infectious diseases that are serious and prevalent in many countries were not included among the physical conditions checklist. While the physical and mental conditions considered in this volume are amongst those most commonly reported in previous population studies, an expansion and disaggregation of these conditions is clearly needed in future studies. At any rate, the burdens of mental disorders included in this volume should be considered an underestimation of the real overall account.

Other limitations involve participation rates and the particular assumptions of the analysis undertaken in this volume, which are extensively discussed in Chapter 2. While the WMH surveys are not free of limitations, the researchers are deeply convinced that these limitations do not override the results as reported here, as considerable caution has been exerted in their interpretation.

Global perspectives

This volume is the result of the countless, continued efforts of a large consortium of researchers, many other collaborating professionals, and, above all, a large cohort of survey participants. Its goal is to improve our knowledge of the many ways mental disorders impose different burdens on human beings. It is our deepest hope that this volume provides clear and relevant new information and that it helps strengthen arguments for the importance of developing interventions to lower the individual and societal burdens of mental disorders throughout the world.

References

Eaton, W. W., Martins, S. S., Nestadt, G., *et al.* (2008). The burden of mental disorders. *Epidemiologic Reviews* **30**, 1–14.

Gustavsson, A., Svensson, M., Jacobi, F., *et al.* (2011). Cost of disorders of the brain in Europe 2010. *European Neuropsychopharmacology* **21**, 718–79.

Kessler, R. C. & Üstün, T. B. (2004). The World Mental Health (WMH) Survey Initiative version of the World Health Organization (WHO) Composite International Diagnostic Interview (CIDI). *International Journal of Methods in Psychiatric Research* **1**, 93–121.

Kessler, R. C. & Üstün, T. B. (2008). *The WHO World Mental Health Surveys: Global Perspectives on the Epidemiology of Mental Disorders*. New York, NY: Cambridge University Press.

Kriegsman, D. M., Penninx, B. W., van Eijk, J. T., Boeke, A. J. P., & Deeg, D. J. H. (1996). Self-reports and general practitioner information on the presence of chronic diseases in community dwelling elderly. A study on the accuracy of patients' self-reports and on determinants of inaccuracy. *Journal of Clinical Epidemiology* **49**, 1407–17.

Leon, A. C., Olfson, M., Portera, L., *et al.* (1997). Assessing psychiatric impairment in primary care with the Sheehan Disability Scale. *International Journal of Psychiatry in Medicine* **27**, 93–105.

Murray, C. J. & López, A. D. (1996). Evidence-based health policy: lessons from the Global Burden of Disease study. *Science* **274**, 740–3.

Murray, C. J., Vos, T., Lozano, R., *et al.* (2012). Disability-adjusted life years (DALYs) for 291 diseases and injuries in 21 regions, 1990–2010: a systematic analysis for the Global Burden of Disease Study 2010. *Lancet* **380**, 197–223.

Nock, M. K., Borges, G., & Ono, Y. (2012). *Suicide: Global Perspective from the WHO World Mental Health Surveys*. New York, NY: Cambridge University Press.

Simon, G. E. & Von Korff, M. (1995). Recall of psychiatric history in cross-sectional surveys: implications for epidemiologic research. *Epidemiologic Reviews* **17**, 221–7.

Suhrcke, M., Arce, R. A., McKee, M., & Rocco, L. (2008). *Economic Costs of Ill Health in the European Region*. Copenhagen: World Health Organization.

Üstün, T. B., Kostanjsek, N., Chatterji, S., & Rehm, J. (2010). *Measuring Health and Disability: Manual for WHO Disability Assessment Schedule (WHODAS 2.0)*. Geneva: World Health Organization.

Von Korff, M. R., Scott, K. M., & Gureje, O. (2009). *Global Perspectives on Mental–Physical Comorbidity in the WHO World Mental Health Surveys*. New York, NY: Cambridge University Press.

Wells, J. E. & Horwood, L. J. (2004). How accurate is recall of key symptoms of depression? A comparison of recall and longitudinal reports. *Psychological Medicine* **34**, 1001–11.

World Bank (1993). *World Development Report 1993: Investing in Health*. Oxford: Oxford University Press.

World Bank (2008). Data and statistics. http://go.worldbank.org/D7SN0B8YU0. Accessed May 12, 2009.

World Health Organization (2008). *The Global Burden of Disease: 2004 Update*. Geneva: WHO.

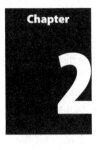

Chapter 2

Methods of the World Mental Health surveys

Ronald C. Kessler, Somnath Chatterji, Steven G. Heeringa,
Beth-Ellen Pennell, Maria V. Petukhova, Gemma Vilagut, and
Alan M. Zaslavsky

The World Mental Health (WMH) Survey Initiative is a World Health Organization (WHO) initiative designed to help countries carry out and analyze epidemiological surveys of the burden of mental disorders in their populations (www.hcp.med.harvard. edu/wmh). Twenty-eight countries have so far completed WMH surveys, and others are in progress. The vast majority of these surveys are nationally representative, although a few are representative of only a single region (e.g., the São Paulo Metropolitan Area in Brazil) or regions (e.g., six metropolitan areas in Japan). Results from 25 surveys carried out in 24 of those countries are reported in this volume. These are all the surveys that have so far been completed and processed, and between them they interviewed a total of 121,899 respondents. The participating countries are grouped into three income levels according to the World Bank (2008). Six of these countries (seven surveys) are classified as low-income or lower-middle-income (Colombia, India–Pondicherry, Iraq, Nigeria, People's Republic of China [PRC]–Beijing/Shanghai, PRC–Shenzhen, Ukraine), six are upper-middle-income (Brazil–São Paulo, Bulgaria, Lebanon, Mexico, Romania, South Africa), and twelve are high-income countries (Belgium, France, Germany, Israel, Italy, Japan, the Netherlands, New Zealand, Northern Ireland, Portugal, Spain, the USA). Some results in this volume are presented stratified by the three income levels.

All WMH surveys use the same standardized procedures for sampling, interviewing, and data analysis. They also all use the same diagnostic interview, the WHO Composite International Diagnostic Interview (CIDI) version 3.0 (Kessler & Üstün 2004, Haro et al. 2008). The CIDI is a fully structured research diagnostic interview designed for use by trained lay

interviewers who do not have clinical experience. It generates diagnoses of mental disorders according to the definitions and criteria of both the International Classification of Diseases (ICD) and Diagnostic and Statistical Manual of Mental Disorders (DSM) systems, although only DSM-IV criteria are used here. Consistent WHO translation, back-translation, and harmonization procedures were used to modify the CIDI for use in each WMH country (Harkness et al. 2008). The same interviewer training materials, training programs, and quality-control monitoring procedures were also used across WMH surveys to guarantee cross-survey comparability of data (Pennell et al. 2008).

The use of these standardized procedures is key to the success of WMH, as the main mission of WMH is to allow countries that might not otherwise be able to implement mental health needs assessment surveys to do so by building on the existing WMH infrastructure. The use of standardized materials reduces costs for each country and makes it easier to implement high-quality surveys by building on tried and true procedures. This applies not only to instrument development and data collection but also to analysis, as WMH uses a centralized data processing and cross-national peer consultation model that allows less experienced collaborators to work with world-class psychiatric epidemiologists and statisticians to analyze, interpret, and write scientific reports about their data.

The current chapter presents information about these standardized materials and procedures. We begin by reviewing the WMH sample design. We then present an overview of the measures that are the focus of this volume. Field procedures are discussed next. The final section discusses the statistical methods used in this volume to assess the burdens of mental disorders.

The WMH sample designs

The sampling procedures used in the WMH surveys are closely related to those originally developed for the World Fertility Survey (WFS) program, one of the first and largest efforts to coordinate a global gathering of survey data (Verma *et al.* 1980). The decisions made in developing sample designs for the WMH surveys drew heavily on the lessons of the WFS experience. Like the WFS and more recent successful international programs of community survey research, the WMH surveys required collaborating countries to employ probability sample designs to select nationally or regionally representative samples of adults for the survey interview. The aim of sampling in the WMH surveys was to obtain a representative sample of the household population in the country or region under study. This usually involved drawing a multistage clustered area probability sample of households in the population and then selecting one, or in some cases two, respondents from each sampled household using probability methods without replacement. These sample designs were standardized across countries based on the principles of probability sampling, but with less emphasis placed on the specific probability sample design features employed across countries, in recognition of the fact that countries varied widely in the information available to develop a sample frame from which the WMH sample could be selected.

In order to achieve the level of coordination in sampling required across countries, we established a WMH Data Collection Coordination Centre at the Institute for Social Research (ISR) at the University of Michigan in the USA. The Survey Research Center (SRC) at ISR is one of the leading academic survey research organizations in the world, with a long history of leadership in the development and implementation of large community surveys (www.src.isr.umich.edu). The Survey Sampling group at SRC, under the direction of Steve Heeringa, supervised WMH sampling, while the Survey Implementation group, under the supervision of Beth-Ellen Pennell, supervised WMH interviewer training and field implementation.

Focusing first on sampling, the SRC group began by developing a list containing a common set of requirements and performance standards that the probability sample design in each WMH survey was required to meet. Unique opportunities available in individual countries were then used to develop a sampling plan that achieved these requirements, and to meet the WMH standards. The staff of the WMH Data Collection Coordination Centre worked closely with local collaborators to develop these sample design plans. The plans were reviewed by a panel of technical experts and revised based on feedback from this panel. Once the design was finalized, day-to-day oversight of implementation was the responsibility of the local research team.

Most WMH countries developed a similar sampling plan that featured multistage area probability sampling. Several countries, however, adopted alternative probability sampling procedures, such as the use of a national registry or combined uses of area probability methods and registry sampling, to achieve the required probability sampling of the designated target population. All these samples, however, were probability samples. No WMH survey used a convenience sample, an interviewer-managed quota sample, or any other non-probability method of sample selection.

The target populations

Probability sample surveys are designed to describe a *target population* of elements that spans a specific geographic space during a specific window of time. Although it might seem obvious how to do this, a number of important considerations arise as soon as one begins to consider the possibilities. Should persons who were temporary residents, guest workers, or those who had legal claim to medical treatment or services be included in the sample? What about people who were incapable of participating in the survey because they were institutionalized, or cognitively or physically impaired, and people living in remote places that would require disproportionate amounts of survey resources to sample and interview? In the end, a decision was made to allow the answers to these questions to vary across countries within a range of options described as follows.

The *survey population* is defined as the subset of the target population that is truly eligible for sampling under the survey design (Groves *et al.* 2004). A decision was needed to decide what restrictions would apply in each participating WMH country to establish a survey population definition that would conform to the survey's scientific objectives, available sample frames, and budget limitations. Multiple dimensions were included here. One of these involved the age range of the sample. WMH was designed to focus on adults. However, the age that defines adulthood (commonly referred to as the "age of majority") varies across countries (most typically either 18 or 21 years old). In addition, some countries decided to impose an upper age limit on the sample (usually 65 years). Other dimensions that defined the survey population involved geographic scope limitations (most typically excluding otherwise eligible people who lived in remote areas of the country), language restrictions, citizenship requirements, and whether to include special populations such as persons living in military barracks and group quarters or persons who were institutionalized at the time of the survey (e.g., hospital patients, prison inmates). These varied somewhat across countries.

Table 2.1 provides a summary of the survey populations and samples for the WMH surveys included in this volume. Starting with the different age limits, the vast majority of the surveys had a minimum age of 18 years. The lowest minimum age was 16 (New Zealand) and the highest was 21 (Israel). For maximum age requirements, Colombia, Mexico, and the regional surveys carried out in Beijing and Shanghai mandated that respondents be no older than 65 or 70 years. Turning to the geographic scope of the survey population, 17 of the 25 surveys defined the geographic scope of their survey population as the entire country. Brazil, India, Japan, Nigeria, and the People's Republic of China restricted their survey populations to specific regions, states/provinces, or cities. Colombia and Mexico conducted national surveys but limited their survey to populations in urban places above a specified population size (e.g., more than 2,500 persons in Mexico).

Sampling frames

Probability sampling requires a sampling frame that provides a high level of coverage for the defined survey population. The sampling frame is defined as the list or equivalent enumeration procedure that identifies all population elements and enables the sampler to assign non-zero selection probabilities to each element (Kish 1965). We carefully reviewed the available choices of sample frames with the collaborators in each WMH country before deciding on a final frame. Options could have included population registries, new or existing area probability sampling frames, postal address lists, voter registration lists, and telephone subscriber lists. The final choice of the frame for each country was determined by a number of factors, including the extent of coverage and statistical efficiency of available frame alternatives, the cost of developing and using the frame for sample selection, and the experience of the data collection organization in the use of the sample frame.

The final sampling frames for the WMH surveys were generally of three types: (1) a database of individual contact information provided in the form of national population registries, voter registration lists, postal address lists, or household telephone directories; (2) a multistage area probability sample frame (Kish 1965); or (3) a hybrid multistage frame that combined area probability methods in the initial stages and a registry or population list in the penultimate and/or final stages of sample selection.

Complex sample designs for the WMH surveys

The goal of all survey sample designs is either to minimize sampling variance and bias for a fixed total cost or to minimize total cost while meeting predetermined analysis objectives. The analysis objectives are typically formulated as fixed targets for the variance and bias components of the total survey error for (a) key survey estimates or (b) the parameter estimates for important population models. In the WMH surveys, there was no single path to this goal. The surveys shared a set of common analysis objectives, primarily centered on the estimation of the population prevalence and correlates of mental disorders. Survey cost structures were highly variable from one country to another, depending on factors such as availability and accessibility of survey infrastructure (government or commercial survey organizations), availability and costs for databases and map materials required to develop sample frames, labor rates for field interviewers and team leaders, and transportation costs for getting trained interviewers to distributed samples of households. Total funding for the surveys also varied widely across countries. In many cases, funding restrictions limited not only the total size of the interviewed sample but also the scope of the survey populations or the use of costly sample design options.

The individual WMH sample designs employed the full range of probability sampling techniques that survey statisticians can use to improve sample precision and reduce costs. Stratification of the samples by geographic regions and demographic characteristics was used to increase sample precision and control sample allocation. Multistage designs with modest clustering in the initial stages of sampling were used to control travel time and expenses. A version of the "double sampling" technique (Cochran 1977) was used in the vast majority of surveys to determine the subsample of initial CIDI respondents

Table 2.1 Sample characteristics by country income level. The WMH surveys.[a]

Country income level	Survey[b]	Sample characteristics[c]	Field dates	Age range	Sample size				Sampling fraction (%) for FB[f]	Response rate[g]
					Part 1	Part 2[d]	Couples sample[e]	Family burden (FB) sample[f]		
I. All countries					121,899	63,678	1,821	43,732		72.0
II. Low/lower-middle										
Colombia	NSMH	All urban areas of the country (approximately 73% of the total national population)	2003	18–65	4,426	2,381		1,287	30	87.7
India–Pondicherry	WMHI	Pondicherry region	2003–5	18–97	2,992	1,373	79			98.8
Iraq	IMHS	Nationally representative	2006–7	18–96	4,332	4,332		4,332	100	95.2
Nigeria	NSMHW	21 of the 36 states in the country, representing 57% of the national population. The surveys were conducted in Yoruba, Igbo, Hausa, and Efik languages	2002–3	18–100	6,752	2,143	394	2,228	33	79.3
PRC[h]–Beijing/Shanghai	B-WMH S-WMH	Beijing and Shanghai metropolitan areas	2002–3	18–70	5,201	1,628				74.7
PRC–Shenzhen	Shenzhen	Shenzhen metropolitan area. Included temporary residents as well as household residents	2006–7	18–88	7,132	2,475	106	7,132	100	80.0
Ukraine[i]	CMDPSD	Nationally representative	2002	18–91	4,724	1,719				78.3
Total					35,559	16,051	579	14,979		
III. Upper-middle										
Brazil–São Paulo	São Paulo Megacity	São Paulo metropolitan area	2005–7	18–93	5,037	2,942	197	5,037	100	81.3
Bulgaria	NSHS	Nationally representative	2003–7	18–98	5,318	2,233	437	1,572	30	72.0
Lebanon	LEBANON	Nationally representative	2002–3	18–94	2,857	1,031	159	770	25	70.0
Mexico	M-NCS	All urban areas of the country (approximately 75% of the total national population)	2001–2	18–65	5,782	2,362		1,728	30	76.6
Romania	RMHS	Nationally representative	2005–6	18–96	2,357	2,357		2,357	100	70.9
South Africa[j]	SASH	Nationally representative	2003–4	18–92	4,315	4,315				87.1
Total					25,666	15,240	793	11,464		

IV. High

Belgium	ESEMeD	Nationally representative. The sample was selected from a national register of Belgium residents	2001–2	18–95	2,419	1,043	27	591	25	50.6
France	ESEMeD	Nationally representative. The sample was selected from a national list of households with listed telephone numbers	2001–2	18–97	2,894	1,436	10	738	25	45.9
Germany	ESEMeD	Nationally representative	2002–3	18–95	3,555	1,323		929	25	57.8
Israel	NHS	Nationally representative	2002–4	21–98	4,859	4,859		4,804	100	72.6
Italy	ESEMeD	Nationally representative. The sample was selected from municipality resident registries	2001–2	18–100	4,712	1,779	27	1,160	25	71.3
Japan	WMHJ2002–2006	Eleven metropolitan areas	2002–6	20–98	4,129	1,682				55.1
Netherlands	ESEMeD	Nationally representative. The sample was selected from municipal postal registries	2002–3	18–95	2,372	1,094		1,451	60	56.4
New Zealand[i]	NZMHS	Nationally representative	2003–4	18–98	12,790	7,312				73.3
Northern Ireland	NISHS	Nationally representative	2004–7	18–97	4,340	1,986		2,501	50	68.4
Portugal	NMHS	Nationally representative	2008–9	18–81	3,849	2,060		556	15	57.3
Spain	ESEMeD	Nationally representative	2001–2	18–98	5,473	2,121	35	1,353	25	78.6
USA	NCS-R	Nationally representative	2002–3	18–99	9,282	5,692	350	3,206	33	70.9
Total					60,674	32,387	449	17,289		

[a] World Bank (2008).

[b] NSMH, The Colombian National Study of Mental Health; WMHI, World Mental Health India; IMHS, Iraq Mental Health Survey; NSMHW, The Nigerian Survey of Mental Health and Wellbeing; B-WMH, The Beijing World Mental Health Survey; S-WMH, The Shanghai World Mental Health Survey; CMDPSD, Comorbid Mental Disorders during Periods of Social Disruption; NSHS, Bulgaria National Survey of Health and Stress; LEBANON, Lebanese Evaluation of the Burden of Ailments and Needs of the Nation; M-NCS, The Mexican National Comorbidity Survey; RMHS, Romania Mental Health Survey; SASH, South Africa Health Study; ESEMeD, The European Study of the Epidemiology of Mental Disorders; NHS, Israel National Mental Health Survey; WMHJ2002–2006, World Mental Health Japan Survey; NZMHS, New Zealand Mental Health Survey; NISHS, Northern Ireland Study of Health and Stress; NMHS, Portugal National Mental Health Survey; NCS-R, The US National Comorbidity Survey Replication.

[c] Most WMH surveys are based on stratified multistage clustered area probability household samples, in which samples of areas equivalent to counties or municipalities in the USA were selected in the first stage followed by one or more subsequent stages of geographic sampling (e.g. towns within counties, blocks within towns, households within blocks) to arrive at a sample of households, in each of which a listing of household members was created and one or two people were selected from this listing to be interviewed. No substitution was allowed when the originally sampled household resident could not be interviewed. These household samples were selected from census area data in all countries other than France (where telephone directories were used to select households) and the Netherlands (where postal registries were used to select households). Several WMH surveys (Belgium, Germany, Italy) used municipal resident registries to select respondents without listing households. The Japanese sample is the only totally unclustered sample, with households randomly selected in each of the 11 metropolitan areas and one random respondent selected in each sample household. Seventeen of the 25 surveys are based on nationally representative household samples.

[d] See the text of the chapter for a discussion of the difference between Part 1 and Part 2 samples. Only 62,971 Part 2 respondents were asked questions about chronic conditions, due to these questions being omitted inadvertently for 429 respondents in Lebanon and 278 in Northern Ireland.

[e] Couples surveys included a subsample of married or cohabiting couples. This was done by selecting a probability subsample of married respondents in the main survey and interviewing the spouse/partner of those respondents. The numbers reported in the column are the numbers of couples, not the numbers of individuals.

[f] Family burden sample. Nineteen surveys asked a probability subsample of respondents about the burdens associated with caring for ill first-degree relatives. This sample is used only in Chapter 13.

[g] The response rate is calculated as the ratio of the number of households in which an interview was completed to the number of households originally sampled, excluding from the denominator households known not to be eligible either because of being vacant at the time of initial contact or because the residents were unable to speak the designated languages of the survey. The weighted average response rate is 72.0%.

[h] PRC, People's Republic of China.

[i] For the purposes of cross-national comparisons we limit the sample to those aged 18+.

who would complete a more intensive set of questions about risk factors. We refer to the questions administered to all respondents as the *part 1* questions and those administered to only a subsample of respondents the *part 2* questions. This two-part approach is discussed in more detail in the next section of this chapter.

The variety of designs used in different WMH surveys is a reflection of the differences in the essential survey conditions faced by the collaborators. With the exception of a small number of studies that sampled adults directly from high-quality population registries, the great majority of WMH surveys used a multistage area probability sampling method. The population registry approach is very attractive when this option is available because it avoids within-household selection and weighting. A few other countries chose a first-stage probability sample of households directly from national postal lists (e.g., the Netherlands) or telephone directories (e.g., France) and then chose random respondents within the selected households. Germany used a two-stage design that involved a first-stage sampling of municipalities and a second-stage sampling of adults from population registries available within each of the selected municipalities. A number of other countries used a similar design but added an intermediate second-stage sampling of electoral or postal districts before selecting eligible adults from a district registry (e.g., Italy) or an enumerated list of residents within selected districts (e.g., Ukraine).

The vast majority of WMH surveys, though, used three-stage or four-stage area probability designs. The three-stage designs began with a primary-stage probability sample of census enumeration districts or neighborhood units selected with probabilities proportional to size, followed by a second-stage sampling of households within the first-stage units, and a third-stage random selection of an eligible adult within the sampled household. Countries that used four-stage designs expanded this same basic approach by beginning with the selection of large county or municipal units and then progressing to selection of area segment blocks, then to households, and then to respondents within households. All WMH surveys that used within-household selection of respondents did so with an objective household selection table method developed by Kish (1949). In a probability subsample of households in some countries, the spouses of selected respondents who were married were also selected to take part in the survey.

It is important to note that considerable effort was required to construct the frames for the WMH samples in countries where pre-existing survey frames did

not exist. In Lebanon, for example, area probability methods were used to build the frame and select a multistage sample, because only limited population data existed in Lebanon. The primary stage of sampling consequently selected area segments (sectors) from a comprehensive list developed by the WMH collaborators, stratified by region and urbanicity. From this list, 342 area segments were selected with probabilities proportional to size. Prior to the second stage of sampling, the Lebanese team sent trained field staff to each selected area segment to create a comprehensive list of all housing units in the segment. Once this enumerative list was completed for each area segment, a second-stage sample was selected of housing units and then of respondents within households.

The WMH guidelines specified a response rate target of 65%, based on a precise method required to calculate the response rate (American Association for Public Opinion Research 2011). This target response rate was achieved by 19 of the surveys, with seven having response rates in the range 70–75%, six in the range 75–80%, and five over 80%. The six surveys that failed to meet the target had response rates in the range 45.9–57.8%. It is noteworthy that these six were all high-income countries (Belgium, France, Germany, Japan, the Netherlands, and Portugal). This is consistent with other evidence that difficulties contacting respondents because they are away from the household are greatest in high-income countries, where people have a higher probability than elsewhere of being away from home in the evening and on weekends, and also that marketing surveys have become so common in high-income countries that the willingness of people to participate in surveys has declined substantially over time (Couper & de Leeuw 2003). Surveys remain sufficiently novel in lower-income countries that response rates are generally higher than in high-income countries. Survey response rates are, of course, also influenced by many other factors, including government privacy rules, population resistance to survey participation, the experience and norms of the chosen data collection organization, and availability of financial resources to invest in incentives or other refusal aversion efforts.

The two-part interview design

As noted above, in all the surveys except four (Iraq, Israel, Romania, and South Africa) the WMH interview was divided into two parts, with the questions in part 1 administered to all respondents and the questions in part 2 administered only to a probability subsample of respondents based on responses to the part 1 questions. The reason for doing this was that the total interview was quite long and sometimes required the interviewer to return to the respondent's household a second or even third time to complete the entire interview. As many respondents did not have any mental disorders, however, we did not need all of these non-cases to achieve maximum statistical power in comparing to cases. This meant that we could realize considerable cost saving by terminating the interview for a probability subsample of non-cases as soon as we learned that they did not meet criteria for any mental disorder. This was accomplished with the two-part interview design. The interview began with a series of basic descriptive warm-up questions and then evaluated lifetime presence of a wide range of core mental disorders. All (100%) of the respondents who met criteria for any of these disorders were continued into part 2, which included questions about a wide range of correlates of the core disorders and also assessed mental disorders of secondary interest. In addition, a probability subsample of the other part 1 respondents (i.e., those who did not meet criteria for any core disorder) were also selected to complete part 2, while interviews with the remaining non-cases were ended after the completion of the part 1 questions.

There has been a good deal of confusion on the part of some journal article reviewers about this two-part design, the most common concern being that the part 2 sample overestimates prevalence because it does not include all non-cases. This concern is unwarranted because the part 2 data are weighted to adjust for the under-sampling of part 1 cases. For example, if we included only a random one-quarter (0.25) of all part 1 non-cases in the part 2 sample in a given country, each of those part 2 non-cases would be assigned a weight of 4.0 (1.0/0.25) to compensate for their under-sampling. This means that if the estimated prevalence of a given lifetime mental disorder was 10% in the part 1 sample it would still be 10% in the weighted part 2 sample. In a similar way, estimates of the correlates of disorder would be expected to be unbiased in the part 2 sample compared to the part 1 sample.

However, the *precision* of these estimates might be lower in the part 2 sample due to the fact that the denominator sample size on which estimates were based would be smaller. Four observations are relevant with regard to precision. First, the precision of estimates increases at a decreasing rate as the number of non-cases increases relative to cases, with the optimal allocation 1:1

(Schlesselman 1982). The number of non-cases selected for the part 2 sample was generally in the range 15–33%, yielding more non-cases than cases of every single disorder in every survey. Second, the part 2 sample was post-stratified (a term explained later in the chapter) in order to adjust for any discrepancies that existed between the measured characteristics of the non-cases selected into part 2 and those not selected into part 2. Third, the certainty selections into part 2 included 100% not only of respondents with any lifetime core disorder but also of any subthreshold manifestation of the core disorders, increasing power to distinguish cases from near-cases. Fourth, probability of selection into part 2 among other non-cases was made in proportion to the number of eligible respondents in the sample household in all surveys that used household sampling. This is a subtle point that edges into the discussion of weighting later in this chapter. Briefly, though, the precision of an estimate is inversely related to the variance of sample weights. Both the probability of selection into part 1 and the conditional probability of selection into part 2 among part 1 respondents contribute to this total weight. The part 1 weight is inversely proportional to the number of eligible respondents in each household due to the fact that we selected only one respondent per household (with the exception of the small couples sample described in the next subsection of this chapter) no matter how many eligible people resided in the household. This led to an over-sampling of people living alone and an under-sampling of people living in married couples, and even more so of people living in households with three or more eligible respondents. The part 1 weight corrects for this differential representation. By sampling non-cases into part 2 with probabilities proportional to the number of eligible household members we were able partially to cancel out the variance in part 1 weights for non-cases. So, for example, while people living alone were over-represented in the part 1 sample (due to having a 100% chance of selection as the household respondent versus a 50% chance for people living with a spouse, a 33% chance for people living with a spouse and one other adult household resident, etc.), they were under-sampled in the selection of non-cases into the part 2 sample, making their proportion in the unweighted part 2 sample closer to their true population proportion than it was in the unweighted part 1 sample. The vast majority of the analyses reported in this volume are based on the part 2 sample. A description of the demographic characteristics of the part 2 sample is presented in Table 2.2. Briefly, mean age of the overall

Table 2.2 Characteristics of the sample by country income level. The WMH surveys (part 2 sample).

Country income level	N	Females		Not married		High school or more		Not working		Age	
		%	(SE)	%	(SE)	%	(SE)	%	(SE)	Mean	(SE)
All countries	63,678	52.0	(0.3)	36.6	(0.3)	57.4	(0.3)	42.0	(0.3)	42.2	(0.1)
Comparison among countries		1.2		20.3*		168.2*		74.6*		184.2*	
Low/lower-middle											
Colombia	2,381	54.5	(1.5)	43.4	(1.7)	46.4	(2.3)	46.4	(2.0)	36.6	(0.3)
India–Pondicherry	1,373	50.0	(1.6)	30.2	(2.1)	47.0	(1.9)	52.1	(1.5)	38.1	(0.6)
Iraq	4,332	49.7	(1.0)	34.4	(1.2)	35.3	(1.1)	59.2	(1.2)	36.9	(0.4)
Nigeria	2,143	51.0	(1.5)	39.7	(1.6)	35.6	(1.3)	31.1	(1.4)	35.8	(0.4)
PRC–Beijing/ Shangai	1,628	47.7	(1.8)	33.4	(1.7)	55.0	(1.6)	41.2	(2.2)	41.2	(0.6)
PRC–Shenzhen	2,475	50.3	(1.6)	46.2	(1.3)	49.4	(1.5)	8.5	(0.6)	29.1	(0.3)
Ukraine	1,719	55.1	(1.3)	34.9	(1.4)	81.9	(1.5)	45.6	(2.1)	46.1	(0.8)
Upper-middle											
Brazil–São Paulo	2,942	52.8	(1.5)	40.2	(1.6)	47.2	(1.3)	35.4	(1.1)	39.1	(0.5)
Bulgaria	2,233	52.2	(1.3)	25.7	(1.6)	64.2	(1.3)	50.4	(1.9)	47.8	(0.6)
Lebanon	1,031	50.5	(2.1)	40.1	(2.7)	40.2	(2.5)	49.3	(2.1)	39.9	(0.8)
Mexico	2,362	52.3	(1.9)	32.7	(1.5)	31.4	(1.7)	41.6	(1.6)	35.2	(0.3)
Romania	2,357	52.4	(1.3)	30.4	(1.2)	49.3	(1.7)	60.7	(1.3)	45.5	(0.5)
South Africa	4,315	53.6	(1.0)	49.7	(1.1)	37.8	(1.1)	65.1	(1.4)	37.1	(0.3)
High											
Belgium	1,043	51.7	(2.4)	30.2	(1.7)	69.7	(3.7)	42.2	(1.4)	46.9	(0.7)
France	1,436	52.2	(1.8)	29.0	(1.8)	–	–	37.9	(1.8)	46.3	(0.7)
Germany	1,323	51.7	(1.4)	36.7	(1.7)	96.4	(0.9)	43.5	(2.1)	48.2	(0.8)
Israel	4,859	51.9	(0.4)	32.2	(0.7)	78.3	(0.7)	39.8	(0.8)	44.4	(0.2)
Italy	1,779	52.0	(1.5)	33.3	(1.6)	39.4	(1.8)	46.1	(1.7)	47.7	(0.6)
Japan	1,682	53.0	(1.9)	31.2	(1.4)	71.6	(1.4)	36.5	(1.8)	51.2	(0.7)
Netherlands	1,094	50.9	(2.2)	27.9	(2.6)	69.7	(1.8)	37.7	(2.6)	45.0	(0.8)
New Zealand	7,312	52.2	(1.0)	34.8	(1.0)	60.4	(1.0)	31.2	(0.9)	44.6	(0.4)
Northern Ireland	1,986	52.2	(1.2)	40.2	(1.8)	88.8	(1.0)	37.4	(1.8)	45.4	(0.6)
Portugal	2,060	51.9	(1.5)	30.4	(1.4)	54.8	(1.7)	40.3	(1.5)	46.5	(0.7)
Spain	2,121	51.4	(1.7)	34.7	(1.5)	41.7	(1.5)	49.6	(1.8)	45.6	(0.7)
USA	5,692	53.1	(1.0)	44.1	(1.2)	83.2	(0.9)	33.2	(1.1)	45.0	(0.5)
Low/lower-middle	16,051	51.1	(0.6)	37.9	(0.6)	47.2	(0.6)	41.9	(0.6)	37.0	(0.2)
Upper-middle	15,240	52.7	(0.6)	38.1	(0.6)	44.4	(0.6)	51.8	(0.7)	40.2	(0.2)
High	32,387	52.2	(0.4)	35.2	(0.4)	69.2	(0.4)	37.5	(0.4)	45.7	(0.2)
Comparison of low/ lower-middle, upper-middle, high		2.1		10.7*		651.8*		179.8*		660.1*	

* Significant at the 0.05 level, two-sided test.

sample was 42.2 years of age, about 52% were female, just over a third of the overall sample individuals were not married, with more than half reporting completed high school or a more advanced educational level, and 42% were not working. As expected, mean age was lower and the education level was lower for low/lower-middle-income and upper-middle-income countries, while the proportion of respondents not working at the time of the interview was substantially lower in the high-income countries (about 38%).

Special subsamples

It is important to note that the 25 surveys are not all included in all chapters, since not all the variable(s) of interest were assessed in all surveys. For example,

Israel and New Zealand are not included in Chapter 3 because these two surveys did not assess parental psychopathology. In Appendix Table 2.1, a complete description of the surveys and information on the demographic characteristics of the participating sample in each of the chapters is shown.

In addition, specific subsamples of respondents were studied in some of the chapters. For instance, in Chapter 8, where the association of serious mental illness with personal earnings is assessed, only the subsample of respondents between 18 to 64 years of age was evaluated.

The WMH surveys include two special subsamples that deserve mention here because they are the focus of two chapters in the volume: the couples sample (Chapter 6) and the family burden sample (Chapter 10). The couples sample consists of 1,821 husband–wife pairs that were built into 11 of the surveys by sampling the spouses of a random sample of the married respondents who completed the WMH interview (Table 2.1). The purpose of creating this couples sample was to facilitate analysis of similarities and differences in the mental health of husbands and wives at the individual level. This rationale and the implications for our analyses are elaborated in Chapter 6. The family burden sample is different from the couples sample in that it did not involve adding new respondents, but rather only asking a special set of questions to a subsample of respondents. This subsample is quite large: a total of 43,732 respondents across 20 of the surveys (Table 2.1). We nonetheless refer to this as a separate sample to highlight the fact that the family burden questions were designed to think of respondents in quite a different way than in the rest of the survey. Specifically, while all other sections of the survey ask respondents about their own mental and physical health problems and we use these reports to estimate the effects of these problems on the various aspects of the lives of these people, the family burden section focuses on the effects of health problems on the family members of the ill person. If we continued to focus on the health problems of our survey respondents in pursuing this line of analysis, we would either have to ask our respondents to estimate the extent to which their health problems affected their family or, in keeping with previous research on family burden, we would have to carry out interviews with the family members of our ill respondents. As we considered the former (i.e., asking ill respondents to estimate the extent to

which their health problems affect their relatives) inadequate to the task and the latter (i.e., interviewing family members) beyond the scope of our study, we settled on a different approach: to think of our respondents as the family members experiencing burden and ask them to tell us about their ill relatives. As detailed in Chapter 10, we did this by asking a probability subsample of WMH survey respondents to enumerate their network of first-degree relatives, to report on the prevalence of mental and physical health problems experienced by these relatives, and to describe to us the various objective and subjective burdens associated with these family health problems.

Non-response surveys

Collaborators in all countries were encouraged to carry out systematic non-response surveys in an effort to evaluate and, to the extent possible, correct for the effects of systematic survey non-response. The basic design of the non-response survey was to select a stratified probability subsample of initial survey non-respondents who were approached one last time and asked to participate in a *brief* interview (typically 10–20 minutes of interview time) that would provide the investigators with basic information about people who were not able to participate in the full survey. Respondents were typically offered a financial incentive to participate in this brief survey. The survey was usually carried out either by telephone or face-to-face. The questions in the survey included a small number of basic sociodemographics (e.g., age, gender, education, marital status) and diagnostic stem questions for diagnoses of core mental and substance disorders. Importantly, identical questions were asked in the main survey. Comparison of responses to these questions in the main sample and the non-respondent sample was used to make inferences about non-response bias, while weighting adjustments described as follows were used to adjust the main sample for these biases.

Weighting

Person-level analysis weights that incorporated sample selection, non-response, and post-stratification factors were constructed for each WMH survey dataset. In a number of cases these weights were developed by survey statisticians on the individual country research teams, while weights were constructed in other cases by the staff of the WMH Data Analysis Coordination Centre at Harvard Medical School (HMS), Boston, USA, using sample design and population control data supplied by the local project teams. The case-specific analysis weights were used in computing estimates of descriptive statistics for the survey population and for estimating the descriptive statistics reported in this volume.

In general, the final analysis weight for each WMH survey respondent was computed as the product of the three weight components:

$$W_{final}, i = W_{sel,i} \cdot W_{nr,i} \cdot W_{psc,i}$$

where:

$W_{sel,i}$ = the selection weight factor for respondent $i = 1, \ldots, n$
$W_{nr,i}$ = the non-response weight adjustment factor for respondent $i = 1, \ldots, n$

and

$W_{psc,i}$ = the post-stratification factor for respondent $i = 1, \ldots n$

The exact sequence of weight calculation steps differed slightly across surveys. In some countries, a separate non-response adjustment step was skipped and the final weight was derived as the product of the sample selection factor and a final, all-encompassing, post-stratification to external population controls.

The sample selection weight was designed to compensate for the differing sampling probabilities for selecting individuals as WMH respondents. The selection weight factor, W_{sel}, is generally the product of the reciprocals of three probabilities: $W_{sel,hh}$, the reciprocal of the multistage probability of selecting the respondent's housing unit selection from the sample frame; $W_{sel,resp}$, the reciprocal of the conditional probability of selecting the WMH respondent at random within the eligible household (Kish 1965); and $W_{sel,Part\ 2}$, the reciprocal of the probability that an eligible WMH survey respondent was subsampled to complete the in-depth part 2 diagnostic section of the WMH interview.

The non-response adjustment weight, W_{nr}, could be computed to account for differential patterns of response across categories of eligible respondents for a country-specific survey. When this weight was applied, non-response adjustments to survey weights were based on endogenous data; that is, on data from the sample frame that was known for both sample respondents and non-respondents. In baseline or cross-sectional surveys such as the WMH studies described here, the data available to develop non-response adjustments is often limited to geographic and possibly demographic information available for respondents and non-respondents in the sample frame, such as population census data collected by the government.

In cases where non-response adjustment was implemented, a non-respondent survey of the sort described previously was used to generate this weight. The non-response sample was first weighted to be representative of all non-respondents using within-household probability of selection weights (see later), and then this weighted subsample was compared to the similarly weighted main sample in an effort to determine if the two samples differed meaningfully on the variables assessed in both samples. When differences of this sort were found, either a weighting class method or a propensity modeling approach (Little & Rubin 2002) was used to develop the adjustment factors.

The weight calculations for most of the WMH survey datasets, however, did not include a separate non-response adjustment. Instead, an adjustment for differential non-response and sample non-coverage of the survey population was integrated into one consolidated adjustment in the post-stratification weighting step, which is described later. In such cases, the factor W_{nr} can be viewed as taking a value of 1.0 in the final composite weight calculation. Readers who are interested in detailed case studies of non-response adjustment weighting for selected WMH datasets are referred to Kessler & Üstün (2004).

The final component in the WMH individual analysis weight is a post-stratification factor, W_{psc}. The post-stratification weighting adjustment differs from the non-response adjustment factors in that post-stratification weighting uses data that are exogenous to the survey design to calibrate the weights for survey estimation. The WMH post-stratification used estimates of population values from external sources such as a recent national census or demographic population estimation program to standardize the sampling weights to known population distribution values, such as the distribution of the population of the cross-classification of age (in categories), gender, and education. The logic of the general procedure used in each country involved forming a matrix of adjustment cells by cross-classifying age, gender, and major geographic regions (data permitting) of the survey population. Within each cell of this matrix, the post-stratification weight factors were computed as the ratio of the external population count for each cell to the sum of computed sample selection weights for the WMH survey cases assigned to that cell:

$$W_{pstrat,c,i} = \frac{\hat{N}_c}{\sum\limits_{i \in c}^{n_c} W_{sel,i} \cdot W_{nr,i}}$$

where:

$W_{pstrat,c,i}$ = the post-stratification factor for all cases in cell c

$\hat{N}_c$ = the WMH country population estimate for cell c

n_c = WMH country sample size in cell c

$W_{sel,i}$ = the composite sample selection weight for case $i = 1, \ldots, n_c$

$W_{nr,i}$ = the non-response adjustment for case $i = 1, \ldots, n_c$

In some countries, it was possible to include much more information than a few sociodemographic and geographic variables, because of the availability of much more detailed population data on a wide range of social and demographic variables that were also assessed in the WMH surveys. In cases of this sort, logistic regression analyses were carried out to compare the WMH survey data, with other weights imposed on the data, to the population data in an effort to pinpoint any variables that were meaningfully discrepant between the two. When the number of such variables was small, a modified post-stratification weighting of the sort described in the last paragraph could have been implemented using post-stratification tables constructed from only those variables. However, when a large number of post-stratification variables were available, we used as many of them as feasible in the post-stratification weighting step. This was based on the logistic regression equation that assigned a predicted probability of participation to each respondent based on a comparison of population data with survey data. This regression-based weighting approach tends to make the weighted sample more representative of the population and in particular to

avoid the risk when fewer variables are controlled of creating discrepancies between the weighted sample and the population on other variables that were originally non-discrepant. A cross-tabulation of many variables, in comparison, would create an excessive number of cells with small or zero sample size. Instead, in the regression-based approach, logistic regression analysis was able to produce a more stable estimate based on a dichotomous outcome that discriminated between the WMH sample and the population in an analysis that included both the sample data and individual-level population data. This prediction equation allowed for interactions among the post-stratification variables and sequentially evaluated a wide range of predictors, arriving at a final model that included core variables (i.e., age, gender, education, geography) and significant discriminating variables. Appropriately weighted predicted probabilities generated from this final equation were used to adjust the final WMH sample to approximate the multivariate distribution of the population on these variables.

Although post-stratification can potentially reduce sampling variances for survey estimates, the primary purpose of weighting is to eliminate potential sources of bias that would be present in an unweighted analysis. Those biases could arise due to differences in the original selection probabilities for respondents, differential non-response (probabilities of observation), and differential sample non-coverage for elements of the target population. However, the pursuit of "unbiasedness" can have a price in the form of increased variance of survey estimates compared to an unweighted estimate based on the same sample size. Weighting effects on standard errors arise due to several factors, including the association between the distributions of the weights and the variables of interest and variance of the weight values assigned to the individual cases. In the process of developing the final analysis weights for the WMH datasets, sensitivity analyses were conducted to determine the effect of extreme weight values on the estimated sampling errors and potential bias of key survey estimates. If sampling variances proved highly sensitive to the most extreme weight values, the computed weights in the extreme lower and upper ranges were trimmed using methods that retained the sum of weights but distributed those weights across cases at each tail of the distribution. This trimming was typically carried out for respondents with the highest and lowest 1–2% of weights, and in extreme cases for those in the highest and lowest 5% of weights. For a detailed example of how this was done in one WMH survey, see Kessler & Üstün (2004).

Sampling error and inference from the WMH surveys data

The WMH surveys are based on a variety of probability sample designs, with each design adapted to the unique resources, experiences, and cost structures of the collaborating countries. Despite the variations in probability sample design, each survey is designed to support robust, design-based estimation of population statistics, such as prevalence of mental health in a chosen survey population.

The survey literature refers to designs like the ones used in the WMH surveys as *complex designs*, a loosely used term meant to denote the fact that the sample incorporates special design features such as stratification, clustering, and differential selection probabilities (i.e., weighting) that analysts must consider in computing sampling errors and confidence intervals for sample estimates of descriptive statistics and model parameters. Standard programs in statistical analysis software packages assume simple random sampling (SRS) or independence of observations in computing standard errors for sample estimates. In general, the SRS assumption results in underestimation of variances of estimates of descriptive statistics and model parameters from surveys with clustered or multistage designs. This means that the confidence intervals based on computed variances that assume independence of observations will be biased (generally too narrow), and design-based inferences will be affected accordingly. This section focuses on sampling error estimation and construction of confidence intervals for WMH survey estimates of descriptive statistics such as means, proportions, ratios, and coefficients for linear and logistic regression models.

Over the past 50 years, advances in survey sampling theory have guided the development of a number of methods for estimating variances from complex sample datasets correctly. Several sampling error programs that implement these complex sample variance estimation methods are available to WMH data analysts. The two most common approaches are the Taylor Series Linearization (TSL) method (and corresponding approximation to its variance) and resampling variance estimation methods such as the Balanced Repeated Replication method and the Jackknife Repeated Replication (JRR) method (Rust 1985). The sampling error estimates presented in the substantive chapters of this volume were, for the most part, estimated in SUDAAN version 9 (Research Triangle Institute 2005) using the Taylor Series Linearization method, although some of the more complex estimates required the use of the JRR method, which we implemented in special SAS macros (SAS Institute Inc. 2008) written by staff of the WMH Data Collection Coordination Centre.

As noted earlier in this chapter in the discussion of the WMH sample designs, the WMH surveys, like most other sample designs in health-related surveys, use stratification and clustering. Stratification is introduced to increase the statistical and administrative efficiency of the sample. Sample elements are selected as clusters in multistage designs to reduce travel costs and improve interviewing efficiency. Disproportionate sampling of population elements may be used to increase the sample sizes for subpopulations of special interest, resulting in the need to employ weighting in the estimation of population prevalence or other descriptive statistics. Relative to simple random sampling, each of these complex sample design features influences the size of standard errors for survey estimates. Figure 2.1 illustrates the effects of these design features on standard errors of estimates. The curve plotted in this figure represents the SRS standard error of an estimate as a function of sample size. At any chosen sample size, the effect of sample stratification is generally a reduction in standard errors relative to SRS. Clustering of sample elements and designs that require weighting for unbiased estimation generally have larger standard errors than an SRS sample of equal size (Kish 1965).

The combined effects of stratification, clustering, and weighting on the standard errors of estimates are termed the *design effect* (D^2) and are measured by the ratio:

$$D^2 = \frac{SE(p)^2_{complex}}{SE(p)^2_{srs}} = \frac{Var(p)_{complex}}{Var(p)_{srs}}$$

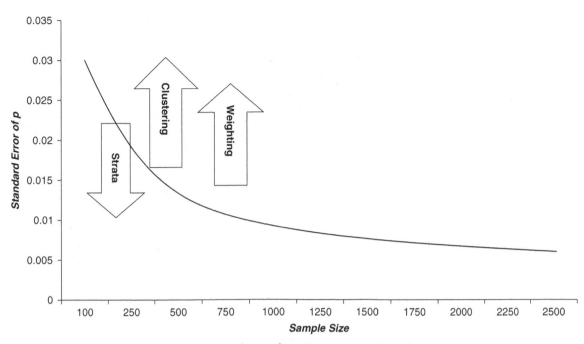

Figure 2.1 Complex sample design effects on standard errors of prevalence estimates (illustration for $p = 0.10$).
Originally appeared in Heeringa, S. G., Wells, J. E., Hubbard, F., *et al.* (2008). Sampling designs and sampling procedures. In R. C. Kessler & T. B. Üstün, eds., *The WHO World Mental Health Surveys: Global Perspectives on the Epidemiology of Mental Disorders.* New York, NY: Cambridge University Press, p. 29. © 2008, World Health Organization, reproduced with permission.

where:

D^2 = the design effect

$Var(p)_{complex}$ = the complex sample design variance of the sample statistic p

$Var(p)_{srs}$ = the simple random variance of p

Table 2.3 provides the design effects for estimates of the lifetime prevalence of the mental disorders that are the main focus of this volume. With only a small number of exceptions, design effects are greater than 1.0 but relatively modest in elevation, with the mean across countries being 1.2 for mood disorders, 1.2 for anxiety disorders, 1.0 for disruptive behavior disorders, 1.1 for substance disorders, and 1.3 for any disorder. The same general patterns hold for 12-month prevalence (see Appendix Table 2.2).

Design effects are for the most part somewhat larger when results are pooled across countries compared to when they are estimated within countries. For example, the range of mean design effects across outcomes in the total sample is 1.3–1.6 compared to 1.0–1.3 for within-country mean design effects. It needs to be remembered, however, that the sample size increases dramatically when data are combined across countries, resulting in substantial decreases in standard errors of estimates despite these relatively small increases in design effects.

Measures

Mental disorders

As noted earlier in this chapter, mental disorders were assessed with the WHO Composite International Diagnostic Interview (CIDI) version 3.0 (Kessler & Üstün 2004), a fully structured lay-administered research diagnostic interview. DSM-IV criteria were used in making diagnoses. There are 21 disorders considered in this volume. They include six mood disorders (bipolar I disorder, bipolar II disorder, dysthymia, major depressive disorder, minor depressive

Table 2.3 Design effects of lifetime prevalence estimates of major mental disorder categories by country income level. The WMH surveys.[a]

Country income level	Mood	Anxiety	Disruptive behavior	Substance	Any disorder
I. All countries	1.5	1.6	1.5	1.3	1.5
II. Cross-national combination of countries					
Low/lower-middle	1.2	1.2	0.9	1.0	1.1
Upper-middle	1.4	1.0	0.9	1.4	1.3
High	1.5	1.8	2.0	1.3	1.7
III. Low/lower-middle					
Colombia	2.3	1.4	1.0	0.5	1.1
India–Pondicherry	0.8	0.9	1.4	1.4	0.8
Iraq	0.9	1.0	0.5	1.3	1.1
Nigeria	1.1	1.7	1.0	0.9	1.5
PRC–Beijing/Shanghai	1.1	1.3	0.8	1.0	1.6
PRC–Shenzhen	1.0	1.6	1.1	–	1.2
PRC (all sites combined)	1.0	1.5	0.9	1.0	1.3
Ukraine	1.4	1.0	1.1	1.1	1.0
IV. Upper-middle					
Brazil–São Paulo	1.6	0.6	0.9	1.4	1.0
Bulgaria	0.6	0.9	1.0	0.6	1.0
Lebanon	1.2	1.0	1.0	1.0	0.7
Mexico	1.7	1.3	0.9	1.1	1.6
Romania	0.9	0.6	1.3	0.4	1.0
South Africa	1.6	1.4	1.1	1.8	2.0
V. High					
Belgium	1.4	2.1	1.3	1.2	1.6
France	0.9	0.9	0.8	0.9	0.8
Germany	1.0	1.8	1.0	1.1	1.9
Israel	1.1	1.1	–	1.2	1.0
Italy	1.1	1.3	1.1	1.1	1.3
Japan (11 cities)	0.5	0.9	0.8	1.0	1.1
Netherlands	1.2	0.7	1.0	1.0	1.1
New Zealand	1.2	1.2	–	1.0	1.3
Northern Ireland	1.5	1.2	0.9	1.4	1.5
Portugal	1.2	1.0	0.9	1.2	1.3
Spain	0.8	1.4	1.0	1.6	1.5
USA	1.8	2.0	1.5	1.2	1.5
VI. Mean D^2 across countries	1.2	1.2	1.0	1.1	1.3

[a] As described in more detail in the text, the design effect (D^2) is the square of the ratio of the standard error of the prevalence estimate using design-based methods, divided by the standard error of the prevalence estimate assuming a simple random sample. D^2 represents the extent to which the design-based sample would have to increase in size to obtain the same standard error as that obtained in a simple random sample of the observed size. For example, the D^2 of 1.1 in Colombia means that the part 2 sample of 2,381 respondents would have to be 2,619 (i.e., 1.1 × 2,381) to achieve a design-based standard error equal in size to the standard error in a simple random sample of 2,381 respondents.
– This group of disorders was not evaluated.

disorder, and subthreshold bipolar disorder), seven anxiety disorders (agoraphobia, generalized anxiety disorder [GAD], panic disorder, post-traumatic stress disorder [PTSD], separation anxiety disorder [SAD], social phobia, specific phobia), four disruptive behavior disorders (attention-deficit/hyperactivity disorder [ADHD], conduct disorder, intermittent explosive disorder, oppositional-defiant disorder), and four

substance disorders (alcohol and drug abuse with or without dependence). In each case, the CIDI assessed lifetime prevalence of the disorder and then obtained retrospective data about age of onset (AOO), 12-month prevalence, and recency.

In many cases we combined subsets of these 21 disorders in order to stabilize estimates. For example, panic disorder and agoraphobia were often combined into a single panic and/or agoraphobia category, while alcohol and drug abuse were often combined into an alcohol and/or drug abuse category. Bipolar I and II and subthreshold bipolar disorder were often combined into a single bipolar disorder variable. In some cases this was done because the individual disorders in the larger composites are comparatively rare, making it necessary to combine them with other disorders to obtain stable estimates. In other cases the combination was based on the desire to simplify models by collapsing predictors with comparable regression coefficients. In some cases, especially those involving subgroup analyses, particular disorders were deleted from the analyses entirely. This kind of deletion was also made in the case of minor depression in a number of chapters, because of the weak associations of minor depression with the outcomes of interest.

A clinical reappraisal study using the DSM-IV Axis I Disorders, Research Version, Non-Patient Edition of the Structured Clinical Interview for DSM-IV (SCID) (First et al. 2002) was carried out in several high-income WMH countries, and generally good concordance was found between diagnoses based on the CIDI and clinical diagnoses based on blinded clinical re-interviews (Haro et al. 2006, 2008). The area under the receiver operator characteristic curve (Hanley & McNeil 1982), a measure of concordance that is relatively insensitive to disorder prevalence (Kraemer et al. 2003), was in the range 0.7–0.8.

Retrospective reports of lifetime mental disorders play a central part in the analyses presented in this volume. It is important, in light of this central role of retrospective reports, that considerable evidence suggests that these reports can be inaccurate (Giuffra & Risch 1994, Simon & Von Korff 1995, Patten 2003, Moffitt et al. 2010). These problems are not unique to interviews about mental disorders. The problems have been recognized by survey methodologists for years, and a considerable amount of methodological research has been carried out to address them (e.g., Turner & Martin 1985, Tanur 1992, Sudman et al. 1996). This research has advanced considerably over the past two decades as cognitive psychologists have become interested in the survey interview as a natural laboratory for studying cognitive processes (Schwarz & Sudman 1994, 1996, Sirken et al. 1999). A number of important insights have emerged from these studies about practical ways to improve the accuracy of retrospective reports. These insights and methods were used in the modified version of the CIDI

developed for use in the WMH surveys (Kessler & Üstün 2004, 2008).

A detailed discussion of these improvements was presented in an earlier volume in this series (Kessler et al. 2012) and will not be repeated here other than to note that the improvements address the following key problems: (1) that respondents often misunderstand the complexity of the task implied in lifetime recall questions, which require careful memory search that is unlikely to be carried out unless respondents are clearly instructed to do so; (2) that respondents might not be motivated to put in the hard work required to think back over their entire lives and answer lifetime recall questions accurately, especially in light of the fact that many CIDI questions deal with potentially embarrassing and stigmatizing experiences; and (3) that respondents might not be able to answer some recall questions accurately, especially those that ask about characteristics of mental disorders that are difficult to remember.

In addition to concerns about the accuracy of lifetime reports about whether or not mental disorders occurred in the past, concerns also can be raised about AOO reports. Previous research has shown that AOO is often difficult to recall accurately even when respondents are motivated to do so (Belli 1998, Prohaska et al. 1998). As retrospective AOO reports play an important part in WMH analyses, a special question series was used to avoid the implausible AOO response patterns found in previous surveys of lifetime mental disorders (Simon & Von Korff 1995). The sequence began with a question designed to emphasize the importance of accurate response: "Can you remember your exact age the very first time you (HAD THE SYNDROME)?" Respondents who answered "no" were probed for a bound of uncertainty by moving up the age range incrementally (e.g., "Was it before you first started school?", "Was it before you became a teenager?", etc.). AOO was set at the upper end of the bound (e.g., age 12 for respondents who reported that onset was before they became teenagers). Experimental research shows that this question sequence yields responses with a much more plausible AOO distribution than the standard CIDI AOO question (Knäuper et al. 1999).

Chronic physical conditions

The WMH also assessed a number of chronic physical conditions. This was done for two purposes: to study the associations of mental disorders as risk factors for the onset and persistence of common physical conditions, and to allow comparisons to be made of the burdens associated with mental and physical disorders. An earlier volume in the WMH series focused on the first of these two purposes (Von Korff *et al.* 2009). We documented in that volume that early-onset mental disorders have very strong associations with the subsequent onset and course of a wide range of commonly occurring physical conditions. While we cannot confirm that these associations are causal with the non-experimental data available in the WMH surveys, it seems quite clear that the associations are prospective and in a number of cases quite powerful. One chapter in the present volume summarizes and extends those previous results about the adverse effects of mental disorders on subsequent physical conditions. But the main use of the physical conditions measures in the current volume is for the second purpose: to allow comparisons to be made of the burdens associated with mental and physical disorders. The outcomes considered in those analyses are described later in this section. For now, though, we focus on the measurement approach used to assess the physical conditions.

We focused on commonly occurring chronic physical conditions that have been shown in previous research to be associated with significant role impairments (Merikangas *et al.* 2007, Ormel *et al.* 2008, Druss *et al.* 2009). These disorders were assessed with two standard chronic conditions checklists based on the list in the US National Health Interview Survey (Schoenborn *et al.* 2003, Centers for Disease Control and Prevention 2004, www.hcp.med.harvard.edu/ncs/replication.php). The first list included symptom-based conditions (e.g., chronic headaches, chronic low back pain). Respondents were asked whether they had ever had each condition and, if so, the age when it first occurred. The second list was of silent conditions (e.g., cancer, hypertension). Respondents were asked whether a health professional had ever told them they had each condition and, if so, the age of being told. In addition, information was obtained on whether reversible conditions were still present in the past 12 months.

Checklists like this have been shown to yield more complete and accurate reports than estimates derived from responses to open-ended questions (Baker *et al.* 2001, Knight *et al.* 2001). Methodological studies in both the USA and the UK have documented good concordance between such condition reports and

medical records (Edwards *et al.* 1994, Baker *et al.* 2001, Revicki *et al.* 2004). The condition reports were grouped into 10 categories to maximize comparability with the categories used in the WHO Global Burden of Disease study (Murray *et al.* 2001). The categories include arthritis, cancer, cardiovascular disorders (heart attack, heart disease, hypertension, stroke), chronic pain conditions (chronic back or neck pain, other chronic pain conditions), diabetes, digestive disorders (stomach or intestinal ulcer, irritable bowel disorder), frequent or severe headaches or migraines, insomnia, neurological disorders (multiple sclerosis, Parkinson's disease, epilepsy, seizure disorders), and respiratory disorders (seasonal allergies, asthma, chronic obstructive pulmonary disease [COPD], emphysema).

Burdens associated with mental disorders

As described in Chapter 1, a wide range of burdens are considered in this volume. Different analytical strategies have been applied, taking into account the timelines of the variables being analyzed. One of these burdens consists of the adverse effects of early-onset mental disorders on important developmental outcomes, such as educational attainment, marital timing and stability, and employment stability. We assessed these outcomes in the WMH surveys by collecting what are known as *event histories* (Caspi *et al.* 1996) for the timing and occurrence of critical events in the domains of education, marriage, and employment.

Another burden, as noted above, consists of effects of mental disorders on subsequent physical conditions. Several specific associations of this sort have been known for many years, such as the association between anxiety disorders and subsequent duodenal ulcers (Tennant 1988) and the association between major depressive disorder and subsequent heart disease (Glassman 2008). The strength of evidence for these various associations varies, as does an understanding of causal mechanisms. The WMH data are limited in their ability to advance our understanding of mechanisms, due to the fact that the WMH surveys are cross-sectional and naturalistic and did not collect information about presumed causal mediators. However, the WMH surveys are useful in that they provide an unprecedented opportunity to examine the generalizability and specificity of associations between mental and later physical conditions in the general population. In terms of generalizability, the WMH data allow us to examine the extent to which predictive associations of mental disorders with later physical conditions are consistent across over two dozen countries. In terms of specificity, the WMH data allow us to determine the extent to which these associations are unique to particular mental disorders (e.g., a specific association of generalized anxiety disorders with ulcers) or are more general across a number of different mental disorders (e.g., non-specific associations of a number of different anxiety disorders with ulcers).

Our analyses of the above-mentioned classes of burdens focus on the effects of *lifetime* mental disorders, as these effects are thought to unfold over the span of many years. A final group of burdens, however, consists of effects of current mental disorders on current role performance and functioning. Included here are effects of mental disorders on income, marital quality, days out of role, disability, and perceived health. A number of different scales are used to assess these outcomes, such as the Conflict Tactics Scale (CTS) (Straus 1979) to assess marital violence and a modified version (Von Korff *et al.* 2008) of the WHO Disability Assessment Schedule 2.0 (WHODAS 2) (Üstün *et al.* 2010) to assess disability. These scales and their measurement are described in the chapters where they are used.

One special scale that assesses functioning is a visual analog scale (VAS) of overall perceived health. This scale was administered to WMH respondents by asking them to take all their physical and mental health problems into consideration and to rate their overall health on a 0-to-100 scale where 0 represents *the worst possible health a person can have* and 100 represents *perfect health*. This kind of VAS of health valuation is widely used in the literature and has been the subject of lively debate regarding advantages (Parkin & Devlin 2006) and disadvantages (Rashidi *et al.* 2006) compared to alternative methods of health valuation. We use this VAS approach to compare the perceived effects of mental and chronic physical disorders on overall health.

Field procedures

Translation

The innovations in CIDI 3.0 measurement were all developed initially in English. One of the fundamental challenges in an undertaking such as the WMH Survey Initiative is to achieve both equivalence in meaning and consistency in measurement across surveys that have multiple languages. This is a special challenge in studying mental disorders, as the symptoms of mental disorders are described and interpreted differently in different cultures (Prince & Tcheng-Laroche 1987, Cheng 2001), making it necessary in some cases to use substantially different terms or even questions in different countries to assess the presence versus absence of these symptoms. Another complexity is that the CIDI source language, English, has a larger lexicon (stock of vocabulary) than any other known language. This can mean that distinctions made in English cannot be matched in one or more target languages. The opposite can also be true with respect to certain areas of lexical or grammatical distinctions, in which the source language may not specify enough detail necessary for translation into a given target language.

WMH collaborators were given guidelines for translation and adaptation of the CIDI aimed at achieving both equivalence in meaning and consistency in measurement across surveys. A detailed discussion of these guidelines is presented elsewhere (Harkness *et al.* 2008) and will not be repeated here. We merely note that these guidelines were modifications of longstanding WHO guidelines for translation and back-translations that were updated by the staff of the WHO Data Collection Coordination Centre under the direction of Beth-Ellen Pennell in collaboration with the WMH Co-Principal Investigators.

Countries were instructed that the central aim of the translation process was to achieve target language versions of the English questionnaire that were *conceptually equivalent* in each of the countries/cultures, rather than attempting literal equivalence in terms of word-for-word translation. It was emphasized that the translation should sound natural in each language (in so far as that is possible in standardized instruments) and should perform in a comparable fashion across the populations and languages. Independent assessors who were experts on cross-national translation reviewed the CIDI translations and found that these aims were generally achieved, but that some of the translations were, at times, too close to the English questionnaire language formulation and structure to sound "natural."

Countries were required to follow a six-step process in achieving these aims. These steps included: (1) forward translation; (2) expert panel review;

(3) independent back-translation; (4) harmonization of vocabulary and formulation across different country versions of a shared language (if appropriate); (5) pretesting and cognitive interviewing; and (6) final revision, creation, and documentation of a final version of the translated questionnaire. A detailed description of each of these steps is presented elsewhere (Harkness *et al.* 2008).

Pretesting

Consistent with best-practice recommendations (Sheatsley 1983, Converse & Presser 1986, Groves *et al.* 2004, Harkness *et al.* 2004, Smith 2004), pretests of the instrument and procedures were carried out in each WMH survey prior to main study implementation. The pretests were designed to mirror the main study in most aspects, except in some cases using experienced interviewers for pretest data collection. Pretest interviews were evaluated by debriefing interviewers to identify potential problem areas with the instrument and survey procedures, checking the distributions of items for high rates of missing data and out-of-range values, and using behavior coding of audiotaped pretest interviews to pinpoint questions that were often misread or often elicited respondent requests for clarification.

Pretesting is especially important in cross-national studies because of the challenges associated with working in many different languages and social contexts (Smith 2004). A separate series of pretests was consequently required in each WMH country. Initial pretests focused on evaluating the translations. Later pretests evaluated the interview schedule and field procedures. The number of the latter pretest rounds varied from one to three, with approximately two-thirds of the countries conducting just one round of pretests and most of the others two rounds. The pretest debriefing sessions identified country-specific difficulties with questionnaire wording and response categories that were modified prior to the beginning of production interviewing. These sessions, along with quantitative analyses of responses, also detected skip-pattern errors in the PAPI (paper and pencil interview) version and programming errors in the CAPI (computer-assisted personal interview) version that were corrected prior to the beginning of production interviewing. The pretests also allowed the investigators to evaluate the adequacy of survey procedures and sample management systems.

Interviewer training and field quality-control monitoring

Although large-scale cross-national surveys have been undertaken for decades (Heath *et al.* 2005 provide a concise history), there is surprisingly little written research on the practical aspects of training and supervising interviewers to achieve high-quality survey data. The necessity of cultural adaptation of survey methods in order to achieve equivalence in measurement across countries is widely recognized (Bulmer 1998, Jowell 1998, Kuechler 1998, Lynn 2003). However, few details are provided in the literature as to how to achieve this equivalence across the many phases of a project's development. In the absence of such standards of practice, many cross-national projects have been left to accept the research traditions of individual countries, which vary widely in methodological rigor. An approach at the other extreme is to implement a "one-size-fits-all" methodology that naively imposes the same procedure and protocols across all countries and cultures based on the assumption that good practice in one culture will be good practice in other cultures (Harkness *et al.* 2002).

The WMH surveys sought to implement an approach between these two extremes by establishing guidelines that set minimum standards for each phase of project implementation but allowed for country-specific adaptations. We saw this earlier in the chapter in the discussion of probability sampling methods that allowed for country-specific variations. The difficulty for the staff of the WMH Data Collection Coordination Centre was determining when variations in approach were necessary and appropriate rather than simply expedient. Staying with the above sampling example, survey organizations in some parts of the world have a tradition of quota sampling and respondent substitution that violates the WMH requirement of probability sampling. This kind of potential conflict between local practice and best practices was found in every phase of the WMH.

A detailed description of the WMH interviewer hiring, training, and data quality-control standards and the ways in which these standards were implemented in the individual WMH countries is presented elsewhere (Pennell *et al.* 2008). These standards were subsequently used by the senior members of the WMH Data Collection Coordination Centre to take the lead in developing internationally recognized guidelines for best practices in cross-national comparative survey research more generally (www.ccsg.isr.umich.edu).

Issues of interviewer recruitment and training, research ethics, field structure, data collection procedures and quality control, and data preparation are all included in these guidelines.

We will not discuss here the many practical decisions made in establishing WMH field procedures, such as the decision to have interviews carried out face-to-face rather than by telephone and the decision to use both paper and pencil and computer-assisted versions of the survey, and to allow individual countries to choose which of the two modes they were able to use, but refer the reader to a detailed discussion of these decisions elsewhere (Pennell *et al.* 2008). It is worth noting, however, that the section on measures made it clear that the CIDI is a complex instrument. Successful implementation of such an instrument requires interviewers to be highly trained. We consequently placed high importance on careful interviewer hiring, training, and quality-assurance monitoring.

Importantly, all countries were required to use the same core training and quality-control procedures appropriately adapted to local circumstances. All interviewers were required to pass a certification test before being approved for production work. In addition, special procedures were developed to monitor interviewer performance during production. Systematic monitoring is critical to survey data quality assurance (Billiet & Loosveldt 1988, Fowler & Mangione 1990). Supervisor re-interview of selected cases, supervisor verification of key survey elements through spot re-contact of respondents, direct observation of interviews, audio-recording, questionnaire review, analysis of performance and production measures, keystroke/trace file analysis (files that record keystrokes and movement of the interviewer through the computerized instrument), and mock interviews/tests of knowledge and practice were all used to monitor interviewer quality. A supervisor-to-interviewer ratio of one supervisor for every 8–10 interviewers was used in the majority of countries that used paper and pencil data collection, to make sure these procedures could be rigorously applied, while lower ratios were used in countries with computer administration based on the greater control over the data collection process afforded by computerized interviewing (Williams 1986, Lavrakas 1993).

Post-processing

All WMH survey data cleaning is carried out collaboratively by the participating country collaborators and the WMH Data Analysis Coordination Centre at Harvard Medical School (HMS) under the supervision of Nancy Sampson, with consultation from Beth-Ellen Pennell. The Centre staff also either oversee or carry out all weighting, post-stratification, imputation of missing values, and scale construction for all WMH surveys, with consultation from Steve Heeringa.

Statistical analysis methods

Quality control

All the data analyses reported in this volume were carried out centrally either by the staff of the WMH Data Analysis Coordination Centre in Boston under the supervision of Nancy Sampson or by the staff of the WMH Regional Coordination Centre at the IMIM (Hospital del Mar Medical Research Institute) in Barcelona, Spain, under the supervision of Gemma Vilagut. The broad design and oversight of these analyses across all chapters was provided by the editors (Alonso, Chatterji, He) in collaboration with Ronald Kessler and Alan Zaslavsky.

Predicting role transitions

Discrete-time survival analysis with person-year used as the unit of analysis (Willett & Singer 1993) is used to study the associations of lifetime mental disorders with role transitions in the domains of education and marriage. The discrete-time approach was chosen over the more traditional Cox proportional hazards analysis approach for two reasons: because our information about timing of role transitions was available only for discrete intervals of time (i.e., years of age); and because the discrete-time approach handles the use of multiple time-varying predictor variables, which is a central feature of our models, much more easily than does the Cox modeling approach (Clayton & Hills 1993).

In these models, each year a respondent is at risk, up to his/her age at the occurrence of the outcome or age at interview (whichever comes first), is represented by a separate observation. The resulting person-year dataset pooled across all respondents is analyzed using logistic regression models with dummy-variable covariates specifying the year of life that each observation represents. Chronological age is used as the time scale. Additional controls are used in models for specific outcomes that are relevant to the outcome. For example, in the model to predict divorce, statistical controls are included for number of years since marriage. Model coefficients are presented as odds ratios, which indicate the relative odds of the outcome in a given year for a person who had a history of a given predictor disorder prior to the outcome compared to a person without the disorder.

An important feature of the analysis of the effects of lifetime mental disorders on these role transitions is that the lifetime disorders are *time-varying*; that is, a given disorder could have started at different ages for different respondents. As a result, in order to maintain the temporal sequence between predictors and outcomes, it is necessary to take timing into consideration in estimating risk-factor models. This is done in the discrete-time survival analysis by coding each year of each respondent's life separately for each lifetime disorder and allowing values to change over time for a single individual depending on the timing of onset of the disorder. For example, the first 19 years of a given respondent's life might be coded as never depressed and the 20th through later years as having a history of depression. This kind of within-person variation in coding is easily achieved in the discrete-time survival approach because each year of each person's life is treated as a separate observational record.

As a detailed exposition of this analysis approach was presented in an earlier volume in this series (Kessler *et al.* 2012), we will not elaborate further on the method other than to note that the basic model always assumes that the associations of predictors with outcomes are constant across years, but this assumption is evaluated in the WMH analyses by including interaction terms in the equation between person-years and predictor disorders. We also examine interactions of predictor disorders with country income level, distinguishing countries classified by the World Bank as low-income or lower-middle-income countries from those classified as upper-middle-income and high-income countries.

Predicting other discrete-time outcomes

Another way in which discrete-time survival models are used is presented in the next chapter (Chapter 3), where we examine the extent to which parental mental disorders predict the subsequent onset of mental disorders in their offspring, and again in Chapter 7, where we examine associations of early-onset mental disorders with the subsequent onset of chronic

physical disorders. In each of these cases, the outcome of interest is a dated discrete outcome, such as first onset of panic disorder at age 25 or the occurrence of a heart attack at age 58. The same discrete-time survival models as described in the previous subsection are used to study the associations of earlier mental disorders (parental mental disorders in Chapter 3 and respondent mental disorders in Chapter 7) with these outcomes. In the case of the Chapter 3 analyses of parental disorders, the predictors are considered time-invariant. That is, we asked respondents whether or not their mother and, separately, their father had each of the disorders considered when the respondent was a child. But we did not ask how old the respondent was when the parent's disorder first started, as pilot work suggested that in most cases respondents reported that the parental disorder was present prior to the respondent's birth and in other cases the respondent was not able to provide dates that they thought were accurate. As a result, we treated the parental disorders as constants in the childhoods of respondents. In the case of the analyses in Chapter 7, in contrast, where respondent mental disorders is used to predict the subsequent onset of respondent chronic physical disorders, we used information provided by respondents on the AOO of their mental disorders to create time-varying predictors of the subsequent onset of temporally secondary physical disorders. Other than for this difference in whether the mental disorders used as predictors are treated as time-invariant (in the case of parental disorders) or as time-varying (in the case of respondent disorders), the logic of the discrete-time survival analyses in Chapters 3 and 7 is identical and consistent with the analyses of the life-course transitions described in the previous subsection of this chapter.

Predicting continuous outcomes

As noted above in the brief description of outcome variables, many of the outcomes we consider here consist of scales of role functioning or other continuous measures that we think are affected by mental disorders. Examples are a measure with a range of 0–30 that assesses the number of days in the past month the respondent was out of role because of health problems, a measure with a range of 0–100 of the perceived impairment in the respondent's social role functioning, the 0–100 VAS measure of perceived health, and even a measure of annual family income that has a range between $0 and $150,000 in the USA and an equivalent range in other currencies in other countries.

One feature that these outcomes have in common is that that they all have skewed distributions that may make ordinary least squares (OLS) regression analysis both biased and inefficient. For example, many people have no earnings, while in the segment of the population that has earnings the proportion with very high earnings is much greater than we would expect in a normal distribution. This problem can be addressed in two ways. First, a two-part modeling approach (Duan *et al.* 1984) can be used where a part 1 logistic regression equation (Hosmer & Lemeshow 2001) is used to predict having a non-zero value in the total sample and a part 2 linear regression equation is used to predict scores in the non-zero range. Individual-level predicted scores can then be estimated by multiplying predicted values based on the two equations.

A problem with this first approach is that non-random variance in prediction errors can lead to bias even when sophisticated transformation methods are used (Manning 1998). A second approach, generalized linear models (GLM), can address that problem by pre-specifying non-linear associations and non-random error structures in one-part models. Such models can sometimes fit highly skewed data better than two-part models (McCullagh & Nelder 1989, Mullahy 1998, Manning & Mullahy 2001). We used both a number of different two-part model specifications and a number of standard GLM specifications in our analysis of continuous outcomes in the WMH analyses. We then selected the best specification using standard empirical model comparison procedures (Buntin & Zaslavsky 2004).

A minor problem with both of the above approaches is that the coefficients in the best-fitting models often have no intuitive interpretation. We address this problem by using simulation to transform the coefficients to more meaningful scales. This is done by generating two estimates of the continuous outcome for each respondent for each coefficient in the best-fitting model based on the coefficients in that model. The first estimate is based on the actual data, while the second estimate is based on a revision of the data in which all respondents are recoded not to have one particular predictor disorder. The first estimate is then subtracted from the second and the sum across respondents is divided by the number of respondents with the focal disorder to arrive at an estimate of the average individual-level change in the outcome associated with that disorder.

Modeling the joint effects of multiple mental disorders

All the analyses reported in this volume focus on the joint effects of multiple mental disorders. We begin with bivariate models for the effect of each mental disorder net of controls with the outcome, and then consider the multivariate associations of the individually significant disorders based on an additive model. A question could be asked whether the *number* of these disorders might not be as important as, or even more important than, the *types* of disorders in predicting the outcomes. There is also the possibility that number and type have distinct associations with the outcomes. In order to investigate this possibility, we estimate a model that includes counts of the number of mental disorders as predictors of the outcomes and we also estimate separate models that include information about both type and number of disorders as predictors. Comparisons of alternative models are made using the Akaike (Burnham & Anderson 2002) and Bayes (Kass & Raftery 1995) information criteria to select a best-fitting model.

It is noteworthy that the models including both type and number as predictors include a separate dummy predictor variable for each disorder, along with a series of dummy predictor variables for number of disorders that began with *two*. A detailed discussion of the logic of this approach is presented elsewhere (Kessler *et al.* 2011) and will only be summarized here. To begin, a model that includes only a series of dummy predictor variables for type of disorder implicitly assumes that the joint effect of the multiple disorders is the sum of the coefficients for the component disorders or, in the case of logistic models, the product of the odds ratios (ORs). A model that includes only a series of dummy variables for number of predictor disorders, in comparison, implicitly allows for interactions in the sense that the coefficients associated with having exactly two or exactly three or exactly *n* disorders can be significantly different from the sum or product of the coefficient associated with having exactly one disorder. However, by excluding information about the content of the disorder, the main effect coefficients for the various component disorders are assumed to be the same.

The model that includes terms for both type and number of predictor disorders, in comparison, allows both for differences in effects of the different disorders and for interactions. Specifically, the coefficients associated with types of disorders can be interpreted as the coefficients of the outcome among individuals who had one and only one specific mental disorder compared to respondents with none of the disorders, while the coefficients associated with number of disorders are offsets (in the case of linear models) or multipliers (in the case of logistic models) of the combination of coefficients associated with the component disorders. For example, assuming that we are using a logistic model to predict a dichotomous outcome (e.g., high-school dropout as an outcome of early-onset mental disorders), if the ORs associated with having a history of early-onset major depression, generalized anxiety disorder, specific phobia, and alcohol abuse are 1.8, 2.0, 2.2, and 2.4, respectively, while the ORs associated with having exactly two, three, and four of these disorders are 1.3, 1.4, and 1.5, respectively, then the predicted OR for a respondent who had the first three of these four disorders would be 11.1 (i.e., $1.8 \times 2.0 \times 2.2 \times 1.4$) compared to a respondent with no disorders, while the predicted OR for a respondent who had only the first and last of these four disorders would be 5.6 (i.e., $1.8 \times 2.4 \times 1.3$).

The simplifying assumption in the type–number model is that the interaction offset or multiplier term varies only with number of disorders. As described elsewhere (Kessler *et al.* 2011), other simplifying assumptions can be made, but our experience exploring several of them is that the assumption made in the type–number model is generally most consistent with the data. Simplifying assumptions of some sort are needed, of course, because it is impossible even in a dataset as large as the WMH series to work with unrestricted models that include a separate coefficient for each of the 2^d logically possibly multivariate profiles made up by cross-classifying d types of mental disorders. If there are 17 different types of mental disorders under consideration, as there are in some of the analyses reported here, 2^{17} is 131,072. It would be impossible to include this large a number of predictors in our models. Data-mining methods exist that could be used to search through this enormous number of combinations to find a stable, significantly predictive set (Kantardzic 2003). However, we did not use this approach because we were more interested in developing models that could give us insights about the importance of individual disorders, which are often obscured in data-mining.

Stacking effect-size estimates across multiple outcomes

One special analysis issue is unique to Chapter 3, where we examine associations of parental mental disorders in predicting the subsequent onset of respondent mental disorders. This is the only chapter in which respondent mental disorders are treated as outcomes rather than as predictors of other outcomes. Given the large number of respondent mental disorders considered, we sought to constrain the very large number of coefficients in the models in order to obtain some parsimony in results. This was done by examining the predictive associations of parental disorders with four broad classes of subsequent respondent disorders (anxiety, mood, disruptive behavior, and substance disorders) rather than with each of the 22 individual respondent disorders considered in the analyses. But rather than create a single variable for, say, whether or not the respondent had *any* of the disorders, we created a more textured data file in which we estimated associations of parental disorders in predicting each individual respondent disorder in such a way as to constrain coefficients to be constant across the outcome disorders. This was accomplished concretely by building a separate discrete-time survival analysis file for each respondent disorder and then *pooling* these data files across a set of disorders. For example, we had seven anxiety disorders in the analysis. A separate person-year data file was created to predict each of those seven outcome disorders using the same set of measures of parental disorders as predictors. All seven of those datasets were then combined into a larger dataset, dummy predictor variables were included in this large dataset to distinguish among the seven outcomes, and a single survival analysis was carried out in it that constrained the coefficients of parental disorders to be constant in predicting each of the seven respondent disorders. We then expanded the model to include interactions between predictors and outcomes to test the validity of the assumption that the coefficients were constant across outcomes. As these tests showed that the assumption of constant coefficients could not be rejected in the vast majority of cases, the constrained version of the models (i.e., the version that assumed constant coefficients across all anxiety disorders and separately across all mood disorders, etc.) was the one we focused on in interpreting results.

Individual and societal levels of analysis

The coefficients described in the earlier parts of this section are all *individual-level* coefficients; that is, coefficients that describe the increased values of a continuous outcome or increased odds of a dichotomous outcome among respondents with versus without the predictor disorder. Individual-level coefficients do not take into consideration how common the predictor disorders are in the population, and consequently they can be used only to describe the relative importance of predictor disorders from the perspective of the individual. We might conclude, for example, that bipolar disorder is worse than specific phobia from an *individual perspective* because the adverse outcomes of an individual with bipolar disorder are worse than those of an individual with specific phobia. However, specific phobia is much more common than bipolar disorder, which means that from a *societal perspective* specific phobia might be associated with more burden than bipolar disorder even though bipolar disorder is the more severe disorder.

It is important to consider both individual and societal perspectives in evaluating the burdens of illness. As noted above, we use unstandardized linear and logistic regression coefficients to describe the individual-level effects. We use the population attributable risk proportion (PARP) to describe societal-level effects (Rockhill *et al.* 1998). PARP can be interpreted in this context as the proportion of respondents with a dichotomous outcome of interest who would not have had this outcome in the absence of a particular set of predictors, if the predictors were causal and the regression equation accurately characterizes the functional form of the associations of the predictors with the outcome (Northridge 1995).

In our case, we calculated PARPs to evaluate the expected effects of either preventing or successfully treating one or more of the mental disorders included as predictors in our regression equations. When we focus on a dichotomous outcome that always happens but varies in time of occurrence (e.g., death) or that varies both in whether it occurs and when it occurs (e.g., a heart attack), PARP can be interpreted as the proportional reduction in time to the event at the population level. In the case of a continuous outcome (e.g., days out of role due to health problems), PARP can be interpreted as the proportion of instances of the outcome that would not have occurred in the absence of the predictor disorders.

In the bivariate case with a dichotomous predictor, we can think of PARP as having two components. The first component is the individual-level association among respondents with the risk factor of interest. Let us say we have a dichotomous measure of an early-onset mental disorder associated with 20% higher risk of teen childbearing than among respondents without the disorder. The individual-level elevated risk would then be 1.2. The second component is the population projection. If the predictor disorder occurs to 10% of the population, the 20% elevation in that subsample means that 10% of the population has a risk of $1.2r$, while the other 90% of the population has a risk of r. If the elevated risk was removed, total risk would be r rather than $1.02r$ (i.e., $1.2r \times 0.1 + 1r \times 0.9$). The proportion of total risk due to the elevation in the high-risk subsample is then roughly 2.0% $[1 - (1/1.02)]$. This would be the estimated value of PARP in this particular case. If the predictor disorder occurred to 20% rather than 10% of the population, PARP would be approximately 4.0%. If the elevation in risk was 50% rather than 20% and it occurred to 20% of the population, PARP would be approximately 9%. The same interpretations apply when the outcome is continuous. For example, we might say that 2% or 4% or p% of all the days out of role in the population are associated with a particular mental disorder.

Calculation of PARP is more complicated when multiple predictors are considered together. In a situation of this sort, PARP is calculated using a simulation method similar to the one described above in the subsection on *Predicting continuous outcomes*. As in that earlier description, coefficients in the best-fitting model are used to predict individual-level outcomes twice for each respondent: once using actual data and a second time assuming that no respondents had one or more of the predictor disorders. The difference between the previously described individual-level method and the calculation of PARP is that the ratio of the *mean* of the two outcome disorder estimates in the *total sample* is used to define PARP. For example, if the expected mean number of days out of role in the past month in the total population is 3.5 and the expected mean in the absence of a series of mental disorders is predicted to be 2.8, the proportion of all days out of role due to those disorders is 20% [i.e., (3.5 − 2.8)/3.5], which is the estimate of PARP.

Design-based estimation

Because the WMH sample designs feature weighting and clustering, significance tests based on the assumption of simple random sampling will be biased. We addressed that problem by using design-based estimation methods that take weighting and clustering into consideration. For simple statistics, such as estimates of prevalence and linear regression coefficients, this was done using the Taylor Series Linearization method (Wolter 1985) implemented in the SUDAAN software system (Research Triangle Institute 2005). For more complex statistics, such as the simulated estimates of disorder effects in GLM models, standard errors were obtained using the Jackknife Repeated Replication method (Wolter 1985) implemented with a SAS macro (SAS Institute Inc. 2008). In this method, each model and each simulation is replicated many times in pseudo-samples to generate a distribution of each coefficient that is then used to calculate an empirical estimate of the standard error of the coefficient. Statistical significance was consistently evaluated using two-sided 0.05 level tests.

Causal inference with cross-sectional non-experimental data

Some reviews of the journal articles on which the empirical chapters in this volume are based criticized us for making causal inferences about the adverse effects of mental disorders based on cross-sectional non-experimental data. In most cases these criticisms were focused narrowly on our use of retrospective lifetime reports to make inferences about the temporal order between lifetime mental disorders and the subsequent occurrence of adverse outcomes. The critics argued that it is illegitimate to use retrospective data in this way because of recall error. As noted earlier in this chapter, data exist to show that recall error of the sort suggested by the critics does, in fact, exist. However, we argue below that the WMH data have considerable value despite the existence of this error.

In a few cases, the critics did not call into question the accuracy of respondent recollections about such things as, say, the age when they first started to have a particular mental disorder or the age they dropped out of school, but rather complained that it is illegitimate to assume that any association documented between an early-onset mental disorder and some subsequent adverse event, such as school dropout (whether based on data collected over time or data reconstructed retrospectively), can be interpreted as due to a causal effect of the mental disorder on the outcome in the absence of an experimental intervention. For example, a controlled treatment study could treat a probability subsample of youth with mental disorders and determine if this intervention led to a subsequent decline in school dropout.

While both of these criticisms are accurate in that the WMH data have the stated limitations, they overlook the critical fact that all research, even the most rigorously implemented experimental research, has limitations. The more important issue is whether the research in question has value despite its limitations. When we consider this issue, as we do below, it becomes clear that the WMH data have considerable value for studying the burdens of mental disorders. We take the two criticisms in turn in making this case.

Retrospective versus prospective data

The criticism about retrospective data has two components. One is that recall bias is so severe that retrospective data cannot be trusted. This argument is patently incorrect, as comparisons of retrospective with prospective reports show that a good deal of useful information can be obtained from retrospective data (Brewin et al. 1993, Hardt & Rutter 2004). Furthermore, innovative data collection methods have been developed by cognitive psychologists working with survey methodologists to improve the accuracy of retrospective recall in surveys (Groves et al. 2004, Glasner & van der Vaart 2009). As noted earlier in this chapter, a number of these methods were used in the WMH surveys.

The second criticism of retrospective data is that such data are not needed in light of the fact that a number of long-term prospective studies exist that can provide the same kinds of information without recall bias. These critics often point to the Dunedin Multidisciplinary Health and Development Study (dunedinstudy.otago.ac.nz) as a prime case in point. The Dunedin study is a prospective cohort study of the 1,037 babies born in the 12 months between April 1, 1972, and Mar 31, 1973, in Dunedin, New Zealand.

These babies were assessed at birth and then again on 11 subsequent occasions (e.g., at ages 3, 5, 7, 9, ... 21, 26, 32), with continuing assessments planned for the future, to study patterns, predictors, and consequences of physical and mental disorders. Other long-term prospective studies include the Christchurch Health and Development Study (www.otago.ac.nz/christchurch/research/healthdevelopment), a study of 1,265 people born in Christchurch, New Zealand, during mid-1977 who have been followed 20 times since baseline; and the 1970 British Cohort Study (www.esds.ac.uk/longitudinal/access/bcs70/l33229.asp), a study of the more than 17,000 babies born in the UK in a particular week in April 1970 who have been followed six times since baseline.

The argument that these kinds of long-term prospective studies make it unnecessary to work with retrospective data has four serious problems. First, long-term prospective studies of mental disorders typically fail to collect data on the lifetime prevalence of mental disorders, but rather focus on point prevalence at each wave of data collection, leaving time gaps (sometimes of more than five years' duration) in assessment (Kim-Cohen *et al.* 2003). This makes it impossible to carry out unbiased prospective studies of the long-term effects of mental disorders, because chronic cases are over-represented, lifetime prevalence is underestimated, and age-of-onset estimates are biased upwards for the cases detected. Retrospective data, collected either in the context of a larger prospective study or in standalone cross-sectional studies, are consequently needed.

Second, long-term prospective studies do not always contain baseline data on all the variables that subsequently come to be of research interest, making it impossible to carry out true prospective studies of these variables. For example, post-traumatic stress disorder (PTSD), while a focus of considerable current interest among psychiatric epidemiologists, was not a focus of interest at the time the baseline Dunedin study was designed. As a result, PTSD was not assessed in the Dunedin study until the tenth follow-up wave, when respondents were 26 years old (Koenen *et al.* 2008), at which time respondents were asked *retrospective questions* about their most traumatic lifetime experience and the PTSD symptoms occurring at the time of that experience as well as in the 12 months before the age-26 interview. The Dunedin researchers then carried out "prospective" analyses examining the associations of early childhood risk factors with

"subsequent" PTSD (Koenen *et al.* 2007). But given that AOO of PTSD was not assessed in the retrospective assessment, the analysis was not truly prospective, as PTSD might have started at an earlier age than the childhood "predictors."

We want to be clear that we agree with the value of using retrospective data in cases of this sort to obtain provisional information about time-lagged associations. That is, in fact, exactly what we did in the WMH surveys. As this example illustrates, though, this is often done more thoughtfully in retrospective than prospective studies due to the fact that researchers who carry out retrospective studies are sensitized to the problems of recall bias and often take great pains to collect data in such a way as to minimize this bias. This was clearly not done in the Dunedin study, as no information was collected on AOO of PTSD.

Third, experiences that occur between the waves of prospective studies often play an important part in analysis. These intercurrent experiences can only be assessed retrospectively, blurring the distinction between retrospective and prospective studies. For example, a widely cited report based on the Dunedin study purported to document a significant gene-by-environment interaction in the association between life events and *subsequent* depression. This was done, however, using retrospective reports about exposure to life events between the ages of 21 (the time of the previous assessment) and 25, from respondents who were interviewed at age 26 to predict major depression in the past 12 months assessed at age 26. There was no way to assess these life events other than retrospectively. Again, this retrospective data collection was carried out with less care than the best retrospective studies (Brown & Harris 2008), as there was no retrospective dating of the onset of the depressive episode. This made it impossible to determine the time lag between exposure to life events and onset of the depressive episode. In fact, it could well have been that the life events most strongly correlated with the depressive episodes were those occurring in the months *after* the onset of the episode that were incorrectly classified as occurring prior to the onset of the episode.

Fourth, even when prospective data exist to address a particular research question, panel attrition can lead to bias in prospective studies. This bias is much less extreme in cross-sectional/retrospective studies because non-response is typically much lower in a single survey than in a series of surveys (de Graaf et al. 2000). Indeed, methodological research shows that retrospective data can yield equally good or, in some cases, even better estimates of longitudinal associations than prospective data when the magnitude of panel attrition bias approaches or exceeds that of recall bias (Tuma & Hannan 1984).

The above four problems, in our view, effectively discredit the argument that the existence of long-term prospective studies makes it unnecessary to consider the kinds of retrospective data available in the WMH surveys. Indeed, recognition of the low external validity of data from available long-term prospective studies (i.e., the fact that the vast majority of respondents in these studies are of Western European descent and live in high-income countries), coupled with recognition of the above problems, makes it clear that parallel analyses of the much more broadly representative retrospective data in the WMH surveys could substantially enrich our understanding of the adverse personal and societal consequences of mental disorders.

Observational versus experimental data

The second criticism, that it is illegitimate to assume that any association documented in an observation study can be interpreted as due to a causal effect (whether the data are cross-sectional or prospective), is deeper than the first. According to this criticism, experimentation is the only legitimate basis for causal inference. The critics who espouse this view complain when any association in the WMH data is described as documenting an "effect" of a predictor on an "outcome."

A considerable amount of theorizing has been done by applied statisticians in recent years to address this criticism (Pearl 2000, Morgan & Winship 2007, Rosenbaum 2009). A careful reading of this literature suggests that even though the criticism has merit, it has to be tempered by two points.

First, causal inference can be treacherous even in experimental studies (Van der Laan & Rose 2011). As a result, it is not clear that one can ever speak unequivocally of an association as an "effect." It is much more sensible to speak of an "estimated" effect or "presumed" effect. This being the case, it is not clear that this way of speaking and of interpreting associations is illegitimate when based on naturalistic data. For example, imagine a study of the family burden associated with having a disabled child. One could certainly imagine carrying out such a study by comparing objective measures of burden in a sample of parents of disabled children versus a sample of parents of healthy children. Importantly, one could not imagine ever carrying out an experiment in which one group of youth was randomly assigned to become disabled and a second group not.

Would it be legitimate to make causal inferences about differences in "outcomes" (if the reader will, for the moment, excuse the use of this term) between the two groups of parents? Perhaps not, as not all disability occurs at random. Some disabled youth, for example, have permanent paralysis and brain damage caused by an automobile accident associated with teenage drunken driving. Teenage drunken driving, in turn, is associated with prior parenting practices (Ryan et al. 2010) that might themselves be independent predictors of family burden. We could try to adjust for these differences between the two sets of families by controlling for parenting practices. Or we could exclude from the analysis all youth with disabilities that are judged not to have occurred "at random." Or we could select a control group that might plausibly be considered equivalent to the group with disability.

Regarding the last possibility, imagine a scenario in which all respondents, both those who are disabled and those not, were selected from youth who had auto accidents associated with drunken driving in which they travelled at the same speed on the same roads in the same early morning hours but differed in that the disabled group went off the road at a place where they hit a telephone pole while the control group went off the road at a place where they missed the telephone pole by mere inches. Would it be legitimate to make causal inferences about differences in the outcomes of these two groups? I would think so, although caution would be needed not to over-interpret the external validity of findings. That is, the burden of having a disabled child of any sort (e.g., a child with Down syndrome) might be much greater in the kinds of families that bring up children who become drunk teenage drivers than in other families.

It is important to note that prospective data collection would be virtually impossible to imagine in a study of the sort described here; that is, assessing the family burden associated with parenting prior to the automobile accident in a large sample of families where a teenage child subsequently has a disabling accident. But the power of this hypothetical study to make causal inference comes from another source: the plausibility of the assumption that the "exposed" group and the "control" group are otherwise identical with respect to both the outcome variables and the determinants of the outcome variables. Prospective observational studies typically use measurement to help support this assumption by controlling for baseline measures of the outcome variable. However, this is not the same as controlling for all the determinants of the outcome variables that might be different in the exposed group and the control group. In some cases, such as the above example of family burden associated with having a disabled child, careful matching of exposed and control groups in a cross-sectional design can usually provide a much firmer basis for causal inference than a prospective design.

The second point that tempers the criticism of causal interpretations of observational data is that these interpretations, at least in the case of the WMH analyses, are always presented as hypotheses to be tested rather than as definitive statements about causal associations. As shown in the literature on retrospective case–control studies, these hypotheses can be of great value in targeting subsequent experimental interventions and shortening the amount of time it takes to make definitive determinations of significant causal effects (Schlesselman 1982).

This use of observational data to help generate causal hypotheses and target interventions is especially important in light of the fact that many more opportunities exist for experimental intervention to prevent or treat mental disorders than could ever be implemented in practice. Some method is needed to help narrow the range of possible experiments. Observational studies are the obvious vehicle for doing this. This is true whether the observational studies are based on prospective data or on cross-sectional data.

Consider as an example the finding that early-onset anxiety disorders are associated with the subsequent onset of adolescent alcohol and drug abuse. The robustness of this finding was suggested long ago in cross-national analyses of community epidemiological survey data in 11 countries using retrospective AOO reports to infer the temporal order between childhood-onset anxiety disorders and adolescent-onset substance disorders (Merikangas *et al.* 1998, Swendsen *et al.* 1998). The association was subsequently confirmed prospectively in two countries (Zimmermann *et al.* 2003, Fergusson *et al.* 2011). This broad consistency of the association argues strongly that it is quite robust. But we know that only a minority of youth with early-onset anxiety

disorders receive timely appropriate treatment for those disorders (Wang *et al.* 2007, Merikangas *et al.* 2011). This raises the question whether efforts to increase detection and effective treatment of early-onset anxiety disorders would be cost-effective in preventing the subsequent onset of adolescent substance abuse.

Note that we did not say that the above series of observational findings *demonstrated* that an intervention to treat early-onset anxiety disorder would be cost-effective in preventing adolescent substance abuse. We posed it as a question. If the association is causal, would the strength of the causal effect be large enough and available treatments sufficiently effective in reducing this effect that such an intervention would be warranted? This question has to be posed and addressed with observational data before it makes sense to launch the complex and expensive intervention needed to evaluate it. The preliminary analysis should use all the approaches to refining estimates of causal effects in observational studies proposed in the statistical literature on this topic (Rosenbaum 2009). The estimate should be made in such a way as to be conservative in light of known biases in observational data. Based on this estimate, and using knowledge about effect sizes in controlled treatment studies, policy simulations could then be carried out to make conservative estimates of the likely cost-effectiveness of such an intervention (Kendall & Kessler 2002). Analyses of this sort are presented in the current volume to assess the individual and societal burdens of mental disorders and the possible cost-effectiveness of interventions aimed at intervening either to prevent or to treat mental disorders.

Overview

This chapter has presented a broad overview of the methods used in the WMH surveys. We showed that the WMH samples are broadly representative of the household population in countries in all parts of the world. This means that we have an unprecedented opportunity to evaluate geographic consistency of findings and to focus on findings that pass the test of geographic consistency. We then presented an overview of the measures that are the focus of this volume, emphasizing the rigor with which we assessed mental disorders and the broad scope of our assessment of the burdens of these disorders. We then discussed WMH field procedures, emphasizing the rigor used at each step of implementation, from initial translation-harmonization of the interview schedule to quality control of data collection and processing. We then discussed the sophisticated statistical methods used to assess the burdens of mental disorders. Finally, we discussed the value of the cross-sectional WMH data for making inferences about the adverse consequences of mental disorders. Make no mistake: we recognize the limitations of the WMH data in making such inferences, but we also recognize the importance of providing provisional information about the enormous societal costs of these disorders throughout the world, the unmet need for treatment of these disorders, and the potential value for individuals and society of expanding interventions to prevent and treat these disorders.

Acknowledgments

Portions of this chapter appeared previously in:

Harkness, J., Pennell, B.-E., Villar, A., *et al.* (2008). Translation procedures and translation assessment in the World Mental Health Survey Initiative. In R. C. Kessler & T. B. Üstün, eds., *The WHO World Mental Health Survey: Global Perspectives on the Epidemiology of Mental Disorders*. New York, NY: Cambridge University Press, pp. 91–113.

Haro, J. M., Arbabzadeh-Bouchez, S., Brugha, T. S., *et al.* (2008). Concordance of the Composite International Diagnostic Interview version 3.0 (CIDI 3.0) with standardized clinical assessments in the WHO World Mental Health surveys. In R. C. Kessler & T. B. Üstün, eds., *The WHO World Mental Health Surveys: Global Perspectives on the Epidemiology of Mental Disorders*. New York, NY: Cambridge University Press, pp. 114–30.

Heeringa, S. G., Wells, J. E., Hubbard, F., *et al.* (2008). Sampling designs and sampling procedures. In R. C. Kessler & T. B. Üstün, eds., *The WHO World Mental Health Surveys: Global Perspectives on the Epidemiology of Mental Disorders*. New York, NY: Cambridge University Press, pp. 14–32.

Kessler, R. C., & Üstün, T. B. (2008). The World Health Organization Composite International Diagnostic Interview. In R. C. Kessler & T. B. Üstün, eds., *The WHO World Mental Health Surveys: Global Perspectives on the Epidemiology of Mental Disorders*. New York, NY: Cambridge University Press, pp. 58–90.

Kessler, R. C., Harkness, J., Heeringa, S. G., *et al.* (2012). Methods of the World Mental Health Surveys. In M. K. Nock, G. Borges, & Y. Ono, eds., *Suicide: Global Perspectives from the WHO World Mental Health Surveys*. New York, NY: Cambridge University Press, pp. 35–62.

Pennell, B.-E., Mneimneh, Z., Bowers, A., *et al.* (2008). Implementation of the World Mental Health surveys. In R. C. Kessler & T. B. Üstün, eds., *The WHO World Mental Health Surveys: Global Perspectives on the Epidemiology of Mental Disorders*. New York, NY: Cambridge University Press, pp. 33–57.

All © World Health Organization. Used with permission.

References

American Association for Public Opinion Research (2011). Standard definitions: final dispositions of case codes and outcome rates for surveys. www.aapor.org. Accessed March 28, 2012.

Baker, M. M., Stabile, M., & Deri, C. (2001). *What Do Self-reported, Objective Measures of Health Measure?* NBER Working Paper Series 8419. Cambridge, MA: National Bureau of Economic Research.

Belli, R. F. (1998). The structure of autobiographical memory and the event history calendar: potential improvements in the quality of retrospective reports in surveys. *Memory* **6**, 383–406.

Billiet, J., & Loosveldt, G. (1988). Interviewer training and quality of responses. *Public Opinion Quarterly* **52**, 190–211.

Brewin, C. R., Andrews, B., & Gotlib, I. H. (1993). Psychopathology and early experience: a reappraisal of retrospective reports. *Psychological Bulletin* **113**, 82–98.

Brown, G. W., & Harris, T. O. (2008). Depression and the serotonin transporter 5-HTTLPR polymorphism: a review and a hypothesis concerning gene-environment interaction. *Journal of Affective Disorders* **111**, 1–12.

Bulmer, M. (1998). The problem of exporting social survey research. *American Behavioral Scientist* **42**, 153–67.

Buntin, M. B., & Zaslavsky, A. M. (2004). Too much ado about two-part models and transformation? Comparing methods of modeling Medicare expenditures. *Journal of Health Economics* **23**, 525–42.

Burnham, K. P., & Anderson, D. R. (2002). *Model Selection and Multimodel Inference: A Practical Information-Theoretic Approach*, 2nd edn. New York, NY: Springer-Verlag.

Caspi, A., Moffitt, T. E., Thornton, A., *et al.* (1996). The life history calendar: a research and clinical assessment method for collecting retrospective event-history data. *International Journal of Methods in Psychiatric Research* **6**, 101–14.

Centers for Disease Control and Prevention (2004). *Health, United States, 2004*. Atlanta, GA: National Center for Health Statistics.

Cheng, A. T. (2001). Case definition and culture: are people all the same? *British Journal of Psychiatry* **179**, 1–3.

Clayton, D., & Hills, M. (1993). *Statistical Models in Epidemiology*. New York, NY: Oxford University Press.

Cochran, W. G. (1977). *Sampling Techniques*. New York, NY: Wiley.

Converse, J., & Presser, S. (1986). *Survey Questions: Handcrafting the Standardized Questionnaire*. Sage Series 63. Thousand Oaks, CA: Sage.

Couper, M. P., & de Leeuw, E. D. (2003). Nonresponse in cross-cultural and cross-national surveys. In J. A. Harkness, F. J. R. Van de Vijver, & P. P. Mohler, eds., *Cross-Cultural Survey Methods*. Hoboken, NJ: Wiley, pp. 155–77.

de Graaf, R., Bijl, R. V., Smit, F., Ravelli, A., & Vollebergh, W. A. (2000). Psychiatric and sociodemographic predictors of attrition in a longitudinal study: the Netherlands Mental Health Survey and Incidence Study (NEMESIS). *American Journal of Epidemiology* **152**, 1039–47.

Druss, B. G., Hwang, I., Petukhova, M., *et al.* (2009). Impairment in role functioning in mental and chronic medical disorders in the United States: results from the National Comorbidity Survey Replication. *Molecular Psychiatry* **14**, 728–37.

Duan, N., Manning, W. G., Morris, C. N., & Newhouse, J. P. (1984). Choosing between the sample-selection model and the multi-part model. *Journal of Business and Economic Statistics* **2**, 283–9.

Edwards, W. S., Winn, D. M., Kurlantzick, V., *et al.* (1994). Evaluation of National Health Interview Survey diagnostic reporting. *Vital and Health Statistics* **2** (120), 1–116.

Fergusson, D. M., Boden, J. M., & Horwood, L. J. (2011). Structural models of the comorbidity of internalizing disorders and substance use disorders in a longitudinal birth cohort. *Social Psychiatry and Psychiatric Epidemiology* **46**, 933–42.

First, M. B., Spitzer, R. L., Gibbon, M., & Williams, J. B. W. (2002). *Structured Clinical Interview for DSM-IV Axis I Disorders, Research Version, Non-Patient Edition (SCID-I/NP)*. New York, NY: Biometrics Research, New York State Psychiatric Institute.

Fowler, F., & Mangione, T. (1990). *Standardized Survey Interviewing: Minimizing Interviewer-Related Error*. Newbury Park, CA: Sage.

Giuffra, L. A., & Risch, N. (1994). Diminished recall and the cohort effect of major depression: a simulation study. *Psychological Medicine* **24**, 375–83.

Glasner, T., & van der Vaart, W. (2009). Applications of calendar instruments in social surveys: a review. *Quality and Quantity* **43**, 333–49.

Glassman, A. (2008). Depression and cardiovascular disease. *Pharmacopsychiatry* **41**, 221–5.

Groves, R. M., Fowler, F. J., Couper, M. P., *et al.* (2004). *Survey Methodology*. Hoboken, NJ: Wiley.

Hanley, J. A., & McNeil, B. J. (1982). The meaning and use of the area under a receiver operating characteristic (ROC) curve. *Radiology* **143**, 29–36.

Hardt, J., & Rutter, M. (2004). Validity of adult retrospective reports of adverse childhood experiences: review of the evidence. *Journal of Child Psychology and Psychiatry* **45**, 260–73.

Harkness, J., Pennell, B.-E., Villar, A., *et al.* (2008). Translation procedures and translation assessment in the World Mental Health survey initiative. In R. C. Kessler & T. B. Üstün, eds., *The WHO World Mental Health Survey: Global Perspectives on the Epidemiology of Mental Disorders*. New York, NY: Cambridge University Press, pp. 91–113.

Harkness, J. A., Van de Vijver, J. R., & Mohler, P. P. (2002). *Cross-Cultural Survey Methods*. New York, NY: Wiley.

Harkness, J. A., Pennell, B.-E., & Schoua-Glusberg, A. (2004). Survey questionnaire translation and assessment. In S. Presser, J. Rothgeb, M. P. Couper, *et al.*, eds., *Methods for Testing and Evaluating Survey Questionnaires*. Hoboken, NJ: Wiley, pp. 453–74.

Haro, J. M., Arbabzadeh-Bouchez, S., Brugha, T. S., *et al.* (2006). Concordance of the Composite International Diagnostic Interview Version 3.0 (CIDI 3.0) with standardized clinical assessments in the WHO World Mental Health surveys. *International Journal of Methods in Psychiatric Research* **15**, 167–80.

Haro, J. M., Arbabzadeh-Bouchez, S., Brugha, T. S., *et al.* (2008). Concordance of the Composite International Diagnostic Interview version 3.0 (CIDI 3.0) with standardized clinical assessments in the WHO World Mental Health surveys. In R. C. Kessler & T. B. Üstün, eds., *The WHO World Mental Health Surveys: Global Perspectives on the Epidemiology of Mental Disorders*. New York, NY: Cambridge University Press, pp. 114–30.

Heath, A., Fisher, S., & Smith, S. (2005). The globalization of public opinion research. *Annual Review of Political Science* **8**, 297–333.

Hosmer, D. W., & Lemeshow, S. (2001). *Applied Logistic Regression*, 2nd edn. New York, NY: Wiley.

Jowell, R. (1998). How comparative is comparative research? *American Behavioral Scientist* **42**, 168–77.

Kantardzic, M. (2003). *Data Mining: Concepts, Models, Methods, and Algorithms*. New York: Wiley.

Kass, R. E., & Raftery, A. E. (1995). Bayes factors. *Journal of the American Statistical Association* **90**, 773–95.

Kendall, P. C., & Kessler, R. C. (2002). The impact of childhood psychopathology interventions on subsequent substance abuse: policy implications, comments, and recommendations. *Journal of Consulting and Clinical Psychology* **70**, 1303–6.

Kessler, R. C., & Üstün, T. B. (2004). The World Mental Health (WMH) Survey Initiative version of the World Health Organization (WHO) Composite International Diagnostic Interview (CIDI). *International Journal of Methods in Psychiatric Research* **13**, 93–121.

Kessler, R. C., & Üstün, T. B. (2008). The World Health Organization Composite International Diagnostic Interview. In R. C. Kessler & T. B. Üstün, eds., *The WHO World Mental Health Surveys: Global Perspectives on the*

Epidemiology of Mental Disorders. New York, NY: Cambridge University Press, pp. 58–90.

Kessler, R. C., Petukhova, M., & Zaslavsky, A. M. (2011). The role of latent internalizing and externalizing predispositions in accounting for the development of comorbidity among common mental disorders. *Current Opinion in Psychiatry* **24**, 307–12.

Kessler, R. C., Harkness, J., Heeringa, S. G., *et al.* (2012). Methods of the World Mental Health Surveys. In M. K. Nock, G. Borges, & Y. Ono, eds., *Suicide: Global Perspectives from the WHO World Mental Health Surveys*. New York, NY: Cambridge University Press, pp. 35–62.

Kim-Cohen, J., Caspi, A., Moffitt, T. E., *et al.* (2003). Prior juvenile diagnoses in adults with mental disorder: developmental follow-back of a prospective–longitudinal cohort. *Archives of General Psychiatry* **60**, 709–17.

Kish, L. (1949). A procedure for objective respondent selection within the household. *Journal of the American Statistical Association* **44**, 380–7.

Kish, L. (1965). *Survey Sampling*. New York, NY: Wiley.

Knäuper, B., Cannell, C. F., Schwarz, N., Bruce, M. L., & Kessler, R. C. (1999). Improving accuracy of major depression age-of-onset reports in the US National Comorbidity Survey. *International Journal of Methods in Psychiatric Research* **8**, 39–48.

Knight, M., Stewart-Brown, S., & Fletcher, L. (2001). Estimating health needs: the impact of a checklist of conditions and quality of life measurement on health information derived from community surveys. *Journal of Public Health Medicine* **23**, 179–86.

Koenen, K. C., Moffitt, T. E., Poulton, R., Martin, J., & Caspi, A. (2007). Early childhood factors associated with the development of post-traumatic stress disorder: results from a longitudinal birth cohort. *Psychological Medicine* **37**, 181–92.

Koenen, K. C., Moffitt, T. E., Caspi, A., *et al.* (2008). The developmental mental-disorder histories of adults with posttraumatic stress disorder: a prospective longitudinal birth cohort study. *Journal of Abnormal Psychology* **117**, 460–6.

Kraemer, H. C., Morgan, G. A., Leech, N. L., *et al.* (2003). Measures of clinical significance. *Journal of the American Academy of Child and Adolescent Psychiatry* **42**, 1524–9.

Kuechler, M. (1998). The survey method: an indispensable tool for social science research everywhere? *American Behavioral Scientist* **42**, 178–200.

Lavrakas, P. J. (1993). *Telephone Survey Methods: Sampling, Selection, and Supervision*. Thousand Oaks, CA: Sage.

Little, R. J. A., & Rubin, D. B. (2002). *Statistical Analysis with Missing Data*, 2nd edn. New York, NY: Wiley.

Lynn, P. (2003). Developing quality standards for cross-national survey research: five approaches. *International Journal of Social Research Methodology* **6**, 323–36.

Manning, S. C. (1998). Configuring compliance: a professional fit. *Journal of American Health Information Management Association* **69**, 36–8.

Manning, W. G., & Mullahy, J. (2001). Estimating log models: to transform or not to transform? *Journal of Health Economics* **20**, 461–94.

McCullagh, P., & Nelder, J. A. (1989). *Generalized Linear Models*, 2nd edn. London: Chapman & Hall.

Merikangas, K. R., Mehta, R. L., Molnar, B. E., *et al.* (1998). Comorbidity of substance use disorders with mood and anxiety disorders: results of the International Consortium in Psychiatric Epidemiology. *Addictive Behaviors* **23**, 893–907.

Merikangas, K. R., Ames, M., Cui, L., *et al.* (2007). The impact of comorbidity of mental and physical conditions on role disability in the US adult household population. *Archives of General Psychiatry* **64**, 1180–8.

Merikangas, K. R., He, J. P., Burstein, M., *et al.* (2011). Service utilization for lifetime mental disorders in U.S. adolescents: results of the National Comorbidity Survey-Adolescent Supplement (NCS-A). *Journal of the American Academy of Child and Adolescent Psychiatry* **50**, 32–45.

Moffitt, T. E., Caspi, A., Taylor, A., *et al.* (2010). How common are common mental disorders? Evidence that lifetime prevalence rates are doubled by prospective versus retrospective ascertainment. *Psychological Medicine* **40**, 899–909.

Morgan, S. L., & Winship, C. (2007). *Counterfactuals and Causal Inference: Methods and Principles for Social Research*. New York, NY: Cambridge University Press.

Mullahy, J. (1998). Much ado about two: reconsidering retransformation and the two-part model in health econometrics. *Journal of Health Economics* **17**, 247–81.

Murray, C. J. L., López, A. D., Mathers, C. D., & Stein, C. (2001). *The Global Burden of Disease 2000 Project: Aims, Methods and Data Sources*. Geneva: World Health Organization.

Northridge, M. E. (1995). Public health methods-attributable risk as a link between causality and public health action. *American Journal of Public Health* **85**, 1202–4.

Ormel, J., Petukhova, M., Chatterji, S., *et al.* (2008). Disability and treatment of specific mental and physical disorders across the world. *British Journal of Psychiatry* **192**, 368–75.

Parkin, D., & Devlin, N. (2006). Is there a case for using visual analogue scale valuations in cost-utility analysis? *Health Economics* **15**, 653–64.

Patten, S. B. (2003). Recall bias and major depression lifetime prevalence. *Social Psychiatry and Psychiatric Epidemiology* **38**, 290–6.

Pearl, J. (2000). *Causality: Models, Reasoning, and Inference*. New York, NY: Cambridge University Press.

Pennell, B.-E., Mneimneh, Z., Bowers, A., *et al.* (2008). Implementation of the World Mental Health surveys. In R. C. Kessler & T. B. Üstün, eds., *The WHO World Mental Health Surveys: Global Perspectives on the Epidemiology of Mental Disorders*. New York, NY: Cambridge University Press, pp. 33–57.

Prince, R., & Tcheng-Laroche, F. (1987). Culture-bound syndromes and international disease classifications. *Cultural Medical Psychiatry* **11**, 3–52.

Prohaska, V., Brown, N. R., & Belli, R. F. (1998). Forward telescoping: the question matters. *Memory* **6**, 455–65.

Rashidi, A. A., Anis, A. H., & Marra, C. A. (2006). Do visual analogue scale (VAS) derived standard gamble (SG) utilities agree with Health Utilities Index utilities? A comparison of patient and community preferences for health status in rheumatoid arthritis patients. *Health and Quality of Life Outcomes* **4**, 25.

Research Triangle Institute (2005). *SUDAAN, Version 9.0.1.* [computer program]. Research Triangle Park, NC: Research Triangle Institute.

Revicki, D. A., Rentz, A. M., Dubois, D., *et al.* (2004). Gastroparesis Cardinal Symptom Index (GCSI): development and validation of a patient reported assessment of severity of gastroparesis symptoms. *Quality of Life Research* **13**, 833–44.

Rockhill, B., Newman, B., & Weinberg, C. (1998). Use and misuse of population attributable fractions. *American Journal of Public Health* **88**, 15–19.

Rosenbaum, P. R. (2009). *Design of Observational Studies.* New York, NY: Springer.

Rust, K. (1985). Variance estimation for complex estimators in sample surveys. *Journal of Official Statistics* **1**, 381–97.

Ryan, S. M., Jorm, A. F., & Lubman, D. I. (2010). Parenting factors associated with reduced adolescent alcohol use: a systematic review of longitudinal studies. *Australian and New Zealand Journal of Psychiatry* **44**, 774–83.

SAS Institute Inc. (2008). *SAS/STAT® Software, Version 9.2 for Unix.* Cary, NC: SAS Institute.

Schlesselman, J. J. (1982). *Case–Control Studies: Design, Conduct, Analysis.* New York, NY: Oxford University Press.

Schoenborn, C. A., Adams, P. F., & Schiller, J. S. (2003). Summary health statistics for the U.S. population: National Health Interview Survey, 2000. *Vital and Health Statistics* **10** (214), 1–83.

Schwarz, N., & Sudman, S., eds. (1994). *Autobiographical Memory and the Validity of Retrospective Reports.* New York, NY: Springer-Verlag.

Schwarz, N., & Sudman, S., eds. (1996). *Answering Questions: Methodology for Determining Cognitive and Communicative Processes in Survey Research.* San Francisco, CA: Jossey-Bass.

Sheatsley, P. B. (1983). Questionnaire construction and item writing. In P. H. Rossi, J. D. Wright, & A. B. Anderson, eds., *Handbook of Survey Research: Quantitative Studies in Social Relations.* New York, NY: Academy Press, pp. 195–230.

Simon, G. E., & Von Korff, M. (1995). Recall of psychiatric history in cross-sectional surveys: implications for epidemiologic research. *Epidemiologic Reviews* **17**, 221–7.

Sirken, M. G., Herrmann, D. J., Schechter, S., *et al.*, eds. (1999). *Cognition and Survey Research.* New York, NY: Wiley.

Smith, T. W. (2004). Developing and evaluating cross-national survey instruments. In S. Presser, J. M. Rothgeb, M. P. Couper, *et al.*, eds., *Methods for Testing and Evaluating Survey Questionnaires.* New York, NY: Wiley, pp. 431–52.

Straus, M. A. (1979). Measuring intrafamily conflict and violence: the Conflict Tactics (CT) Scale. *Journal of Marriage and Family* **41**, 75–88.

Sudman, S., Bradburn, N., & Schwarz, N. (1996). *Thinking About Answers: the Application of Cognitive Processes to Survey Methodology.* San Francisco, CA: Jossey-Bass.

Swendsen, J. D., Merikangas, K. R., Canino, G. J., *et al.* (1998). The comorbidity of alcoholism with anxiety and depressive disorders in four geographic communities. *Comprehensive Psychiatry* **39**, 176–84.

Tanur, J. M. (1992). *Questions about Questions: Inquiries Into the Cognitive Bases of Surveys.* New York, NY: Russell Sage Foundation.

Tennant, C. (1988). Psychosocial causes of duodenal ulcer. *Australian and New Zealand Journal of Psychiatry* **22**, 195–201.

Tuma, N., & Hannan, M. (1984). *Social Dynamics.* Orlando, FL: Academic Press.

Turner, C., & Martin, E. (1985). *Surveying Subjective Phenomena.* New York, NY: Russell Sage Foundation.

Üstün, T. B., Kostanjsek, N., Chatterji, S., & Rehm, J. (2010). *Measuring Health and Disability: Manual for WHO Disability Assessment Schedule (WHODAS 2.0).* Geneva: World Health Organization.

Van der Laan, M. J., & Rose, S., eds. (2011). *Targeted Learning: Causal Inference for Observational and Experimental Data.* New York, NY: Springer.

Verma, V., Scott, C., & O'Muircheartaigh, C. (1980). Sample designs and sampling errors for the World Fertility Survey. *Journal of the Royal Statistical Society* **143**, 431–73.

Von Korff, M., Crane, P. K., Alonso, J., *et al.* (2008). Modified WHODAS-II provides valid measure of global disability but filter items increased skewness. *Journal of Clinical Epidemiology* **61**, 1132–43.

Von Korff, M. R., Scott, K. M., & Gureje, O. (2009). *Global Perspectives on Mental–Physical Comorbidity in the WHO World Mental Health Surveys.* New York, NY: Cambridge University Press.

Wang, P. S., Angermeyer, M., Borges, G., *et al.* (2007). Delay and failure in treatment seeking after first onset of mental disorders in the World Health Organization's World Mental Health Survey Initiative. *World Psychiatry* **6**, 177–85.

Willett, J. B., & Singer, J. D. (1993). Investigating onset, cessation, relapse, and recovery: why you should, and how you can, use discrete-time survival analysis to examine event occurrence. *Journal of Consulting and Clinical Psychology* **61**, 952–65.

Williams, B. J. (1986). Suggestions for the application of advanced technology in Canadian collection operations. *Journal of Official Statistics* **2**, 555–60.

Wolter, K. M. (1985). *Introduction to Variance Estimation.* New York, NY: Springer-Verlag.

World Bank (2008). Data and statistics. http://go.worldbank.org/D7SN0B8YU0. Accessed May 12, 2009.

Zimmermann, P., Wittchen, H. U., Hofler, M., *et al.* (2003). Primary anxiety disorders and the development of subsequent alcohol use disorders: a 4-year community study of adolescents and young adults. *Psychological Medicine* **33**, 1211–22.

Parent psychopathology and offspring mental disorders

Katie A. McLaughlin, Anne M. Gadermann, Irving Hwang,
Nancy A. Sampson, Laura Helena Andrade, José Miguel Caldas
de Almeida, Yanling He, Aimee Nasser Karam, Samuel D. Murphy,
and Ronald C. Kessler

Introduction

Parent psychopathology is known to be strongly associated with elevated risk of mental disorders in offspring (Downey & Coyne 1990, Beidel & Turner 1997, Merikangas *et al.* 1998b, Lieb *et al.* 2002, Clark *et al.* 2004, Bornovalova *et al.* 2010). This risk has been shown to be transmitted through both genetic and environmental mechanisms (Downey & Coyne 1990, Kendler *et al.* 1992, Kendler *et al.* 2003, Hettema *et al.* 2005). From the perspective of the current volume, this finding can be interpreted as meaning that one of the adverse societal costs of mental disorder is the creation of future cases of mental disorders in subsequent generations. A central unresolved question in this literature, though, is whether having a parent with a mental disorder creates a generalized vulnerability to psychopathology that increases risk of a wide range of offspring disorders, or whether particular parent disorders are associated with particular offspring disorders (Bornovalova *et al.* 2010). A number of studies have addressed this issue by examining the familial aggregation of mental disorders, suggesting that some disorders "breed true" in families (e.g., parental anxiety is associated with an increased risk for offspring anxiety: Biederman *et al.* 2006) and that within-disorder associations (corresponding parental and offspring disorders) are generally larger than cross-disorder associations (Lieb *et al.* 2000, 2002, Clark *et al.* 2004). But the pattern of associations differs somewhat by disorder (Kendler *et al.* 1997, Biederman *et al.* 2006), and much of this research examined only a single or a limited number of parent disorders at a time, without accounting for comorbidity among parent disorders (Beidel &

Turner 1997, Merikangas *et al.* 1998b, Lieb *et al.* 2002, Biederman *et al.* 2006). Failure to account for comorbidity may have artificially inflated estimates of the associations between specific parent and offspring disorders. Indeed, evidence from a national sample found that the familial aggregation of some common mental disorders was substantially attenuated when comorbidity among parent disorders was taken into consideration (Kendler *et al.* 1997). Several small family studies have reported a similar result, although with less consistency (Merikangas *et al.* 1998a, Low *et al.* 2008).

An additional problem in previous research on this issue of intergenerational continuity of psychopathology is that the few studies that considered comorbidity among parent disorders assumed additive associations across these disorders in predicting offspring disorders; that is, that there were no interactions among parent disorders in predicting continuity into the next generation. Given emerging evidence that significant sub-additive interactions consistently exist both among more general measures of childhood adversities in predicting subsequent mental disorders (Green *et al.* 2010, Kessler *et al.* 2010) and among temporally primary mental disorders in predicting secondary comorbid disorders (Kessler *et al.* 2011), this assumption of additivity in the effects of parent disorders needs to be reconsidered.

Another limitation of previous studies in this area is that most of them have been conducted in the USA or Europe. Cross-national differences in results consequently have not previously been examined. Yet there is reason to believe that the associations of parental psychopathology with offspring psychopathology

---

The Burdens of Mental Disorders, ed. Jordi Alonso, Somnath Chatterji, and Yanling He. Published by
Cambridge University Press. © World Health Organization 2013.

might differ across countries. For example, stigmatization of individuals with psychopathology generalizes to the family (Lefley 1989), and this may be more pronounced in countries where the collective representation of the family has greater social implications (Tsang *et al.* 2003). This can lead families to conceal their relatives' mental disorder, because it is perceived as shameful (Chang & Horrocks 2006) or as a punishment for collective family misdeeds (Hsiao & Van Riper 2010). A potential consequence is greater social isolation of the family in these kinds of cultural contexts (Tsang *et al.* 2003, Lauber & Rossler 2007), which may impact children's risk for psychopathology. Other factors that may differ cross-nationally and influence the strength of associations between parent and offspring disorders are access to mental health treatment and delay and failure in treatment seeking for both social and economic reasons. Treatment access is lower and delays in treatment seeking are higher in developing countries (Wang *et al.* 2007, Bruckner *et al.* 2011), which may force families to provide care for a mentally ill family member and result in children being exposed to a mentally ill parent for longer periods of time.

The WHO World Mental Health (WMH) surveys provide a unique and unparalleled opportunity both to examine the associations between multiple parent disorders and offspring disorders and to evaluate whether the pattern of associations is similar across the wide range of countries in the WMH surveys.

Methods

Sample

The analysis focuses on all the surveys considered in this volume other than those in two countries (Israel and New Zealand) that did not assess parent psychopathology. The total sample size in the remaining 23 surveys is 104,253. See Chapter 2 for a description of these surveys. It is noteworthy that parent psychopathology was assessed in part 2 of these surveys, which include a total of 51,509 respondents. As detailed in Chapter 2, the part 2 sample was weighted in each survey to be representative of the original full survey so as to correct for the over-sampling of part 1 cases. See Chapter 2 for a more detailed discussion of this issue.

Measures

Parent psychopathology was assessed with an expanded version of the Family History Research Diagnostic

Criteria Interview (Endicott *et al.* 1978, Kendler *et al.* 1991). Respondents were asked to report parent disorders that were present during at least some part of the respondents' childhoods. The disorders assessed included major depressive episodes, panic disorder, generalized anxiety disorder (GAD), substance dependence, and antisocial personality disorder, as well as parent suicide attempt and suicide death. We distinguished between paternal and maternal disorders.

The respondent mental disorders considered in this chapter include all those described in Chapter 2 other than minor depression. However, these outcome disorders were pooled into aggregate measures of respondent anxiety, mood, disruptive behavior, and substance disorders. See the discussion in Chapter 2 about the procedures used to carry out this pooling. For present purposes it is sufficient to note that the resulting coefficients tell us the average association of each parental disorder with each of the four sets of respondent disorders averaged across the respondent disorders in the class.

Statistical analysis

Associations between parent psychopathology and lifetime occurrence of respondent disorders were estimated in a series of discrete-time survival models that used person-year as the unit of analysis. Again, see Chapter 2 for a description of these methods. Controls were included in the models for country, respondent age at interview, and sex. Analysis began with a series of bivariate models in which each type of parent disorder was considered individually as a predictor of respondent disorders. This was followed by a series of multivariate models in which all parent disorders were considered simultaneously in predicting respondent disorders. Subsequent models then examined the associations of either (1) number of parental disorders, or (2) both number and type of parental disorders, with respondent disorders. As noted in Chapter 2, all these models began by using a consolidated set of 20 separate person-year data files, each focused on a single respondent outcome disorder, which forced the estimated slopes of respondent disorders on parent disorders to be constant across outcomes. We then disaggregated this consolidated set of files to estimate separate models to predict first onset of disorders within each of four broad disorder classes (mood, anxiety, substance, and disruptive behavior disorders).

The population attributable risk proportion (PARP) of respondent disorders predicted by parent disorders was computed for the best-fitting multivariate model using simulation methods that generated individual-level predicted probabilities of the outcome disorders from the coefficients in the model with and without coefficients for parent disorders. As noted in Chapter 2, PARP can be interpreted as the proportion of the observed outcomes that would not have occurred in the absence of one or more predictors under the model based on the assumption that the regression coefficients in the model represents causal effects of the predictor. See Chapter 2 for a discussion of the computation of PARP. The survival coefficients and their standard errors were exponentiated and are presented as odds ratios (OR) with 95% confidence intervals (95% CI). As in all other chapters throughout this volume, adjustments for the weighting and clustering of the sample design were made by calculating standard errors of prevalence estimates and survival coefficients using a design-based estimation method, in this case the Taylor Series Linearization method (Wolter 1985), implemented in the SUDAAN software system (Research Triangle Institute 2005). Multivariate significance was evaluated with Wald χ^2 tests based on design-corrected coefficient variance–covariance matrices. Statistical significance was consistently evaluated using 0.05 level two-sided tests.

Results

Preliminary analysis

We first conducted preliminary tests to determine whether the associations between parent and offspring mental disorders differed depending on which parent (i.e., mother or father) had the disorder, how many parents had the disorder (i.e., one or both), and whether the respondent was male or female. These analyses showed that the associations consistently differed depending on whether one parent or both parents had a disorder, with the exception of parent suicide death. All subsequent models therefore included separate dummy variables coding whether one or both parents had each disorder and whether either parent had died by suicide. Distinguishing between whether a respondent's mother or father had the disorder influenced only the associations involving parent substance abuse, so an additional predictor was included in the final specification to distinguish maternal from paternal

substance abuse. Sex of the respondent did not interact with any of the measures of parent disorders. We also evaluated whether parent suicide attempt and death contributed unique information in predicting offspring psychopathology or whether they could be combined into a single indicator of suicidality. These analyses suggested that both indicators had unique associations with offspring disorder outcomes, and they were retained as separate variables in all analyses. Parent suicide death was the only type of parent psychopathology entered as a time-varying covariate, as information was not available on the respondent's age when each parent disorder started. All we knew was that the parent disorder was present for at least some of the time during the years the respondent was a child, and we coded these disorders as time-invariant predictors.

Bivariate associations of parent disorders with offspring disorders

We examined the associations of parent disorders with offspring disorder in bivariate models that considered only one type of parent disorder at a time. In the combined sample, all parent disorders were significant predictors of lifetime onset of offspring DSM-IV/CIDI disorders in pooled models that combined estimates across all offspring disorders (Table 3.1). ORs were in the range 1.5–2.9 for one parent having a given disorder and 2.2–4.6 for both parents having the disorder. In all cases, the odds were higher if both parents had the disorder than only one. A similar pattern was observed in bivariate models predicting each of the four disorder classes (mood, anxiety, substance, and disruptive behavior disorders). Each type of parent disorder significantly predicted each of the four types of offspring disorders with the exception of parent suicide death. Within-class associations (e.g., parent depression predicting offspring mood disorders; parent anxiety disorders predicting offspring anxiety disorders) were somewhat higher than across-class associations (e.g., parent depression predicting offspring substance disorders). However, this pattern was not pronounced and there were notable exceptions to it, such as parent GAD having an OR as large as that of parent depression in predicting offspring mood disorders, and parent GAD as well as parent depression both having higher ORs than parent antisocial personality disorder in predicting offspring disruptive behavior disorders.

Table 3.1 Bivariate associations of parent psychopathology with subsequent onset of offspring lifetime mental disorders. The WMH surveys.[a]

Types of parent disorder	Offspring disorders									
	Mood disorder		Anxiety disorder		Disruptive behavior disorder		Substance disorder		Any disorder	
	OR	(95% CI)	OR	(95% CI)	OR	(95% CI)	OR	(95% CI)	OR	(95% CI)
I. Major depressive episode										
Exactly 1 parent	2.6*	(2.3–2.9)	2.8*	(2.5–3.2)	3.6*	(3.0–4.2)	2.5*	(2.1–3.0)	2.8*	(2.5–3.1)
Both parents	4.0*	(2.8–5.6)	4.1*	(2.9–5.8)	5.2*	(3.4–8.1)	2.5*	(1.3–4.7)	4.0*	(2.9–5.4)
χ^2_2	307.9*		389.0*		253.5*		113.6*		451.8*	
II. Generalized anxiety										
Exactly 1 parent	2.7*	(2.4–3.0)	3.0*	(2.7–3.3)	41.9*	(34.0–51.7)	2.4*	(2.0–2.8)	2.9*	(2.6–3.2)
Both parents	4.0*	(3.1–5.2)	4.6*	(3.6–5.9)	6303.1*	(2455.3–16181.2)[b]	4.4*	(2.9–6.5)	4.6*	(3.7–5.8)
χ^2_2	449.0*		619.2*		1234.5*		169.8*		710.0*	
III. Panic disorder										
Exactly 1 parent	2.3*	(2.1–2.5)	2.6*	(2.4–2.8)	2.8*	(2.4–3.2)	2.2*	(2.0–2.5)	2.5*	(2.3–2.6)
Both parents	3.1*	(2.5–3.9)	4.1*	(3.3–5.0)	4.6*	(3.5–6.2)	3.2*	(2.4–4.3)	3.7*	(3.1–4.4)
χ^2_2	479.8*		730.7*		278.5*		201.5*		782.9*	
IV. Substance abuse										
Exactly 1 parent – mother	2.2*	(1.7–2.7)	2.1*	(1.7–2.6)	3.2*	(2.4–4.3)	3.2*	(2.5–4.0)	2.5*	(2.1–3.0)
Exactly 1 parent – father	1.8*	(1.6–2.0)	1.8*	(1.7–2.0)	2.4*	(2.0–2.9)	2.4*	(2.1–2.7)	2.0*	(1.8–2.2)
Both parents	2.3*	(1.6–3.2)	3.0*	(2.3–4.1)	3.7*	(2.6–5.2)	4.3*	(3.0–6.1)	3.1*	(2.4–4.1)
χ^2_3	221.3*		309.0*		156.2*		364.5*		445.3*	
V. Antisocial personality disorder										
Exactly 1 parent	2.1*	(1.9–2.4)	2.4*	(2.1–2.7)	3.5*	(2.9–4.2)	2.6*	(2.3–3.0)	2.5*	(2.3–2.8)
Both parents	2.0*	(1.1–3.8)	2.8*	(1.5–5.1)	4.0*	(2.4–6.7)	3.7*	(2.1–6.6)	3.0*	(1.8–5.0)
χ^2_2	142.2*		267.0*		189.0*		209.0*		368.7*	
VI. Suicide attempt										
Exactly 1 parent	1.8*	(1.6–2.0)	1.8*	(1.6–2.0)	2.3*	(1.9–2.8)	1.8*	(1.5–2.2)	1.8*	(1.6–2.1)
Both parents	2.2*	(1.0–4.8)	2.3*	(1.0–5.4)	3.5*	(1.6–7.5)	1.0	(0.4–2.3)	2.2*	(1.1–4.4)
χ^2_2	90.9*		79.1*		73.7*		39.1*		113.2*	
VII. Suicide (death from suicide)[c]										
Any	1.6*	(1.1–2.2)	1.3	(0.9–2.0)	1.2	(0.4–3.5)	1.6	(0.8–3.3)	1.5*	(1.0–2.0)
χ^2_1	7.0*		1.6		0.1		2.1		4.9*	

[a] Assessed in the part 2 sample. Models control for country, person-year, age, and sex.
[b] Although the number of respondents who reported that both their parents had GAD is small, the consistency of these respondents having multiple behavior disorders is so great that the association between both-parent GAD and offspring behavior disorders is statistically significant despite the instability of the OR and CI.
[c] Parent death from suicide is a time-varying predictor; all other parent disorders are considered time-invariant.
* Significant at the 0.05 level, two-sided test.

We next estimated this series of bivariate models separately for high-income, upper-middle-income, and low/lower-middle-income countries (Appendix Table 3.1). The pattern of associations observed in each of the three country groups was quite similar to the pattern in the total sample. Each type of parent disorder was associated with each type of offspring disorder, with the exception of parent suicide death. The one notable difference was that having two parents with a particular disorder was not associated consistently with greater odds of offspring disorder than having only one parent with a given disorder. For example, in low/lower-middle-income countries, having two parents with a suicide attempt was not associated with any offspring disorder outcomes, and having two parents with depression, substance abuse, or antisocial personality disorder was not associated with offspring substance disorders. Because the magnitude of the ORs for some of these associations was relatively large (e.g., the OR for the association of having two parents with antisocial personality disorder with offspring substance disorder was 3.2), this pattern most likely reflects inadequate power due to the small number of respondents in low/lower-middle-income countries who reported having two parents with each of these disorders. Indeed, only 24 respondents with a lifetime mental disorder reported having two parents with major depression in these countries, 10 reported having two parents with GAD, 94 reported having two parents with panic disorder, 6 reported having two parents with substance abuse, 8 reported having two parents with antisocial personality disorder, and 5 reported suicide attempts in both parents. As a result, estimates of having two parents with a disorder at the level of country income groups are relatively unstable and are not presented here.

Multivariate associations of parent mental disorders with subsequent offspring disorders

The bivariate associations observed in the total sample were uniformly attenuated in the additive multivariate model, which examines all parent disorders as predictors of offspring disorders simultaneously (Table 3.2). Five of the seven types of parent psychopathology were significantly associated with offspring mental disorders in the pooled model (ORs in the range 1.3–1.9

for one parent and 1.5–2.2 for both parents). Neither parent suicide attempt nor suicide death was associated with offspring disorders in this model. The odds of offspring disorder were higher if both parents had the disorder only in the cases of parent panic disorder and substance abuse. A test for the joint associations of all parent disorders in this model was significant ($\chi^2_{14} = 1437.5$, $p < 0.001$).

When the pooled additive multivariate model was estimated separately in each of the three country groups, the overall patterns of associations were largely similar, with a few exceptions (Appendix Table 3.2). Parent suicide death and suicide attempt were unassociated with offspring disorders in all country groups. Having two parents with a disorder was associated with greater odds of offspring disorder for all parent disorders in high-income countries, but only for panic and substance abuse in upper-middle-income countries and for panic, depression, and antisocial personality disorder in low/lower-middle-income countries. Finally, parent GAD was not associated with offspring disorder in low/lower-middle-income countries. The joint associations of all parent disorders in predicting offspring disorder were significant in high-income ($\chi^2_{14} = 1188.2$, $p < 0.001$), upper-middle-income ($\chi^2_{14} = 328.2$, $p < 0.001$), and low/lower-middle-income countries ($\chi^2_{14} = 485.2$, $p < 0.001$).

Disaggregation of the additive multivariate model by type of offspring disorders in the total sample revealed little variation (Table 3.2). All types of parent psychopathology other than suicide attempt and suicide death predicted offspring mood, anxiety, and disruptive behavior disorders. The one exception was offspring substance disorders, where parent GAD and depression were not significant predictors. The joint associations of all parent disorders as a set were significant in predicting all four classes of offspring disorders ($\chi^2_{14} = 641.0–1,263.6$, $p < 0.001$). Within-class associations were generally stronger than across-class associations, with two exceptions. First, parent GAD and panic disorder were stronger predictors than parent depression of offspring mood disorders. Second, parent panic disorder was as strong a predictor as parent antisocial personality disorder of offspring disruptive behavior disorders. A similar pattern of associations was observed when these models were estimated separately in each of the three country groups. Parent suicide attempt and suicide death were largely not associated with offspring

Table 3.2 Multivariate associations of parent psychopathology with subsequent onset of offspring lifetime mental disorders based on an additive model. The WMH surveys.[a]

Types of parent disorder	Offspring disorders									
	Mood disorder		Anxiety disorder		Disruptive behavior disorder		Substance disorder		Any disorder	
	OR	(95% CI)	OR	(95% CI)	OR	(95% CI)	OR	(95% CI)	OR	(95% CI)
I. Major depressive episode										
Exactly 1 parent	1.3*	(1.2–1.5)	1.3*	(1.2–1.5)	1.4*	(1.2–1.8)	1.2	(1.0–1.6)	1.3*	(1.2–1.5)
Both parents	1.5*	(1.0–2.3)	1.4	(0.9–2.1)	1.2	(0.8–1.9)	0.8	(0.3–1.8)	1.3	(0.9–1.9)
χ^2_2	16.9*		18.6*		10.5*		3.6		18.9*	
II. Generalized anxiety										
Exactly 1 parent	1.6*	(1.4–1.8)	1.7*	(1.5–1.9)	1.7*	(1.4–2.1)	1.2	(1.0–1.5)	1.6*	(1.4–1.7)
Both parents	1.5*	(1.0–2.1)	1.5*	(1.1–2.2)	1.7*	(1.1–2.5)	1.5	(0.8–2.7)	1.5*	(1.0–2.1)
χ^2_2	38.9*		67.7*		24.6*		4.4		59.2*	
III. Panic disorder										
Exactly 1 parent	1.8*	(1.7–2.0)	2.0*	(1.8–2.1)	1.9*	(1.7–2.2)	1.7*	(1.5–2.0)	1.9*	(1.7–2.0)
Both parents	1.9*	(1.5–2.5)	2.4*	(2.0–3.0)	2.2*	(1.6–3.0)	2.2*	(1.6–3.1)	2.2*	(1.8–2.7)
χ^2_2	168.9*		267.1*		96.6*		63.0*		291.6*	
IV. Substance abuse										
Exactly 1 parent – mother	1.2	(0.9–1.5)	1.1	(0.9–1.4)	1.6*	(1.1–2.2)	2.0*	(1.5–2.7)	1.4*	(1.1–1.7)
Exactly 1 parent – father	1.3*	(1.2–1.5)	1.3*	(1.2–1.4)	1.5*	(1.2–1.9)	1.9*	(1.6–2.2)	1.4*	(1.3–1.6)
Both parents	1.4*	(1.0–2.0)	1.7*	(1.3–2.2)	1.8*	(1.3–2.6)	3.0*	(2.2–4.3)	1.9*	(1.4–2.4)
χ^2_3	33.5*		35.4*		22.1*		122.2*		82.1*	
V. Antisocial personality disorder										
Exactly 1 parent	1.3*	(1.2–1.5)	1.5*	(1.3–1.7)	1.9*	(1.5–2.3)	1.5*	(1.3–1.7)	1.5*	(1.4–1.7)
Both parents	1.0	(0.6–1.7)	1.4	(0.9–2.2)	1.6	(0.9–2.6)	1.6	(0.8–3.2)	1.5	(1.0–2.2)
χ^2_2	15.3*		47.7*		32.7*		28.9*		64.2*	
VI. Suicide attempt										
Exactly 1 parent	1.1	(0.9–1.2)	1.0	(0.9–1.2)	1.1	(0.9–1.4)	1.1	(0.9–1.3)	1.1	(0.9–1.2)
Both parents	1.1	(0.6–2.0)	0.9	(0.4–1.8)	1.0	(0.5–2.1)	0.3*	(0.1–0.8)	0.8	(0.4–1.5)
χ^2_2	1.5		0.2		0.9		5.9		1.6	
VII. Suicide (death from suicide)[b]										
Any	1.3	(1.0–1.9)	1.2	(0.8–1.7)	1.0	(0.3–2.8)	1.5	(0.8–2.9)	1.3	(0.9–1.7)
χ^2_1	2.8		0.6		0.0		1.6		2.5	
Global χ^2_{14}	842.8*		1,263.6*		891.3*		641.0*		1,437.5*	

[a] Assessed in the part 2 sample. Models include dummy variables for all parent mental disorders and control for country, person-year, age, and sex.
[b] Parent death from suicide is a time-varying predictor; all other parent disorders are not time-varying.
* Significant at the 0.05 level, two-sided test.

disorders in all country groups; parent suicide death was associated with offspring mood disorders in upper-middle-income countries and with disruptive behavior disorders in low/lower-middle-income countries. Parent depression and GAD were unassociated with offspring substance disorders, with the exception of high-income countries for GAD. In low/lower-middle-income countries, parental antisocial personality disorder was associated only with offspring anxiety and disruptive behavior disorders. The joint associations of all parent disorders in predicting offspring disorder were significant for all disorder classes in high-income (χ^2_{14} = 638.1–1084.4, p < 0.001), upper-middle-income (χ^2_{14} = 152.2–300.2, p < 0.001), and low/lower-middle-income countries (χ^2_{14} = 254.1–1161.0, p < 0.001).

Associations of number of parent disorders with subsequent offspring disorders

In the total sample, a generally increasing association was observed between number of parent disorders and odds of offspring disorders in the pooled model, with ORs ranging from 1.9 for exactly 1 maternal disorder to 3.6 for 5 and 3.0 for 6+ maternal disorders (Table 3.3). The ORs increased from 1.6 for exactly 1 paternal disorder to 2.8 for exactly 4 paternal disorders and then decreased to 1.9–2.0 for 5 and 6+ paternal disorders. The joint associations of number of parental disorders with pooled offspring disorders was significant for both maternal (χ^2_6 = 580.8, p < 0.001) and paternal (χ^2_6 = 346.7, p < 0.001) disorders.

Disaggregation of this model shows a similar pattern in predicting each class of offspring disorders (i.e., mood, anxiety, substance, and disruptive behavior disorders), with joint associations of both maternal and paternal number of disorders significant in predicting each class of offspring disorders (χ^2_5 = 114.9–515.7, p < 0.001). A monotonic dose–response relationship between number of parent disorders and odds of offspring disorders exists for maternal disorders predicting offspring substance disorder.

The same generally increasing association between number of parent disorders and odds of offspring disorders was observed in the pooled model across country groups for maternal and paternal disorders (Appendix Table 3.3). In high-income countries, the ORs ranged from 1.8 for exactly 1 maternal disorder to 3.2–3.6 for 5 and 6+ maternal disorders, and the ORs increased from 1.8 for exactly

1 paternal disorder to 3.7 for exactly 4 paternal disorders, and then decreased to 1.8–2.0 for 5 and 6+ paternal disorders. In upper-middle-income countries, the ORs ranged from 2.0 for exactly 1 maternal disorder to 3.3 for 4+ maternal disorders, and the ORs increased from 1.4 for exactly 1 paternal disorder to 2.2 for exactly 3 paternal disorders, and then decreased to 1.1 for 4+ paternal disorders. Finally, in low/lower-middle-income countries, the ORs ranged from 2.2 for exactly 1 maternal disorder to 3.8 for 3+ maternal disorders, and the ORs increased from 1.5 for exactly 1 paternal disorder to 2.5 for 4+ paternal disorders. In all three country groups, the joint associations of number of parental disorders with pooled offspring disorders were significant for both maternal (χ^2_{3-6} = 111.4–377.9, p < 0.001) and paternal (χ^2_{4-6} = 49.7–328.0, p < 0.001) disorders.

Disaggregation of this model shows a similar pattern in predicting each class of offspring disorders, with joint associations of both maternal and paternal number of disorders significant in predicting offspring mood (χ^2_{3-4} = 15.2–214.3, p < 0.001), anxiety (χ^2_{3-5} = 26.5–356.5, p < 0.001), disruptive behavior (χ^2_{3-4} = 20.3–161.3, p < 0.001), and substance disorders (χ^2_{2-4} = 12.7–148.7, p < 0.001–0.002) in all three country groups.

Associations of type–number of parent disorders with subsequent offspring disorders

We next estimated a series of multivariate models that included information about both type and number of parent disorders to predict offspring disorders (Table 3.4). In the total sample, each type of parent disorder was significantly associated with odds of offspring disorders in the pooled model (ORs in the range 1.4–2.1 for one parent and 1.5–3.0 for both parents), controlling for number of disorders. Types of parent disorders were significant as a set after controlling for number of disorders (χ^2_{14} = 670.0, p < 0.001). The ORs associated with parent disorder types in this model were generally higher than in the additive model. This means that the additivity assumption led to a downward bias in the estimated associations of parent disorders with offspring disorders in the earlier model. This bias occurred because the ORs associated with number of parent disorders were significant as a set (χ^2_5 = 74.1, p < 0.001 for maternal disorders;

Table 3.3 Multivariate associations between number of parent mental disorders and subsequent onset of offspring lifetime mental disorders. The WMH surveys.[a]

Number of parent disorders	Offspring disorders									
	Mood disorder		Anxiety disorder		Disruptive behavior disorder		Substance disorder		Any disorder	
	OR	(95% CI)	OR	(95% CI)	OR	(95% CI)	OR	(95% CI)	OR	(95% CI)
I. Number of maternal disorders[b]										
1	1.8*	(1.7–2.0)	2.0*	(1.9–2.2)	1.9*	(1.7–2.3)	1.8*	(1.6–2.1)	1.9*	(1.8–2.1)
2	2.2*	(1.8–2.6)	2.1*	(1.8–2.5)	2.5*	(2.0–3.1)	2.0*	(1.6–2.6)	2.2*	(1.9–2.5)
3	3.0*	(2.5–3.6)	3.3*	(2.7–3.9)	4.2*	(3.3–5.3)	2.4*	(1.7–3.4)	3.2*	(2.7–3.7)
4	2.2*	(1.6–3.1)	2.5*	(1.8–3.4)	4.7*	(3.1–7.3)	3.3*	(2.2–5.0)	2.8*	(2.1–3.8)
5	2.8*	(1.7–4.6)	3.2*	(2.3–4.6)	3.7*	(2.1–6.4)	4.3*	(2.0–9.5)	3.6*	(2.4–5.3)
6+									3.0*	(1.1–7.9)
χ^2_6	349.8*		515.7*		249.6*		156.5*		580.8*	
II. Number of paternal disorders[b]										
1	1.5*	(1.4–1.7)	1.6*	(1.5–1.7)	1.8*	(1.5–2.0)	1.8*	(1.6–2.0)	1.6*	(1.5–1.7)
2	1.7*	(1.4–2.0)	2.0*	(1.7–2.4)	2.5*	(1.9–3.3)	2.1*	(1.8–2.6)	2.0*	(1.8–2.3)
3	2.1*	(1.6–2.8)	2.2*	(1.7–2.8)	2.7*	(2.0–3.6)	1.9*	(1.2–3.0)	2.2*	(1.7–2.7)
4	2.4*	(1.7–3.3)	2.6*	(1.9–3.6)	2.8*	(2.0–4.0)	2.7*	(1.6–4.5)	2.8*	(2.0–3.8)
5									1.9*	(1.1–3.4)
6+									2.0*	(1.1–3.6)
χ^2_6	140.1*		253.0*		114.9*		126.0*		346.7*	
Global χ^2_{12}	922.1*		1,113.6*		685.1*		508.7*		1,417.7*	

[a] Assessed in the part 2 sample. Models include dummy variables for number of parent mental disorders and control for country, person-year, age, and sex.
[b] For number of parent disorders, the last odds ratio represents the odds of the number or more. For example, for mood disorders, the last odds ratio for maternal disorders represents 5 or more maternal disorders.
* Significant at the 0.05 level, two-sided test.

Table 3.4 Multivariate associations of types and number of parent mental disorders and offspring mental disorders. The WMH surveys.[a]

					Offspring disorders								
	Mood disorder		Anxiety disorder		Disruptive behavior disorder		Substance disorder		Any disorder	
	OR	(95% CI)	OR	(95% CI)	OR	(95% CI)	OR	(95% CI)	OR	(95% CI)
Types of parent disorder										
I. Major depressive episode										
Exactly 1 parent	1.8*	(1.5–2.1)	1.9*	(1.7–2.3)	1.8*	(1.4–2.3)	1.5*	(1.1–2.0)	1.8*	(1.6–2.1)
Both parents	2.6*	(1.8–3.9)	3.0*	(2.1–4.4)	2.1*	(1.2–3.6)	1.1	(0.5–2.8)	2.6*	(1.9–3.7)
X^2_2	53.9*		91.0*		22.7*		8.8*		82.9*	
II. Generalized anxiety										
Exactly 1 parent	2.0*	(1.7–2.3)	2.3*	(2.0–2.6)	2.1*	(1.6–2.7)	1.5*	(1.2–1.9)	2.1*	(1.8–2.3)
Both parents	2.8*	(1.9–4.0)	3.4*	(2.3–5.0)	3.1*	(1.9–5.1)	2.5*	(1.2–4.9)	3.0*	(2.1–4.3)
X^2_2	85.4*		366.3*		38.5*		11.6*		123.7*	
III. Panic disorder										
Exactly 1 parent	2.0*	(1.8–2.2)	2.2*	(2.0–2.4)	2.0*	(1.8–2.4)	1.8*	(1.6–2.1)	2.0*	(1.9–2.2)
Both parents	2.4*	(1.9–3.1)	3.5*	(2.8–4.3)	2.9*	(2.1–4.1)	2.7*	(1.8–3.8)	3.0*	(2.5–3.6)
X^2_2	217.6*		366.3*		98.2*		71.5*		362.4*	
IV. Substance abuse										
Exactly 1 parent – mother	1.7*	(1.3–2.3)	1.7*	(1.4–2.2)	2.0*	(1.3–2.9)	2.2*	(1.7–3.0)	1.9*	(1.5–2.4)
Exactly 1 parent – father	1.4*	(1.3–1.6)	1.4*	(1.3–1.6)	1.6*	(1.3–2.0)	2.0*	(1.7–2.3)	1.5*	(1.4–1.7)
Both parents	2.0*	(1.4–2.8)	2.6*	(1.9–3.5)	2.3*	(1.6–3.5)	3.6*	(2.5–5.3)	2.6*	(2.0–3.4)
X^2_3	70.6*		90.1*		37.3*		121.1*		156.6*	
V. Antisocial personality disorder										
Exactly 1 parent	1.6*	(1.4–1.9)	1.9*	(1.7–2.1)	2.3*	(1.8–2.8)	1.8*	(1.5–2.1)	1.9*	(1.7–2.1)
Both parents	1.8*	(1.0–3.2)	2.8*	(1.7–4.5)	2.9*	(1.8–4.8)	2.5*	(1.3–4.6)	2.6*	(1.7–3.9)
X^2_2	46.9*		104.0*		58.2*		44.3*		155.9*	
VI. Suicide attempt										
Exactly 1 parent	1.4*	(1.2–1.6)	1.4*	(1.2–1.6)	1.4*	(1.1–1.7)	1.2	(1.0–1.5)	1.4*	(1.2–1.5)
Both parents	1.9	(1.0–3.8)	1.9	(0.9–3.8)	1.8	(0.8–4.0)	0.5	(0.2–1.2)	1.5	(0.9–2.8)
X^2_2	23.9*		24.2*		7.6*		5.7		32.6*	

Table 3.4 (cont.)

	Offspring disorders									
	Mood disorder		Anxiety disorder		Disruptive behavior disorder		Substance disorder		Any disorder	
	OR	(95% CI)	OR	(95% CI)	OR	(95% CI)	OR	(95% CI)	OR	(95% CI)
VII. Suicide (death from suicide)[b]										
Any	1.5*	(1.1–2.2)	1.4	(0.9–2.1)	1.1	(0.4–3.3)	1.8	(0.9–3.4)	1.5*	(1.1–2.1)
χ^2_1	6.1*		2.7		0.1		2.9		6.8*	
VIII. Global tests for types										
Global χ^2_{14}	419.8*		553.7*		201.8*		227.2*		670.0*	
χ^2_{12} for difference among types	51.8*		81.4*		28.6*		47.4*		64.2*	
Number of parent disorders										
I. Number of maternal disorders[c]										
2	0.7*	(0.6–0.9)	0.6*	(0.5–0.7)	0.7*	(0.6–1.0)	0.8	(0.6–1.1)	0.6*	(0.5–0.8)
3	0.5*	(0.4–0.7)	0.4*	(0.3–0.6)	0.6*	(0.4–1.0)	0.6*	(0.4–1.0)	0.5*	(0.4–0.6)
4	0.3*	(0.2–0.4)	0.2*	(0.1–0.3)	0.4*	(0.2–0.9)	0.5	(0.3–1.0)	0.3*	(0.2–0.4)
5	0.2*	(0.1–0.4)	0.1*	(0.1–0.2)	0.2*	(0.1–0.4)	0.4*	(0.1–1.0)	0.2*	(0.1–0.3)
6+									0.1*	(0.0–0.3)*
χ^2_5	45.9*		84.0*		19.4*		6.7		74.1*	
II. Number of paternal disorders[c]										
2	0.7*	(0.6–0.9)	0.7*	(0.6–0.9)	0.8	(0.6–1.1)	0.8	(0.6–1.0)	0.7*	(0.6–0.8)
3	0.5*	(0.4–0.7)	0.4*	(0.3–0.6)	0.5*	(0.3–0.8)	0.4*	(0.3–0.8)	0.4*	(0.3–0.6)
4	0.3*	(0.2–0.5)	0.3*	(0.2–0.5)	0.3*	(0.1–0.6)	0.5	(0.2–1.0)	0.4*	(0.2–0.6)
5			0.1*	(0.1–0.2)					0.2*	(0.1–0.3)
6+									0.1*	(0.1–0.2)
χ^2_5	36.2*		63.0*		12.3*		10.2*		70.5*	
III. Global test for number										
Global χ^2_{10}	62.3*		105.4*		23.7*		12.9		103.9*	

[a] Assessed in the part 2 sample. Models include dummy variables for both type and number of parent mental disorders and control for country, person-year, age, and sex.

[b] Parent death from suicide is a time-varying predictor; all other parent disorders are not time-varying.

[c] For number of parent disorders, the last odds ratio represents the odds of the number or more. For example, for mood disorders, the last odds ratio for maternal disorders represents 5 or more maternal disorders. No variable for exactly one parent disorder is included in the model, as this value is redundant with the information on types of disorders.

* Significant at the 0.05 level, two-sided test.

$\chi^2_5 = 70.5$, $p < 0.001$ for paternal disorders) and consistently less than 1.0 in the pooled model that included terms for both type and number of disorders. This pattern of associations suggests the presence of *sub-additive* interactions among comorbid parent disorders: that is, a situation in which the positive associations of parent disorders predicting offspring disorders decrease as the number of comorbid parent disorders increases. A similar pattern of significant sub-additive interactions was observed in high-income and upper-middle-income countries for maternal disorders ($\chi^2_{3-5} = 19.2$–47.4, $p < 0.001$) and in all three country groups for paternal disorders ($\chi^2_{3-5} = 10.5$–54.9, $p < 0.001$–0.015). The only instance for which the sub-additive pattern of associations was not significant was for maternal disorders in low/lower-middle-income countries ($\chi^2_2 = 4.3$, $p = 0.12$) (Appendix Table 3.4).

Disaggregation of this model in the total sample showed that the same basic pattern of associations exists in predicting all four classes of offspring disorders. Specifically, every type of parent disorder was associated with elevated odds of offspring mood disorders, all types other than suicide death with offspring anxiety and disruptive behavior disorders, and all types other than suicide attempt and suicide death with offspring substance disorders. Significant sub-additive interactions among parent disorders occurred for both maternal and paternal disorders in predicting all classes of offspring disorder, with the exception of maternal and paternal disorders predicting offspring substance disorders. With regard to the ORs associated with types of parent disorders, patterns of within-class and between-class coefficients were similar to those in the additive model.

Further disaggregation by country group revealed a very similar pattern in all three country groups. Sub-additive interactions among parent disorders were observed for both maternal and paternal disorders in predicting all classes of offspring disorders, although in upper-middle-income and low/lower-middle-income countries there were too few respondents who reported more than three parent disorders to fully examine these interactions, particularly in predicting substance and disruptive behavior disorders. The only differences observed across country groups were that parent depression did not predict offspring substance disorders in high-income and upper-middle-income countries, nor disruptive behavior disorders in upper-middle-income countries; parent substance abuse did not predict offspring mood disorders, and parent GAD did not predict offspring substance abuse, in upper-middle-income countries; and parent GAD predicted only mood disorders in low/lower-middle-income countries (Appendix Table 3.4).

Population-level associations of parental disorders with subsequent offspring disorders

Population attributable risk proportions (PARPs) based on the most complex multivariate model show that parent disorders explain, in a predictive sense, 12.4% of all offspring disorders (9.8% of offspring mood disorders, 13.0% of anxiety disorders, 17.3% of disruptive behavior disorders, and 11.4% of substance disorders) (Table 3.5). Parent panic has the largest disorder-specific PARP (5.5% for all disorders, and 4.4–7.2% for disorder classes), whereas parent suicide attempt and death have the lowest PARPs. Disaggregation of results by country income level reveals remarkable consistency across country groups in a number of broad patterns. The highest PARP in all country groups is associated with parent disorders predicting offspring disruptive behavior disorders. Parent panic has the largest disorder-specific PARP in all country groups (5.2–6.1% of all disorders), and parent suicide attempt and death have the lowest (0.07–1.4% of all disorders). PARPs are relatively comparable in high-income and upper-middle-income countries and smaller in low/lower-middle-income countries (80% of comparisons). The PARP of all parent disorders predicting all offspring disorder is 8.7% in low/lower-middle-income, 13.6% in upper-middle-income, and 13.6% in high-income countries.

Discussion

This study provides novel information about the relationship between parent psychopathology and offspring mental disorders using data from a coordinated set of surveys conducted in 22 countries around the world. Study results indicated that each parent disorder examined, with the exception of suicide, was associated with increased risk for every class of offspring mental disorder. This pattern was evident even after controlling for the presence of comorbid parent disorders as well as for number of parent disorders. Although we found within-class associations involving

Table 3.5 Population attributable risk proportions (PARPs) of offspring mental disorders due to parent psychopathology by country income level. The WMH surveys.

Types of parent disorder	Offspring disorders				
	Mood disorder	Anxiety disorder	Disruptive behavior disorder	Substance disorder	Any disorder
	PARP (%)	PARP (%)	PARP (%)	PARP (%)	PARP (%)
I. All countries					
Major depressive episode	2.2	3.1	3.8	1.4	2.6
Generalized anxiety	2.9	4.0	5.0	1.8	3.4
Panic disorder	4.5	6.2	7.2	4.4	5.5
Substance abuse	2.0	2.6	5.0	5.0	3.2
Antisocial personality disorder	1.2	2.1	4.5	2.3	2.2
Suicide attempt	0.85	1.0	1.5	0.46	0.98
Suicide (death from suicide)	0.09	0.04	0.02	0.12	0.07
Any	9.8	13.0	17.3	11.4	12.4
II. Low/lower-middle-income countries					
Major depressive episode	2.1	2.9	3.0	0.83	2.2
Generalized anxiety	1.1	1.2	0.78	0.01	0.96
Panic disorder	5.7	6.5	7.2	3.7	5.7
Substance abuse	0.78	0.83	2.1	2.4	1.3
Antisocial personality disorder	0.38	1.1	1.5	1.3	0.97
Suicide attempt	0.30	−0.04	−0.20	0.29	0.13
Suicide (death from suicide)	0.00	0.06	0.30	0.12	0.09
Any	8.1	9.5	11.0	7.1	8.7
III. Upper-middle-income countries					
Major depressive episode	2.2	3.5	4.5	.92	2.8
Generalized anxiety	3.7	4.7	5.5	1.9	4.3
Panic disorder	4.9	6.7	9.9	4.6	6.1
Substance abuse	1.6	1.6	6.2	5.1	2.8
Antisocial personality disorder	1.3	1.6	3.3	2.4	2.0
Suicide attempt	0.86	1.1	0.78	−0.38	0.87
Suicide (death from suicide)	0.21	0.07	−0.07	−0.03	0.07
Any	11.0	13.7	19.9	11.7	13.6

Table 3.5 (cont.)

Types of parent disorder	Offspring disorders				
	Mood disorder	Anxiety disorder	Disruptive behavior disorder	Substance disorder	Any disorder
	PARP (%)	PARP (%)	PARP (%)	PARP (%)	PARP (%)
IV. High-income countries					
Major depressive episode	2.1	2.7	3.2	1.2	2.5
Generalized anxiety	3.5	4.8	6.1	2.2	4.2
Panic disorder	3.7	5.8	6.1	4.7	5.2
Substance abuse	2.8	3.7	5.7	6.2	4.3
Antisocial personality disorder	1.5	2.6	6.0	2.6	2.8
Suicide attempt	1.2	1.4	2.2	0.54	1.4
Suicide (death from suicide)	0.11	0.04	−0.13	0.20	0.08
Any	10.2	14.0	18.5	12.8	13.6

The model presented in Table 3.4 was used to estimate the PARPs. Each row displays the proportion of disorder onsets in the population that are attributable to each parental disorder. The final row of the table shows the proportion of disorder onsets in the population that are attributable to all parental disorders jointly.

pure parent disorders generally to be higher than across-class associations, this pattern was weak. We also found consistent evidence of sub-additive interactions, which means that the joint ORs of multiple parent disorders with offspring disorders are for the most part significantly less than the product of the ORs associated with the component pure disorders. At a population level, parent disorders were associated with a meaningful (7.1–19.9% across country and outcome disorder groups), although not overwhelming, proportion of all offspring disorders. To our knowledge, we provided the first estimates of the population-level influence of parent psychopathology on offspring disorders.

The cross-national population-based nature of our data is unique and consequently may have produced results that are more generalizable than those reported from smaller and more selected samples. Nonetheless, these findings should be interpreted in light of study limitations. Most notably, parent disorders were assessed via informant reports made by their grown children. Although known to provide useful information about the presence of mental disorders

in relatives (Kendler & Roy 1995, Prescott *et al.* 2005), this method of collecting information is susceptible to recall error and bias (Roy *et al.* 1996), with respondents who have a psychiatric disorder more likely than those without to report psychopathology in their family members (Kendler *et al.* 1991, Milne *et al.* 2009). Because previous research suggests that respondents with a mental disorder are more likely than unaffected siblings to report *that same disorder* in a parent (Kendler *et al.* 1991), any such bias would have inflated within-class associations in the current study. However, our results indicate less familial aggregation of specific disorder classes than prior studies (Low *et al.* 2008). Second, the survey only assessed parent disorders present during the respondent's childhood. This likely resulted in under-reporting of parent disorders, given that respondents may not have had a full appreciation of parental symptoms. If respondents consequently reported only the most severe parent disorders, this may have inflated estimates of parent–offspring disorder associations. On the other hand, lack of information on parent disorders occurring later in the respondent's life likely produced conservative estimates of the associations between parent and offspring disorders. Third, the WMH surveys do not have a genetically informative design, making it impossible to estimate the heritability of specific disorders or determine the proportion of parent–offspring disorder associations that were due to genetic versus environmental factors. Fourth, we focused only on a small number of common parent disorders rather than on more severe but uncommon disorders (e.g., psychotic disorders). Because familial transmission is likely to be most evident for severe disorders (Merikangas *et al.* 1998b), inclusion of less severe parent disorders would have attenuated associations with offspring disorders. Finally, although PARP is a joint function of the prevalence of parent disorder and the strength of association with offspring disorders, we did not distinguish between these two factors in our comparisons across country groups. Examination of these joint effects at a disaggregated country level represents an important area for future research.

Within the context of these limitations, our results are consistent with those of previous studies in documenting significant associations between parent and offspring disorders. Indeed, we found that virtually every type of parent mental disorder was associated with elevated odds of every class of offspring disorder. This was true even after accounting for type and number of comorbid parent disorders. Because the controls for number of disorders can be interpreted as pooled interactions (Green *et al.* 2010), the net associations of individual parent disorders with offspring disorders in the model that controls number of disorders can be interpreted as the estimated associations of *pure* parent disorders (i.e., comparisons between parents who had a history of only that one disorder versus parents who had no disorders) with offspring disorders. This means that pure parent disorders have relatively pervasive associations with offspring disorders.

We found less familial aggregation of specific disorder classes than many prior studies (Merikangas *et al.* 1998b, Lieb *et al.* 2000, Lieb *et al.* 2002), with little specificity in the associations of particular parent disorders with particular offspring disorders other than a modest pattern of within-class associations being larger than across-class associations. This pattern is indirectly consistent with research suggesting that most genetic liability factors are associated with a propensity to experience internalizing and externalizing pathology rather than with elevated risk of specific

disorders (Kendler *et al.* 1997, 2003, Hicks *et al.* 2004). Other data consistent with this general pattern have been reported, such as a finding that parent depression was associated with increased risk for a wide range of offspring disorders (Lieb *et al.* 2002) and that numerous parent disorders were associated with offspring social phobia (Lieb *et al.* 2000). Although other studies found more specificity in the intergenerational transmission of particular disorders, including anxiety disorders (Beidel & Turner 1997, Biederman *et al.* 2006), substance use disorders (Merikangas *et al.* 1998b), disruptive behavioral disorders (Clark *et al.* 2004), and major depression (Lieb *et al.* 2002), the majority of these studies were based on relatively small samples and examined only a single or limited number of parent disorders. The few previous studies with sufficient sample sizes that included controls for comorbid disorders have typically found a more generalized pattern of intergenerational transmission of mental disorders similar to the pattern found here (Kendler *et al.* 1997, Hicks *et al.* 2004, Bornovalova *et al.* 2010).

This pattern raises important questions about why parent psychopathology is a relatively non-specific risk factor for offspring disorders. One possibility is that parents with mental disorders not only transmit genetic vulnerability to their offspring, but also are more likely than parents without psychopathology to engage in negative parenting behaviors that do not vary substantially by type of parent disorder (Downey & Coyne 1990, Lieb *et al.* 2000, Chen & Johnston 2007). Consistent with this possibility, parent psychopathology has been associated in several studies with a wide range of maladaptive family-related adversities, such as maltreatment and family violence (Conron *et al.* 2009, Green *et al.* 2010, Kessler *et al.* 2010). These adversities, in turn, have been shown to be robust and relatively non-specific risk factors of adult mental disorders (Green *et al.* 2010, Kessler *et al.* 2010).

Our findings that the associations of maternal and paternal psychopathology with offspring disorders were relatively similar, that these associations did not vary by sex of offspring, and that the odds of offspring disorder were consistently higher when both parents had a disorder rather than only one parent are all broadly consistent with previous research (Dierker *et al.* 1999, Lieb *et al.* 2002). Although parent–offspring associations within disorder classes were found to be generally stronger than across-class associations, these patterns were weak and had some exceptions, such as parent GAD and panic disorder predicting offspring mood disorders more strongly than parent depression. Most of these deviations are consistent with evidence from behavior genetics research that genetic liability factors broadly predispose individuals to develop internalizing pathology (Kendler et al. 2003) and that similar genetic factors underlie GAD and depression (Kendler et al. 1992) as well as GAD and panic disorder (Hettema et al. 2005). We also found that parent depression and GAD were associated with offspring disruptive behavior disorders as strongly as parent antisocial personality disorder. This pattern is similar to the previous finding of a high degree of familial co-aggregation between depressive and disruptive behavioral disorders (Biederman et al. 2001).

We provide the first population-based estimates of the proportion of offspring disorders that are associated with parent disorders. These findings suggest that parent disorders are associated with a meaningful proportion of disorder onsets, with little variation across country income groups in the overall pattern of associations. This finding that parent disorders are associated with the highest proportion of offspring disruptive behavior disorder onsets in all country groups is consistent with previous research showing that the PARPs associated with a broader range of childhood adversities related to family maladjustment, including maltreatment and parental criminal behavior, are highest for disruptive behavior disorders (Green et al. 2010, Kessler et al. 2010). Parent panic disorder has the largest disorder-specific PARP in all country groups. Although previous research has consistently documented elevated rates of panic disorder in children of parents with the disorder (Weissman 1993, Weissman et al. 1993), we are unaware of previous research linking panic disorder to a wider range of mental health problems in offspring. The only meaningful difference across countries is that the PARPs are higher in high-income and upper-middle-income countries as compared to low/lower-middle-income countries. Although the overall magnitude of this difference was small (13.6% for high- and upper-middle-income countries versus 8.7% for low/lower-middle-income countries for any disorder), the PARPs associated with parent disorders were consistently lowest in low/lower-middle-income countries. Smaller PARPs in low/lower-middle-income countries might be due to the fact that there are larger family networks involved in child rearing that buffer against

the effects of parent psychopathology on children, a possibility that warrants further investigation in future research.

The pervasive pattern of sub-additive interactions among comorbid parent disorders in predicting offspring disorders reported here represents a unique contribution of the WMH surveys to the study of the intergenerational transmission of mental disorders. This pattern mirrors associations observed among a wide range of childhood adversities in predicting subsequent first onset of mental disorders (Green et al. 2010, Kessler et al. 2010), as well as associations among temporally primary disorders in predicting the subsequent first onset of other secondary disorders (Kessler et al. 2011). It is important to recognize that these negative interactions do not mean that additional parent disorders are associated with *decreased* risk of offspring disorders, but that increases in risk occur at a decreasing rate. This can be seen most clearly in Table 3.3, where we find that the ORs associated with high parent comorbidity are elevated but not dramatically higher than the ORs associated with lower numbers of parent disorders. We observed these sub-additive interactions for all disorder classes in offspring other than for the association of maternal disorders with offspring substance disorders.

Implications

Our findings suggest that future behavior genetics studies should both assess comorbid parent disorders and utilize appropriate statistical models to account for the non-additive associations of comorbid parent disorders with offspring disorders. To the extent that the sub-additive interactions reflect causal effects of parent disorders, this pattern implies that intervening to treat any single parent disorder in the presence of comorbidity would likely have little effect on offspring disorder, as odds of offspring disorder are not markedly lower in the presence of a small compared to large number of parent disorders. Effective interventions to prevent offspring disorders would consequently require intervening so as to protect the child from the full range of parent disorders. Given that parent disorders are robust predictors of offspring disorders across all the disorder classes and country groups considered here, it is important to recognize the potential public health importance of such interventions, not only to improve the functioning of mentally ill parents but also to reduce the intergenerational transmission of mental disorders.

Acknowledgments

Portions of this chapter are based on McLaughlin, K. A., Gadermann, A. M., Hwang, I., et al. (2012). Parent psychopathology and offspring mental disorders in the WHO World Mental Health Surveys. *British Journal of Psychiatry* **200**, 290–9. © 2012. The Royal College of Psychiatrists. Reproduced with permission.

References

Beidel, D. C., & Turner, S. M. (1997). At risk for anxiety: I. Psychopathology in the offspring of anxious parents. *Journal of the American Academy of Child and Adolescent Psychiatry* **36**, 918–24.

Biederman, J., Faraone, S. V., Hirshfeld-Becker, D. R., et al. (2001). Patterns of psychopathology and dysfunction in high-risk children of parents with panic disorder and major depression. *American Journal of Psychiatry* **158**, 49–57.

Biederman, J., Petty, C., Faraone, S. V., et al. (2006). Effects of parental anxiety disorders in children at high risk for panic disorder: a controlled study. *Journal of Affective Disorders* **94**, 191–7.

Bornovalova, M. A., Hicks, B. M., Iacono, W. G., & McGue, M. (2010). Familial transmission and heritability of childhood disruptive disorders. *American Journal of Psychiatry* **167**, 1066–74.

Bruckner, T. A., Scheffler, R. M., Shen, G., et al. (2011). The mental health workforce gap in low- and middle-income countries: a needs-based approach. *Bulletin of the World Health Organization* **89**, 184–94.

Chang, K. H., & Horrocks, S. (2006). Lived experiences of family caregivers of mentally ill relatives. *Journal of Advanced Nursing* **53**, 435–43.

Chen, M., & Johnston, C. (2007). Maternal inattention and impulsivity and parenting behaviors. *Journal of Clinical Child and Adolescent Psychology* **36**, 455–68.

Clark, D. B., Cornelius, J., Wood, D. S., & Vanyukov, M. (2004). Psychopathology risk transmission in children of parents with substance use disorders. *American Journal of Psychiatry* **161**, 685–91.

Conron, K. J., Beardslee, W., Koenen, K. C., Buka, S. L., & Gortmaker, S. L. (2009). A longitudinal study of maternal depression and child maltreatment in a national sample of families investigated by child protective services. *Archives of Pediatrics & Adolescent Medicine* **163**, 922–30.

Dierker, L. C., Merikangas, K. R., & Szatmari, P. (1999). Influence of parental concordance for psychiatric disorders on psychopathology in offspring. *Journal of the American Academy of Child and Adolescent Psychiatry* **38**, 280–8.

Downey, G., & Coyne, J. C. (1990). Children of depressed parents: an integrative review. *Psychological Bulletin* **108**, 50–76.

Endicott, J., Andreasen, N., & Spitzer, R. L. (1978). *Family History Research Diagnostic Criteria*. New York, NY: Biometrics Research, New York State Psychiatric Institute.

Green, J. G., McLaughlin, K. A., Berglund, P. A., et al. (2010). Childhood adversities and adult psychiatric disorders in the national comorbidity survey replication I: associations with first onset of DSM-IV disorders. *Archives of General Psychiatry* **67**, 113–23.

Hettema, J. M., Prescott, C. A., Myers, J. M., Neale, M. C., & Kendler, K. S. (2005). The structure of genetic and environmental risk factors for anxiety disorders in men and women. *Archives of General Psychiatry* **62**, 182–9.

Hicks, B. M., Krueger, R. F., Iacono, W. G., McGue, M., & Patrick, C. J. (2004). Family transmission and heritability of externalizing disorders: a twin-family study. *Archives of General Psychiatry* **61**, 922–8.

Hsiao, C.-Y., & Van Riper, M. (2010). Research on caregiving in Chinese families living with mental illness: a critical review. *Journal of Family Nursing* **16**, 68–100.

Kendler, K. S., & Roy, M. A. (1995). Validity of a diagnosis of lifetime major depression obtained by personal interview versus family history. *American Journal of Psychiatry* **152**, 1608–14.

Kendler, K. S., Silberg, J. L., Neale, M. C., et al. (1991). The family history method: whose psychiatric history is measured? *American Journal of Psychiatry* **148**, 1501–4.

Kendler, K. S., Neale, M. C., Kessler, R. C., Heath, A. C., & Eaves, L. J. (1992). Major depression and generalized anxiety disorder. Same genes, (partly) different environments? *Archives of General Psychiatry* **49**, 716–22.

Kendler, K. S., Davis, C. G., & Kessler, R. C. (1997). The familial aggregation of common psychiatric and substance use disorders in the National Comorbidity Survey: a family history study. *British Journal of Psychiatry* **170**, 541–8.

Kendler, K. S., Prescott, C. A., Myers, J., & Neale, M. C. (2003). The structure of genetic and environmental risk factors for common psychiatric and substance use disorders in men and women. *Archives of General Psychiatry* **60**, 929–37.

Kessler, R. C., McLaughlin, K. A., Green, J. G., et al. (2010). Childhood adversities and adult psychopathology in the WHO World Mental Health Surveys. *British Journal of Psychiatry* **197**, 378–85.

Kessler, R. C., Ormel, J., Petukhova, M., et al. (2011). Development of lifetime comorbidity in the World Health Organization World Mental Health Surveys. *Archives of General Psychiatry* **68**, 90–100.

Lauber, C., & Rossler, W. (2007). Stigma towards people with mental illness in developing countries in Asia. *International Review of Psychiatry* **19**, 157–78.

Lefley, H. P. (1989). Family burden and family stigma in major mental illness. *American Psychologist* **44**, 556–60.

Lieb, R., Wittchen, H. U., Hofler, M., et al. (2000). Parental psychopathology, parenting styles, and the risk of social phobia in offspring: a prospective-longitudinal community study. *Archives of General Psychiatry* **57**, 859–66.

Lieb, R., Isensee, B., Hofler, M., Pfister, H., & Wittchen, H. U. (2002). Parental major depression and the risk of depression and other mental disorders in offspring: a prospective-longitudinal community study. *Archives of General Psychiatry* **59**, 365–74.

Low, N. C., Cui, L., & Merikangas, K. R. (2008). Specificity of familial transmission of anxiety and comorbid disorders. *Journal of Psychiatric Research* **42**, 596–604.

Merikangas, K. R., Stevens, D. E., Fenton, B., *et al.* (1998a). Co-morbidity and familial aggregation of alcoholism and anxiety disorders. *Psychological Medicine* **28**, 773–88.

Merikangas, K. R., Stolar, M., Stevens, D. E., *et al.* (1998b). Familial transmission of substance use disorders. *Archives of General Psychiatry* **55**, 973–9.

Milne, B. J., Caspi, A., Crump, R., *et al.* (2009). The validity of the family history screen for assessing family history of mental disorders. *American Journal of Medical Genetics Part B: Neuropsychiatric Genetics* **150**B, 41–9.

Prescott, C. A., Sullivan, P. F., Myers, J. M., *et al.* (2005). The Irish Affected Sib Pair Study of Alcohol Dependence: study methodology and validation of diagnosis by interview and family history. *Alcoholism: Clinical and Experimental Research* **29**, 417–29.

Research Triangle Institute (2005). *SUDAAN, Version 9.0.1.* [computer program]. Research Triangle Park, NC: Research Triangle Institute.

Roy, M. A., Walsh, D., & Kendler, K. S. (1996). Accuracies and inaccuracies of the family history method: a multivariate approach. *Acta Psychiatrica Scandinavica* **93**, 224–34.

Tsang, H. W. H., Tam, P. K. C., Chan, F., & Cheung, W. M. (2003). Stigmatizing attitudes towards individuals with mental illness in Hong Kong: implications for their recovery. *Journal of Community Psychology* **31**, 383–96.

Wang, P. S., Angermeyer, M., Borges, G., *et al.* (2007). Delay and failure in treatment seeking after first onset of mental disorders in the World Health Organization's World Mental Health Survey Initiative. *World Psychiatry* **6**, 177–85.

Weissman, M. M. (1993). Family genetic studies of panic disorder. *Journal of Psychiatric Research* **27** (Suppl 1), 69–78.

Weissman, M. M., Wickramaratne, P., Adams, P. B., *et al.* (1993). The relationship between panic disorder and major depression: a new family study. *Archives of General Psychiatry* **50**, 767–80.

Wolter, K. M. (1985). *Introduction to Variance Estimation.* New York, NY: Springer-Verlag.

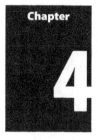

Associations between mental disorders and early termination of education

Joshua Breslau, Sing Lee, Adley Tsang, Michael C. Lane,
Sergio Aguilar-Gaxiola, Jordi Alonso, Matthias C. Angermeyer,
Yueqin Huang, Johan Ormel, José Posada-Villa, and David R. Williams

Introduction

Education is one of the most important domains in which mental disorders may have effects that extend across the life course. Most individuals who will have a disorder during their lifetime will have their first disorder during childhood or adolescence, when they are still of school age (Kim-Cohen *et al.* 2003, Kessler *et al.* 2007). The impairments associated with these disorders are likely to disrupt the ability of students to function in school settings, which demand a certain level of rule-following, effort, and focused attention (Farkas 2003). Students who do not perform well in school because of problems with discipline or academic achievement may be more likely to withdraw from schooling entirely or, in more extreme cases, may be expelled from school (Rumberger 2004). Early termination of schooling is associated with a wide range of limitations in adulthood that include diminished financial security, occupational achievement, self-esteem, marital opportunity, and other later-life opportunities (Featherman 1980, Koivusilta *et al.* 2001, Fronstin *et al.* 2005, Freudenberg & Ruglis 2007). At the societal level, the human capital lost from early termination of education can constrain economic development and impose higher health and social welfare costs (World Bank 2002).

Recent reviews of research in the USA (Breslau 2010) and Europe (Suhrcke & de Paz Nieves 2011) suggest that among the health conditions that affect children and adolescents, mental health conditions have the largest population-level effects on educational attainment. Prior epidemiological studies examined associations between early-onset mental disorders and the successful completion of educational

milestones, such as graduating from high school or completing a four-year post-secondary degree. In these studies, all broad categories of mental disorder were found to be associated with lower likelihood of completing one or more educational milestones, and these associations persisted after accounting for familial and other childhood determinants of educational attainment (Kessler *et al.* 1995, Johnson *et al.* 1999, Miech *et al.* 1999, Woodward & Fergusson 2001, Fergusson & Woodward 2002). Given the high co-morbidity among disorders, several of these studies attempted to discern whether the associations of mental disorders with educational attainment reflect distinct effects of all types of disorders or whether they result from the effect of a smaller set of disorders. Evidence from these analyses pointed to disruptive behavior disorders, conduct disorder, and attention-deficit/hyperactivity disorder (ADHD) as the ones with the most severe adverse effects on educational attainment (Miech *et al.* 1999, McLeod & Kaiser 2004, Breslau *et al.* 2011). However, as all these studies were conducted in high-income countries, broader cross-national evidence on the associations between mental disorders and educational attainment is lacking. Given the wide cross-national variation in school systems and average levels of educational attainment (Buchmann & Hannum 2001), the generalizability of existing results to other countries cannot be taken for granted.

An earlier WMH analysis examined associations between mental disorders and subsequent educational attainment in the first 16 WMH surveys (Lee *et al.* 2009). While the general pattern of associations was similar across the countries examined in that study,

The Burdens of Mental Disorders, ed. Jordi Alonso, Somnath Chatterji, and Yanling He. Published by Cambridge University Press. © World Health Organization 2013.

differences were found between high- versus low- and middle-income countries. Most notably, prior substance use disorders were found to be associated with non-completion of all stages of education in high-income countries, with anxiety, mood, and disruptive behavior disorders associated with early termination of secondary education. For lower-income countries, in comparison, the associations of early-onset mental disorders with educational attainment were generally weaker and were significant only for disruptive behavior disorders and substance use disorders predicting early termination of secondary education.

Methods

Sample

The current chapter expands on the above analyses by presenting data on the associations of early-onset mental disorders with educational attainment in 24 of the 25 WMH surveys considered in this volume. The survey in France was excluded, because complete information on education was not obtained in that survey. The sample studied consisted of 62,242 respondents from the part 2 sample: 16,051 in low/lower-middle-income countries, 15,240 in upper-middle-income countries, and 30,951 in high-income countries.

Measures

Although respondents in all countries were asked how many years of education they completed, the number of years that constitutes primary, secondary, and tertiary education varies across countries. As a result, we recoded respondent reports into country-specific stages of educational attainment. For example, we required eight years of education to define completion of primary school in the USA but only five years in the People's Republic of China (PRC), as these differences reflect the different numbers of years of primary school in these countries.

The analysis was then carried out for the following set of educational milestones across countries: completing primary education in the total sample; completing secondary education among those who completed primary education; entering (i.e., completion of at least one year of) tertiary education among those who completed secondary education; and completing tertiary education among those who started it. To maintain consistency with the earlier

WMH analyses of educational attainment, we considered 20 of the DSM-IV disorders assessed in the WMH surveys (minor depression was the only disorder mentioned in Chapter 2 that was omitted), but combined some of these disorders to stabilize estimates. Specifically, we combined panic disorder and agoraphobia into a single either-or-both measure and we combined bipolar I, bipolar II, and subthreshold bipolar disorders into a single measure of bipolar disorder.

Statistical analysis

Associations of mental disorders with subsequent termination of education were analyzed using the discrete-time survival analysis approach described in Chapter 2, with disorders considered as predictors only if they occurred prior to the time at which the termination of education is presumed to have occurred.

Statistical controls were included in this analysis for factors that are likely to influence both mental disorders and educational attainment and might therefore confound the estimates of their association. These controls included birth cohort, parental education, family environment (parental mental disorder, divorce, and parental death), childhood adversities indicative of poor family functioning (being beaten by caretakers, rape or sexual assault, parental neglect), and nativity (whether the respondent, their parents, and grandparents were born in the country in which the respondent was interviewed).

To estimate the total impact of mental disorders on educational attainment we used the simulation methods described in Chapter 2 to calculate population attributable risk proportions (PARPs). Discrete-time survival models were estimated taking account of variations in key covariates across the countries. For example, race or ethnic background and foreign versus native birth are important predictors of mental health and educational attainment in some countries, including the USA and New Zealand, but there are not enough data to include these characteristics as predictors in the analysis in most other countries. These models were used to estimate the prevalence of termination of each educational milestone with and without the effect of mental disorders. We calculated the percent change in the prevalence of early termination when the removal of the effect of mental disorders was simulated using those model results. Positive percentages indicate the percent increase in completion of an educational milestone when the effect of mental disorders is removed. In interpreting these results it is important to keep in mind that the PARP depends on two parameters that both might vary independently across countries, the prevalence of the disorder and the strength of its association with the outcome, net of controlled factors.

Results

Prevalence of early termination of education

The proportions of people completing each educational milestone among those who completed the previous milestone are presented for the three categories of country income level in Figure 4.1. Termination of education prior to completion of primary school (i.e., the first educational milestone according to each country's educational system), which includes people who never had any schooling, is more prevalent in low/lower-middle-income (18.7%) and upper-middle-income (18.6%) countries than in high-income countries (8.7%). This is also true of early termination of secondary education (47% in low/lower-middle-income countries, 50.5% in upper-middle-income countries, 26% in high-income countries). The prevalence of early termination does not follow this pattern across country income levels for the two later educational milestones, college entry and college graduation. The proportion of high

school graduates who did not enter college is 37% in low/lower-middle-income countries, 53% in upper-middle-income countries and 45% in high-income countries, while the proportion of college entrants who terminated prior to college graduation is 54% in low/lower-middle-income countries, 41% in upper-middle-income countries, and 47% in high-income countries.

Association of mental disorders with termination of education

Results from summary models that examined associations of prior history of each of four categories of disorder (anxiety, mood, disruptive behavior, and substance disorders) and number of comorbid disorders with the educational outcomes using discrete-time survival methods are presented in Table 4.1. Note that prior analyses not reported here distinguished among types of disorders within each of the four classes and investigated the possible existence of dose–response relationships between number of disorders in the class and educational outcomes. The less complex model presented here was found in those analyses to capture the main associations of temporally prior mental disorders with subsequent educational attainment. Minor depression was excluded from these analyses, based on evidence in the preliminary models that minor depression does not predict reduced educational attainment.

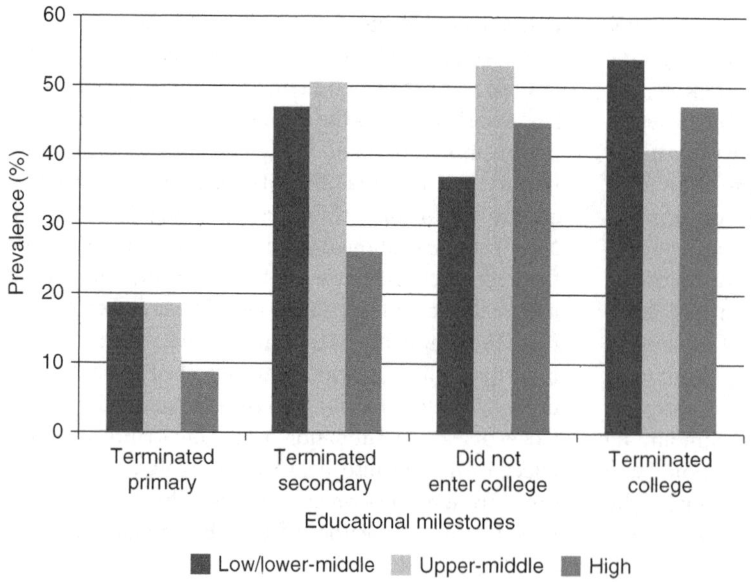

Figure 4.1 Early termination of education prior to completion of four educational milestones by country income level. The WMH surveys.

Table 4.1 Mental disorders as predictors of non-completion of four educational milestones by country income level. The WMH surveys.

Country income level	Non-completion of primary school			Non-completion of secondary education			Non-entry into tertiary education			Non-completion of tertiary education		
	OR	(95% CI)	X^2	OR	(95% CI)	X^2	OR	(95% CI)	X^2	OR	(95% CI)	X^2
Low/lower-middle												
Mood disorders	1.5	(0.4–6.2)	0.3	0.9	(0.5–1.4)	0.4	0.7	(0.5–1.2)	1.3	0.9	(0.6–1.4)	0.1
Anxiety disorders	0.9	(0.6–1.5)	0.1	1.0	(0.8–1.2)	0.0	0.6*	(0.4–0.9)	6.9	0.9	(0.7–1.3)	0.4
Disruptive behavior disorders	1.7*	(1.0–3.1)	3.8	1.2	(1.0–1.5)	3.5	1.0	(0.7–1.3)	0.1	0.9	(0.6–1.1)	1.0
Substance disorders	2.0	(0.7–6.1)	1.5	1.7	(1.0–3.1)	3.5	0.5*	(0.3–0.9)	5.4	1.1	(0.7–1.9)	0.2
Any 1 disorder	1.1	(0.8–1.4)	0.5	1.0	(0.8–1.1)	0.3	1.0	(0.8–1.2)	0.1	1.1	(0.9–1.3)	0.5
Any 2 disorders	1.2	(0.7–2.1)	0.3	1.4*	(1.0–1.9)	3.9	0.9	(0.6–1.4)	0.2	0.9	(0.7–1.3)	0.4
3+ disorders	0.1*	(0.0–0.6)	7.3	1.5	(1.0–2.4)	3.1	1.1	(0.6–1.8)	0.1	1.0	(0.6–1.7)	0.0
Upper-middle												
Mood disorders	1.5	(0.9–2.6)	2.8	1.5*	(1.2–2.0)	9.1	1.0	(0.7–1.6)	0.0	1.0	(0.6–1.7)	0.0
Anxiety disorders	1.0	(0.8–1.2)	0.1	1.2	(1.0–1.4)	3.6	1.2	(0.8–1.6)	0.8	1.0	(0.7–1.5)	0.0
Disruptive behavior disorders	1.1	(0.8–1.5)	0.3	1.3*	(1.0–1.6)	5.2	1.1	(0.7–1.6)	0.1	1.3	(0.8–2.0)	1.0
Substance disorders	1.7	(0.6–4.4)	1.1	1.2	(0.9–1.7)	1.4	1.0	(0.7–1.5)	0.0	1.1	(0.7–1.6)	0.2
Any 1 disorder	1.0	(0.8–1.2)	0.0	1.0	(0.9–1.1)	0.3	1.0	(0.8–1.2)	0.0	1.3	(1.0–1.7)	2.6
Any 2 disorders	1.2	(0.8–1.6)	0.8	1.1	(0.9–1.3)	0.5	1.0	(0.7–1.4)	0.0	1.3	(0.9–1.9)	2.3
3+ disorders	1.8*	(1.1–3.0)	6.2	1.8*	(1.3–2.5)	13.8	1.4	(0.9–2.4)	2.0	1.1	(0.6–2.2)	0.1
High												
Mood disorders	2.0*	(1.3–3.1)	11.2	1.5*	(1.3–1.7)	25.4	1.0	(0.9–1.2)	0.1	1.1	(1.0–1.3)	1.7
Anxiety disorders	1.0	(0.8–1.3)	0.1	1.3*	(1.2–1.4)	26.1	1.1	(0.9–1.2)	0.8	1.1	(1.0–1.3)	3.4
Disruptive behavior disorders	1.2	(0.8–1.8)	0.6	1.8*	(1.5–2.1)	39.6	1.1	(0.9–1.3)	0.5	1.4*	(1.2–1.7)	16.9
Substance disorders	12.8*	(5.5–29.7)	35.5	2.8*	(2.3–3.3)	134.8	1.4*	(1.2–1.6)	17.3	1.4*	(1.2–1.6)	17.4
Any 1 disorder	0.9	(0.7–1.1)	1.1	1.2*	(1.1–1.3)	12.8	1.1	(1.0–1.2)	3.5	1.0	(0.9–1.2)	0.4
Any 2 disorders	1.2	(0.8–1.8)	0.6	1.6*	(1.4–1.8)	45.6	1.0	(0.9–1.2)	0.0	1.2*	(1.0–1.4)	6.0
3+ disorders	1.6	(1.0–2.5)	3.4	2.2*	(1.9–2.6)	115.6	1.2*	(1.1–1.4)	7.2	1.3*	(1.1–1.5)	10.3

* Significant at the 0.05 level, two-sided test.

Early termination of primary school education is significantly associated with having one or more prior disruptive behavior disorders in low/lower-middle-income countries (OR = 1.7, 95% CI 1.0–3.1) and with having one or more prior mood and substance use disorders in high-income countries (OR = 12.8, 95% CI 5.5–29.7), and, in all three groups of countries, the association of substance disorders with termination is stronger than that for other categories of disorder (1.7 to 12.8). Across all three groups of countries, having only one disorder is not associated with higher risk of termination of primary education compared with those with no disorders. In the low/lower-middle-income countries, having three or more disorders is associated with a low probability of terminating primary education. In contrast, in the two higher-income groups of countries, the association with termination emerges only at fairly high levels of comorbidity.

The associations of mental disorders with early termination of education are strongest and most consistent across types of disorder during secondary school in upper-middle-income and high-income countries. In the upper-middle-income countries in particular, mood (OR = 1.5, 95% CI 1.2–2.0) and disruptive behavior disorders (OR = 1.3, 95% CI 1.0–1.6) are significantly associated with termination of secondary education, but, interestingly, substance use disorders are not. In this group of countries we did not observe a steady increase in risk of termination of secondary education with increasing comorbidity. In the high-income countries, all four categories of disorder are significantly associated with termination of secondary school, with the magnitude of the association lowest for anxiety disorders (OR = 1.3) and strongest for substance use disorders (OR = 2.8). Having just one disorder is associated with higher likelihood of termination in this group of countries, and likelihood of termination increases with higher numbers of comorbid disorders. Indeed, the association of disorder with termination was observed only among those with relatively high levels of comorbidity, suggesting that there may be synergistic interactions among co-occurring disorders. In the low/lower-middle-income countries, none of the disorder categories is individually associated with termination of secondary education, but termination is more common among those with two or more disorders, again suggesting synergistic interactions between disorders.

For both of the post-secondary educational milestones, college entry and college graduation, we observe stronger associations of mental disorders with early termination of education in the high-income countries than in the other two groups of countries. In the high-income countries, substance use disorders are associated with early termination at both of these milestones (OR = 1.4 in both), and disruptive behavior disorders are associated only with termination of college prior to graduation (OR = 1.4, 95% CI 1.2–1.7); increasing comorbidity is associated with higher likelihood of termination. This pattern is not observed for the other country groups. In the low/lower-middle-income countries only two of the associations are statistically significant and both are *negative*, indicating that people with these disorders (anxiety and substance disorders) are less likely to terminate their post-secondary education than people who do not have these disorders. In the upper-middle-income countries none of the associations reach statistical significance for either of the post-secondary educational milestones, suggesting that among those who reach this level of educational attainment, mental disorders are not important determinants of academic progression. It is striking that in this large sample we observed no statistically significant elevation in the likelihood of early termination of education associated with high levels of comorbidity, i.e., three or more mental disorders, in either the low/lower-middle-income countries or the upper-middle-income countries.

Estimating the societal impact of mental disorders on educational attainment

Results shown in Table 4.2 suggest that the societal effects of mental disorders on early termination are modest and vary both across countries and across the four milestones. Of the 92 estimates, only 30 suggest that the prevalence of completion of an educational milestone would be increased by 1% or more by the removal of the effect of mental disorders. Many of the effects are very small and some of these are negative, indicating that in that country the dominant pattern is contrary to the one found in the USA of mental disorders predicting early termination of education. Notably, the population attributable risk proportions (PARPs)

Table 4.2 Population attributable risk proportions (PARPs) of early termination of education due to mental disorders by country income level. The WMH surveys.

Country income level	Primary education	Secondary education	College entry	College graduation
	PARP (%)	PARP (%)	PARP (%)	PARP (%)
Low/lower-middle				
Colombia	1.2	1.1	0.78	0.56
India–Pondicherry	1.3	1.8	1.4	1.3
Iraq	0.05	0.05	0.05	0.04
Nigeria	0.08	0.08	0.05	0.04
PRC–Beijing/Shanghai	−0.14	−0.22	−0.17	−0.08
PRC–Shenzhen	−1.0	−1.3	−1.0	−0.26
Ukraine	0.75	1.4	1.6	1.4
Upper-middle				
Brazil–São Paulo	2.6	2.5	1.3	1.0
Bulgaria	−0.12	−0.10	−0.08	−0.07
Lebanon	−0.06	−0.08	−0.08	−0.07
Mexico	0.11	0.10	0.08	0.36
Romania	0.65	0.78	0.50	0.47
South Africa	0.41	0.73	0.47	0.21
High				
Belgium	0.29	0.34	0.29	0.25
Germany	−0.15	−0.22	−0.20	−0.04
Israel	0.15	0.39	0.41	0.39
Italy	0.39	0.30	0.19	0.16
Japan	−0.16	−0.33	−0.30	−0.29
Netherlands	2.2	2.3	2.2	1.8
New Zealand	2.7	5.0	3.2	2.3
Portugal	1.1	1.0	0.81	0.78
Spain	1.2	1.0	1.0	0.87
USA	3.4	3.8	2.8	1.9

for the PRC–Shenzhen sample are consistently negative, suggesting that mental disorders are associated with lower-than-average rates of educational termination in that sample.

Discussion

Two main findings on the association between mental disorders and early termination of education at the societal level are worthy of discussion. First, across countries the PARPs are generally stronger for the earlier educational milestones, primary and secondary school completion, than for the later milestones, college entry and college graduation. This may occur because selection effects have a stronger impact on the population at risk for higher levels of education. For instance, the people who enter college are less likely to have disorders because those with disorders were selected out earlier and have low rates

of college entry, although the low PARP values even at earlier levels of education show that this sort of exclusion is relatively weak. Nonetheless, the finding of higher PARPs at lower levels of education is important, because it means that the bulk of the impact of mental disorders on education occurs early in life. Efforts to reduce this impact should consequently focus on children in the primary and secondary school years. There are exceptions to this rule, such as the relatively high PARPs for the later educational milestones in New Zealand. Whether these large PARPs are due to lingering effects of disorders that began in childhood or to disorders with onset closer in time to the person's termination of education is an important question for future research.

Second, the PARPs also tend to be somewhat larger in high-income than in middle-income and low/lower-middle-income countries. This finding is likely due partly to the lower prevalence of disorders in the latter countries, but it also reflects the weaker associations of mental disorders with education in low/lower-middle-income countries than in high-income countries. One reason the individual-level associations of mental disorders with education are weaker in low/lower-middle-income countries may be that the labor market for jobs requiring higher education is comparatively small, which means that the decision to continue investing in education rather than terminate education and enter the labor market would be affected by many factors other than mental disorders (Hunt 2008, Borges *et al* 2011). In fact, it is possible that individuals with mental disorders may stay in school because their impairments limit other options for employment.

As with the other life-course outcomes examined in this volume, the analyses presented here are limited by the fact that the data were collected retrospectively, relying on respondent recall, rather than prospectively, where the timing of onset of disorders and termination of education could be precisely and independently assessed. There are some known biases associated with retrospective reports. The task of recalling symptoms over the course of a lifetime is more difficult for older respondents than for younger respondents, simply because they have to remember across longer periods of time. In addition, there is evidence that respondents whose current mental health is poor are more likely to report having had poor mental health in the past than respondents whose current mental health is good. Because of this recall bias, the respondents who report disorders are more likely to have more severe and persistent disorders compared to the actual group of people with a lifetime disorder in the general population. These biases may result in overestimating the impact of mental disorders on educational attainment.

There is also likely to be some error in the way the timing of termination of education was assessed. The WHO Composite International Diagnostic Interview (CIDI) collected information on education by simply asking respondents the highest level of education they completed. The respondent's age at the last year of education was not directly assessed but had to be assigned in order to establish the temporal ordering relative to the onset of the mental disorders. This assignment was done by assuming that respondents progressed through their educational careers at an orderly pace, without taking breaks or being held back or accelerated. The assumption of an orderly academic progression might result in some disorders being classified as having onset subsequent to termination of education, even though these disorders could have occurred prior to termination. If so, our findings would be biased towards a smaller association between mental disorders and termination.

Implications

The evidence in this cross-national study strongly suggests that there are long-term life-course effects of mental disorders that deserve further research attention. It is important to note that studies that focus exclusively on current functioning, such as work performance or income, are likely to underestimate the impact of mental disorders because they elide the cumulative impacts of disorders that begin in childhood and influence life opportunities. For instance, studies of current income adjust for potential confounding by educational attainment because educational attainment is associated with both mental disorders and income. However, by 'adjusting out' the effect of educational attainment, those studies do not include the effects that mental disorders may already have had on the life course.

Although cultural values about the importance of mental health relative to competing social issues are likely to vary widely across countries, our findings suggest that few countries, whether they be high-income or upper-middle-income, can afford to forgo the opportunity to develop early interventions and treatments for mental disorders in order to minimize their costly burden on society and vulnerable citizens. Lastly, a focus on termination of education may also bring to the attention of education departments and school administrators the importance of tackling problems such as substance use and impulse control disorders with mental health interventions. This is especially salient in low/lower-middle-income countries, where suicide and psychiatric diseases are highly stigmatized and priority for mental health research and programs is low.

The WMH survey results should provide motivation for future intervention and observational studies that aim to better understand the involvement of mental disorders in complex life-course trajectories.

How do mental disorders affect educational attainment?

A number of different pathways through which mental disorders might adversely affect educational attainment have been suggested in the literature. One of the key mediators of interest in these pathways is academic achievement, as measured by grades or scores on achievement tests (Duncan *et al.* 2007). Students with low achievement are less likely to continue schooling (Rumberger 2004), perhaps because they perceive smaller returns from continued academic efforts (Heckman *et al.* 2006). Mental disorders might affect academic achievement in a number of ways. Depression or anxiety may undermine students' motivation to achieve or the effort that they devote to their work (Fletcher 2008, Quiroga & Janosz 2009). The attention problems that are characteristic of attention-deficit/hyperactivity disorder (ADHD) may limit a student's ability to focus on learning activities (Biederman *et al.* 2008). The association between attention problems at the time of entry into school and later achievement has been found in several longitudinal studies (Duncan *et al.* 2007, Breslau *et al.* 2009). The disruptive behaviors that characterize conduct disorder may lead to frequent disciplinary problems and disconnection from school (Rapport *et al.* 1999).

With regard to the treatment of early-onset mental disorders associated with termination of education, several issues are noteworthy. The school environment provides unparalleled contact with youth and hence creates an ideal opportunity for teachers to work with parents and use a multi-domain developmental approach in the early identification of children in need of attention (e.g., Cohen *et al.* 1988, Linares *et al.* 1991). Some commentators have argued that interventions should not focus on clinical disorders alone, but rather should screen for subclinical emotional and behavioral problems before affected children come to the attention of teachers (Lloyd *et al.* 1991). These problems may manifest as learning difficulties, an inability to build or maintain satisfactory interpersonal relationships, inappropriate behavior under normal circumstances, a general pervasive mood of unhappiness, or a tendency to develop physical symptoms or fears associated with personal or school problems (Kutash *et al.* 2011). Clearly, early identification is an important strategy because of the early age at which the impact of mental disorders occurs (Swaim *et al.* 1989, Kazdin & Johnson 1994). However, screening is also likely to identify many more students suspected to have potential mental health problems than can possibly be treated, given existing resources. Moreover, screening carries a risk of over-pathologization and stigma during sensitive periods of child development (Barret & Pahl 2006). Research that identifies the particular pathways through which mental disorders affect education has the promise of refining our ability to screen for potential problems so that the benefits clearly outweigh the costs.

Acknowledgments

Portions of this chapter are based on Lee, S., Tsang, A., Breslau, J., *et al.* (2009). Mental disorders and termination of education in high-income and low- and middle-income countries: epidemiological study. *British Journal of Psychiatry* **194**, 411–17. © 2009. The Royal College of Psychiatrists. Reproduced with permission.

References

Barrett, P. M., & Pahl, K. M. (2006). School-based intervention: examining a universal approach to anxiety management. *Australian Journal of Guidance and Counselling* **16**, 55–75.

Biederman, J., Petty C. R., Fried R., *et al.* (2008). Educational and occupational underattainment in adults with attention-deficit/hyperactivity disorder: a controlled study. *Journal of Clinical Psychiatry* **69**, 1217–22.

Borges, G., Medina-Mora, M. E., Benjet, C., *et al.* (2011). Influence of mental disorders on school dropout in Mexico. *Pan American Journal of Public Health* **30**, 477–83.

Breslau, J. (2010). *Health in Childhood and Adolescence and High School Dropout*. Santa Barbara, CA: California Dropout Research Project, 17.

Breslau, J., Miller, E., Breslau N., *et al.* (2009). The impact of early behavior disturbances on academic achievement in high school. *Pediatrics* **123**, 1472–6.

Breslau, J., Miller, E., Joanie Chung W. J., & Schweitzer J. B. (2011). Childhood and adolescent onset psychiatric disorders, substance use, and failure to graduate high school on time. *Journal of Psychiatric Research* **45**, 295–301.

Buchmann, C., & Hannum E. (2001). Education and stratification in developing countries: a review of theories and research. *Annual Review of Sociology* **27**, 77–102.

Cohen, N. J., Kershner, J., & Wehrspann, W. (1988). Correlates of competence in a child psychiatric population. *Journal of Consulting and Clinical Psychology*, **56**, 97–103.

Duncan, G., Dowsett C., Claessens A., *et al.* (2007). School readiness and later achievement. *Developmental Psychology* **43**, 1428–46.

Farkas, G. (2003). Cognitive skills and noncognitive traits and behaviors in stratification processes. *Annual Review of Sociology* **29**, 541–62.

Featherman, D. L. (1980). Schooling and occupational careers: constancy and change in worldly success. In O. G. Brim & J. Kagan, eds., *Constancy and Change in Human Development*. Cambridge, MA: Harvard University Press, pp. 675–738.

Fergusson, D. M., & Woodward, L. J. (2002). Mental health, educational, and social role outcomes of adolescents with depression. *Archives of General Psychiatry* **59**, 225–31.

Fletcher, J. M. (2008). Adolescent depression: diagnosis, treatment, and educational attainment. *Health Economics* **17**, 1215–35.

Freudenberg, N., & Ruglis, J. (2007). Reframing school dropout as a public health issue. *Preventing Chronic Disease* **4**, A107.

Fronstin, P., Greenberg, D. H., & Robins, P. K. (2005). The labor market consequences of childhood maladjustment. *Social Science Quarterly* **86**, 1170–95.

Heckman, J. J., Stixrud J., & Urzua S. (2006). The effects of cognitive and noncognitive abilities on labor market outcomes and social behavior. *Journal of Labor Economics* **24**, 411–82.

Hunt, F. (2008). *Dropping Out from School: a Cross Country Review*. Falmer: Consortium for Research on Educational Access, Transitions and Equity (CREATE).

Johnson, J. G., Cohen, P., Dohrenwend, B. P., Link, B. G., & Brook, J. S. (1999). A longitudinal investigation of social causation and social selection processes involved in the association between socioeconomic status and psychiatric disorders. *Journal of Abnormal Psychology*. **108**, 490–9.

Kazdin, A. E., & Johnson, B. (1994). Advances in psychotherapy for children and adolescents: interrelations of adjustment, development and intervention. *Journal of School Psychology* **32**, 217–46.

Kessler, R. C., Foster, C. L., Saunders, W. B., & Stang, P. E. (1995). Social consequences of psychiatric disorders, I: educational attainment. *American Journal of Psychiatry* **152**, 1026–32.

Kessler, R. C., Amminger, G. P., Aguilar-Gaxiola, S., *et al.* (2007). Age-of-onset of mental disorders: a review of recent literature. *Current Opinion in Psychiatry* **20**, 359–64.

Kim-Cohen, J., Caspi A., Moffitt, T. E., *et al.* (2003). Prior juvenile diagnoses in adults with mental disorder:

developmental follow-back of a prospective longitudinal cohort. *Archives of General Psychiatry* **60**, 709–17.

Koivusilta, L. K., Rimpela, A. H., Rimpela, M., & Vikat, A. (2001). Health behavior-based selection into educational tracks starts in early adolescence. *Health Education Research* **16**, 201–14.

Kutash, K., Duchnowski, A. J., & Green, A. L. (2011). School-based mental health programes for students who have emotional disturbances: academic and social emotional outcomes. *School Mental Health* **3**, 191–208.

Lee, S., Tsang, A., Breslau, J., *et al.* (2009). Mental disorders and termination of education in high-income and low- and middle-income countries: epidemiological study. *British Journal of Psychiatry* **194**, 411–17.

Linares, L. O., Leadbeater, B. J., Kato, P. M., & Jaffe, L. (1991). Predicting school outcomes for minority group adolescent mothers: can subgroups be identified? *Journal of Research on Adolescence* **1**, 379–400.

Lloyd, J. W., Kauffman, J. M., Landrum, T. J., & Roe, D. L. (1991). Why do teachers refer pupils for special education? An analysis of referral records. *Exceptionality* **2**, 115–26.

McLeod, J. D., & Kaiser, K. (2004). Childhood emotional and behavioral problems and educational attainment. *American Sociological Review* **69**, 636–58.

Miech, R. A., Caspi, A., Moffitt, T. E., Wright, B. E., & Silva, P. A. (1999). Low socioeconomic status and mental disorders: a longitudinal study of selection and causation during young adulthood. *American Journal of Sociology* **104**, 1096–131.

Quiroga, C., & Janosz, M. (2009). Paths toward school dropout: mechanisms linking adolescent depression symptoms, self-perceived academic competence, and achievement. Montreal: University of Montreal.

Rapport, M., Scanlan, S. W., & Denney, C. B. (1999). Attention-deficit/hyperactivity disorder and scholastic achievement: a model of dual developmental pathways. *Journal of Child Psychology and Psychiatry* **40**, 1169–83.

Rumberger, R. (2004). Why students drop out of school. In G. Orfield, ed., *Dropouts in America: Confronting the Graduation Rate Crisis*. Cambridge, MA: Harvard Education Press, pp. 131–56.

Suhrcke, M., & de Paz Nieves, C. (2011). *The Impact of Health and Health Behaviours on Educational Outcomes in High-Income Countries: A Review of the Evidence*. Copenhagen: WHO Regional Office for Europe.

Swaim, R. C., Oetting, E. R., Edwards, R. W., & Beauvais, F. (1989). Links from emotional distress to adolescent drug use: a path model. *Journal of Consulting and Clinical Psychology* **57**, 227–31.

Woodward, L. J., & Fergusson, D. M. (2001). Life course outcomes of young people with anxiety disorders in adolescence. *Journal of the American Academy of Child and Adolescent Psychiatry* **40**, 1086–93.

World Bank (2002). Lifelong learning in the global knowledge economy: challenges for developing countries. http://www1.worldbank.org/education/stuttgart_conference/download/news_paper_oct_2002.pdf. Accessed March 28, 2012.

Chapter 5

Mental disorders, marriage, and divorce

Joshua Breslau, Elizabeth Miller, Robert Jin, Laura Helena Andrade,
Somnath Chatterji, Maria Elena Medina-Mora, and Rajesh Sagar

Introduction

The burden of mental disorders may extend across the adult life course through effects on marital relationships. Across cultures, marriages are universally celebrated life-cycle events and marital relationships are basic units of economic, social, and cultural organization. It is perhaps not surprising in light of this that a large body of research, based mainly on studies in high-income Western countries, suggests that marriage has a broad range of benefits (Ribar 2004) that include better physical and mental health, economic well-being and stability (Zagorsky 2005, Bardasi & Taylor 2008), and life satisfaction (Easterlin 2003). Theoretical explanations for these effects emphasize the social support that spouses provide each other, the motivation a marriage provides individuals to moderate substance use and other risky behavior, and the ability to specialize in particular activities that a marital partnership affords. There is also evidence of contrasting effects of divorce. Evidence suggests that divorce leads to psychological distress, reduced income, and low child well-being (Amato 2000). To the extent that mental disorders interfere with a person's ability to marry or increase the likelihood of divorcing if they do marry, mental disorders would impose a life-course burden on individuals, with serious implications for society at large. However, given that becoming married might be protective against the onset of mental disorders, and that widowhood and divorce might be causal risk factors for the onset of mental disorders, great care is needed in sorting out the effects of marital status on mental disorder when trying to estimate the effects of mental disorders on marital status.

The best practical way to sort out the potentially reciprocal effects of mental disorders and marital status on each other would be to examine time-lagged associations. Only one study that we are aware of has examined predictive associations between a broad range of mental disorders and subsequent likelihood of becoming married. That study, based on a national sample of the US population, found evidence of countervailing effects at different ages of marriage (Forthofer *et al.* 1996). Early-onset mental disorders were associated with increased probability of marriage prior to age 18, whereas mental disorders as a whole were associated with decreased probability of marriage at ages 18 and older. It is noteworthy in this regard that marriage prior to age 18, defined as child marriage by the WHO, is strongly predictive of divorce and may have adverse rather than beneficial effects (Loughran & Zissimopoulos 2004), whereas marriages that take place at ages 18 and older are associated with benefits.

A number of studies have examined other measures of mental health as predictors of marriage, but the results have not been consistent. Several studies have found that higher scores on scales of non-specific distress are associated with lower likelihood of subsequent marriage (Mastekaasa 1992, Horwitz *et al.* 1996, Hope *et al.* 1999), but other studies have not found evidence of this predictive association (Kim & McKenry 2002, Simon 2002, Lamb *et al.* 2003). No association between alcohol problems and marriage was found in either of two studies that examined that relationship (Horwitz *et al.* 1996, Simon 2002). None of these studies considered variations across age at marriage. The evidence regarding mental health measures as predictors of divorce are more consistent. Studies have found that married individuals with mental disorders have high rates of divorce (Kessler *et al.* 1998), and that high levels of distress (Mastekaasa 1994, Simon 2002, Wade & Pevalin 2004, Bulloch *et al.* 2009) and high levels of alcohol use (Collins *et al.* 2007) both predict elevated risk of divorce.

The Burdens of Mental Disorders, ed. Jordi Alonso, Somnath Chatterji, and Yanling He. Published by
Cambridge University Press. © World Health Organization 2013.

The WMH surveys provide an opportunity to assess the impact of mental disorders on marital relationships from a broad cross-national perspective. These surveys allow examining the associations between mental disorders and the subsequent likelihood of getting married, and also whether the above-mentioned pattern, previously reported in the United States, where the association between mental disorders and marriage varied by age at marriage, holds in this large cross-national sample. The WMH surveys also allow us to examine a number of issues that have not previously been addressed in population-based data. First, no prior studies have had the breadth of assessment of mental disorders included in the WHO Composite International Diagnostic Interview (CIDI), particularly with respect to disruptive behavior disorders. For instance, violence associated with intermittent explosive disorder (IED) may be likely to lead to divorce, but this disorder has not been assessed in previous epidemiological studies of mental disorders and marital relationships.

Second, the large sample size also allows us to explore how the impact of mental disorders might be magnified or suppressed by the co-occurrence of other disorders. Co-occurring disorders might have a synergistic, or supra-additive, interaction in which the impact of each disorder on marriage or divorce is magnified when the disorder co-occurs with other disorders compared to when it occurs in isolation. For instance, alcohol use may trigger or exacerbate violent behavior associated with IED, so that the combination of these two disorders would have a stronger relationship with divorce than either occurring separately. It is also conceivable that interactions among co-occurring disorders might be antagonistic, with each additional disorder contributing a smaller increment in risk. For instance, we might expect that panic disorder or depression would each have a negative impact on marital relationships, but that in a person who has depression, the added impact of panic disorder might be relatively small.

Third, the diversity of the sample, which includes high-income, upper-middle-income, and low/lower-middle-income countries, allows us to test whether the association between mental disorders and marriage is consistent across a wide range of settings. Societal patterns of marriage and divorce vary dramatically. The age at first marriage, for instance, tends to be much later in high-income countries than in low/lower-middle-income countries. The social acceptability of divorce also varies dramatically. Whether these cultural and socioeconomic variations alter the relationship between mental disorders and marital relationships has not previously been examined.

Methods

Sample

In this chapter, we used data from the 20 WMH surveys that included information on the timing of first marriage to examine associations between mental disorders and the subsequent likelihood of getting married ($n = 46,126$). Information on the timing of disorders and marriage is used to ensure that the onset of disorders preceded the marriage. The excluded surveys are those in Iraq, Israel, Northern Ireland, Portugal, and South Africa. Information was also included in 13 of the 20 surveys on whether the respondent's first marriage ended in divorce (the additionally excluded surveys were in Belgium, France, Germany, Italy, the Netherlands, New Zealand, and Spain), with a total sample size of 30,020 individuals. We use these data to examine whether mental disorders with onsets prior to the age at divorce are associated with divorce among people who were ever married.

Measures

The outcome variables in this chapter were age at first marriage and age at divorce. The set of mental disorders considered here differs somewhat from those in other chapters, because of the mix of disorders assessed in the subset of surveys that contained information on timing of marriage and divorce. Unlike a number of other chapters, we distinguished between major depression and dysthymia, based on the thinking that chronic minor depression, as indicated by a diagnosis of dysthymia, might be more important than episodic major depression when it comes to predicting marriage and, even more so, divorce. We also distinguished between panic disorder and agoraphobia and between substance abusers who did versus did not have a history of dependence. Bipolar I and II disorders were combined with subthreshold bipolar disorder into a single measure. Other disorders that were assessed in other chapters but not here were omitted because they were included in too few of the subset of surveys considered here to allow for powerful analysis.

Statistical analysis

As with other chapters in this section of the volume, data were analysed using the discrete-time survival analysis methods described in Chapter 2. The associations of lifetime mental disorders with subsequent first marriage were analysed in models in which age at first marriage was the outcome, mental disorders were the predictors of primary interest, and demographic factors (age, sex, educational attainment, and country), were included as statistical controls. The mental disorders were entered as time-varying predictors using information on age at onset. This means that disorders were only considered as potential predictors of marriage if their onset occurred prior to the age at which the respondent was first married, thereby limiting the possibility that our results are biased due to reverse causality, i.e., the impact of marriage on subsequent mental disorders. The models provide estimates of the difference in the probability of getting married between two people who are similar with respect to their demographics but differ in that one has a history of mental disorder and the other does not.

The associations between mental disorders and divorce were analyzed in a similar way. Discrete-time survival models were estimated in the sample of people who had at least one marriage. Age at divorce was the outcome and mental disorders occurring prior to that age were the predictors of primary interest. Statistical controls were entered to adjust for factors known to be related to divorce: sex, age, educational attainment, years since marriage, months dating prior to marriage, and country.

We were also interested in whether the associations of mental disorders with marriage and divorce were the same when disorders occurred in isolation (e.g., when a person had major depressive disorder and no other mental disorders) and when disorders co-occurred (e.g., when a person had major depressive disorder and a substance use disorder). This is a critical issue because we know from many previous surveys that mental disorders tend to co-occur and that the overall burden of disorders is related to the combination of disorders a person has had. It was not known, however, how comorbid disorders interact to affect marriage and divorce. This issue was examined using models described in Chapter 2 in which the individual disorders and the number of co-occurring disorders are entered simultaneously. If the number of co-occurring disorders is statistically significant in this model, then the association between individual disorders and the outcome (marriage or divorce) is not the same when disorders co-occur as when they occur in isolation. If the association is significant and positive, then the interaction between the disorders is *synergistic* – the combination is greater than the individual parts. If the association is significant and negative, then the interaction is *antagonistic* – the combination is less than the individual parts.

Results

Prevalence of marriage and divorce

Table 5.1 shows the prevalence of marriage and the proportion of first marriages that ended in divorce or separation across the WMH sample. The prevalence of marriage is broken down into three categories based on age. "Early" marriage was defined as marriage before the age of 18 years, corresponding to the WHO definition of child marriage (UNICEF 2007, Raj 2010). Early marriage ranged in prevalence from lows of 0.2% in Japan, 0.4% in Germany, and 0.6% in the two surveys in the People's Republic of China (PRC) to highs of 10.7% in Brazil–São Paulo, 12.3% in Mexico, and 13.8% in India. "On-time" marriage was defined as marriage occurring between age 18 and the age at which 75% of first marriages in that specific country had occurred. The prevalence of on-time marriage among people who had not married early ranged from 31% in Colombia to 65.5% in Ukraine. Of people who did not marry early or on time, the proportion who married late ("late" marriage: i.e., at any age above "on-time" for each country) ranged from 24.4% in Colombia to 75.4% in Ukraine.

The prevalence of divorce or separation among first marriages was 17.9% in the 12 countries for which data were available, but there was wide variation across these countries. Divorce and separation were relatively uncommon in India (2.5%), Lebanon (4.4%), and the PRC studies (8.1% and 5.0%) and much more common in Colombia (25.0%), Ukraine (25.6%), Brazil–São Paulo (28.0%), and the United States (39.6%).

Mental disorders and marriage

The relationship between mental disorders and first marriage is presented in Table 5.2. The first column, labeled "adjusted bivariate model," shows associations between each individual disorder and marriage, adjusting for sex, age, country, and educational attainment,

Table 5.1 Prevalence of early, on-time, and late marriage, and divorce or separation, by country income level. The WMH surveys.[a]

Country income level	Early marriage		On-time marriage		Late marriage		Divorce or separation	
	%	(SE)	%	(SE)	%	(SE)	%	(SE)
All countries	5.3	(0.1)	51.0	(0.3)	58.5	(0.6)	17.9	(0.3)
Low/lower-middle								
Colombia	6.3	(0.9)	31.0	(1.7)	24.4	(2.0)	25.0	(1.7)
India–Pondicherry	13.8	(1.0)	51.8	(2.1)	74.4	(4.6)	2.5	(0.4)
Nigeria	7.4	(0.6)	45.8	(1.5)	69.3	(3.7)	19.9	(1.2)
PRC–Beijing/Shanghai	0.6	(0.2)	56.7	(1.8)	71.7	(4.0)	8.1	(1.1)
PRC–Shenzhen	0.6	(0.3)	37.4	(1.2)	67.8	(2.8)	5.0	(0.6)
Ukraine	3.8	(0.7)	65.5	(1.7)	75.4	(2.6)	25.6	(1.6)
Upper-middle								
Brazil–São Paulo	10.7	(0.9)	52.2	(1.2)	66.0	(2.9)	28.0	(1.6)
Bulgaria	8.7	(0.6)	61.5	(1.5)	66.8	(2.7)	10.2	(1.1)
Lebanon	9.9	(1.2)	44.9	(2.3)	55.1	(4.7)	4.4	(1.0)
Mexico	12.3	(1.0)	48.1	(1.5)	48.4	(2.7)	11.8	(0.9)
Romania	5.8	(0.7)	58.3	(1.3)	68.8	(1.8)	12.1	(0.8)
High								
Belgium	1.2	(0.4)	54.5	(2.0)	58.9	(3.4)	N/A	(N/A)
France	2.2	(0.7)	48.5	(2.8)	50.4	(4.1)	N/A	(N/A)
Germany	0.4	(0.2)	39.3	(2.2)	44.4	(2.4)	N/A	(N/A)
Italy	2.6	(0.4)	55.9	(1.6)	58.4	(3.0)	N/A	(N/A)
Japan	0.2	(0.1)	57.7	(1.8)	67.2	(3.8)	9.7	(1.1)
Netherlands	1.5	(0.6)	47.5	(2.2)	59.4	(4.4)	N/A	(N/A)
New Zealand	1.3	(0.2)	51.6	(1.1)	52.6	(1.8)	N/A	(N/A)
Spain	1.9	(0.4)	52.2	(1.6)	59.7	(3.6)	N/A	(N/A)
USA	6.5	(0.5)	53.9	(1.2)	58.9	(2.0)	39.6	(1.1)

[a] Early marriage = marriage prior to age 18; on-time marriage = marriage between 18 and country-specific 75th percentile of age at marriage among those not married before 18; late marriage = marriage after the 75th percentile of age at marriage among those not married before the 75th percentile of age at marriage. Divorce or separation is given as the proportion of people who were ever married. Information on the timing of divorce was not available (N/A) from Belgium, France, Germany, Italy, the Netherlands, New Zealand, and Spain.

with each disorder examined in a separate model. Results of this model show whether people with each disorder are more or less likely to get married, but they do not take account of co-occurring disorders. The results show that people with mental disorders are less likely to get married. Of the 18 disorders examined, all but two are associated with a lower likelihood of marriage, as indicated by an odds ratio (OR) less than or equal than 1.0, and 14 of the associations reach statistical significance. The disorders significantly associated with marriage include all 10 anxiety and mood disorders considered here (ORs ranging from 0.6 to 0.9) and all four substance use disorders (ORs ranging from 0.6 to 0.8). Interestingly, none of the disruptive behavior disorders is significantly associated with subsequent likelihood of becoming married.

The second column, labeled "multivariate model," shows the results when all 18 disorders are considered simultaneously. As expected, the ORs are attenuated relative to the previous model, with 8 of the 18 disorders maintaining significant associations with marriage. Mood disorders have the strongest associations with marriage in this model, with ORs ranging from 0.7 to 0.8, followed by substance disorders, with ORs ranging from 0.7 to 1.0. Conduct disorder, which was not associated with marriage prior to adjustment for co-occurring disorders, is positively associated with marriage (OR = 1.2, 95% CI 1.0–1.3) after this adjustment.

The multivariate model in Table 5.2 was expanded to test several hypotheses about variation in the association between mental disorders and marriage. First, in order to test whether these associations vary when disorders co-occur, a variable representing the *number of co-occurring disorders* was added to the model. If this variable were significant, it would indicate that disorders do not have the same association with marriage when they co-occur as they have when they

Table 5.2 Association between premarital mental disorders and marriage status and the age of first marriage. The WMH surveys.[a]

| Types of disorder | Model 1. Adjusted bivariate model | | Model 2. Multivariate model | | Model 3. Multivariate model by age period[b] | | | | | |
| | Marriage | | Marriage | | Early marriage | | On-time marriage | | Late marriage | |
	OR	(95% CI)	OR	(95% CI)	OR	(95% CI)	OR	(95% CI)	OR	(95% CI)
Mood disorders										
Bipolar	0.7*	(0.6–0.8)	0.8*	(0.7–0.9)	1.1	(0.6–2.1)	0.8	(0.7–1.0)	0.7*	(0.5–0.9)
Dysthymia	0.6*	(0.5–0.7)	0.8*	(0.7–0.9)	1.0	(0.5–2.1)	0.9	(0.7–1.1)	0.7	(0.6–1.0)
Major depressive disorder	0.6*	(0.6–0.7)	0.7*	(0.6–0.7)	1.1	(0.8–1.5)	0.8*	(0.7–0.8)	0.7*	(0.6–0.8)
Anxiety disorders										
Agoraphobia	0.8*	(0.7–0.9)	0.9	(0.8–1.1)	0.9	(0.5–1.5)	0.9	(0.7–1.1)	0.6*	(0.4–0.9)
Generalized anxiety	0.7*	(0.6–0.8)	0.8*	(0.8–0.9)	1.1	(0.7–1.9)	0.9	(0.8–1.0)	0.9	(0.7–1.2)
Panic disorder	0.7*	(0.6–0.8)	0.9	(0.8–1.0)	0.8	(0.5–1.2)	1.0	(0.8–1.1)	0.8	(0.7–1.1)
Post-traumatic stress	0.7*	(0.6–0.7)	0.8*	(0.7–0.9)	0.9	(0.6–1.5)	0.9	(0.8–1.1)	0.8	(0.6–1.1)
Separation anxiety	0.8*	(0.7–0.8)	0.9*	(0.8–0.9)	0.8	(0.6–1.1)	0.9	(0.8–1.0)	0.8	(0.6–1.1)
Social phobia	0.8*	(0.8–0.9)	1.0	(0.9–1.0)	0.9	(0.7–1.1)	0.9	(0.8–1.0)	1.0	(0.9–1.2)
Specific phobia	0.9[c]	(0.9–1.0)	1.0	(1.0–1.1)	1.3*	(1.1–1.6)	1.0	(1.0–1.1)	0.8*	(0.7–0.9)
Disruptive behavior disorders										
Attention-deficit/hyperactivity	0.9	(0.8–1.0)	1.0	(0.9–1.2)	0.5*	(0.3–0.8)	1.1	(0.9–1.3)	1.1	(0.7–1.7)
Conduct disorder	1.0	(0.9–1.1)	1.2[c]	(1.0–1.3)	1.4	(0.9–2.2)	1.0	(0.9–1.2)	1.3	(0.9–1.8)
Intermittent explosive disorder	1.0	(0.9–1.1)	1.1	(1.0–1.2)	0.9	(0.6–1.5)	1.1	(1.0–1.2)	0.9	(0.7–1.2)
Oppositional-defiant disorder	0.9	(0.8–1.0)	1.1	(0.9–1.2)	0.9	(0.5–1.6)	0.9	(0.7–1.1)	1.3	(0.8–2.1)
Substance disorders										
Alcohol abuse	0.8*	(0.8–0.9)	1.0	(0.9–1.1)	1.0	(0.4–2.5)	0.9	(0.8–1.0)	0.7*	(0.6–0.9)
Alcohol abuse with dependence	0.6*	(0.6–0.7)	0.7*	(0.7–0.8)	1.2	(0.3–5.1)	0.8*	(0.7–0.9)	0.8	(0.6–1.1)
Drug abuse	0.7*	(0.7–0.8)	0.9	(0.8–1.0)	1.0	(0.3–3.8)	0.7*	(0.6–0.8)	1.2	(0.9–1.6)
Drug abuse with dependence	0.6*	(0.5–0.7)	0.8	(0.7–1.0)	2.1	(0.4–10.4)	0.9	(0.6–1.1)	0.8	(0.5–1.3)

[a] ORs estimated in discrete-time survival models with statistical controls for sex, age, country, and educational attainment.
[b] Early marriage = marriage prior to age 18; on-time marriage = between age 18 and country-specific 75th percentile of age at marriage among those not married before 18; late marriage = above country-specific 75th percentile of age at marriage.
[c] Bound of confidence interval rounds to 1, but p-value < 0.05.
* Significant at the 0.05 level, two-sided test.

occur in isolation. However, in this case, the number of co-occurring disorders was not significantly related to marriage ($\chi^2_4 = 1.5$, $p = 0.83$).

To what extent do the associations described above depend on demographic factors, and to what extent are they homogeneous across the population? To explore this question we tested a series of models with all the possible statistical interactions of mental disorders with suspected sources of variation: sex, country income level (low/lower-middle, upper-middle, and high according to World Bank classifications from 2008: see Chapter 2), and time of marriage (early, on-time, and late, as defined above). The interaction models were compared with respect to how well they fit the data with the multivariate model with no interaction terms using both the Bayes and Akaike information criteria, which assess model fit corrected for model complexity. From among these models, the best-fitting model was one that included a statistical interaction between disorders and time period of marriage. Results from this model are shown in the rightmost three columns of Table 5.2.

Associations between disorders and marriage are generally null (i.e., OR not statistically distinguishable from 1) for early age at marriage, but negative associations come to predominate at later ages. ORs for early marriage are nearly equally divided between those less than and those greater than 1.0. Only two reach statistical significance: a weak positive association (OR = 1.3, 95% CI 1.1–1.6) between specific phobia and early marriage, and a strong negative association (OR = 0.5, 95% CI 0.3–0.8) between attention-deficit/hyperactivity disorder (ADHD) and early marriage. Three ORs less than 1.0, indicating lower odds of marriage, reach statistical significance for on-time marriage and five reach statistical significance for late marriage. Major depressive disorder and alcohol abuse are significantly associated with lower likelihood of both on-time and late marriage.

Mental disorders and divorce

Table 5.3 shows results from a parallel series of survival models that was estimated to examine the association between mental disorders and the likelihood that respondents' first marriages ended in divorce or separation. These results were obtained in models using only those respondents who had been married. In the adjusted bivariate models all 18 mental disorders are significantly associated with divorce after adjustment for sex, age, country, years since marriage, months dating prior to marriage, and educational attainment. The adjusted bivariate ORs ranged from 1.2 to 1.8. There is some attenuation of these associations when all 18 disorders are examined simultaneously in the multivariate model, but 17 of the 18 ORs remain greater than 1, indicating higher risk for divorce, with eight reaching statistical significance. Statistically significant ORs are in the range 1.2–1.6.

Contrary to the results regarding marriage, there is evidence that the associations between specific disorders and divorce are modified by the number of co-occurring disorders. Accounting for the specific associations of each of the 18 individual disorders with divorce, the number of co-occurring disorders is significantly associated with divorce ($\chi^2_4 = 9.6$, $p = 0.047$). The ORs associated with having two, three, or four disorders are not different than 1, indicating that the joint effects of an individual's first four co-occurring disorders on divorce are additive. The OR associated with having five or more disorders is significantly less than 1 (OR = 0.6, 95% CI 0.4–0.9), indicating that at high levels of comorbidity the increment of risk for divorce associated with additional disorders declines substantially.

As with the analysis of marriage, we examined variation in the relationship between disorders and other predictors of divorce. All possible statistical interactions of disorders with years since first marriage, months dating prior to marriage, sex, age period, and income level of country were tested. The main effects model was found to have the best fit according to both Akaike and Bayes information criteria.

Societal impact of mental disorders on marriage and divorce

Discrete-time survival models for marriage and divorce were used to simulate changes in the prevalence of marriage and divorce due to mental disorders, under the assumption that the associations in these models represent causal effects (Table 5.4). The estimated population attributable risk proportions (PARPs) are useful because they combine information on the prevalence and strength of association with the outcome for each disorder into a single term that can be compared across individual disorders and with other factors affecting marriage and divorce. Specific phobia accounts for an increase of 3.6% in the prevalence of early marriage and

71

Table 5.3 Association between premarital mental disorders and the age of first divorce in all countries. The WMH surveys.[a]

Types of disorder	Adjusted bivariate		Multivariate		Multivariate with number of disorders	
	OR	(95% CI)	OR	(95% CI)	OR	(95% CI)
Mood disorders						
Bipolar	1.6*	(1.2–2.1)	1.2	(0.9–1.6)	1.3	(1.0–1.7)
Dysthymia	1.5*	(1.2–1.9)	1.0	(0.7–1.3)	1.0	(0.8–1.3)
Major depressive disorder	1.6*	(1.5–1.8)	1.6*	(1.4–1.8)	1.5*	(1.3–1.7)
Anxiety disorders						
Agoraphobia	1.6*	(1.3–2.0)	1.4 [b]	(1.0–1.8)	1.3 [b]	(1.0–1.7)
Generalized anxiety	1.4*	(1.2–1.8)	1.2	(0.9–1.5)	1.1	(0.9–1.4)
Panic disorder	1.4*	(1.1–1.6)	1.1	(0.9–1.3)	1.1	(0.9–1.3)
Post-traumatic stress	1.7*	(1.4–2.1)	1.5*	(1.2–1.8)	1.4*	(1.2–1.7)
Separation anxiety	1.5*	(1.3–1.8)	1.4*	(1.2–1.7)	1.3*	(1.1–1.5)
Social phobia	1.4*	(1.2–1.6)	1.3*	(1.2–1.5)	1.1	(1.0–1.3)
Specific phobia	1.3*	(1.2–1.5)	1.2 [b]	(1.0–1.3)	1.1 [b]	(1.0–1.3)
Disruptive behavior disorders						
Attention-deficit/hyperactivity	1.6*	(1.2–2.0)	1.1	(0.8–1.5)	1.1	(0.9–1.4)
Conduct disorder	1.7*	(1.3–2.3)	1.4	(1.0–2.0)	1.3	(0.9–1.8)
Intermittent explosive disorder	1.2*	(1.1–1.4)	1.1	(0.9–1.3)	1.0	(0.8–1.2)
Oppositional-defiant disorder	1.8*	(1.4–2.2)	1.3	(0.9–1.7)	1.2	(0.9–1.5)
Substance disorders						
Alcohol abuse	1.7*	(1.5–1.9)	1.6*	(1.4–1.9)	1.4*	(1.2–1.7)
Alcohol abuse with dependence	1.8*	(1.5–2.2)	1.0	(0.8–1.3)	1.2	(0.9–1.6)
Drug abuse	1.8*	(1.4–2.2)	1.6*	(1.2–2.2)	1.3	(0.9–1.7)
Drug abuse with dependence	1.7*	(1.3–2.4)	0.7	(0.5–1.2)	0.9	(0.6–1.4)
Number of disorders						
Exactly 2 disorders	–	–	–	–	1.0	(0.8–1.2)
Exactly 3 disorders	–	–	–	–	0.9	(0.7–1.1)
Exactly 4 disorders	–	–	–	–	1.0	(0.7–1.3)
5+ disorders	–	–	–	–	0.6*	(0.4–0.9)

[a] OR estimated in discrete-time survival models with statistical adjustment for sex, age, country, years since marriage, months dating prior to marriage, and educational attainment.
[b] Bound of confidence interval rounds to 1.0, but p-value < 0.05.
* Significant at the 0.05 level, two-sided test.

a decrease of 1.2% in the prevalence of late marriage. Major depressive disorder and alcohol abuse are associated with decreases in the prevalence of on-time or late marriage of over 1%.

The same three disorders have the largest population attributable risks for divorce. Specific phobia, major depression, and alcohol abuse are associated with the largest proportions of divorces (1.3%, 4.0%, and 2.9%, respectively). Post-traumatic stress disorder (PTSD) is associated with a slightly smaller population attributable risk than specific phobia, 1.0% of divorces.

Taken together, the estimated impact of mental disorders is a 1.9% increase in the prevalence of early marriage, reductions in on-time and late marriage of 2.7% and 6.7% respectively, and a 12% increase in the prevalence of divorce.

Discussion

The World Mental Health Survey Initiative offered an opportunity to examine relationships between mental disorders, marriage, and divorce on a much broader international scale than any previous studies. The

Table 5.4 Population attributable risk proportions (PARPs) of marriages and divorces due to mental disorders. The WMH surveys.[a]

Types of disorder	Marriages [b]			Divorces
	Early	On-time	Late	
	PARP (%)	PARP (%)	PARP (%)	PARP (%)
Mood disorders				
Bipolar	0.1	−0.1	−0.3	0.3
Dysthymia	0.0	−0.1	−0.2	−0.1
Major depressive disorder	0.3	−1.0	−2.2	4.0
Anxiety disorders				
Agoraphobia	−0.2	0.0	−0.3	0.4
Generalized anxiety	0.2	−0.1	−0.1	0.2
Panic disorder	−0.3	0.0	−0.2	0.1
Post-traumatic stress	−0.1	−0.1	−0.3	1.0
Separation anxiety	−0.6	−0.1	−0.2	0.9
Social phobia	−0.6	−0.4	0.0	0.6
Specific phobia	3.6	0.1	−1.2	1.3
Disruptive behavior disorders				
Attention-deficit/hyperactivity	−0.9	0.1	0.1	0.0
Conduct disorder	0.5	0.0	0.1	0.3
Intermittent explosive disorder	−0.1	0.1	−0.1	−0.1
Oppositional-defiant disorder	−0.1	−0.1	0.1	0.2
Substance disorders				
Alcohol abuse	0.0	−0.3	−1.2	2.9
Alcohol abuse with dependence	0.1	−0.2	−0.3	0.3
Drug abuse	0.0	−0.4	0.2	0.5
Drug abuse with dependence	0.2	−0.1	−0.1	−0.2
Any disorder	1.9	−2.7	−6.7	12.0

[a] PARPs estimated as the change in predicted prevalence of the outcome when the effects of premarital mental disorders are removed from the population. Positive percentages indicate increases in the outcome associated with the presence of the disorder.
[b] Early marriage = marriage prior to age 18; on-time marriage = between age 18 and country-specific 75th percentile of age at marriage among those not married before 18; late marriage = above country-specific 75th percentile of age at marriage.

evidence suggests that the patterns which have been identified in high-income Western countries hold much more generally across the wide variations in economic, cultural, and social conditions in the diverse group of WMH countries. Although the countries differ dramatically in the prevalence of marriage and divorce, the relationships of mental disorders with marriage and divorce are relatively stable. A previous study which examined the consistency of risk factors for divorce in the USA also found that the risk factors for divorce are very similar across historical periods despite wide variation in the rates of divorce (Teachman 2002). The cross-national sample is not truly global, and there are likely to be exceptions to these findings, but the consistency of these relationships is striking. The findings suggest that marital relationships are an important component of the public health burden of mental disorders. PARP calculations suggest that mental disorders account for a small but meaningful proportion of marriages and divorces.

The evidence suggests that mental disorders reduce the amount of time people spend in marital relationships both by reducing the likelihood that they will marry and by increasing the likelihood that they will divorce or separate after marrying. No single disorder or group of disorders accounts for the pattern of associations. Rather, a mix of anxiety, mood, and substance use disorders remain significant predictors of marital outcomes in multivariate models. Of the disorders examined, mood disorders and substance dependence are most strongly associated with lower likelihood of marriage. Major depression, PTSD, and alcohol or drug abuse (with or without dependence) are the disorders most strongly associated with divorce. This mix of disorders suggests that there may be multiple distinct pathways through which mental disorders affect marital relationships.

What might account for these findings? Marriage and divorce are both affected by many factors occurring at different points in the life course, and mental disorder may play a role during several key periods. The negative associations of mental disorders with marriage (on-time and late marriages, to be specific) may arise from the cumulative impact of early-onset mental disorders on educational attainment or impairment in functioning in young adulthood when marital partnerships are forming. Stigma, negative perceptions of people with disorders by potential partners, may also play a role (Link & Phelan 2001). With respect to divorce, both direct and indirect effects of mental disorders may occur. The direct effects would arise from difficulties that people with mental disorders have in managing interpersonal relationships over time. For instance, mental disorders may account for the relationship that has been observed between frequent intoxication and subsequent divorce (Collins et al. 2007). Indirect effects may arise from impairments in other domains, such as work performance, that have secondary effects on the fulfillment of marital role expectations.

Exceptions to the rule

There are two important exceptions to the general pattern of negative associations between mental disorders and subsequent marriage. First, the disruptive behavior disorders are not associated with lower likelihood of marriage, contrasting with all other groups of disorders. In fact, in the multivariate model which adjusts for co-occurring disorders, there is a statistically significant positive relationship between conduct disorder and marriage. One possible explanation for this finding is that the disinhibition that underlies some of the symptoms of conduct disorder also contributes to the likelihood of marrying. These individuals may interact with more potential marriage partners and be more likely to form intimate relationships. This finding is also balanced against the finding that conduct disorder is one of the most powerful predictors of divorce. Another disruptive behavior disorder, ADHD, which is associated with impaired rather than disinhibited interpersonal relationships, is strongly negatively associated with early marriage.

ADHD has not been assessed in prior epidemiological studies of the consequences of mental disorder for marital relationships. A recent case–control study of adolescent girls with ADHD reported significant problems in formation of romantic relationships (Babinski et al. 2011).

Second, as previous studies in the USA have found (Kessler et al. 1998), the association between mental disorders and marriage varies across age at marriage. Prior to age 18, associations of mental disorders with marriage are generally quite weak, with the exceptions of the *positive* association between specific phobia and marriage and the *negative* association between ADHD and marriage mentioned above. The negative association between mental disorders and marriage emerges in the on-time and late marriages. Previous researchers commenting on evidence of a positive association between mental disorders and early marriage have suggested that distressed adolescents may be motivated to marry in order to escape stressful home environments (Quinton & Rutter 1988). These patterns reinforce concerns about child marriages (UNICEF 2005, Raj et al. 2009, Raj 2010), suggesting that individuals in these marriages may bring pre-existing social and psychological vulnerabilities into these relationships, setting up poor marital outcomes.

Mental comorbidity, marriage, and divorce

The significant associations between each individual mental disorder and marriage are not particularly strong, ranging from 0.7 to 0.9 in the multivariate model. However, comorbidity among these disorders is high, and the overall impact of mental disorders depends not only on the outcomes associated with individual disorders but on the effects of combinations of disorders. In this study, we found no significant interactions among co-occurring disorders, ruling out both synergistic and antagonistic effects. Rather, the evidence suggests that the joint impact of multiple co-occurring disorders is additive, i.e., that the cumulative impact is simply the sum of the impacts of the individual disorders (mathematically the product of the odds ratios associated with the individual disorders). This implies that the total impact of disorders on marriage for a person with multiple co-occurring disorders may be quite large. For instance, at late ages of marriage, the odds of becoming married for a person with a history of specific phobia, major depression, and alcohol abuse would be $0.8 \times 0.7 \times 0.7 = 0.4$, relative to a person with no disorder. Additivity of effects also implies that removing the effect of any single disorder would have an equally positive impact for individuals with complex psychopathology involving multiple disorders as for individuals with a single disorder.

There is some evidence of a departure from additivity in the joint effects of multiple co-occurring disorders on divorce, but only at very high levels of comorbidity which affect a small portion of the population. Associations with divorce are roughly additive for the first four premarital disorders. The increment of risk associated with an additional disorder is only reduced for the fifth or higher-number disorders. For instance, the predicted relative odds of divorce in a first marriage for a person with a premarital history of the same three disorders examined above – specific phobia, major depression, and alcohol abuse – compared to a person with no premarital disorder would be $1.1 \times 1.4 \times 1.5 \times 0.9 = 2.1$. If, in addition, this person also had panic disorder and PTSD, the predicted odds of first divorce relative to someone with no disorder would be the same: $1.1 \times 1.4 \times 1.5 \times 1.1 \times 1.4 \times 0.6 = 2.1$.

Limitations

Several limitations of this study should be noted. First, assessments of mental disorders are based on retrospective reports and are thus likely to be underestimates of the actual prevalence of disorders. Second, reporting accuracy may differ across countries due to differences in the extent to which mental disorders are stigmatized. Statistical adjustment for variations across individual countries minimizes the likelihood that this type of variation affects the pooled cross-national results. Third, the survey data did not allow for separate analysis of the impact of mental disorders on formation of relationships on the one hand and entry into marriage on the other. Future studies that make this distinction could advance understanding of how particular disorders disrupt romantic relationships.

Evidence of an adverse impact on marital relationships adds to evidence regarding the impact of mental disorders on a range of adverse events across the lifespan, including early termination of education (Lee *et al.* 2009) and lower earnings (Levinson *et al.* 2010), as described in Chapters 4 and 8 of this volume, respectively. The impact of mental disorders on marital relationships may also have intergenerational effects because of the influence of divorce on the

early life conditions for children. Findings that were originally reported in the USA have now been reported in cross-national studies, suggesting that mental disorders disrupt life-course trajectories across a very wide range of cultural and social settings.

Implications

Taken together, mental disorders account for a small but meaningful reduction in the proportion of people who marry, and an increase in the proportion of people who divorce in their first marriage. These estimates are based on the assumption that the coefficients reported in Tables 5.2 and 5.3 represent causal effects of disorders on marriage or divorce. While the models from which these coefficients were derived are covariate-adjusted, this assumption is unlikely to hold. Therefore, estimates of the population attributable risk should be taken as heuristic upper bounds to the likely societal effects of disorders on marriage and divorce.

Notably, about half of the societal impact of mental disorders on divorce is due to two disorders, major depression and alcohol abuse. These two disorders also have among the largest population attributable risks for on-time and late marriage. Clinical and/or public health interventions that aim to reduce the negative impact of disorders on marital relationships might be best targeted at these conditions. Current intervention programs that target major depression or alcohol abuse should also consider assessing intervention effects on marital relationships.

Acknowledgments

Portions of this chapter are based on Breslau, J., Miller, E., Jin, R., *et al.* (2011). A multinational study of mental disorders, marriage, and divorce. *Acta Psychiatrica Scandinavica* 124, 474–86. © 2011. John Wiley & Sons A/S.

References

Amato, P. R. (2000). The consequences of divorce for adults and children. *Journal of Marriage and the Family* 62, 1269–87.

Babinski, D. E., Pelham, W. E., Molina, B. S., *et al.* (2011). Late adolescent and young adult outcomes of girls diagnosed with ADHD in childhood: an exploratory investigation. *Journal of Attention Disorders* 15, 204–14.

Bardasi, E., & Taylor, M. (2008). Marriage and wages: a test of the specialization hypothesis. *Economica* 75, 569–91.

Bulloch, A. G., Williams, J. V., Lavorato, D. H., & Patten, S. B. (2009). The relationship between major depression and marital disruption is bidirectional. *Depression and Anxiety* **26**, 1172–7.

Collins, R. L., Ellickson, P. L., & Klein, D. J. (2007). The role of substance use in young adult divorce. *Addiction* **102**, 786–94.

Easterlin, R. A. (2003). Explaining happiness. *Proceedings of the National Academy of Sciences of the USA* **100**, 11176–83.

Forthofer, M. S., Kessler, R. C., Story, A. L., & Gotlib, I. H. (1996). The effects of psychiatric disorders on the probability and timing of first marriage. *Journal of Health and Social Behavior* **37**, 121–32.

Hope, S., Rodgers, B., & Power, C. (1999). Marital status transitions and psychological distress: longitudinal evidence from a national population sample. *Psychological Medicine* **29**, 381–9.

Horwitz, A. V., White, H. R., & Howell-White, S. (1996). Becoming married and mental health: a longitudinal study of a cohort of young adults. *Journal of Marriage and the Family* **58**, 895–907.

Kessler, R. C., Walters, E. E., & Forthofer, M. S. (1998). The social consequences of psychiatric disorders, III: probability of marital stability. *American Journal of Psychiatry* **155**, 1092–6.

Kim, H. K., & McKenry, P. C. (2002). The relationship between marriage and psychological well-being: a longitudinal analysis. *Journal of Family Issues* **23**, 885–911.

Lamb, K. A., Lee, G. R., & Demaris, A. (2003). Union formation and depression: selection and relationship effects. *Journal of Marriage and the Family* **65**, 953–62.

Lee, S., Tsang, A., Breslau, J., *et al.* (2009). Mental disorders and termination of education in high-income and low- and middle-income countries: epidemiological study. *British Journal of Psychiatry* **194**, 411–17.

Levinson, D., Lakoma, M. D., Petukhova, M., *et al.* (2010). Associations of serious mental illness with earnings: results from the WHO World Mental Health surveys. *British Journal of Psychiatry* **197**, 114–21.

Link, B., & Phelan, J. (2001). Conceptualizing stigma. *Annual Review of Sociology* **27**, 363–85.

Loughran, D. S., & Zissimopoulos, J. M. (2004). *Are There Gains to Delaying Marriage? The Effect of Age at First Marriage on Career Development and Wages.* Labor and Population Working Paper Series, WR-207. Santa Monica, CA: Rand.

Mastekaasa, A. (1992). Marriage and psychological well-being: some evidence on selection into marriage. *Journal of Marriage and the Family* **54**, 901–11.

Mastekaasa, A. (1994). Psychological well-being and marital dissolution: selection effects. *Journal of Family Issues* **15**, 208–28.

Quinton, D., & Rutter, M. (1988). *Parenting Breakdown: the Making and Breaking of Inter-Generational Links.* Brookfield, VT: Gower.

Raj, A. (2010). When the mother is a child: the impact of child marriage on the health and human rights of girls. *Archives of Disease in Childhood* **95**, 931–5.

Raj, A., Saggurti, N., Balaiah, D., & Silverman, J. G. (2009). Prevalence of child marriage and its impact on the fertility and fertility control behaviors of young women in India. *Lancet* **373**, 1883–9.

Ribar, D. C. (2004). *What Do Social Scientists Know About the Benefits of Marriage? A Review of Quantitative Methodologies.* Discussion Papers Series 998. Bonn: Institute for the Study of Labor.

Simon, R. W. (2002). Revisiting the relationships among gender, marital status, and mental health. *American Journal of Sociology* **107**, 1065–96.

Teachman, J. D. (2002). Stability across cohorts in divorce risk factors. *Demography* **39**, 331–51.

UNICEF (2005). *Early Marriage: a Harmful Traditional Practice.* New York, NY: UNICEF.

UNICEF (2007). Protecting against abuse, exploitation and violence: child marriage. http://www.unicef.org/progressforchildren/2007n6/index_41843.htm. Accessed December 2012.

Wade, T. J., & Pevalin, D. J. (2004). Marital transitions and mental health. *Journal of Health and Social Behavior* **45**, 155–70.

Zagorsky, J. L. (2005). Marriage and divorce's impact on wealth. *Journal of Sociology* **41**, 406–24.

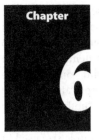

Chapter

6

Premarital mental disorders and risk for marital violence

Elizabeth Miller, Joshua Breslau, Maria V. Petukhova, John Fayyad,
Jen Green, Lola Kola, Soraya Seedat, Maria Carmen Viana,
Jordi Alonso, and Graça Cardoso

Introduction

Perpetration of, and victimization by, physical violence in marital relationships (marital violence) are associated with mental disorders. While much of the literature on family and domestic violence has focused on the mental health *consequences* of experiencing interpersonal violence, a growing number of studies point to the potential role of mental disorders in increasing risk for marital violence (Riggs *et al.* 2000, Kessler *et al.* 2001, Lorber & O'Leary 2004, O'Leary *et al.* 2008, Whisman & Schonbrun 2009). Studies on risk for violence perpetration, especially among males, have found a higher prevalence of substance abuse, depression, antisocial behavior, and poor impulse control than in the general population (Kessler *et al.* 2001, Lorber & O'Leary 2004, Rosen *et al.* 2005). In several cross-sectional studies, female victims report a high prevalence of mood and anxiety disorders. While such mood disorders are presumed to be consequences of violence victimization, it is possible that some of these mood disorders were present prior to marriage, that is, preceding the onset of marital violence (Riggs *et al.* 2000, Cano *et al.* 2003, Stith *et al.* 2004, Lehrer *et al.* 2006, Hellmuth & McNulty 2008, Kim *et al.* 2008, Leaman 2008, O'Leary, *et al.* 2008, Whisman & Schonbrun 2009). Identifying which particular mental disorders or class of disorders are associated with increased risk for marital violence victimization and perpetration could inform clinical screening and safety assessments.

This chapter focuses specifically on assessing the burden of mental disorders on risk for marital violence. Examining the contribution of mental disorders to risk for marital violence also requires consideration of how

spousal characteristics may influence such risk for violence. Respondent mental disorders are likely to be correlated with spouse's mental disorders, such that an association found between a respondent's mental disorder and risk for marital violence may in fact miss the role of the spouse's mental disorders in increasing such risk. A related challenge when examining marital violence using self-report on surveys is a high likelihood of under-reporting due to social desirability biases. While the methods employed for the World Mental Health (WMH) surveys tried to ensure respondent privacy, spouses were not infrequently present during the interview. Thus, for analyses of marital violence, having spousal reports may also corroborate and enhance individual self-reports of marital violence.

Methods

Sample

This chapter utilizes a unique subsample embedded within a number of the country-specific WMH surveys: a subsample of married couples. This subsample was obtained in 11 countries of the 25 surveys by administering the WMH interview to a probability subsample of the spouses of married respondents. This couples sample is invaluable for addressing the question of the role of mental disorders on risk for marital violence. Both partners answered an identical set of questions about their own perpetration of, and victimization by, physical violence in their current marriage (see Chapter 2 for description of these surveys). Having reports of violence from both members of spousal pairs may help address the challenges of

---

The Burdens of Mental Disorders, ed. Jordi Alonso, Somnath Chatterji, and Yanling He. Published by
Cambridge University Press. © World Health Organization 2013.

under-reporting associated with self-report. In addition, both members of each couple completed the same assessment of mental disorders. As spousal history of mental disorders is likely to modify the effects of an individual's premarital mental disorders on their risk for marital violence, these data offer the opportunity to take spousal characteristics into account. A total of 1,821 heterosexual couples were interviewed (see Table 2.1 for the countries involved and the sample sizes in each country). The vast majority (95%) of these couples were married, while the remainder reported "living with someone in a marriage-like relationship." As the bulk of research on mental disorders and marital violence has been conducted in Western high-income and upper-middle-income countries, having couples samples from a set of more diverse countries offers the opportunity to assess whether the associations between mental disorders and marital violence are consistent across countries.

Given the small sample size used in most of the analyses in this chapter, low/lower-middle-income countries and upper-middle-income countries (Brazil, Bulgaria, People's Republic of China–Shenzhen, India–Pondicherry, Lebanon, and Nigeria) were grouped together in a single category and compared with high-income countries (Belgium, France, Italy, Spain, and USA).

Measures

Marital violence was assessed using questions based on the modified Conflict Tactics Scale (Straus *et al.* 1996). Interviewers provided each respondent with a written list of specific violent behaviors and asked whether any of these actions ever occurred in their current marriage. The question was: "People handle disagreements in many different ways. Over the course of your relationship, how often have you ever done any of these things on this list to your current (spouse/partner) – often, sometimes, rarely or never?" Marital violence was defined as "pushed, grabbed or shoved, threw something, slapped or hit." A report other than "never," "don't know," or "refused" was coded as having ever experienced marital violence perpetration in the current marriage. Marital violence victimization used the same examples, phrased as "how often has your current (spouse/partner) done any of these things to you?"

Answering positively to any of the victimization or perpetration items was coded as having experienced "any" marital violence. Those responding positively to either perpetration or victimization items were coded as "perpetrator only" and "victim only." Those responding that they had both perpetrated violence and been victimized were coded as "both perpetrator and victim."

Given the comparatively small sample size used in this analysis, it was necessary to use an extreme approach in collapsing disorders into two very broad categories of internalizing disorders (all the anxiety and mood disorders assessed in the WMH surveys) and externalizing disorders (all the disruptive behavior disorders and substance disorders assessed in the WMH surveys). Having onset of any one or more of the disorders in each of these two broad categories prior to the age at current marriage was coded as "any disorder" of that type.

Statistical analysis

Prevalence estimates for marital violence were calculated separately for women and men within each country and for all 11 countries together based on individual reports. In the couples sample, marital violence was considered present if reported by either member of a couple. Assortative mating by premarital mental disorders was assessed by examining the presence of any mental disorder (internalizing and externalizing) in one spouse as predictor of the presence of mental disorders in the other spouse, prior to the current marriage. The overall approach to statistical analyses is described in greater detail in Chapter 2. In general, however, logistic regression models were used to estimate associations between premarital-onset mental disorders and marital violence. Preliminary models analyzed all internalizing and externalizing disorders as predictors of marital violence. The best-fitting model based on standard fit criteria (the Akaike and Bayes information criteria) was found to be one that included binary variables for presence of any internalizing and any externalizing disorder. This model was then used in simulations to estimate the proportion of cases of marital violence that may be attributable to mental disorders with adjustments for country, age at start of current marriage, age at start of current marriage squared, years in the marriage, and education of both spouses.

Results

Prevalence of marital violence

In 80% of couples, both spouses reported that there was no marital violence (Table 6.1). Among those couples in which any marital violence was reported, three-quarters disagreed on the spouses' respective roles in the violence, i.e., who had perpetrated and who had been victimized. Notably, for 65% of couples in which one respondent endorsed any violence, violence was denied by the spouse.

Table 6.1 Concordance of spouse reports of marital violence and role. The WMH surveys (couples sample).

	%	(SE)
Agree, no violence	80.0	(1.0)
Agree on violence and role	5.0	(0.5)
Agree on violence, disagree on role	2.0	(0.3)
Disagree, one spouse denies violence	13.0	(0.8)

Given this discordance in reporting of violence among couples, both individual and couples reports of marital violence are compared in Table 6.2. The prevalence of marital violence is similar when assessed by individual reports in the entire sample from 11 countries (n = 8,766, top panel) and in the couples sample only (n = 3,642, middle panel): the prevalence of any marital violence is similar for both women (13.8% vs. 13.7%) and men (13.4% vs. 12.7%). The distribution of categories of violence (any, both perpetrator and victim, perpetrator only, victim only) is also similar across these two samples. This finding suggests that the couples sample is similar to the total WMH sample in these countries with respect to marital violence.

The bottom panel of Table 6.2 shows the prevalence of marital violence in the couples sample when taking the response of the spouse who endorsed any marital violence to "enhance" the respondent's report. That is, when a respondent reported no violence, but the spouse reported any violence (whether victimization, perpetration, or both), the respondent was coded as having experienced violence (the spouse report was taken as the true response). In the couples sample, using this

Table 6.2 Prevalence of marital violence ever in current marriage. The WMH surveys.

	Female			Male			Total		
	N	%	(SE)	N	%	(SE)	N	%	(SE)
Individual reports of violence in all married individuals in 11 countries									
Any violence	777	13.8	(0.7)	627	13.4	(0.6)	1,404	13.6	(0.5)
Both	330	5.6	(0.4)	266	5.5	(0.4)	596	5.6	(0.3)
Perpetrator only	238	4.2	(0.4)	255	5.3	(0.5)	493	4.8	(0.3)
Victim only	209	4.0	(0.4)	106	2.5	(0.4)	315	3.3	(0.3)
(n)	(4,696)			(4,070)			(8,766)		
Individual reports of violence in the couples sample									
Any violence	288	13.7	(1.0)	277	12.7	(0.9)	565	13.1	(0.7)
Both	130	5.6	(0.7)	116	4.9	(0.5)	246	5.2	(0.4)
Perpetrator only	64	3.7	(0.7)	117	5.0	(0.6)	181	4.4	(0.4)
Victim only	94	4.4	(0.5)	44	2.8	(0.5)	138	3.5	(0.4)
(n)	(1,821)			(1,821)			(3,642)		
Couples' reports of violence in the couples sample[a]									
Any violence	404	19.8	(1.1)	404	20.2	(1.1)	808	20.0	(0.9)
Both	174	8.1	(0.7)	171	8.1	(0.7)	345	8.1	(0.6)
Perpetrator only	85	4.8	(0.7)	158	7.3	(0.6)	243	6.1	(0.5)
Victim only	145	6.9	(0.7)	75	4.8	(0.7)	220	5.8	(0.5)
(n)	(1,821)			(1,821)			(3,642)		

[a] Reports of violence by either spouse.

approach of enhancing individual reports with spousal reports of any violence, the prevalence increases to 20.0% from 13.1% (the overall prevalence of any marital violence based on individual reports).

Premarital mental disorders and marital violence

To examine the role of internalizing and externalizing premarital mental disorders in predicting any marital violence (i.e., marital violence as reported by either spouse), a series of models were constructed with statistical adjustments for age at start of current marriage, years in the marriage, education, and country (Table 6.3). We focused on associations involving dichotomous measures of having any internalizing and any externalizing disorders rather than more complex models of disorder counts. When any marital violence was examined, all four odds ratios (ORs) were greater than 1, indicating higher risk of marital violence, but only premarital externalizing disorders significantly predicted marital violence among men (OR = 1.7, 95% CI 1.2–2.3). Male premarital externalizing disorders were related to two subtypes

of marital violence: cases where both spouses reported being perpetrators (OR = 1.9, 95% CI 1.2–3.1) and cases where only the male was a perpetrator (OR = 2.2, 95% CI 1.4–3.5). Female internalizing disorders were significantly related to being in a relationship in which both members of the couple were perpetrators of violence (OR = 1.6, 95% CI 1.0–2.4).

Spousal concordance for premarital mental disorders

The couples sample offered the opportunity to assess whether premarital mental disorders are associated with marital violence because of spousal selection. For instance, women's internalizing disorders and marital violence could be associated because women with internalizing disorders might be more likely to marry men with externalizing disorders; that is, the effect of internalizing disorders on risk for marital violence may not be a direct one. Logistic regression models were specified in the couples sample to estimate associations between husbands' and wives' premarital internalizing and externalizing disorders, with statistical controls for number of years in the relationship, country,

Table 6.3 Odds ratios and population attributable risk proportions (PARPs) from multivariate models of marital violence due to premarital mental disorders by sex. The WMH surveys (couples sample).[a]

Violence	Disorder	Female				Male			
					Test for joint significance of both disorder variables				Test for joint significance of both disorder variables
		OR	(95% CI)	PARP (%)	χ^2_2	OR	(95% CI)	PARP (%)	χ^2_2
Any	Any disorder	–	–	5.0	3.2	–	–	10.4	12.3*
	Any externalizing	1.2	(0.9–1.7)	1.5	–	1.7*	(1.2–2.3)	8.5	–
	Any internalizing	1.2	(0.9–1.6)	3.6	–	1.1	(0.8–1.5)	2.1	–
Both	Any disorder	–	–	13.0	7.5*	–	–	14.6	6.9*
	Any externalizing	1.4	(0.8–2.2)	2.7	–	1.9*	(1.2–3.1)	11.3	–
	Any internalizing	1.6*	(1.0–2.4)	10.5	–	1.2	(0.8–1.9)	3.8	–
Perpetrator only	Any disorder	–	–	–14.0	3.1	–	–	11.1	14.6*
	Any externalizing	1.2	(0.7–2.2)	2.9	–	2.2*	(1.4–3.5)	9.8	–
	Any internalizing	0.6	(0.3–1.1)	–17.4	–	1.1	(0.7–1.9)	1.6	–
Victim only	Any disorder	–	–	4.3	2.7	–	–	–5.3	0.8
	Any externalizing	0.8	(0.4–1.6)	–1.1	–	1.0	(0.5–2.0)	1.1	–
	Any internalizing	1.4	(0.9–2.0)	5.3	–	0.8	(0.5–1.3)	–6.4	–

[a] Violence as reported by either spouse.
* Significant at the 0.05 level, two-sided test.

Table 6.4 Wives' and husbands' internalizing and externalizing disorders predicted by spouses' disorders. The WMH surveys (couples sample).[a]

Dependent variable	Predictor	OR	(95% CI)	X^2_2
Wife's externalizing	Husband's externalizing	2.1*	(1.4–3.3)	–
	Husband's internalizing	1.2	(0.8–1.9)	–
	All husband's disorders	–	–	13.5*
Wife's internalizing	Husband's externalizing	1.1	(0.7–1.6)	–
	Husband's internalizing	1.6*	(1.1–2.3)	–
	All husband's disorders	–	–	7.4*
Husband's externalizing	Wife's externalizing	2.2*	(1.4–3.4)	–
	Wife's internalizing	1	(0.7–1.6)	–
	All wife's disorders	–	–	12.4*
Husband's internalizing	Wife's externalizing	1.2	(0.8–1.8)	–
	Wife's internalizing	1.5*	(1.1–2.2)	–
	All wife's disorders	–	–	8.3*

[a] All models control for country, years in the relationship, education (wife's and husband's), age at the start of the relationship (wife's and husband's).
* Significant at the 0.05 level, two-sided test.

education, and age at start of the relationship (Table 6.4). Both internalizing and externalizing disorders sort along similar types: women with internalizing disorders are more likely to be married to men with internalizing disorders (OR = 1.5, 95% CI 1.1–2.2) and women with externalizing disorders are more likely to be married to men with externalizing disorders (OR = 2.2, 95% CI 1.4–3.4).

Couples' premarital mental disorders and marital violence

Given the potential confounding that arises due to marital selection (assortative mating) as noted above, premarital mental disorders and associations with marital violence were examined by using a dataset in which each couple served as a single observation. Premarital externalizing and internalizing disorders in each spouse were examined as predictors of any marital violence, with statistical adjustment for age at start of marriage (for both husband and wife), years in the marriage, husband's and wife's education, and country. While all four ORs were greater than 1, meaning likelihood of higher risk of marital violence among those with pre-existing disorders, only one – husband's externalizing disorders – was statistically significant (OR = 1.7, 95% CI 1.3–2.1) (Table 6.5).

As specific combinations of spousal disorders prior to marriage could increase risk for marital violence (beyond the additive associations shown in Table 6.3),

Table 6.5 Multivariate models predicting any violence. Population attributable risk proportions (PARPs) of any violence due to premarital mental disorders. The WMH surveys (couples sample).[a]

Disorders	OR	(95% CI)	PARP (%)
All disorders	–	–	17.2
All externalizing disorders	–	–	11.4
Husband's externalizing	1.7*	(1.3–2.1)	9.5
Wife's externalizing	1.3	(0.9–1.7)	2.0
All husband's disorders	–	–	11.0
All internalizing disorders	–	–	6.4
Husband's internalizing	1.1	(0.9–1.4)	1.6
Wife's internalizing	1.2	(1.0–1.6)	4.8
All wife's disorders	–	–	6.7
Husband's internalizing, wife's externalizing	–	–	3.5
Husband's externalizing, wife's internalizing	–	–	14.1

[a] Controlling for country, age at start of relationship (both husband's and wife's), age at start of relationship squared, years in the relationship, husband's and wife's education.
* Significant at the 0.05 level, two-sided test.

models with statistical interactions between husband and wife disorders were specified. The main effects model had consistently better fit compared to the interaction models.

Table 6.6 Population attributable risk proportions (PARPs) of marital violence due to premarital mental disorders, individual educational attainment, and length of current marriage, by country income status. The WMH surveys.

Individual educational attainment / Length of marriage	Premarital mental disorders	All countries	Low/ lower-middle	High/ upper-middle
		PARP (%)	PARP (%)	PARP (%)
Low education	All disorders	21.8	16.1	26.3
	Husband's externalizing	11.6	7.9	15.1
	Wife's externalizing	−0.4	−1.4	0.9
	Husband's internalizing	4.6	4.4	3.7
	Wife's internalizing	7.1	5.4	8.1
High education	All disorders	10.2	13.7	9.5
	Husband's externalizing	5.3	6.5	3.9
	Wife's externalizing	7.2	12.8	5.9
	Husband's internalizing	−2.0	−5.6	−1.2
	Wife's internalizing	−0.3	−1.6	1.0
Married 10 years or less	All disorders	29.3	16.9	30.8
	Husband's externalizing	19.0	13.3	16.6
	Wife's externalizing	4.0	−0.4	8.5
	Husband's internalizing	−0.7	2.4	0.2
	Wife's internalizing	8.5	2.1	7.1
Married 11 years or more	All disorders	8.6	15.5	5.7
	Husband's externalizing	4.4	5.3	3.6
	Wife's externalizing	0.8	0.8	1.0
	Husband's internalizing	1.4	4.8	0.0
	Wife's internalizing	2.1	4.5	1.2
Total	All disorders	17.2	15.4	17.4
	Husband's externalizing	9.5	7.8	9.2
	Wife's externalizing	2.0	0.3	3.3
	Husband's internalizing	1.6	4.0	0.7
	Wife's internalizing	4.8	3.7	4.8

Marital violence attributable to premarital mental disorders

The model reported in Table 6.6 was used to estimate population attributable risk proportions (PARPs), which are intended to estimate the contribution of premarital mental disorders to risk for marital violence at a population level. Taking all 11 countries together, 17.2% of cases of marital violence were associated with premarital mental disorders, of which male externalizing disorders accounted for over half (9.5%). When comparing low/lower-middle-income with high-income and upper-middle-income countries, the contribution of mental disorders to risk for marital violence as estimated by PARPs was similar (15.4% and 17.4%, respectively).

Some subgroup variations in PARPs did emerge. Educational attainment was particularly important in high- and upper-middle-income countries, where mental disorders prior to marriage contributed to nearly three times as great a proportion of marital violence among respondents with low levels of education compared to those with high levels of education (26.3% vs. 9.5%). In low/lower-middle-income countries there was little variation in PARP across levels of education (16.1% vs. 13.7%).

Similarly, among respondents in the high- and upper-middle-income countries with less than 10 years in the current marriage, the presence of any mental disorders prior to marriage was associated with a PARP of 30.8% compared to 5.7% among respondents married for more than 10 years. This variation based on length of time in the current marriage was not found in low/lower-middle-income countries (16.9% vs. 15.5%). That is, in high-income and upper-middle-income settings, among those respondents with shorter duration of current marriages (adjusted for age) almost a third of cases of marital violence were associated with premarital mental disorders.

Discussion

This chapter has focused on how the couples sample can help to disentangle the potential contribution of premarital mental disorders to risk for marital violence, recognizing the significant contribution of spousal characteristics to the likelihood of mental disorders being present in a respondent and his or her spouse prior to their marriage. The critical time frame to analyze the burden of mental disorders on marital violence is to assess the presence or absence of mental disorders at the time of the current marriage. Having both respondent and spousal reports strengthens this analysis in several significant ways.

First, the couples sample reflects a diverse set of countries where marital violence and mental disorders were assessed with the same survey instrument. This cross-national study expands the scope of previous research on mental health and marital violence, which has been largely studied in high-income Western countries. Second, this representative sample offers the opportunity to calculate population attributable risk proportions (PARPs) to estimate the contribution of premarital mental disorders to risk for marital violence at a population level. Third, only premarital disorders were examined as predictors of marital violence, excluding disorders that might have occurred as a result of marital violence. And finally, data on both members of married couples allowed for combination of spousal reports in the assessment of marital violence *and* statistical adjustment for the potential contribution of spouse's mental disorders.

Where there was any marital violence, couples tended not to agree. Specifically, in three-quarters of the couples in which one member reported marital violence, reports were discordant on whether there was any violence at all as well as on the role of each spouse in the violence. Combining reports from spouses (when the respondent reported no violence) raised the estimated prevalence of marital violence in the sample by more than 50%, from 13.1% to 20%. The higher estimate from enhancing individual reports with spousal reports of any violence may be closer to the true prevalence of marital violence. As severity of violence was not assessed, it is also possible that the discordant reports represent incidents of lesser severity which only one member of a couple recollects. However, given the sensitivity of discussing marital violence, it is likely that this reporting of marital violence remains an underestimate for several reasons.

First, both members of couples, including victims, may avoid disclosure of marital violence because of the undesirability in their social context (Ellsberg *et al.* 2001). Second, the marital violence measure was limited to acts of physical violence, missing reports of sexual violence or emotional abuse. Third, as this is a representative sample of current marriages only, marriages that were of short duration were underrepresented. If marital violence is associated with divorce, then the sample of current marriages is likely to have proportionally fewer marriages with marital violence. Fourth, the presence of a spouse or family member in some of the interviews may have dissuaded respondents from disclosing violence as they were taking the survey.

The availability of both partners' mental disorder history allowed for assessing the role of marital selection (Dufort 1994, Krueger *et al.* 1998, Maes *et al.* 1998, Merikangas *et al.* 2003), through statistical adjustment for spousal premarital mental disorders. By distinguishing between wife and husband mental health histories in predicting marital violence, a significant gender difference emerged in the association of premarital mental disorders with marital violence. These couples' data suggest that the primary contribution of premarital mental disorders to marital violence is through male externalizing disorders.

Assortative mating is a key issue when considering the impact of mental disorders on a couple's likelihood of having violence in their relationship. The impact of mental disorders on violence in one partner may depend on mental disorders in the other partner. For instance, people with externalizing disorders may be at higher risk if married to a partner with an externalizing disorder rather than a partner with no disorder or an internalizing disorder (Ehrensaft 2008). Marriages between men with externalizing disorders and women with internalizing disorders may be at particularly high risk for marital violence (Kim & Capaldi 2004). Unlike what was expected based on these hypothesized synergies, statistical interactions between disorders in spouses did not emerge. The influence of male externalizing disorders on risk for marital violence thus appears to be of similar magnitude regardless of the history of mental health problems in the spouse.

One pathway that connects externalizing disorders with marital violence emerges in the family violence research literature on the intergenerational continuity of violence. Childhood exposure to family violence (including childhood physical and sexual abuse as well as exposure to interparental violence) is associated with violence in adult relationships (Hotaling & Sugarman 1986, Straus *et al.* 1996, Ehrensaft *et al.* 2003, Stith *et al.* 2004, Ehrensaft 2008, Gil-Gonzalez *et al.* 2008, Herrenkohl *et al.* 2010, Simons & Wurtele, 2010), and also with increased risk for early-onset mental disorders (Kessler *et al.* 1997, Dube *et al.* 2001, Levendosky *et al.* 2002, Ehrensaft *et al.* 2003, Afifi *et al.* 2008, Green *et al.* 2010, McLaughlin *et al.* 2010). It is important to note, however, that associations of early-childhood adverse experiences with adolescent and adult mental disorders are not specific to externalizing disorders.

Internalizing disorders in women contribute less to the likelihood of marital violence compared with externalizing disorders in men. The association with wife's internalizing disorders was barely significant and not of large magnitude; the PARP was much smaller than the PARP for male externalizing disorders (4.8% compared with 9.5%). Such variations in PARPs also suggest that the pathways by which premarital mental disorders increase risk for marital violence are likely to vary by type of disorder and gender.

Population attributable risk differed in notable ways across countries. Differences across levels of education and by duration of current marriage were noted in high-income and upper-middle-income, but not in low/lower-middle-income countries. In low/lower-middle-income countries, disparities in educational status may be less pronounced than in higher-income countries, and lower educational status may not be as significant a marker for social disadvantage as it is in high/upper-middle-income countries. In addition, in high- and upper-middle-income countries, divorce may be more common and marital violence may be one reason that married couples divorce. This would lead to greater selection out of the population of married individuals among people in marriages with violence in the high/upper-middle-income versus low/lower-middle-income countries. What is notable about the cross-country variations, however, is actually the consistency of the attributable risk for any marital violence that is associated with husbands' externalizing disorders across these varied country settings. This suggests that, at least for this subset of disorders, a common pathway is likely where early disruptive and impulsive behavior patterns continue into adult intimate relationships.

These analyses of the couples sample should be interpreted in light of several limitations. Retrospective self-reports (even with spousal reports incorporated) may introduce significant biases. For instance, respondents may have forgotten events or made errors in the timing of events. Inaccuracies are especially likely in reported ages of onset (Kazemian & Farrington 2005), although the distributions of age of onset of mental disorders reported in other studies using these data are consistent with distributions found in prospective studies (Lahey *et al.* 1999, Maughan *et al.* 2004), suggesting that recall bias may not have as significant a role in this regard. Moreover, systematic reviews on the use of retrospective surveys have revealed that despite the limitations, participants in retrospective studies are generally able to recall experiences from as far back as childhood and adolescence with sufficient accuracy to provide useful information (Brewin *et al.* 1993, Hardt & Rutter 2004).

Implications

Husbands' externalizing disorders appear to be the primary mental health component contributing to risk for marital violence across both low/lower-middle-income and high- and upper-middle-income countries after accounting for other mental disorders and spousal selection. Premarital mental disorders appear to be less predictive of marital violence risk for females than for males. How male externalizing disorders appear to increase risk for marital violence, and explanations for the gender difference, merits further study.

These findings support exploring the potential for early mental health interventions in addressing subsequent risk for violence in marital relationships. First, the association between husbands' externalizing disorders and marital violence suggests that early identification and treatment of externalizing disorders among males in school, clinical, and community settings may be one strategy to reduce risk for marital violence. Second, a related strategy for reducing risk for marital violence may involve working with batterer treatment as well as substance abuse programs to engage clients in specific skill-building to address and reduce violence in their relationships. It is important to note in this regard that while there was not an apparent distinction between the impact of substance use disorders and that of other externalizing disorders (e.g., conduct disorder) on marital violence, these conditions are behaviorally quite distinct and may require tailored treatment approaches. In contrast, identification and treatment of internalizing disorders, while important, is less likely to result in reductions in marital violence.

One final implication of these findings for violence prevention is that the contribution of premarital mental disorders to risk for marital violence appears to be quite modest, suggesting that multiple other factors contribute to the complex etiology of violence in intimate relationships. These social and cultural factors likely include unequal power dynamics, gender inequity, and social norms that condone violence within relationships. Based on these findings, targeted mental health interventions for individuals at risk for marital violence in their intimate relationships should be considered only one strategy among many for the prevention of marital violence. While these findings do support exploring the role for early mental health interventions in addressing subsequent risk for marital violence, the overall global impact on marital violence prevention may be limited.

Acknowledgments

Portions of this chapter are based on Miller, E., Breslau, J., Petukhova, M., *et al.* (2011). Premarital mental disorders and physical violence in marriage: cross-national study of married couples. *British Journal of Psychiatry* **199**, 330–7. © 2011. The Royal College of Psychiatrists. Reproduced with permission.

References

Afifi, T. O., Enns, M. W., Cox, B. J., *et al.* (2008). Population attributable fractions of psychiatric disorders and suicide ideation and attempts associated with adverse childhood experiences. *American Journal of Public Health* **98**, 946–52.

Brewin, C. R., Andrews, B., & Gotlib, I. H. (1993). Psychopathology and early experience: a reappraisal of retrospective reports. *Psychological Bulletin* **113**, 82–98.

Cano, A., Scaturo, D. J., Sprafkin, R. P., *et al.* (2003). Family support, self-rated health, and psychological distress. *Primary Care Companion to the Journal of Clinical Psychiatry* **5**, 111–17.

Dube, S. R., Anda, R. F., Felitti, V. J., *et al.* (2001). Childhood abuse, household dysfunction, and the risk of attempted suicide throughout the life span: findings from the Adverse Childhood Experiences Study. *JAMA* **286**, 3089–96.

Dufort, B. (1994). Gamete dealers. *Bulletin of Medical Ethics* **97**, 21–2.

Ehrensaft, M. K. (2008). Intimate partner violence: persistence of myths and implications for intervention. *Child and Youth Services Review* **30**, 276–86.

Ehrensaft, M. K., Cohen, P., Brown, J., *et al.* (2003). Intergenerational transmission of partner violence: a 20-year prospective study. *Journal of Consulting and Clinical Psychology* **71**, 741–53.

Ellsberg, M., Heise, L., Pena, R., *et al.* (2001). Researching domestic violence against women: methodological and ethical considerations. *Studies in Family Planning* **32**, 1–16.

Gil-Gonzalez, D., Vives-Cases, C., Ruiz, M. T., *et al.* (2008). Childhood experiences of violence in perpetrators as a risk factor of intimate partner violence: a systematic review. *Journal of Public Health* **30**, 14–22.

Green, J. G., McLaughlin, K. A., Berglund, P. A., *et al.* (2010). Childhood adversities and adult psychiatric disorders in the National Comorbidity Survey Replication I: associations with first onset of DSM-IV disorders. *Archives of General Psychiatry* **67**, 113–23.

Hardt, J., & Rutter, M. (2004). Validity of adult retrospective reports of adverse childhood experiences: review of the evidence. *Journal of Child Psychology and Psychiatry* **45**, 260–73.

Hellmuth, J. C., & McNulty, J. K. (2008). Neuroticism, marital violence, and the moderating role of stress and behavioral skills. *Journal of Personality and Social Psychology* **95**, 166–80.

Herrenkohl, T. I., Kosterman, R., Mason, W. A., *et al.* (2010). Effects of childhood conduct problems and family adversity on health, health behaviors, and service use in early adulthood: tests of developmental pathways involving adolescent risk taking and depression. *Developmental Psychopathology* **22**, 655–65.

Hotaling, G. T., & Sugarman, D. B. (1986). An analysis of risk markers in husband to wife violence: the current state of knowledge. *Violence and Victims* **1**, 101–24.

Kazemian, L., & Farrington, D. P. (2005). Comparing the validity of prospective, retrospective, and official onset for different offending categories. *Journal of Quantitative Criminology* **21**, 127–47.

Kessler, R. C., Davis, C. G., & Kendler, K. S. (1997). Childhood adversity and adult psychiatric disorder in the US National Comorbidity Survey. *Psychological Medicine* **27**, 1101–19.

Kessler, R. C., Molnar, B. E., Feurer, I. D., *et al.* (2001). Patterns and mental health predictors of domestic violence in the United States: results from the National Comorbidity Survey. *International Journal of Law and Psychiatry* **24**, 487–508.

Kim, H. K., & Capaldi, D. M. (2004). The association of antisocial behavior and depressive symptoms between partners and risk for aggression in romantic relationships. *Journal of Family Psychology* **18**, 82–96.

Kim, H. K., Laurent, H. K., Capaldi, D. M., *et al.* (2008). Men's aggression toward women: a 10-year panel study. *Journal of Marriage and Family* **70**, 1169–87.

Krueger, R. F., Moffitt, T. E., Caspi, A., *et al.* (1998). Assortative mating for antisocial behavior: developmental and methodological implications. *Behavioral Genetics* **28**, 173–86.

Lahey, B., Miller, T., Gordon, R., & Riley, A. (1999), Developmental epidemiology of the disruptive behavior disorders. In H. Quay & A. Hogan, eds., *Handbook of the Disruptive Behavior Disorders*. New York, NY: Plenum Press, pp. 23–48.

Leaman, T. R. (2008). Nettle reaction in a foal. *Veterinary Record* **162**, 164.

Lehrer, J. A., Buka, S., Gortmaker, S., *et al.* (2006). Depressive symptomatology as a predictor of exposure to intimate partner violence among US female adolescents and young adults. *Archives of Pediatric and Adolescent Medicine* **160**, 270–6.

Levendosky, A. A., Huth-Bocks, A., & Semel, M. A. (2002). Adolescent peer relationships and mental health functioning in families with domestic violence. *Journal of Clinical Child and Adolescent Psychology* **31**, 206–18.

Lorber, M. F., & O'Leary, K. D. (2004). Predictors of the persistence of male aggression in early marriage. *Journal of Family Violence* **19**, 329–38.

Maes, H. H., Neale, M. C., Kendler, K. S., *et al.* (1998). Assortative mating for major psychiatric diagnoses in two population-based samples. *Psychological Medicine* **28**, 1389–401.

Maughan, B., Rowe, R., Messer, J., *et al.* (2004). Conduct disorder and oppositional defiant disorder in a national sample: developmental epidemiology. *Journal of Child Psychology and Psychiatry* **45**, 609–21.

McLaughlin, K. A., Green, J. G., Gruber, M. J., *et al.* (2010). Childhood adversities and adult psychiatric disorders in the National Comorbidity Survey Replication II: associations with persistence of DSM-IV disorders. *Archives of General Psychiatry* **67** (2), 124–132.

Merikangas, K. R., Zhang, H., Avenevoli, S., *et al.* (2003). Longitudinal trajectories of depression and anxiety in a prospective community study: the Zurich Cohort Study. *Archives of General Psychiatry* **60**, 993–1000.

O'Leary, K. D., Smith Slep, A. M., Avery-Leaf, S., *et al.* (2008). Gender differences in dating aggression among multiethnic high school students. *Journal of Adolescent Health* **42**, 473–9.

Riggs, D. S., Caulfield, M. B., & Street, A. E. (2000). Risk for domestic violence: factors associated with perpetration and victimization. *Journal of Clinical Psychology* **56**, 1289–316.

Rosen, K. H., Stith, S. M., Few, A. L., *et al.* (2005). A qualitative investigation of Johnson's typology. *Violence and Victims* **20**, 319–34.

Simons, D. A., & Wurtele, S. K. (2010). Relationships between parents' use of corporal punishment and their children's endorsement of spanking and hitting other children. *Child Abuse and Neglect* **34**, 639–46.

Stith, S. M., Smith, D. B., Penn, C. E., *et al.* (2004). Intimate partner physical abuse perpetration and victimization risk factors: a meta-analytic review. *Aggression and Violent Behavior*, **10**, 65–98.

Straus, M. A., Hamby, S. L., Boney-McCoy, S., & Sugarman, D. B. (1996). The Revised Conflict Tactics Scales (CTS2). *Journal of Family Issues* **17**, 283–316.

Whisman, M. A., & Schonbrun, Y. C. (2009). Social consequences of borderline personality disorder symptoms in a population-based survey: marital distress, marital violence, and marital disruption. *Journal of Personality Disorders* **23**, 410–15.

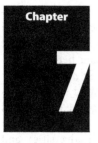

Chapter

7

Early-onset mental disorders and their links to chronic physical conditions in adulthood

Kate M. Scott, Ben Wu, Kathleen Saunders, Corina Benjet, Yanling He, Jean-Pierre Lépine, Hisateru Tachimori, and Michael Von Korff

Introduction

Mental disorders often first occur early in life. When they are severe, long-lasting, or recurring, they can have enduring influence on many aspects of people's lives. We know from earlier research (Kessler *et al.* 1995, 1997, 1998, Ettner *et al.* 1997, Jayakody *et al.* 2012), and from the research presented in this volume, that early-onset mental disorders are linked to subsequent poor social, educational, marital, and occupational outcomes. What is less clear is whether chronic physical conditions occurring later in life might be among the negative outcomes associated with early-onset mental disorders.

How might early-onset mental disorders come to be associated with chronic physical conditions? One possibility is through behavioral pathways. People with mental disorders are known to be more likely to smoke, to be sedentary, to be heavy drinkers, and to have a range of cardiovascular risk factors (Davidson *et al.* 2001, Scott *et al.* 2006). Because health-related behaviors are often established early in life, there is the potential for early-onset disorders to influence the choices individuals make in relation to smoking, drinking, and diet, in part as a way of regulating depressed mood or anxiety, or coping with stress. Psychological factors such as personality and mood have a major impact on the stress we experience because they influence whether an experience is perceived as stressful or not (Lazarus & Folkman 1984).

In fact, stress per se, not just the perception of it but also the biological response to it, may be fundamental to how mental disorders, especially early-onset or recurrent mental disorders, influence chronic physical conditions. Two main physiological systems are involved in our reaction to stress – the autonomic nervous system (through the sympathetic–adrenal–medullary [SAM] axis) and the neuroendocrine system (through the hypothalamic–pituitary–adrenal [HPA] axis). Some degree of dysregulation of these systems, resulting in over- or under-activity of the hormones involved (e.g., cortisol, epinephrine, and norepinephrine), has been associated with both depression and anxiety disorders (Heim & Nemeroff 1999, Goodyer 2007). If this pattern of dysregulated stress response occurs early in life and becomes an established way of responding to stress, it may have adverse effects on the metabolic, cardiovascular, and immune systems, and so influence physical disease development (Miller *et al.* 2002, Musselman *et al.* 2007, Steptoe 2007a, Scott 2009).

Although we tend to think of mental disorders as being the consequence of stressful life experiences, it has been suggested that they may also constitute a source of stress. The experience of depression and post-traumatic stress disorder, for example, involves rumination on or reliving adverse experience, thus contributing to stress exposure (McEwen 2003). In fact, mental disorders such as depression have been hypothesized to contribute to allostatic load (McEwen 1998). Allostatic load is a term used to indicate the cumulative biological "wear and tear" that occurs through a chronic imbalance in the hormonal mediators of the stress response, particularly those involved in the HPA axis. It has been linked with a range of adverse metabolic, cardiovascular, immune, and cognitive effects (Miller *et al.* 2002, Chrousos & Kino 2007). We also know from other research that it is the stressors occurring early in life that have the most potential to contribute to allostatic load, because that is when the physiological systems responsible for

---

responding to stress are most sensitive to disruption and subsequent dysregulation (Heim *et al.* 2000, Teicher *et al.* 2002, Sanchez 2006). Early-onset mental disorders, particularly in cases where these become persistent or recurring, may therefore contribute to dysregulation of the HPA axis, and/or contribute in other ways to allostatic load, and thereby affect the development of chronic physical conditions occurring later in adulthood (Scott 2009).

There is extensive prospective evidence for an association of depression and anxiety with coronary heart disease onset (Hemingway 1999, Rozanski *et al.* 1999, Krantz & McCeney 2002, Rugulies 2002, Rudisch & Nemeroff 2003, Wulsin & Singal 2003, Suls & Bunde 2005, Nicholson *et al.* 2006, Steptoe 2007b, van der Kooy *et al.* 2007, Goldston & Baillie 2008), reasonable evidence for an association of depression with subsequent onset of diabetes (Eaton *et al.* 1996, van den Akker *et al.* 2004, Engum 2007, Musselman *et al.* 2007), and some evidence for prospective links between either anxiety or depression and other chronic physical conditions (Everson *et al.* 1998, Jonas & Mussolino, 2000, Evans *et al.* 2005, Van Puymbroeck *et al.* 2007, Chida *et al.* 2008, Goodwin *et al.* 2009). However, in all of these studies, depression or anxiety was measured during adulthood, usually mid-life, and typically using symptom screening scales. We are not aware of prior studies that have investigated early-onset mental disorders in this context. This is partly because the requisite data have not been available. For example, prospective studies that have diagnostic information on mental disorders do not yet have cohorts that are old enough to have developed some of the major chronic physical conditions such as heart disease. Older cohorts lack diagnostic information on mental disorders occurring earlier in life. Although the WMH surveys are limited by their cross-sectional nature, their information on the onset timing of mental disorders and of physical conditions allows the utilization of a prospective analytical approach within a survival framework. This helps establish the temporal priority of the proposed mental disorder predictors.

In the following analysis we investigate not just early-onset mental disorders as predictors of adult-onset physical conditions, but also childhood familial adversities as additional predictors. Our first reason for including childhood adversities is to be able to ascertain whether early-onset mental disorders are associated with later physical health independent of childhood adversities. Childhood adversities are now

thought to be associated with physical health outcomes, and clearly they are also associated with mental disorders (Green *et al.* 2010), so they have the potential to confound any observed associations between mental and physical health (Goodwin *et al.* 2004). Our second reason for including childhood adversities is because the WMH surveys are one of the few datasets with comprehensive information on both mental disorders and a range of childhood adversities, and so offer a rare opportunity to ascertain the relative strength of these two sets of predictors in their association with later physical health.

A further feature of the analysis reported here is that we investigated a *range* of physical outcomes: heart disease, adult-onset asthma, diabetes, arthritis, chronic back or neck pain, frequent or severe headaches. This is in contrast to pevious studies of associations between depression or anxiety and subsequent physical ill health, which have usually focused on a single physical condition outcome (typically, heart disease). Studies of single outcomes do not allow consideration of whether mental disorders have specific or generic relationships with physical condition onsets (Goodwin *et al.* 2009), which has important implications for the consideration of mechanisms. One recent study evaluated links between mental health problems in childhood and physical conditions occurring between ages 18 and 23 in Finnish men (Goodwin *et al.* 2009), but the age of that sample greatly limited the type of physical conditions that could be considered.

Methods

Sample

We used only 13 of the WMH surveys in the analyses reported in this chapter (Colombia, Mexico, United States, Belgium, France, Germany, Italy, the Netherlands, Spain, Japan, Northern Ireland, Portugal, and Romania), with a total sample size of 25,715. The remaining surveys could not be included because they did not collect either data on age of onset of physical conditions or data on childhood adversity. Only individuals from the part 2 sample were included, because chronic conditions were only evaluated in this subsample in most of the countries.

Measures

As detailed in Chapter 2, the physical conditions considered here as dependent variables were assessed using a checklist adapted from the US National Health Interview Survey. The *medical diagnoses* or *silent conditions* were ascertained by the following question: "Did a doctor or other health professional ever tell you that you had ... heart disease; asthma; diabetes or high blood sugar?" *Symptom-based conditions* were ascertained with the question: "Have you ever had ... arthritis or rheumatism; chronic back or neck problems; frequent or severe headaches?" For all conditions reported, respondents were asked how old they were when they were first diagnosed with the condition (for the medical diagnoses) or first experienced the condition (for the symptomatic conditions). The six physical conditions assessed in this chapter are: arthritis, asthma, chronic back or neck pain, diabetes, frequent or severe headache, and heart disease. Selection of these physical outcomes was based on consideration of whether there was existing research on their links with temporally prior mental disorders, together with consideration of the frequency of the physical conditions in the WMH surveys dataset.

We considered only a limited set of the mental disorders assessed in the WMH surveys. Specifically, we focused on major depressive disorder and on a subset of anxiety disorders (generalized anxiety disorder, panic disorder and/or agoraphobia, post-traumatic stress disorder, and social phobia). The rationale for this narrow focus is that prior WMH survey analyses showed that these were the disorders considered in the WMH surveys that are most strongly associated with the physical conditions assessed in the surveys (Scott *et al.* 2007, Von Korff 2009). Those earlier analyses also demonstrated that despite the variation in frequency of both mental disorders and physical conditions across WMH surveys, the associations between mental disorders and physical conditions are remarkably consistent across countries, thus justifying our decision to pool analyses across countries.

The childhood adversities considered here include physical abuse, sexual abuse, neglect, parental death, parental divorce, other parental loss, parental mental disorder, parental substance use disorder, parental criminal behavior, family violence, and family economic adversity. The aim was to assess the occurrence of childhood adversities occurring in the context of the family (not all possible childhood adversities), with the thought that these are more likely to be sustained over long periods of time and so to have chronic health effects. Those respondents who reported that

the experience occurred before the age of 18 and met the criteria specified for a given adversity were coded as having experienced childhood family adversity. Assessment of the adversities is detailed in earlier publications (Scott *et al.* 2008, Von Korff 2009) and in Appendix 7.

Statistical analysis

As in many previous chapters in this volume, the associations of childhood adversities and early-onset mental disorders with subsequent onset of adult physical conditions were studied using discrete-time survival analyses based on retrospectively reported reports about age of onset of both mental and physical disorders. This method is discussed in Chapter 2. The start of the period at risk of the physical conditions was set at age 20. That is, the small number of people who reported that a given physical condition that we studied had an onset before age 21 were excluded from analysis. Models predicted first onset of each physical condition, with number and type of childhood adversities and early-onset (< 21 years of age) depressive/anxiety disorders coded as time-varying predictors. Specific childhood adversities, specific early-onset mental disorders, and the number of childhood adversities (none, one, two, and three or more) were the predictor variables. People with no childhood adversities and people with no early-onset depression or anxiety disorders served as the reference groups. Childhood adversities and early-onset mental disorders were included in the models first separately and then simultaneously to investigate the extent to which they were independently associated with subsequent onset of each physical condition.

As in earlier chapters, all associations are expressed as odds ratios (ORs) that measure the relative odds of the physical condition occurring as a function of the prior mental disorder after adjustment for age, sex, and country. The main analyses were repeated additionally controlling for education, but as the results were consistently similar to those not controlling for education, the simpler model results are reported here. Models of asthma and heart disease additionally controlled for prior history of smoking (ever, never, current). We also assessed for the interaction of childhood adversities with early-onset mental disorders in predicting the onset of each physical condition, but these interaction effects are not reported because they were not significant. Only main effects are reported. Country was included in all analyses as a stratifying variable, which adjusted for between-country differences in prevalence of the outcome disorders.

Results

Bivariate associations of mental disorders and adversities with adult-onset physical conditions

All five early-onset mental disorders are associated with the onset of each of the three chronic pain conditions in adulthood (arthritis, chronic back or neck pain, and frequent or severe headaches) in bivariate models, with ORs in the range 1.5–2.2 (Table 7.1). With regard to the medical conditions, four of the five early-onset mental disorders are associated with the subsequent onset of asthma and heart disease, but no disorder is associated with the onset of diabetes.

Table 7.1 also shows associations between specific childhood adversities and onset of each physical health outcome. Physical abuse is the only childhood adversity associated with onset of all six chronic disease outcomes, while sexual abuse, parental mental disorder, parental substance use disorder, violence in the family, and criminal behavior are associated with onset of five of the six health outcomes. The associations between individual adversities and physical conditions are generally modest in magnitude, with almost all ORs 2.0 or less. The exception is the association of sexual abuse with later heart disease (OR = 3.0, 95% CI 2.0–4.4).

Multivariate associations of mental disorders and adversities with adult-onset physical conditions

After adjustment for childhood adversities, early-onset depressive/anxiety disorders ("any") are associated with the onset of five physical conditions in adulthood (Table 7.2), with ORs ranging from 1.4 for arthritis to 1.8 for frequent or severe headaches. Table 7.2 shows a dose–response relationship between the number of childhood adversities experienced and the likelihood of later physical condition onset, with exactly two childhood adversities associated with four of the six physical condition outcomes (ORs in the range 1.4–1.5), and three or more childhood adversities

associated with all six physical conditions after adjustment for early-onset mental disorders (ORs in the range 1.5–1.9).

Discussion

In this analysis, based on 13 of the WMH countries, we found that early-onset mental disorders are independently associated with five of the six adult-onset chronic physical conditions studied (the exception being diabetes) after adjustment for childhood adversities. A history of three or more childhood adversities is also independently associated with all six of the physical conditions after adjustment for mental disorders. The strength of associations between each set of predictors (mental disorders and childhood adversities) and the physical outcomes is similar.

The study is clearly limited by its cross-sectional nature, which can result in biased recall of the occurrence of mental disorders (generally under-reporting due to forgetting) (Wells & Horwood 2004) and biased recall of age of onset of mental disorders (Simon & Von Korff 1995). We were also unable to take into account the severity of the mental disorders or the childhood adversities. These associations should therefore be considered as "averages," which may underestimate the strength of association between the more severe adversities or mental disorders occurring at critical childhood developmental stages. A further limitation is that the medical conditions were assessed on the basis of self-report, although there is generally good agreement between self-report of medical diagnoses and physician or medical-record confirmation of those diagnoses (Kriegsman et al. 1996, Baumeister et al. 2010). We are reassured by the fact that the early-onset mental disorders are as strongly associated with the diagnosed medical conditions as they are with the symptomatic pain conditions; this is noteworthy because there is greater potential for current mood state to amplify associations between a history of mental disorder and report of symptomatic pain conditions than report of diagnosed medical conditions (Vassend & Skrondal 1999, Kolk et al. 2002). Finally, there may be sample selection biases operating, due to non-respondents having poorer mental or physical health or differential selection out of the population through early mortality. These sample selection factors would probably lead to downward (conservative) bias in estimating the strength of associations.

Table 7.1 Association of specific early-onset mental disorders and childhood adversities with the subsequent onset of chronic physical conditions in adulthood. The WMH surveys.[a]

	Arthritis		Asthma		Back/neck pain		Diabetes		Headache		Heart disease	
	OR	(95% CI)	OR	(95% CI)	OR	(95% CI)	OR	(95% CI)	OR	(95% CI)	OR	(95% CI)
Early-onset mental disorders (< 21 years)												
Major depressive disorder	1.5*	(1.3–1.8)	2.1*	(1.5–2.8)	1.5*	(1.4–1.8)	1.3	(1.0–1.6)	1.7*	(1.4–2.0)	1.5*	(1.0–2.2)
Generalized anxiety	1.8*	(1.5–2.2)	1.8*	(1.2–2.6)	2.2*	(1.9–2.6)	1.1	(0.7–1.8)	1.8*	(1.4–2.2)	1.2	(0.7–1.9)
Panic disorder/agoraphobia	1.6*	(1.3–2.0)	1.8*	(1.2–2.7)	1.7*	(1.4–2.0)	1.6	(1.0–2.5)	1.8*	(1.5–2.2)	2.0*	(1.4–2.9)
Post-traumatic stress	1.7*	(1.3–2.2)	2.0*	(1.2–3.3)	2.1*	(1.7–2.6)	1.1	(0.7–1.7)	1.8*	(1.3–2.3)	2.3*	(1.6–3.3)
Social phobia	1.6*	(1.4–1.8)	1.3	(0.9–1.8)	1.6*	(1.4–1.8)	1.2	(0.9–1.7)	1.8*	(1.5–2.1)	1.7*	(1.3–2.2)
Childhood adversities												
Physical abuse	1.4*	(1.2–1.7)	1.8*	(1.3–2.6)	1.7*	(1.5–1.9)	1.5*	(1.2–2.0)	1.6*	(1.4–1.8)	1.5*	(1.2–1.9)
Sexual abuse	1.6*	(1.2–2.0)	1.3	(1.0–1.9)	1.6*	(1.2–2.1)	1.5	(0.6–1.6)	1.8*	(1.4–2.2)	3.0*	(2.0–4.4)
Neglect	1.7*	(1.4–2.0)	1.2	(0.8–1.9)	1.5*	(1.2–1.8)	1.2	(0.9–1.6)	1.5*	(1.3–1.8)	1.8*	(1.4–2.5)
Parental death	1.0	(0.9–1.1)	1.2*	(1.0–1.5)	1.0	(0.9–1.2)	1.0	(0.8–1.2)	1.1	(0.9–1.2)	1.2*	(1.0–1.5)
Parental divorce	1.0	(0.8–1.2)	1.0	(0.6–1.6)	1.2	(1.0–1.4)	1.2	(0.9–1.6)	1.1	(0.9–1.4)	1.7*	(1.3–2.2)
Other parental loss	1.3*	(1.1–1.6)	1.2	(0.9–1.6)	1.2*	(1.1–1.4)	1.5*	(1.1–2.1)	1.2*	(1.0–1.5)	1.3	(1.0–1.7)
Parental mental disorder	1.4*	(1.2–1.6)	1.5*	(1.1–2.1)	1.5*	(1.3–1.7)	1.2	(0.9–1.6)	1.5*	(1.3–1.8)	1.4*	(1.1–1.8)
Parental substance use disorder	1.4*	(1.2–1.7)	1.5	(1.0–2.1)	1.4*	(1.2–1.6)	1.5*	(1.1–2.0)	1.4*	(1.2–1.7)	1.5*	(1.1–2.1)
Parental criminal behavior	1.4*	(1.1–1.7)	1.5	(1.0–2.4)	1.4*	(1.1–1.7)	1.7*	(1.2–2.4)	1.5*	(1.2–1.9)	2.0*	(1.4–2.7)
Family violence	1.4*	(1.2–1.7)	1.4*	(1.1–1.9)	1.5*	(1.3–1.7)	1.3	(1.0–1.6)	1.4*	(1.3–1.7)	1.3*	(1.0–1.7)
Family economic adversity	1.0	(0.9–1.2)	1.0	(0.7–1.4)	1.1	(1.0–1.3)	1.5*	(1.1–2.1)	1.2	(0.9–1.4)	1.2	(0.9–1.6)

[a] Bivariate models: each early-onset mental disorder (= first onset < 21 years of age) and childhood adversity was estimated as a predictor of the physical condition onset in a separate discrete-time survival model controlling for person-year, age cohorts, age cohorts, sex, and country. Models for heart disease and asthma additionally adjust for smoking status.
* Significant at the 0.05 level, two-sided test.

Table 7.2 Association of early-onset mental disorders and number of childhood adversities with subsequent onset of chronic physical conditions in adulthood. The WMH surveys.[a]

	Arthritis	Asthma	Back/neck pain	Diabetes	Headache	Heart disease
	OR (95% CI)	OR (95% CI)	OR (95% CI)	OR (95% CI)	OR (95% CI)	OR (95% CI)
Any early-onset mental disorder (< 21 years)	1.4* (1.3–1.6)	1.6* (1.2–2.1)	1.6* (1.5–1.8)	1.2 (1.0–1.5)	1.8* (1.6–2.0)	1.6* (1.3–1.9)
Exactly 1 childhood adversity	1.1 (0.9–1.2)	1.1 (0.9–1.4)	1.1* (1.0–1.3)	1.2 (1.0–1.5)	1.4* (1.2–1.5)	1.2 (1.0–1.5)
Exactly 2 childhood adversities	1.4* (1.2–1.6)	1.2 (0.9–1.7)	1.4* (1.3–1.6)	1.0 (0.8–1.3)	1.5* (1.3–1.8)	1.4* (1.1–1.8)
3+ childhood adversities	1.5* (1.3–1.7)	1.5* (1.1–2.0)	1.6* (1.4–1.8)	1.5* (1.1–1.9)	1.8* (1.5–2.0)	1.9* (1.5–2.4)

[a] Multivariate model: a dummy variable representing any early-onset mental disorder (= first onset < 21 years of age) and dummy variables for the number of childhood adversities were entered simultaneously in the discrete-time survival model, controlling for person-year, age cohorts, sex, and country. Models for heart disease and asthma additionally adjust for smoking status.
* Significant at the 0.05 level, two-sided test.

Given these limitations, this study should be considered exploratory in nature. A more definitive study will require prospective data, although such data will not be forthcoming for some decades because it requires a large sample of individuals with diagnostic information on mental disorders in childhood followed up over the lifetime of the study participants. We note that our findings are consistent with results of prospective research where these are available. For example, the odds ratio we observe of 1.5 between early-onset major depressive disorder and heart disease onset is within the 1.50–2.00 range obtained in meta-analyses of prospective associations between depression and subsequent heart disease (Wulsin & Singal 2003, Nicholson et al. 2006). The ORs of 1.8–2.1 we observe between anxiety or depressive disorders and asthma are consistent with the ORs from 1.4–2.5 found in the prospective studies examining associations between depression or anxiety and the subsequent report or diagnosis of asthma (Chida et al. 2008). Similarly, the associations between early-onset mental disorders and chronic pain we find in our data (ORs in the range 1.5–2.2) are consistent with prospective studies of this relationship reporting ORs of 1.6–2.2 (Van Puymbroeck et al. 2007). The lack of association between mental disorders and diabetes in this study contrasts with other research where a relationship has been observed (Eaton et al. 1996, Engum 2007), but the relationship between mental disorders and

diabetes has been less consistently found than the relationship between mental disorders and heart disease.

The limitations noted above notwithstanding, these results are potentially important. Early-onset mental disorders have not been investigated previously in terms of their links with later physical conditions. These findings support the possibility that early-onset mental disorders may shape biological and behavioral responses in such a way as to increase risks of a range of chronic physical conditions in later life (Scott 2009). As mentioned in the introduction to this chapter, early-onset depression or anxiety may constitute a kind of endogenous stressor, contributing directly to allostatic load. This may occur because the experience of severe depression or anxiety is itself a highly stressful experience that could have similar physiological effects to the chronic experience of an external stressor (McEwen 2003). It is also likely that depression and anxiety disorders add to allostatic load through exacerbation of risky health behaviors. Behaviors such as smoking, heavy consumption of alcohol, and overeating can be part of an individual's way of coping with depression or anxiety, but they then have negative physiological consequences which increase risk of disease (Hertzman 1999, McEwen 2003).

Another emerging theory about how mental disorders could influence physical disease development views chronic mental disorders as syndromes of accelerated aging (Simon *et al.* 2006, Kirkpatrick *et al.* 2008, Wolkowitz *et al.* 2008). The recent research on telomere attrition is now giving this theory considerable impetus. Telomeres are DNA protein complexes that cap the ends of chromosomes, providing chromosomal stability and integrity (Blackburn 2000, Aviv *et al.* 2003, Chan & Blackburn 2004). With each cell division in somatic cells the telomere is not fully replicated, eventually whittling down to a critical threshold, at which point no further replication can happen (Aviv *et al.* 2003, Chan & Blackburn 2004). Telomere length is thereby considered an indicator of the biological age of a cell and its future replicative potential (Aviv *et al.* 2003). In epidemiological research telomere length has been associated with a wide range of chronic physical conditions and their risk factors (Jeanclos *et al.* 1998, Aviv & Aviv 1999, von Zglinicki *et al.* 2000, Samani *et al.* 2001, Brouilette *et al.* 2003, 2007, Panossian *et al.* 2003, Benetos *et al.* 2004, Gardner *et al.* 2005, Valdes *et al.* 2005, 2007, Demissie *et al.* 2006, Fitzpatrick *et al.* 2007). Mental disorders and chronic stress are hypothesized to be among the causes of accelerated attrition. The mediating biological processes are probably oxidative stress and inflammation, and both of these have been associated with mental disorders (Irie *et al.* 2003, Khanzode *et al.* 2003, Irwin & Miller 2007). Moreover, recent data have found cross-sectional links of telomere length with mood disorders (Simon *et al.* 2006), schizophrenia (Kao *et al.* 2008, Yu *et al.* 2008), and other chronic stressors (Epel *et al.* 2004, 2006).

It is interesting that childhood adversities and early-onset mental disorders have independent associations with physical condition onset. These two types of early life difficulty may be influencing different biological or behavioral pathways, or they may simply combine to have additive effects, with early-onset mental disorders perhaps augmenting the effects of early childhood maltreatment or adversity. Disentangling the respective effects of childhood adversities and early-onset mental disorders will be the work of future studies using prospective data.

A further reason why these results are noteworthy is that they suggest that the influence of early-onset mental disorders (and of childhood adversities) is broad in its scope: that is, it extends to a range of common chronic physical conditions. So even though the strength of individual associations is relatively modest, the fact that each predictor is associated with a range of highly prevalent outcomes greatly expands the potential population impact of these links.

There are many compelling reasons to be concerned that individuals with mental disorders receive timely and effective treatment. If the results presented in this chapter are confirmed in other studies, and if the associations prove to be causal, they suggest we can now add a further reason to lobby for early detection and treatment of mental disorders: because they may increase the risk of poor physical health later in life.

Acknowledgments

This chapter builds on and expands the analyses performed in Scott, K. M., Von Korff, M., Angermeyer, M. C., *et al.* (2011). Association of childhood adversities and early-onset mental disorders with adult-onset chronic physical conditions. *Archives of General Psychiatry* **68**, 838–44. © 2011. American Medical Association.

References

Aviv, A., & Aviv, H. (1999). Telomeres and essential hypertension. *American Journal of Hypertension* **12**, 427–32.

Aviv, A., Levy, D., & Mangel, M. (2003). Growth, telomere dynamics and successful and unsuccessful human aging. *Mechanisms of Ageing Development* **124**, 829–37.

Baumeister, H., Kriston, L., Bengel, J., & Härter, M. (2010). High agreement of self-report and physician-diagnosed somatic conditions yields limited bias in examining mental-physical comorbidity. *Journal of Clinical Epidemiology* **63**, 558–65.

Benetos, A., Gardner, J. P., Zureik, M., *et al.* (2004). Short telomeres are associated with increased carotid atherosclerosis in hypertensive subjects. *Hypertension* **43**, 182–5.

Blackburn, E. H. (2000). Telomere states and cell fates. *Nature* **408**, 53–6.

Brouilette, S., Singh, R. K., Thompson, J. R., Goodall, A. H., & Samani, N. J. (2003). White cell telomere length and risk of premature myocardial infarction. *Arteriosclerosis, Thrombosis and Vascular Biology* **23**, 842–6.

Brouilette, S. W., Moore, J. S., McMahon, A. D., *et al.* (2007). Telomere length, risk of coronary heart disease, and statin treatment in the West of Scotland Primary Prevention Study: a nested case–control study. *Lancet* **369**, 107–14.

Chan, S. R. W. L., & Blackburn, E. H. (2004). Telomeres and telomerase. *Philosophical Transactions of the Royal Society of London B: Biological Sciences* **359**, 109–21.

Chida, Y., Hamer, M., & Steptoe, A. (2008). A bidirectional relationship between psychosocial factors and atopic disorders: a systematic review and meta-analysis. *Psychosomatic Medicine* **70**, 102–16.

Chrousos, G. P., & Kino, T. (2007). Glucocorticoid action networks and complex psychiatric and/or somatic disorders. *Stress* **10**, 213–19.

Davidson, S., Judd, F., Jolley, D., *et al.* (2001). Cardiovascular risk factors for people with mental illness. *Australian and New Zealand Journal of Psychiatry* **35**, 196–202.

Demissie, S., Levy, D., Benjamin, E. J., *et al.* (2006). Insulin resistance, oxidative stress, hypertension, and leukocyte telomere length in men from the Framingham Heart Study. *Aging Cell* **5**, 325–30.

Eaton, W. W., Armenian, H., Gallo, J., Pratt, L., & Ford, D. E. (1996). Depression and risk for onset of type II diabetes. A prospective population-based study. *Diabetes Care* **19**, 1097–102.

Engum, A. (2007). The role of depression and anxiety in onset of diabetes in a large population-based study. *Journal of Psychosomatic Research* **62**, 31–8.

Epel, E. S., Blackburn, E. H., Lin, J., *et al.* (2004). Accelerated telomere shortening in response to life stress. *Proceedings of the National Academy of Sciences of the USA* **101**, 17312–15.

Epel, E. S., Lin, J., Wilhelm, F. H., *et al.* (2006). Cell aging in relation to stress arousal and cardiovascular disease risk factors. *Psychoneuroendocrinology* **31**, 277–87.

Ettner, S. L., Frank, R. G., & Kessler, R. C. (1997). The impact of psychiatric disorders on labor market outcomes. *Industrial and Labor Relations Review* **51**, 64–81.

Evans, D. L., Charney, D. S., Lewis, L., *et al.* (2005). Mood disorders in the medically ill: scientific review and recommendations. *Biological Psychiatry* **58**, 175–89.

Everson, S. A., Roberts, R. E., Goldberg, D. E., & Kaplan, G. A. (1998). Depressive symptoms and increased risk of stroke mortality over a 29-year period. *Archives of Internal Medicine* **158**, 1133–8.

Fitzpatrick, A. L., Kronmal, R. A., Gardner, J. P., *et al.* (2007). Leukocyte telomere length and cardiovascular disease in the cardiovascular health study. *American Journal of Epidemiology* **165**, 14–21.

Gardner, J. P., Li, S., Srinivasan, S. R., *et al.* (2005). Rise in insulin resistance is associated with escalated telomere attrition. *Circulation* **111**, 2171–7.

Goldston, K., & Baillie, A. J. (2008). Depression and coronary heart disease: a review of the epidemiological evidence, explanatory mechanisms and management approaches. *Clinical Psychology Review* **28**, 289–307.

Goodwin, R. D., Fergusson, D. M., & Horwood, L. J. (2004). Asthma and depressive and anxiety disorders among young persons in the community. *Psychological Medicine* **34**, 1465–74.

Goodwin, R. D., Sourander, A., Duarte, C. S., *et al.* (2009). Do mental health problems in childhood predict chronic physical conditions among males in early adulthood? Evidence from a community-based prospective study. *Psychological Medicine* **39**, 301–11.

Goodyer, I. M. (2007). The hypothalamic–pituitary–adrenal axis: cortisol, DHEA and mental and behavioral function. In A. Steptoe, ed., *Depression and Physical Illness*. Cambridge: Cambridge University Press, pp. 280–298.

Green, J. G., McLaughlin, K. A., Berglund, P. A., *et al.* (2010). Childhood adversities and adult psychiatric disorders in the National Comorbidity Survey Replication I: associations with first onset of DSM-IV disorders. *Archives of General Psychiatry* **67**, 113–23.

Heim, C., & Nemeroff, C. B. (1999). The impact of early adverse experiences on brain systems involved in the pathophysiology of anxiety and affective disorders. *Biological Psychiatry* **46**, 1509–22.

Heim, C., Newport, D. J., Heit, S., *et al.* (2000). Pituitary–adrenal and autonomic responses to stress in women after sexual and physical abuse in childhood. *JAMA* **284**, 592–7.

Hemingway, H. (1999). Psychological factors in the aetiology and prognosis of coronary heart disease: systematic review of prospective cohort studies. *BMJ* **318**, 1460–7.

Hertzman, C. (1999). The biological embedding of early experience and its effects on health in adulthood. *Annals of the New York Academy of Sciences* **896**, 85–95.

Irie, M., Asami, S., Ikeda, M., & Kasai, H. (2003). Depressive state relates to female oxidative DNA damage via neutrophil activation. *Biochemical and Biophysical Research Communications* **311**, 1014–18.

Irwin, M. R., & Miller, A. H. (2007). Depressive disorders and immunity: 20 years of progress and discovery. *Brain, Behavior and Immunity* **21**, 374–83.

Jayakody, R., Danziger, D., & Kessler, R. C. (2012). Early-onset psychiatric disorders and male socioeconomic status. *Social Science Research* **27**, 371–87.

Jeanclos, E., Krolewski, A., Skurnick, J., *et al.* (1998). Shortened telomere length in white blood cells of patients with IDDM. *Diabetes* **47**, 482–6.

Jonas, B. S., & Mussolino, M. E. (2000). Symptoms of depression as a prospective risk factor for stroke. *Psychosomatic Medicine* **62**, 463–71.

Kao, H. T., Cawthon, R. M., Delisi, L. E., *et al.* (2008). Rapid telomere erosion in schizophrenia. *Molecular Psychiatry* **13**, 118–19.

Kessler, R. C., Foster, C. L., Saunders, W. B., & Stang, P. E. (1995). Social consequences of psychiatric disorders, I: educational attainment. *American Journal of Psychiatry* **152**, 1026–32.

Kessler, R. C., Berglund, P. A., Foster, C. L., *et al.* (1997). Social consequences of psychiatric disorders, II: teenage parenthood. *American Journal of Psychiatry* **154**, 1405–11.

Kessler, R. C., Walters, E. E., & Forthofer, M. S. (1998). The social consequences of psychiatric disorders, III: probability of marital stability. *American Journal of Psychiatry* **155**, 1092–6.

Khanzode, S. D., Dakhale, G. N., Khanzode, S. S., Saoji, A., & Palasodkar, R. (2003). Oxidative damage and major depression: the potential antioxidant action of selective serotonin re-uptake inhibitors. *Redox Report* **8**, 365–70.

Kirkpatrick, B., Messias, E., Harvey, P. D., Fernandez-Egea, E., & Bowie, C. R. (2008). Is schizophrenia a syndrome of accelerated aging? *Schizophrenia Bulletin* **34**, 1024–32.

Kolk, A. M., Hanewald, G. J., Schagen, S., & Gijsbers van Wijk, C. M. (2002). Predicting medically unexplained physical symptoms and health care utilization: a symptom-perception approach. *Journal of Psychosomatic Research* **52**, 35–44.

Krantz, D. S., & McCeney, M. K. (2002). Effects of psychological and social factors on organic disease: a critical assessment of research on coronary heart disease. *Annual Review of Psychology* **53**, 341–69.

Kriegsman, D. M., Penninx, B. W., van Eijk, J. T., Boeke, A. J. P., & Deeg, D. J. H. (1996). Self-reports and general practitioner information on the presence of chronic diseases in community dwelling elderly: a study on the accuracy of patients' self-reports and on determinants of inaccuracy. *Journal of Clinical Epidemiology* **49**, 1407–17.

Lazarus, R. S., & Folkman, S. (1984). *Stress, Appraisal and Coping*. New York, NY: Springer.

McEwen, B. S. (1998). Protective and damaging effects of stress mediators. *New England Journal of Medicine* **338**, 171–9.

McEwen, B. S. (2003). Mood disorders and allostatic load. *Biological Psychiatry* **54**, 200–7.

Miller, G. E., Cohen, S., & Ritchey, A. K. (2002). Chronic psychological stress and the regulation of proinflammatory cytokiness: a glucocorticoid resistence model. *Health Psychology* **21**, 536–41.

Musselman, D., Bowling, A., Gilles, N., et al. (2007). The interrelationship of depression and diabetes. In A. Steptoe, ed., *Depression and Physical Illness*. Cambridge: Cambridge University Press, pp. 165–94.

Nicholson, A., Kuper, H., & Hemingway, H. (2006). Depression as an aetiologic and prognostic factor in coronary heart disease: a meta-analysis of 6362 events among 146 538 participants in 54 observational studies. *European Heart Journal* **27**, 2763–74.

Panossian, L. A., Porter, V. R., Valenzuela, H. F., et al. (2003). Telomere shortening in T cells correlates with Alzheimer's disease status. *Neurobiology of Aging* **24**, 77–84.

Rozanski, A., Blumenthal, J. A., & Kaplan, J. (1999). Impact of psychological factors on the pathogenesis of cardiovascular disease and implications for therapy. *Circulation* **99**, 2192–217.

Rudisch, B., & Nemeroff, C. B. (2003). Epidemiology of comorbid coronary artery disease and depression. *Biological Psychiatry* **54**, 227–40.

Rugulies, R. (2002). Depression as a predictor for coronary heart disease. a review and meta-analysis. *American Journal of Preventative Medicine* **23**, 51–61.

Samani, N. J., Boultby, R., Butler, R., Thompson, J. R., & Goodall, A. H. (2001). Telomere shortening in atherosclerosis. *Lancet* **358**, 472–3.

Sanchez, M. M. (2006). The impact of early adverse care on HPA axis development: nonhuman primate models. *Hormones and Behavior* **50**, 623–31.

Scott, K. M. (2009), The development of mental–physical comorbidity. In M. Von Korff, K. M. Scott, & O. Gureje, eds., *Global Perspectives on Mental–Physical Comorbidity in the WHO World Mental Health Surveys*. New York, NY: Cambridge University Press, pp. 97–107.

Scott, K. M., Oakley Browne, M. A., McGee, M. A., et al. (2006). Mental–physical comorbidity in Te Rau Hinengaro: the New Zealand Mental Health Survey. *Australian and New Zealand Journal of Psychiatry* **40**, 882–8.

Scott, K. M., Bruffaerts, R., Tsang, A., et al. (2007). Depression-anxiety relationships with chronic physical conditions: results from the World Mental Health surveys. *Journal of Affective Disorders* **103**, 113–20.

Scott, K. M., Von Korff, M., Alonso, J., et al. (2008). Childhood adversity, early-onset depressive/anxiety disorders, and adult-onset asthma. *Psychosomatic Medicine* **70**, 1035–43.

Simon, G. E., & Von Korff, M. (1995). Recall of psychiatric history in cross-sectional surveys: implications for epidemiologic research. *Epidemiology Review* **17**, 221–7.

Simon, N. M., Smoller, J. W., McNamara, K. L., et al. (2006). Telomere shortening and mood disorders: preliminary support for a chronic stress model of accelerated aging. *Biological Psychiatry* **60**, 432–5.

Steptoe, A. (2007a). *Depression and Physical Illness* Cambridge University Press, Cambridge.

Steptoe, A. (2007b). Depression and the development of coronary heart disease. In A. Steptoe, ed., *Depression and Physical Illness*. Cambridge: Cambridge University Press, pp. 53–86.

Suls, J., & Bunde, J. (2005). Anger, anxiety, and depression as risk factors for cardiovascular disease: the problems and implications of overlapping affective dispositions. *Psychology Bulletin* **131**, 260–300.

Teicher, M. H., Andersen, S. L., Polcari, A., Anderson, C. M., & Navalta, C. P. (2002). Developmental neurobiology of childhood stress and trauma. *Psychiatric Clinics of North America* **25**, 397–426, vii–viii.

Valdes, A. M., Andrew, T., Gardner, J. P., et al. (2005). Obesity, cigarette smoking, and telomere length in women. *Lancet* **366**, 662–4.

Valdes, A. M., Richards, J. B., Gardner, J. P., et al. (2007). Telomere length in leukocytes correlates with bone mineral density and is shorter in women with osteoporosis. *Osteoporosis International* **18**, 1203–10.

van den Akker, A. M., Schuurman, A., Metsemakers, J., & Buntinx, F. (2004). Is depression related to subsequent diabetes mellitus? *Acta Psychiatrica Scandinavica* **110**, 178–83.

van der Kooy, K. K., van Hout, H., Marwijk, H., *et al.* (2007). Depression and the risk for cardiovascular diseases: systematic review and meta analysis. *International Journal of Geriatric Psychiatry* **22**, 613–26.

Van Puymbroeck, C. M., Zautra, A. J., & Harakas, P. P. (2007), Chronic pain and depression: twin burdens of adaptation. In A. Steptoe, ed., *Depression and Physical Illness*. Cambridge: Cambridge University Press, pp. 145–164.

Vassend, O., & Skrondal, A. (1999). The role of negative affectivity in self assessment of health: a structural equation approach. *Journal of Health Psychology* **4**, 465–82.

Von Korff, M. R. (2009). Global perspectives on mental-physical comorbidity. In M. R. Von Korff, K. M. Scott, & O. Gureje, eds., *Global Perspectives on Mental–Physical Comorbidity in the WHO World Mental Health Surveys*. New York, NY: Cambridge University Press, pp. 1–11.

von Zglinicki, T., Serra, V., Lorenz, M., *et al.* (2000). Short telomeres in patients with vascular dementia: an indicator of low antioxidative capacity and a possible risk factor? *Laboratory Investigation* **80**, 1739–47.

Wells, J. E., & Horwood, L. J. (2004). How accurate is recall of key symptoms of depression? A comparison of recall and longitudinal reports. *Psychological Medicine* **34**, 1001–11.

Wolkowitz, O. M., Epel, E. S., & Mellon, S. (2008). When blue turns to grey: do stress and depression accelerate cell aging? *World Journal of Biological Psychiatry* **9**, 2–5.

Wulsin, L. R., & Singal, B. M. (2003). Do depressive symptoms increase the risk for the onset of coronary disease? A systematic quantitative review. *Psychosomatic Medicine* **65**, 201–10.

Yu, W. Y., Chang, H. W., Lin, C. H., & Cho, C. L. (2008). Short telomeres in patients with chronic schizophrenia who show a poor response to treatment. *Journal of Psychiatry and Neuroscience* **33**, 244–7.

Chapter

8

Association between serious mental illness and personal earnings

Daphna Levinson, Maria V. Petukhova, Michael Schoenbaum,
Guilherme Borges, Ronny Bruffaerts, Giovanni de Girolamo,
Yanling He, Oye Gureje, Mark A. Oakley Browne, and Ronald C. Kessler

Introduction

Previous research on the societal burden of mental disorders in terms of disability-adjusted life years (DALYs) (Murray & López 1996) and as a fraction of national budgets (Gabriel & Liimatainen 2000) has emphasized the importance of indirect costs associated with reduced rates of labor force participation (Zhang *et al.* 2009), unemployment among those in the labor force (Chatterji *et al.* 2007), and under-employment among those who are employed (Kessler *et al.* 2008b). The most commonly used approach to study these labor market costs is the *human capital approach* (Tarricone 2006). This approach is based on the observation that wages and salaries are paid in direct return for productive services, making earnings a good indicator of the human capital accumulated by the individual and making earnings-equivalent time forgone because of an illness a good representation of the indirect costs of that illness to the employer. Although a considerable body of empirical research has used the human capital approach to document adverse societal effects of mental disorders, this research has been carried out largely in a few developed countries (Kessler *et al.* 1999, Chatterji *et al.* 2007). Yet the WMH data show clearly that mental disorders are common throughout the world (Kessler *et al.* 2008a). The purpose of the current chapter is to use the WMH data to make estimates of the human capital costs of mental disorders in the WMH countries in terms of personal earnings. We focus on serious mental illness (SMI) because previous research has shown that earnings and long-term work incapacity are both much more strongly related to SMI than to less serious forms of mental illness (Shiels *et al.* 2004, Kessler *et al.* 2008b).

Methods

Sample

The analysis is based on 23 WMH surveys considered in this volume. The two excluded surveys are Romania and Ukraine. The Romanian survey was excluded because there was a skip error in the survey section on personal earnings. The Ukrainian survey was excluded because personal earnings were not assessed in that survey. As mentioned in Chapter 2, all countries were classified according to the World Bank 2008 classification as low/lower-middle-income countries, upper-middle-income countries, and high-income countries. Results are reported separately for each of these three segments of the overall sample. Analyses are limited to the part 2 sample, as earnings were assessed in part 2, and to respondents of working age, which we defined for purposes of this analysis as 18–64 years of age, for a total of 52,275 respondents across all the participating surveys.

Measures

All part 2 respondents were asked to report their personal earnings in the past 12 months before taxes. Respondents were instructed to count only wages and other stipends from employment, not pensions, investments, or other financial assistance or income. As in most community surveys, the item-level non-response rate for this question was non-trivial (with a range of 0.8–27.9% and an interquartile range [IQR] of 2.7–8.7% across surveys). Regression-based multiple imputation (Rubin 1987) was used to impute missing values using information collected in the survey on such predictors

The Burdens of Mental Disorders, ed. Jordi Alonso, Somnath Chatterji, and Yanling He. Published by Cambridge University Press. © World Health Organization 2013.

of earnings as education, employment status, other relevant sociodemographics (e.g., age, sex, marital status), and household size. SMI was not significantly related to having a missing value on the earnings variable in the vast majority of countries, while in the remaining countries the associations had inconsistent signs (e.g., positively in Portugal, South Africa, and the USA; negatively in Northern Ireland and India). Earnings reports were divided by median within-country values to pool across countries, but retain information about between-country differences in earnings variation. This transformed score was the outcome in regression analyses estimated simultaneously across all countries for associations of 12-month SMI with earnings.

Prior to carrying out this analysis, earnings distributions were compared for respondents with and without SMI. The earnings distributions among respondents with any earnings were divided for this purpose into four categories by defining *low* earnings as less than half the within-country median, *low-average* earnings as up to the median, *high-average* earnings as up to twice the median, and *high* earnings as greater than two times the median. The regression analyses were then carried out using a dummy variable for SMI as the predictor of primary interest. The outcome was the transformed earnings score. Control variables included sociodemographics (age, sex), country (22 dummy variables to distinguish respondents across the 23 surveys), substance disorders, and interactions between sex and all other predictors. The sex interactions were included because previous research has shown that the predictors of earnings are different for males and females (Rice & Miller 1998, Kessler et al. 2008b).

As noted in Chapter 2, a wide range of mental disorders were assessed in the WMH surveys. We focused on disorders present in the 12 months before interview to carry out the analyses reported in this chapter. These analyses were carried out first in the USA at the request of the US government's National Institute of Mental Health (NIMH) to update estimates of the effects of recent mental disorders on earnings in the US population. That update analysis was designed to extend two earlier reports from the 1980s (Rice et al. 1990) and 1990s (Harwood et al. 2000). Consistent with those earlier reports, the US analysis focused on anxiety, mood, and disruptive behavior disorders and excluded, but controlled for, substance disorders (Kessler et al. 2008b). An earlier cross-national replication of the US analysis was carried out in a smaller number of WMH surveys (Levinson et al. 2010). We expand that analysis in the current chapter to the full set of WMH surveys available at the time this volume was prepared.

SMI was defined following previous WMH analyses (Demyttenaere et al. 2004) as either meeting criteria for bipolar I disorder or having any other 12-month DSM-IV diagnosis along with evidence of serious role impairment. Serious role impairment was defined as either having a score in the severe range on one or more of the Sheehan Disability Scales (Leon et al. 1997), which assess disability in work role performance, household maintenance, social life, or intimate relationships, or attempting suicide at some time in the 12 months before the WMH surveys.

Statistical analysis

A major statistical problem in estimating regression equations of this sort is that the earnings distribution is highly skewed, with a meaningful minority of the sample in each country reporting no earnings and a much higher proportion of other respondents having high earnings than would be found in a normal distribution. This makes ordinary least squares (OLS) regression analysis both biased and inefficient. Earlier analyses of the association between mental illness and earnings by other researchers addressed this problem by using either weighted least squares (WLS) regression analysis (Rice et al. 1990) or a two-part model (Duan et al. 1984), where a part 1 logistic regression model (Hosmer & Lemeshow 2001) predicted having any earnings and a part 2 linear regression model (OLS with a logarithmic transformation of the dependent variable) predicted amount earned among respondents with any earnings (Harwood et al. 2000). Individual-level predictions from these two models were multiplied and transformed with a correction adjustment to predict earnings for each respondent.

Although two-part models have several desirable features compared to WLS regression, the multiplication and transformation of individual-level estimates is highly sensitive to model mis-specification (Manning 1998). As noted in Chapter 2, generalized linear models (GLM: McCullagh & Nelder 1989) address this problem (Mullahy 1998) by using pre-specified non-linear relationships and suitably specified error structures to estimate one-part models that fit highly skewed earnings data better than two-part models (Manning & Mullahy 2001). We consequently used GLM and compared model fit to the fit of two-part models as well as conventional OLS regression analysis (with linear, square root, and logarithmic link functions). The best-fitting specification was chosen using standard empirical model comparison procedures (Buntin & Zaslavsky 2004).

The final best-fitting model was a one-part GLM that assumed a logarithmic link function between predictors and the outcome with prediction error variance proportional to the predicted values (Appendix 8, Appendix Table 8.1). Because this model used a non-linear transformation of the outcome in conjunction with an interaction between SMI and sex, model-based simulation was needed to interpret the coefficients (Appendix Table 8.2). This was done by predicting earnings twice for each respondent from the model coefficients, once using the actual characteristics of the respondent and a second time recoding all respondents with SMI to assume that they did not have SMI. Individual-level differences between these estimates were averaged across all respondents with SMI to estimate the mean individual-level decrease in earnings associated with SMI. Societal-level estimates were then obtained by multiplying this individual-level estimate by the prevalence of SMI to generate estimates of population attributable risk proportion (PARP). As described in Chapter 2, PARP represents the proportional reduction in total earnings we might expect at the population level that would be prevented if SMI were eliminated, based on the assumption that the regression coefficient for SMI represents a causal effect on earnings.

Demographic rate standardization (Schempf & Becker 2006) was then used to decompose the societal-level estimates into components due to the associations of SMI with the probability of having any earnings and with the amount earned by those with any earnings. Because the WMH sample design featured weighting and clustering, the standard errors of the model coefficients and the simulated estimates were obtained using the design-based Jackknife Repeated Replication (JRR) method (Wolter 1985). In this method, each model and each simulation is replicated many times in pseudo-samples to generate a distribution of each coefficient that is then used to calculate an empirical estimate of the standard error of the coefficient. Multivariate significance was estimated using design-adjusted Wald χ^2 tests (Engle 1983). Statistical significance was consistently evaluated using two-sided tests at the 0.05 level of significance.

Results

Sample distributions

Consistent with their official distributions in census data on the populations of the participating countries, the age distribution of the sample is different across low/lower-middle-income, upper-middle-income, and high-income countries ($\chi^2_6 = 669.0$, $p < 0.001$) (Table 8.1). The largest proportion of respondents in the age ranges 18–24 (27.5%) and 25–39 (42.0%) are in low/lower-middle-income countries compared to upper-middle-income (22.0% and 39.6%) and high-income countries (15.4% and 34.9%). The opposite trend is found for the older age groups, with the largest proportion of respondents for the age groups 40–54 (33.9%) and 55–64 (15.8%) in high-income countries, compared to upper-middle-income (27.1% and 11.2%) and low/lower-middle-income countries (21.8% and 8.7%).

Women have a somewhat older age distribution than men in upper-middle-income countries ($\chi^2_3 = 15.8$, $p = 0.002$), but there are no significant sex differences in the age distributions in low/lower-middle-income and high-income countries ($\chi^2_3 = 1.4$–6.8, $p = 0.08$-.70). SMI prevalence is estimated to be significantly different across the country income groups in the total sample, with the highest prevalence in high-income countries (4.4% in high-income, 4.2% in upper-middle-income, and 2.0% in low/lower-middle-income countries, $\chi^2_2 = 155.4$, $p < 0.001$). The same trend is found separately among men (3.4% vs. 2.7% vs. 1.6%, $\chi^2_2 = 100.9$, $p < 0.001$). SMI prevalence is also estimated to be significantly different across country income groups among women ($\chi^2_2 = 55.9$, $p < 0.001$), but with the highest prevalence in upper-middle-income countries (5.6%) followed by high-income (5.4%) and low/lower-middle-income countries (2.4%). SMI is estimated to be significantly more common among women than men in the three country income groups ($\chi^2_1 = 6.6$-61.7, $p < 0.001$-0.011).

Earnings distributions among respondents with and without SMI

The proportion of respondents with non-zero earnings is significantly lower among those with than without SMI in all three country income groups (44.0% vs. 66.1%, $t = 7.2$, $p < 0.001$ in low/lower-middle-income countries, 51.2% vs. 57.6%, $t = 2.8$,

Table 8.1 Distributions of age, gender, and serious mental illness (SMI) by country income level. The WMH surveys.

	Country income level																
	Low/lower-middle						Upper-middle						High					
	Women		Men		Total		Women		Men		Total		Women		Men		Total	
	%	(SE)	%	(SE)	%	(SE)	%	(SE)	%	(SE)	%	(SE)	%	(SE)	%	(SE)	%	(SE)
Age, years[a]																		
18–24	28.5	(0.9)	26.5	(0.8)	27.5	(0.6)	20.6	(0.7)	23.5	(0.9)	22.0	(0.6)	15.0	(0.5)	15.7	(0.5)	15.4	(0.4)
25–39	40.5	(0.8)	43.6	(1.0)	42.0	(0.6)	40.2	(0.8)	39.1	(1.0)	39.6	(0.6)	35.1	(0.5)	34.8	(0.6)	34.9	(0.4)
40–54	22.0	(0.7)	21.6	(0.8)	21.8	(0.5)	26.9	(0.7)	27.4	(0.9)	27.1	(0.6)	34.0	(0.5)	33.9	(0.6)	33.9	(0.4)
55–64	9.0	(0.5)	8.3	(0.5)	8.7	(0.4)	12.3	(0.5)	10.0	(0.6)	11.2	(0.4)	15.9	(0.4)	15.6	(0.4)	15.8	(0.3)
12-month serious mental illness[b]	2.4	(0.3)	1.6	(0.2)	2.0	(0.2)	5.6	(0.3)	2.7	(0.3)	4.2	(0.2)	5.4	(0.2)	3.4	(0.2)	4.4	(0.1)
(n)	(7,186)		(6,292)		(13,478)		(6,982)		(4,714)		(11,696)		(15,528)		(11,573)		(27,101)	

[a] Significance of age differences was evaluated with Wald design-based χ^2 tests. The age distribution is significantly different across the three country income groups in the total sample ($\chi^2_6 = 669.0$, $p < 0.001$) and separately among men ($\chi^2_6 = 385.4$, $p < 0.001$) and women ($\chi^2_6 = 331.1$, $p < 0.001$). Men and women also have significantly different age distributions in upper-middle-income countries ($\chi^2_3 = 15.8$, $p = 0.002$), but not in low/lower-middle-income ($\chi^2_3 = 6.8$, $p = 0.08$) or high-income countries ($\chi^2_3 = 1.4$, $p = 0.70$).

[b] The estimated prevalence of serious mental illness differs significantly across the country income groups in the total sample ($\chi^2_2 = 155.4$, $p < 0.001$) and separately among men ($\chi^2_2 = 100.9$, $p < 0.001$) and women ($\chi^2_2 = 55.9$, $p < 0.001$). Men and women also differ in prevalence of serious mental illness in low/lower-middle-income ($\chi^2_1 = 6.6$, $p = 0.011$), upper-middle-income ($\chi^2_1 = 48.2$, $p < 0.001$), and high-income countries ($\chi^2_1 = 61.7$, $p < 0.001$).

$p = 0.006$ in upper-middle-income countries, and 71.3% vs. 80.1%, $t = 6.4$, $p < 0.001$ in high-income countries) (Table 8.2). Similar differences are found when we look separately at men ($t = 6.3–7.6$, $p < 0.001$) and women ($t = 3.2–6.1$, $p \leq 0.001$) in high-income and low/lower-middle-income countries. In upper-middle-income countries this trend is non-significant for men ($t = 0.3$, $p = 0.78$) and women ($t = 1.1$, $p = 0.27$). The overall differences are due to the proportions of respondents with low and low-average earnings being significantly higher among those with than without SMI in low/lower-middle-income countries (low-average only: 45.4% vs. 35.9%, $t = 3.8$, $p < 0.001$) and in high-income countries (38.6% vs. 23.2%, $t = 11.9$, $p < 0.001$ low earnings; 32.4% vs. 29.2%, $t = 2.3$, $p = 0.019$ low-average earnings), and the proportions of respondents with high-average and high incomes being significantly higher among those without than with SMI in low/lower-middle-income countries (high earnings only: 24.3% vs. 17.8%, $t = 3.8$, $p < 0.001$) and in high-income countries (29.3% vs. 20.6%, $t = 6.7$, $p < 0.001$ high-average earnings; 18.4% vs. 8.3%, $t = 11.9$, $p < 0.001$ high earnings). A similar pattern is found in upper-middle-income countries, but the only significant finding is that proportions of respondents with low-average earnings are higher among those with than without SMI (39.6% vs. 30.6%, $t = 2.5$, $p = 0.014$). Furthermore, roughly similar patterns are found when we look separately at women and men in the three country income groups.

Individual-level regression models of the association between SMI and earnings

The model-based simulations estimate that SMI is associated with a reduction in earnings equal to 29% of the median within-country earnings in high-income countries and 31% in low/lower-middle-income countries. In upper-middle-income countries this association (reduction in earnings of 36%) is not statistically significant for the total sample, but only among women (reduction in earnings equal to 59% of the median within-country earnings in upper-middle-income countries) (Table 8.3). The association is considerably larger among men than women in low/lower-middle-income countries (61% vs. 11%, $t = 3.0$, $p = 0.003$) and in high-income countries (48% vs. 17%, $t = 4.3$, $p < 0.001$). Decomposition shows that 58% of the total association between SMI and earnings in low/lower-middle-income countries, 8% in upper-middle-income

countries, and 31% in high-income countries is due to reduced probability of having any earnings among people with SMI. Although the difference is non-significant, this component is smaller for men than for women in low/lower-middle-income countries and in high-income countries (45% vs. 96%, $t = 0.8$, $p = 0.45$, and 29% vs. 34%, $t = 0.6$, $p = 0.57$). A larger component of the total association, 61% of the total in high-income countries and 90% in upper-middle-income countries, is due to the lower mean level of earnings among people with than without SMI who have any earnings. In low/lower-middle-income countries 33% of the total association is due to the lower mean level of earnings among people with than without SMI who have any earnings. This component is comparable for men and women in high-income countries (61% vs. 60%, $t = 0.1$, $p = 0.90$) but smaller for women than for men in low/lower-middle-income countries (3% vs. 42%, $t = 0.7$, $p = 0.49$).

Country-specific individual-level and societal-level projections

It is instructive to compare results across countries and to put the individual-level estimates into perspective by considering them in their natural metrics projected to the societal level. This was done by estimating the coefficients in the best-fitting model separately in each of the 23 surveys, expressing the estimates in terms of mean rather than median earnings, multiplying these estimates by the prevalence of SMI, and then multiplying this product by the population size of the country in the age range of the sample to obtain societal-level estimates (Table 8.4). SMI is associated with a reduction in earnings in 19 out of the 22 countries (the exceptions being Brazil–São Paulo, Iraq, and Lebanon), with a weighted average value of 17.5% of mean earnings in low/lower-middle-income countries, 5.0% of mean earnings in upper-middle-income countries, and 21.7% of mean earnings in high-income countries (the first and last being statistically significant). Between-country differences in these individual-level estimates are not significant in upper-middle-income countries ($\chi^2_4 = 4.3$, $p = 0.37$) or in high-income countries ($\chi^2_{11} = 18.2$, $p = 0.08$), but differ across low/lower-middle-income countries ($\chi^2_5 = 23.4$, $p < 0.001$), with much lower estimates in Iraq and PRC–Shenzhen (−1.4% and 8.1%) than in the other countries (17.9–45.4%). At the societal level, the estimate averages 0.4% in low/lower-middle-income countries, 0.2% of all

Table 8.2 Earnings distributions for respondents with and without serious mental illness (SMI) by country income level. The WMH surveys.[a]

	Country income level																	
	Low/lower-middle						Upper-middle						High					
	Female		Male		Total		Female		Male		Total		Female		Male		Total	
	%	(SE)	%	(SE)	%	(SE)	%	(SE)	%	(SE)	%	(SE)	%	(SE)	%	(SE)	%	(SE)
Any earnings																		
Total sample	51.6	(0.9)	80.1	(0.7)	65.7	(0.6)	46.0	(0.8)	69.7	(1.0)	57.3	(0.7)	73.5	(0.5)	86.1	(0.5)	79.7	(0.4)
Serious mental illness	34.2*	(2.8)	59.2*	(2.7)	44.0*	(3.0)	43.5	(2.3)	69.0	(2.3)	51.2*	(2.2)	68.4*	(1.6)	75.9*	(1.6)	71.3*	(1.3)
Others	52.0*	(0.9)	80.4*	(0.7)	66.1*	(0.6)	46.2	(0.9)	69.7	(1.0)	57.6*	(0.7)	73.8*	(0.6)	86.5*	(0.5)	80.1*	(0.4)
Low earnings among the employed																		
Total sample	20.9	(1.0)	17.0	(0.8)	18.6	(0.6)	32.6	(1.2)	25.7	(1.1)	28.6	(0.9)	32.4	(0.6)	16.2	(0.6)	23.8	(0.4)
Serious mental illness	20.4	(1.2)	14.0	(3.5)	17.0	(2.3)	28.6	(2.5)	23.1	(2.4)	26.3	(2.1)	43.2*	(1.6)	32.0*	(1.6)	38.6*	(1.2)
Others	20.9	(1.0)	17.1	(0.8)	18.6	(0.6)	32.8	(1.3)	25.8	(1.1)	28.7	(0.9)	31.8*	(0.7)	15.7*	(0.6)	23.2*	(0.5)
Low-average earnings among the employed																		
Total sample	41.7	(1.3)	32.3	(0.9)	36.0	(0.7)	34.1	(1.3)	28.6	(1.2)	30.9	(1.0)	35.5	(0.6)	23.8	(0.6)	30.9	(0.5)
Serious mental illness	44.5	(2.0)	46.3*	(1.8)	45.4*	(2.4)	45.8*	(4.3)	30.6	(3.6)	39.6*	(3.5)	36.3	(1.6)	26.8	(1.7)	32.4*	(1.3)
Others	41.6	(1.3)	32.2*	(0.9)	35.9*	(0.7)	33.5*	(1.4)	28.5	(1.3)	30.6*	(1.0)	35.4	(0.7)	23.7	(0.6)	29.2*	(0.5)
High-average earnings among the employed																		
Total sample	19.2	(1.0)	22.4	(0.8)	21.2	(0.6)	14.9	(1.0)	20.3	(1.0)	18.0	(0.7)	24.0	(0.6)	33.4	(0.7)	29.0	(0.4)
Serious mental illness	21.0	(0.8)	18.7	(4.2)	19.8	(2.7)	11.3	(2.4)	19.6	(3.3)	14.7	(1.9)	16.2*	(1.1)	27.1*	(1.8)	20.6*	(1.2)
Others	19.2	(1.0)	22.5	(0.8)	21.2	(0.6)	15.1	(1.1)	20.3	(1.0)	18.2	(0.7)	24.4*	(0.6)	33.6*	(0.7)	29.3*	(0.5)

High earnings among the employed

	Total sample		Serious mental illness		Others				
Total sample	18.2	(1.0)	28.2	(1.0)	24.2	(0.7)	18.4	(1.1)	25.4	(1.3)	22.4	(0.9)	8.1	(0.4)	26.7	(0.6)	18.0	(0.4)
Serious mental illness	14.2	(1.3)	21.0*	(1.0)	17.8*	(1.6)	14.3	(2.3)	26.6	(2.0)	19.4	(1.8)	4.3*	(0.6)	14.2*	(1.1)	8.3*	(0.7)
Others	18.2	(1.0)	28.3*	(1.0)	24.3*	(0.7)	18.6	(1.2)	25.4	(1.3)	22.6	(1.0)	8.4*	(0.4)	27.1*	(0.7)	18.4*	(0.4)
X^2_3	1.8		4.4		8.0#		6.1		0.6		6.0		59.0#		43.0#		166.3#	
(n)	(7,186)		(6,292)		(13,478)		(6,982)		(4,714)		(11,696)		(15,528)		(11,573)		(27,101)	

[a] Low earnings were defined as less than half the within-country median among those with any earnings, low-average earnings as up to the median, high-average earnings as up to twice the median, and high earnings as greater than twice the median.

* Significant difference between respondents with serious mental illness and other respondents at the 0.05 level, two-sided test.

Significant difference at the 0.05 level between the earnings distributions of respondents with and without serious mental illness among those with non-zero earnings.

Table 8.3 Simulated associations of serious mental illness (SMI) with reduced earnings at the individual level by sex and country income level. The WMH surveys.

	Country income level																	
	Low/lower-middle						Upper-middle						High					
	Female		Male		Total		Female		Male		Total		Female		Male		Total	
	Est	(SE)	Est	(SE)	Est	(SE)	Est	(SE)	Est	(SE)	Est	(SE)	Est	(SE)	Est	(SE)	Est	(SE)
Overall association																		
Association between SMI and earnings in the total sample[a]	0.11	(0.06)	0.61*	(0.15)	0.31*	(0.08)	0.59*	(0.26)	−0.17	(0.33)	0.36	(0.21)	0.17*	(0.02)	0.48*	(0.07)	0.29*	(0.03)
Component effects																		
Effect of SMI on probability of non-zero earnings[b]	0.08*	(0.03)	0.18*	(0.08)	0.12*	(0.04)	0.04	(0.05)	−0.04	(0.05)	0.02	(0.03)	0.08*	(0.01)	0.12*	(0.02)	0.10*	(0.01)
Estimated effect of SMI on earnings given non-zero earnings[a]	0.01	(0.16)	0.43	(0.23)	0.23	(0.15)	1.2	(0.72)	−0.13	(0.45)	0.63	(0.47)	0.15*	(0.03)	0.39*	(0.08)	0.24*	(0.04)
Decomposition of overall effect[c]																		
Due to difference in probability of non-zero earnings	0.96	(0.64)	0.45*	(0.22)	0.58*	(0.21)	0.08	(0.11)	0.50	(1.4)	0.08	(0.16)	0.34*	(0.06)	0.29*	(0.07)	0.31*	(0.05)
Due to difference in earnings given non-zero earnings	0.03	(0.53)	0.42*	(0.20)	0.33	(0.18)	0.85*	(0.18)	0.52	(1.4)	0.90*	(0.22)	0.60*	(0.06)	0.61*	(0.07)	0.61*	(0.05)
Due to the interaction between the two components	0.01	(0.11)	0.13*	(0.04)	0.09*	(0.04)	0.07	(0.08)	−0.03	(0.08)	0.03	(0.06)	0.07*	(0.01)	0.10*	(0.01)	0.09*	(0.01)

[a] The estimates reported in these rows summarize the results of individual-level simulations based on the coefficients in the best-fitting multiple regression model. These are proportions over the median within-country earnings and are presented as percentages in the corresponding text.

[b] The estimates reported in this row were calculated as the ratio of the average income of the simulated average income among those employed minus the ratio of the simulated average income of the total sample to the average income among those employed.

[c] Demographic rate standardization (Schempf & Becker 2006) was then used to decompose the societal-level estimates into components due to the associations of serious mental illness with probability of having any earnings and with the amount earned by those with any earnings. These proportions are expressed as percentages in the text.

* Significant at the 0.05 level, two-sided test.

Table 8.4 Simulated association of serious mental illness (SMI) with reduced earnings at the individual and the societal level by country income level. The WMH surveys.

Country income level	Serious mental illness Prevalence		The associations expressed as a percentage of mean national earnings[a]				The associations expressed in local currency[b]			
			Individual level[c]		Societal level[d]		Individual level		Societal level (in billions)	
	%	(SE)	Estimate	(SE)	Estimate	(SE)	Estimate	(SE)	Estimate	(SE)
Low/lower-middle										
Colombia	4.1	(0.4)	17.9*	(3.6)	0.7*	(0.2)	945,898*	(189,646)	881.7*	(176.8)
India–Pondicherry	1.0	(0.2)	20.4	(11.0)	0.2	(0.1)	9,013	(4,844)	1.2	(0.6)
Iraq	2.9	(0.4)	–1.4	(5.9)	0.0	(0.2)	–36,538	(151,517)	–14.4	(59.6)
Nigeria	0.5	(0.2)	34.0*	(16.4)	0.2*	(0.1)	23,883*	(11,548)	6.0*	(2.9)
PRC–Beijing/Shanghai	0.7	(0.2)	45.4*	(8.2)	0.3*	(0.1)	8,758*	(1,590)	0.9*	(0.2)
PRC–Shenzhen	0.9	(0.2)	8.1	(12.4)	0.1	(0.1)	2,594	(3,945)	0.0	(0.1)
Upper-middle										
Brazil–São Paulo	9.3	(0.7)	–0.7	(9.1)	–0.1	(0.8)	–100	(1,279)	–0.1	(1.3)
Bulgaria	1.5	(0.3)	14.7	(16.4)	0.2	(0.2)	372	(417)	0.0	(0.0)
Lebanon	4.1	(0.7)	–7.6	(8.0)	–0.3	(0.3)	–572	(607)	–0.1	(0.1)
Mexico	2.2	(0.2)	6.2	(5.6)	0.1	(0.1)	2,151	(1,924)	2.5	(2.2)
South Africa	3.2	(0.3)	16.4	(10.6)	0.5	(0.4)	4,222	(2,735)	3.4	(2.2)
High										
Belgium	4.9	(1.0)	22.5*	(6.6)	1.1*	(0.3)	189,701*	(55,322)	59.0*	(17.2)
France	3.8	(0.5)	33.0*	(9.8)	1.2*	(0.4)	36,905*	(10,934)	49.0*	(14.5)
Germany	2.7	(0.4)	32.0*	(7.7)	0.8*	(0.2)	11,929*	(2,872)	16.8*	(4.0)
Israel	3.7	(0.3)	24.8*	(3.2)	0.9*	(0.1)	20,097*	(2,575)	2.5*	(0.3)
Italy	1.3	(0.2)	4.5	(8.4)	0.1	(0.1)	1,306,888	(2,446,642)	619.6	(1,159.4)
Japan	1.2	(0.4)	13.4	(28.0)	0.2	(0.3)	491,016	(1,021,578)	4.9	(10.3)
Netherlands	4.4	(0.7)	18.4*	(7.5)	0.8*	(0.3)	8,800*	(3,571)	4.2*	(1.7)
New Zealand	5.0	(0.3)	27.1*	(5.5)	1.3*	(0.3)	9,233*	(1,871)	1.0*	(0.2)
Northern Ireland	6.8	(0.8)	32.0*	(5.1)	2.2*	(0.4)	5,343*	(854)	0.4*	(0.1)
Portugal	4.0	(0.5)	12.8	(7.9)	0.5	(0.3)	1,206	(748)	0.3	(0.2)
Spain	1.9	(0.3)	25.8*	(5.8)	0.5*	(0.1)	509,311*	(114,483)	255.4*	(57.4)
USA	6.8	(0.3)	15.4*	(3.5)	1.0*	(0.2)	5,061*	(1,167)	61.5*	(14.2)

Table 8.4 (cont.)

Country income level	Serious mental illness Prevalence		The associations expressed as a percentage of mean national earnings[a] Individual level[c]		Societal level[d]		The associations expressed in local currency[b] Individual level		Societal level (in billions)	
	%	(SE)	Estimate	(SE)	Estimate	(SE)	Estimate	(SE)	Estimate	(SE)
Pooled										
Low/lower-middle income	2.0	(0.2)	17.5*	(3.8)	0.4*	(0.1)				
Upper-middle income	4.2	(0.2)	5.0	(5.8)	0.2	(0.2)				
High income	4.4	(0.1)	21.7*	(2.2)	1.0*	(0.1)				

[a] Results are expressed here in terms of mean earnings, whereas they are expressed in terms of median earnings in Table 8.3 because this transformation was considered the one that makes most sense as the basis for constraining model coefficients to be constant across countries. The mean is used here because it is the natural metric for interpreting the substantive meaning of results. To clarify the interpretation: if 4.4% of respondents in high-income countries have serious mental illness and serious mental illness is associated with a 21.7% reduction in earnings, then this level of loss in this segment of the population represents $0.217 \times 0.044 = 1.0\%$ of all national earnings.

[b] The local currencies are francs in Belgium, francs in France, marks in Germany, shekels in Israel, lira in Italy, yen in Japan, guilders in the Netherlands, dollars in New Zealand, pound sterling in Northern Ireland, euro in Portugal, pesetas in Spain, dollars in the USA, reals in Brazil, lev in Bulgaria, pounds in Lebanon, pesos in Mexico, rand in South Africa, pesos in Colombia, rupees in India, dinar in Iraq, naira in Nigeria, and yuan in People's Republic of China (PRC).

[c] Estimates do not differ significantly across either high-income countries ($\chi^2_{11} = 18.2$, $p = 0.08$) or upper-middle-income countries ($\chi^2_4 = 4.3$, $p = 0.37$), but differ significantly across low/lower-middle-income countries ($\chi^2_5 = 23.4$, $p < 0.001$) based on design-based χ^2 tests.

[d] Estimates differ significantly across low/lower-middle-income countries ($\chi^2_5 = 18.8$, $p < 0.01$) and high-income countries ($\chi^2_{11} = 74.3$, $p < 0.001$), but not upper-middle-income countries ($\chi^2_4 = 3.3$, $p = 0.51$) based on design-based χ^2 tests.

* Significant at the 0.05 level, two-sided test.

national earnings in upper-middle-income countries, and 1.0% of all national earnings in high-income countries (the first and last being statistically significant). Between-country differences are statistically significant in low/lower-middle-income countries ($\chi^2_5 = 18.8$, $p < 0.01$), with lower estimates in Iraq and PRC–Shenzhen (0.0–0.1%) than in the other countries (0.2–0.7%), and in high-income countries ($\chi^2_{11} = 74.3$, $p < 0.001$), with lower estimates in Italy, Japan, Portugal, and Spain (0.1–0.5%) than in the other countries (0.8–2.2%). Between-country differences in the societal-level estimates are not statistically significant in upper-middle-income countries ($\chi^2_4 = 3.3$, $p = 0.51$).

Discussion

We found that SMI is associated with a reduction in population-level earnings equivalent to 0.4% in low/lower-middle-income countries, 0.2% of all national earnings in upper-middle-income countries, and 1.0% of all national earnings in high-income countries. We are aware of no other comparable studies of the societal costs of mental disorders with which these estimates can be compared, other than US studies that are broadly consistent with the results reported here for the US WMH sample (Rice et al. 1990, Harwood et al. 2000) and one previous WMH report that used a subset of the countries analyzed in this chapter (Levinson et al. 2010).

To put these values into perspective we use the US context as an example. The 1.0% decrement in societal-level earnings associated with SMI in high-income countries (the same as the US-specific estimate) is equal to $61.5 billion, which would cover the costs of college (including tuition, fees, room and board) for about half of all full-time college students in the USA (Leonhardt 2010). Alternatively, this amount of money would be enough to pay for universal preschool for all three- and four-year-olds in the USA. The 0.4% decrement in societal-level earnings associated with SMI in low/lower-middle-income countries, in comparison, is equivalent to roughly two-thirds of the annual budget of the US National Institutes of Health, the primary US government agency for health-related research. These comparisons make it clear that mental disorders are associated with massive losses of productive human capital not only at the individual level (29–36% of median national earnings, 5–22% of mean national earnings) but also at the societal level in the WMH countries.

Controlled intervention trials have shown that employment rates and earnings among the employed can both be increased among people with severe and persistent mental illness (SPMI), the vast majority of whom have a history of psychosis, using such methods as prevocational training and supported employment (Crowther et al. 2001, Latimer 2005). It is important to note, though, that only a minority of people with SMI have SPMI (Kessler et al. 1996). Little is known about the effects of treatment on occupational outcomes among the much larger proportion of people with SMI who do not have SPMI, the majority of whom suffer from chronic anxiety or behavior disorders or recurrent depression. The fact that low earnings, among people who have earnings, accounts for a larger component of the total effect of SMI on earning than having no earnings raises the question whether outpatient interventions for employed people with non-serious mental illness might be a useful remedy. A handful of controlled studies have documented that such interventions can reduce job loss and sickness absence (Rost et al. 2004, Wang et al. 2007), but we are aware of no controlled intervention studies that have documented an effect on earnings among the employed. Long-term follow-up would likely be required to document such an effect. A useful preliminary step might be to examine naturalistic longitudinal data to increase our understanding of the occupational career dynamics associated with non-serious mental illness and the extent to which the high unemployment rate of people with SMI is due to a high long-term unemployment rate versus a high short-term circulating unemployment rate. Intervention implications differ depending on the mix of these two kinds of unemployment, which cannot be distinguished with the data examined here.

An important issue to consider in doing this is that the 12-month SMI we treated as the primary predictor in this analysis might have started many years earlier and affected current earnings through a more direct effect in the form of low education. It is relevant in this regard that we have already seen in Chapter 4 that early-onset mental disorders do, in fact, predict low education. It is also possible, of course, that low education is a risk factor for SMI and that part of the presumed effect of SMI on low earnings is really due to effects of low education or some other unmeasured common causes on both outcomes. Again, this possibility cannot be considered with a model of the sort estimated in this chapter. Such an investigation requires a life-course perspective to be taken to focus on time-lagged associations of temporally primary mental disorders with later earnings, adjusting for effects of education and other possibly important common causes. Retrospective data can be used to approximate an analysis of that sort. The results of such an analysis are presented in the next chapter.

Acknowledgments

Portions of this chapter are based on Levinson, D., Lakoma, M. D., Petukhova, M., *et al.* (2010). Associations of serious mental illness with earnings: results from the WHO World Mental Health surveys. *British Journal of Psychiatry* 197, 114–21. © 2010. The Royal College of Psychiatrists. Reproduced with permission.

References

Buntin, M. B., & Zaslavsky, A. M. (2004). Too much ado about two-part models and transformation? Comparing methods of modeling Medicare expenditures. *Journal of Health Economics* 23, 525–42.

Chatterji, P., Alegria, M., Lu, M., & Takeuchi, D. (2007). Psychiatric disorders and labor market outcomes: evidence from the National Latino and Asian American Study. *Health Economics* 16, 1069–90.

Crowther, R. E., Marshall, M., Bond, G. R., & Huxley, P. (2001). Helping people with severe mental illness to obtain work: systematic review. *BMJ* 322, 204–8.

Demyttenaere, K., Bruffaerts, R., Posada-Villa, J., *et al.* (2004). Prevalence, severity, and unmet need for treatment of mental disorders in the World Health Organization World Mental Health surveys. *JAMA* 291, 2581–90.

Duan, N., Manning, W., Morris, C., & Newhouse, J. (1984). Choosing between the sample-selection model and the multi-part model. *Journal of Business and Economic Statistics* 2, 283–9.

Engle, R. F. (1983). Wald, likelihood ratio, and Lagrange multiplier tests in econometrics. In Z. Griliches, & M. D. Intriligator, eds., *Handbook of Econometrics, Volume I*. New York, NY: Elsevier, pp. 796–801.

Gabriel, P., & Liimatainen, M. R. (2000). *Mental Health in the Workplace*. Geneva: International Labour Office.

Harwood, H., Ameen, A., Denmead, G., *et al.* (2000). *The Economic Cost of Mental Illness, 1992*. Rockville, MD: National Institute of Mental Health.

Hosmer, D. W., & Lemeshow, S. (2001). *Applied Logistic Regression*, 2nd edn. New York, NY: Wiley.

Kessler, R. C., Berglund, P. A., Zhao, S., *et al.* (1996). The 12-month prevalence and correlates of serious mental illness (SMI). In R. W. Manderscheid & M. A. Sonnenschein, eds., *Mental Health, United States, 1996*. Washington, DC: US Government Printing Office, pp. 59–70.

Kessler, R. C., Barber, C., Birnbaum, H. G., *et al.* (1999). Depression in the workplace: effects on short-term disability. *Health Affairs* 18, 163–71.

Kessler, R. C., Aguilar-Gaxiola, S., Alonso, J., *et al.* (2008a). Prevalence and severity of mental disorders in the World Mental Health Survey Initiative. In R. C. Kessler, & T. B. Üstün, eds., *The WHO World Mental Health Surveys: Global Perspectives on the Epidemiology of Mental Disorders*. New York, NY: Cambridge University Press, pp. 534–40.

Kessler, R. C., Heeringa, S., Lakoma, M. D., *et al.* (2008b). Individual and societal effects of mental disorders on earnings in the United States: results from the National Comorbidity Survey Replication. *American Journal of Psychiatry* 165, 703–11.

Latimer, E. (2005). Economic considerations associated with assertive community treatment and supported employment for people with severe mental illness. *Journal of Psychiatry and Neuroscience* 30, 355–9.

Leon, A. C., Olfson, M., Portera, L., Farber, L., & Sheehan, D. V. (1997). Assessing psychiatric impairment in primary care with the Sheehan Disability Scale. *International Journal of Psychiatry in Medicine* 27, 93–105.

Leonhardt, D. (2010) What does $60 billion buy? *New York Times*. http://economix.blogs.nytimes.com/2010/12/05/what-does-60-billion-buy/. Accessed March 28, 2012.

Levinson, D., Lakoma, M. D., Petukhova, M., *et al.* (2010). Associations of serious mental illness with earnings: results from the WHO World Mental Health surveys. *British Journal of Psychiatry* 197, 114–21.

Manning, W. G. (1998). The logged dependent variable, heteroscedasticity, and the retransformation problem. *Journal of Health Economics* 17, 283–95.

Manning, W. G., & Mullahy, J. (2001). Estimating log models: to transform or not to transform? *Journal of Health Economics* 20, 461–94.

McCullagh, P., & Nelder, J. (1989). *Generalized Linear Models*. London: Chapman & Hall.

Mullahy, J. (1998). Much ado about two: reconsidering retransformation and the two-part model in health econometrics. *Journal of Health Economics* 17, 247–81.

Murray, C. J. L., & López, A. D. (1996). *The Global Burden of Disease: A Comprehensive Assessment of Mortality and Disability from Diseases, Injuries and Risk Factors in 1990 and Projected to 2020*. Cambridge, MA: Harvard University Press.

Rice, D. P., & Miller, L. S. (1998). Health economics and cost implications of anxiety and other mental disorders in the United States. *British Journal of Psychiatry Supplement* 173, 4–9.

Rice, D. P., Kelman, S., Miller, L. S., & Dunmeyer, S. (1990). *The Economic Costs of Alcohol and Drug Abuse and Mental Illness: 1985*. Washington, DC: US Department of Health and Human Services.

Rost, K., Smith, J. L., & Dickinson, M. (2004). The effect of improving primary care depression management on employee absenteeism and productivity: a randomized trial. *Medical Care* **42**, 1202–10.

Rubin, D. B. (1987). *Multiple Imputation for Nonresponse in Surveys*. New York, NY: Wiley.

Schempf, A., & Becker, S. (2006). On the application of decomposition methods. *American Journal of Public Health* **96**, 1899; author reply 1899–901.

Shiels, C., Gabbay, M. B., & Ford, F. M. (2004). Patient factors associated with duration of certified sickness absence and transition to long-term incapacity. *British Journal of General Practice* **54**, 86–91.

Tarricone, R. (2006). Cost-of-illness analysis. What room in health economics? *Health Policy* **77**, 51–63.

Wang, P. S., Simon, G. E., Avorn, J., *et al.* (2007). Telephone screening, outreach, and care management for depressed workers and impact on clinical and work productivity outcomes: a randomized controlled trial. *JAMA* **298**, 1401–11.

Wolter, K. M. (1985). *Introduction to Variance Estimation*. New York, NY: Springer-Verlag.

Zhang, X., Zhao, X., & Harris, A. (2009). Chronic diseases and labour force participation in Australia. *Journal of Health Economics* **28**, 91–108.

Early-onset mental disorders and adult household income

Norito Kawakami, Wai Tat Chiu, Somnath Chatterji, Ron de Graaf, Herbert Marschinger, William LeBlanc, Sing Lee, and Ronald C. Kessler

Introduction

Chapter 8 showed that recent serious mental illness (SMI) is closely associated with low earnings. There are a number of plausible causal pathways that might account for this association. One of them was examined in Chapter 4: that early-onset mental disorders might lead to lower educational attainment, which in turn has long been known to be a powerful cause of low earnings. A process of this sort was hypothesized by Morgan & David in 1963. It is also possible that some mental disorders reduce motivation or the ability to work (Sanderson & Andrews 2006), give rise to impairments in interpersonal functioning (Tyrer 2007), or lead to discrimination (Sharac et al. 2010), all of which can reduce an individual's chances of occupational advancement. Mental disorders are also responsible for a meaningful proportion of all occupational disabilities (Henderson et al. 2011). In addition, it is possible that the cross-sectional associations documented in Chapter 8 between recent SMI and recent earnings are caused by the adverse effects of low earnings on mental disorders rather than, or in addition to, the adverse effects of mental disorders on earnings. Consistent with this possibility, causal effects of low income on mental disorders have been documented in quasi-experimental studies of job loss (Dooley et al. 1996) and in time-series studies of associations between the unemployment rate and the suicide rate (Jones 1991).

The only way to definitively determine actual causation from all of the above competing possibilities would be to launch a large-scale, long-term experiment on the effects on earnings or efforts to prevent or treat mental disorders. However, as such an experiment would be impractical, suggestive evidence is the best we are likely to get in the near future. Perhaps the most obvious type of such evidence comes from controlled treatment effectiveness trials, which document significant short-term effects of mental disorder treatments on decreases in work disability and unemployment (Lo Sasso et al. 2006, Wang et al. 2007). However, such studies are incapable of estimating the long-term effects of mental disorders, as treatment is withheld from control groups in these types of studies for only a period of weeks or months.

Plausible provisional estimates of the magnitude of long-term effects of mental disorders would nonetheless be useful for public policy purposes (Greenberg et al. 1993). One way to obtain such estimates would be to take advantage of the fact that most common mental disorders start in childhood or adolescence (Kessler et al. 2007), and to use prospective naturalistic epidemiological data to study long-term associations between early-onset mental disorders and subsequent earnings, controlling as best as possible for the effects of potential confounders. Several such studies have been carried out. A recent US study, for example, found that retrospectively recalled emotional problems before age 17 predicted a 20% reduction in household income among adults aged 25–53 (Smith & Smith 2010). Two prospective studies in New Zealand found that recurrent depression at ages 16–21 predicted unemployment and low income at ages 21–25 (Fergusson et al. 2007), and that mental disorders at ages 18–25 predicted poor workforce participation and low income at age 30 (Gibb et al. 2010). Finally, a longitudinal UK study found that psychological problems developed by age 16 predicted a 28% reduction in household income at age 50 (Goodman et al. 2011).

Such results, while compelling, are limited to a small number of high-income countries and a few measures of early-onset mental disorders. No large-scale prospective

---

The Burdens of Mental Disorders, ed. Jordi Alonso, Somnath Chatterji, and Yanling He. Published by Cambridge University Press. © World Health Organization 2013.

epidemiological studies with appropriate time intervals and measures have been conducted to provide more complete estimates in most countries. However, a rough approximation is possible by using the cross-sectional data available from the WMH surveys, where we can examine associations of retrospective reports about early-onset mental disorders with subsequent income. These are the data presented in this chapter. We examined retrospectively reported lifetime disorders as of the age when each respondent completed education, to establish a temporal priority of disorders before income. We used household income rather than personal earnings alone as the outcome because the former is the more relevant outcome for policy purposes than the latter. But we also disaggregated the total associations between early-onset mental disorders with total family income into indirect effects through the main proximal determinants of family income: employment, earnings among the employed, marriage, spousal employment among the married, spousal earnings among those with an employed spouse, and other income. We looked at level of education in order to determine whether early-onset mental disorders predict subsequent income above and beyond their effects on education.

Methods

Sample

The analyses reported in this chapter are based on 23 of the 25 WMH surveys considered in this volume. The surveys in France and South Africa were excluded because of unavailability of data on either disabilities or earnings. The outcome of primary interest, household income, was assessed in part 2 of the sample. Only those respondents of working age, which we defined for the purposes of this analysis as between 18 and 64 years old, were included. Respondents who were students or retired were excluded from this analysis, resulting in a final sample of $n = 44,527$ respondents. New Zealand and Ukraine were additionally excluded from the earnings analysis because information on earnings was not collected in either of those surveys, leading to a reduction in sample size to $n = 37,741$ for that analysis.

Measures

Respondents were asked if they were employed or self-employed at any time in the past 12 months. Those who responded positively were asked about personal earnings, which were defined as including only wages and other stipends from employment, excluding pensions, investments, financial assistance, and other sources of income. We also assessed spousal earnings and separately assessed all "other" household income. As in most community surveys, the item-level non-response rate for questions on income and earnings was non-trivial (range 0.8–18.3%; interquartile range 2.2–7.0%). Regression-based imputation was used to impute these missing values. Mental disorders were not strongly related to missing income/earnings data.

Reported income and earnings were divided by median within-country values in order to pool across countries while retaining information about between-country differences in income/earnings variations. These transformed scores were used as outcomes in regression analyses calculated simultaneously across all countries for associations of lifetime mental disorders as of the respondent's age upon completing education (henceforth referred to as *early-onset* disorders) with income and earnings, controlling for sex, education, time since completing education, and country.

All mental disorders assessed in the WMH surveys are included in this chapter other than minor depression, but the three separate bipolar disorders (bipolar I, bipolar II, and subthreshold bipolar disorder) were combined into a single measure as bipolar disorder. As noted in the introduction to this chapter, we recognize that later-onset mental disorders might also influence subsequent income, but we wanted to err on the side of caution in establishing the temporal priority of disorders with later income, leading to conservative estimates of predictive associations between mental disorders and subsequent income and earnings. In addition to coding years of education as a continuous variable, educational attainment was classified in a country-specific scheme that included categories for no education, less than secondary education, completed secondary education, some post-secondary school, completed junior college or associate degree, completed some college beyond junior/associate college, and completed a college or university degree.

Statistical analysis

As noted in Chapter 8, a major statistical problem in estimating regression equations to predict income and earnings is that the distributions are highly skewed. A meaningful minority of people report no income or earnings and a much higher proportion of other respondents have higher income/earnings than would be found in a normal distribution. These distributional characteristics make the ordinary least squares (OLS) regression analysis both biased and inefficient. As described in more detail in Chapter 2, this problem can be addressed by using either two-part models (Goodman *et al.* 2011) or one-part generalized linear models (GLMs) with non-linear link functions and complex error structures (McCullagh & Nelder 1989). Given a previous experience in which we found that one-part models work better than two-part models in predicting earnings (Levinson *et al.* 2010) and after confirming by means of a preliminary analysis that the same is true for total family income, the formal analysis of the comparative model fit (Buntin & Zaslavsky 2004) was restricted to one-part GLMs. This analysis showed that models with either log link function and variance proportional to the mean (total and other household income) or linear link function and constant variance (personal and spousal earnings) provided the best fit (see Appendix Table 9.1). Logistic regression models were used to predict dichotomous (yes/no) measures of work disability, employment among those not disabled, marriage, and spousal employment among the married.

Given the evidence of substantial comorbidity among the mental disorders assessed in the WMH surveys (Kessler *et al.* 2011), we evaluated a number of non-additive model specifications among comorbid disorders. After determining a best-fitting model, the population attributable risk proportion (PARP) was calculated to represent the proportional reduction in total income that would be prevented if early-onset mental disorders were eliminated, based on the assumption that the regression coefficients represent causal effects (Northridge 1995). (See Chapter 2 for a discussion of PARPs and a description of estimation methods.) The design-based Jackknife Repeated Replication method (Wolter 1985) was used to estimate standard errors due to weighting and clustering of data in a series of SAS (SAS Institute Inc. 2008) macros. Statistical significance was consistently evaluated using 0.05-level, two-sided design-based tests.

Results

Prevalence of early-onset mental disorders
Preliminary analyses found that the lifetime prevalence of any early-onset disorder is highest in

high-income countries (21.5%), intermediate in upper-middle-income countries (17.1%), and lowest in low/lower-middle-income countries (11.7%). Disorder-specific prevalence estimates generally follow the same cross-national pattern (Table 9.1). See Appendix Tables 9.2 and 9.3 for sex-specific prevalence estimates.

Association of early-onset mental disorders with subsequent income and earnings
The best-fitting model for total household income is an additive model with a separate coefficient for each of the 15 mental disorders and two disorder subtypes (i.e., the subset of alcohol and drug abuse cases that also meet criteria for dependence). We also considered non-additive models including a model for number of disorders (henceforth referred to as the *number-of-disorders model*) and a series of more complex non-additive models with interactions between number and types of disorders (see Appendix Tables 9.4–9.5). Although the additive model was the best-fitting model overall, the number-of-disorders model was the best-fitting model in most of the subgroups described below. Therefore, the coefficients for both models are shown below.

While the additive model was significant mainly in predicting total household income (χ^2_{17} = 60.5, $p < 0.001$), only two disorders (agoraphobia and specific phobia) were found to be individually significant (Table 9.2, part I). These significant coefficients are both negative, with a fairly consistent sign pattern across disorders (13 of 17 coefficients). As the model for total income is based on a log link function, exponentiated coefficients can be interpreted as ratios of expected incomes among respondents without predictor disorders. Negative coefficients represent ratios less than 1.0. The −0.04 coefficient for specific phobia and −0.17 for agoraphobia represent income ratios of 0.96 and 0.83, respectively. The coefficients in the number-of-disorders model had a significant monotonic pattern where high comorbidity (four or more disorders) was associated with a household income approximately 16% (1 − the antilog of the regression coefficient of −0.18) lower than the national median (Table 9.2, part II).

Decomposition shows that early-onset mental disorders also significantly predict five of the seven components of income considered here. Two of these are continuous outcomes (Table 9.2): low personal

Table 9.1 Lifetime prevalence estimates of early-onset mental disorders among respondents who were in the age range 18–64 at the time of interview, by country income level. The WMH surveys.

	All countries		Low/ lower-middle		Upper-middle		High	
	%	(SE)	%	(SE)	%	(SE)	%	(SE)
Mood disorders								
Bipolar	0.8	(0.0)	0.3	(0.0)	0.6	(0.1)	1.3	(0.1)
Major depressive disorder or dysthymia	3.2	(0.1)	1.8	(0.1)	2.5	(0.2)	4.7	(0.2)
Anxiety disorders								
Agoraphobia	0.6	(0.0)	0.6	(0.1)	0.8	(0.1)	0.5	(0.0)
Generalized anxiety	0.9	(0.1)	0.4	(0.1)	0.6	(0.1)	1.3	(0.1)
Panic disorder	0.7	(0.0)	0.4	(0.1)	0.5	(0.1)	1.1	(0.1)
Post-traumatic stress	1.2	(0.1)	0.2	(0.0)	0.8	(0.1)	2.0	(0.1)
Separation anxiety[a]	3.5	(0.1)	2.4	(0.2)	2.9	(0.2)	4.6	(0.2)
Social phobia	3.5	(0.1)	1.2	(0.1)	2.6	(0.2)	6.1	(0.2)
Specific phobia	7.7	(0.2)	6.1	(0.3)	7.7	(0.3)	9.3	(0.3)
Disruptive behavior disorders								
Attention-deficit/hyperactivity[b]	2.1	(0.1)	0.5	(0.1)	1.6	(0.2)	4.2	(0.3)
Conduct disorder[c]	2.5	(0.2)	1.2	(0.2)	1.4	(0.2)	4.2	(0.3)
Intermittent explosive disorder	2.8	(0.1)	1.7	(0.1)	2.0	(0.2)	5.0	(0.3)
Oppositional-defiant disorder[d]	3.0	(0.2)	3.2	(0.4)	1.5	(0.2)	3.9	(0.3)
Substance disorders								
Alcohol abuse[e]	2.5	(0.1)	0.8	(0.1)	1.6	(0.2)	3.9	(0.2)
Alcohol abuse with dependence	0.5	(0.0)	0.2	(0.0)	0.3	(0.1)	0.8	(0.1)
Drug abuse[e]	1.4	(0.1)	0.2	(0.1)	0.6	(0.1)	3.1	(0.2)
Drug abuse with dependence	0.4	(0.0)	0.0	(0.0)	0.2	(0.1)	0.9	(0.1)
Number of disorders								
Exactly 1 disorder	10.9	(0.2)	8.9	(0.4)	11.1	(0.5)	12.3	(0.3)
Exactly 2 disorders	3.4	(0.1)	1.9	(0.1)	3.6	(0.2)	4.5	(0.2)
Exactly 3 disorders	1.5	(0.1)	0.6	(0.1)	1.5	(0.1)	2.2	(0.1)
Exactly 4 disorders	0.6	(0.0)	0.2	(0.0)	0.5	(0.1)	1.0	(0.1)
5+ disorders	0.8	(0.1)	0.1	(0.0)	0.4	(0.1)	1.5	(0.1)
(n)	(37,741)		(12,162)		(8,055)		(17,524)	

[a] Age is restricted to ≤ 44 for India, Lebanon, Belgium, Germany, Italy, the Netherlands, and Spain; age is restricted to ≤ 39 for Nigeria and PRC–Beijing/Shanghai.
[b] Age is restricted to ≤ 44 for Colombia, India, Bulgaria, Lebanon, Mexico, Belgium, Germany, Italy, the Netherlands, Portugal, Spain, and USA.
[c] Age is restricted to ≤ 44 for Colombia, India, Bulgaria, Lebanon, Mexico, Belgium, Germany, Italy, the Netherlands, Portugal, Spain, and USA; age is restricted to ≤ 39 for Nigeria and PRC–Beijing/Shanghai.
[d] Age is restricted to ≤ 44 for Colombia, Mexico, Belgium, Germany, Italy, the Netherlands, Portugal, Spain, and USA.
[e] With or without dependence.

earnings among the employed ($\chi^2_{17} = 67.4$, $p < 0.001$) and, in the number-of-disorders model, low spousal earnings among married people with employed spouses ($\chi^2_5 = 15.1$, $p = 0.010$). The other three are dichotomous outcomes (Table 9.3): increased probability of work disability ($\chi^2_{17} = 558.6$, $p < 0.001$), decreased probability of employment if not disabled ($\chi^2_{17} = 102.0$, $p < 0.001$), and decreased probability of

being married ($\chi^2_{17} = 103.2$, $p < 0.001$). The association with work disability is by far the strongest of these five, with 12 significant coefficients for individual disorders. The sign pattern shows that most early-onset mental disorders predict most components of low household income, and that high comorbidity consistently has especially strong associations with these outcomes.

Table 9.2 Regressions of total family income and continuous income component measures on type and number of early-onset mental disorders among respondents who were in the age range 18–64 at the time of interview. The WMH surveys.[a]

	Total household income		Personal earnings among the employed		Spouse earnings among those with an employed spouse		Other household income	
	Coeff	(SE)	Coeff	(SE)	Coeff	(SE)	Coeff	(SE)
Part I. Types of disorder[b]								
Mood disorders								
Bipolar disorder	−0.08	(0.05)	−0.02	(0.06)	−0.03	(0.08)	0.09	(0.09)
Major depressive disorder or dysthymia	−0.02	(0.02)	−0.06*	(0.02)	0.01	(0.04)	0.11*	(0.04)
Anxiety disorders								
Agoraphobia	−0.17*	(0.06)	−0.25*	(0.06)	−0.22	(0.13)	−0.01	(0.09)
Generalized anxiety	−0.04	(0.05)	−0.02	(0.05)	0.04	(0.10)	−0.03	(0.08)
Panic disorder	−0.02	(0.05)	−0.07	(0.07)	−0.08	(0.07)	0.11	(0.08)
Post-traumatic stress	−0.07	(0.04)	0.00	(0.05)	0.01	(0.06)	−0.13	(0.09)
Separation anxiety	−0.03	(0.03)	−0.02	(0.04)	−0.02	(0.05)	0.05	(0.06)
Social phobia	−0.02	(0.02)	−0.01	(0.03)	−0.00	(0.04)	−0.07	(0.04)
Specific phobia	−0.04*	(0.02)	−0.05	(0.03)	−0.09*	(0.04)	0.02	(0.04)
Disruptive behavior disorders								
Attention-deficit/hyperactivity	0.03	(0.03)	0.03	(0.04)	−0.03	(0.09)	−0.02	(0.09)
Conduct disorder	−0.02	(0.04)	−0.03	(0.04)	0.07	(0.08)	−0.03	(0.07)
Intermittent explosive disorder	0.04	(0.03)	0.05	(0.03)	0.00	(0.06)	−0.03	(0.06)
Oppositional-defiant disorder	0.05	(0.03)	0.04	(0.05)	−0.04	(0.07)	0.16*	(0.07)
Substance disorders								
Alcohol abuse[c]	−0.04	(0.03)	0.01	(0.04)	−0.03	(0.06)	−0.14*	(0.07)
Alcohol abuse with dependence	−0.08	(0.06)	−0.08	(0.06)	−0.08	(0.11)	−0.04	(0.12)
Drug abuse[c]	−0.03	(0.04)	−0.08	(0.05)	−0.10	(0.09)	0.10	(0.09)
Drug abuse with dependence	0.01	(0.07)	0.01	(0.08)	0.03	(0.13)	−0.04	(0.13)
χ^2_{17}[d]	60.5*		67.4*		21.9		27.8*	
χ^2_{16}[e]	29.6*		44.4*		11.2		26.5*	
Part II. Number of disorders[b]								
Exactly 1 disorder	−0.02	(0.02)	−0.02	(0.02)	−0.03	(0.03)	0.00	(0.03)
Exactly 2 disorders	−0.02	(0.02)	−0.01	(0.03)	0.01	(0.04)	−0.03	(0.04)
Exactly 3 disorders	−0.08*	(0.03)	−0.10*	(0.03)	−0.11	(0.07)	0.06	(0.06)
Exactly 4 disorders	−0.18*	(0.04)	−0.09	(0.06)	−0.18	(0.10)	−0.01	(0.08)
5+ disorders	−0.18*	(0.04)	−0.17*	(0.05)	−0.26*	(0.07)	0.07	(0.07)
χ^2_5[d]	40.0*		22.4*		15.1*		2.7	
(n)	(37,741)		(25,460)		(18,213)		(37,741)	

[a] Based on GLM multiple regression models with controls for country, sex, level of education, and time since completing education estimated in all countries. The equations for total household income and other income use a log link function and Poisson error variance structure, while the equations for personal earnings among the employed and spouse earnings among those with an employed spouse use a linear link function and normally distributed error structure. Exponentiated values of the log link function coefficients can be interpreted as the ratio of expected incomes among respondents with versus without the predictor disorder. For example, coefficients of −0.05, −0.10, −0.15, and −0.20 represent mean income ratios of 0.95, 0.90, 0.86, and 0.82 among respondents with versus without the predictor disorder. The linear link function coefficients, in comparison, can be interpreted as the mean income difference between respondents with versus without the predictor disorder.
[b] The results in parts I and II are for two different models. The first model has a separate dummy predictor variable for each mental disorder assessed in the surveys. The second model includes a set of dummy predictor variables for the number of disorders the respondent had without distinguishing types of disorders. We also investigated models that included predictors for both type and number of disorders as well as models that included interactions between type and number of disorders, but the less complex models shown here out-performed those other models.
[c] With or without dependence.
[d] Joint significance of the coefficients associated with the disorders assessed in the model.
[e] Significance of differences among the coefficients associated with the disorders assessed in the model.
* Significant at the 0.05 level, two-sided test.

Table 9.3 Logistic regressions of dichotomous income component measures on type and number of early-onset mental disorders among respondents who were in the age range 18–64 at the time of interview. The WMH surveys.[a]

	Disabled		Employed		Married		Spouse employed among the married	
	OR	(95% CI)	OR	(95% CI)	OR	(95% CI)	OR	(95% CI)
Part I. Mental disorders[b]								
Mood disorders								
Bipolar	2.5*	(1.8–3.5)	0.7*	(0.5–0.9)	0.7*	(0.5–0.9)	0.8	(0.5–1.4)
Major depression or dysthymia	2.0*	(1.7–2.3)	0.9	(0.8–1.0)	0.7*	(0.6–0.8)	1.1	(0.9–1.3)
Anxiety disorders								
Agoraphobia	2.1*	(1.5–3.0)	0.7	(0.5–1.0)	0.6*	(0.5–0.9)	0.6	(0.4–1.0)
Panic disorder	1.5*	(1.1–2.0)	0.7*	(0.6–1.0)	0.8	(0.6–1.1)	1.0	(0.6–1.6)
Generalized anxiety	1.9*	(1.4–2.4)	0.6*	(0.5–0.8)	0.9	(0.7–1.2)	1.0	(0.7–1.6)
Post-traumatic stress	2.0*	(1.6–2.5)	0.8	(0.7–1.1)	1.0	(0.8–1.4)	0.8	(0.6–1.2)
Separation anxiety	1.3*	(1.0–1.6)	1.0	(0.8–1.1)	1.0	(0.8–1.1)	1.0	(0.8–1.4)
Social phobia	1.4*	(1.2–1.7)	0.9*	(0.8–1.0)	0.8*	(0.7–1.0)	1.3*	(1.1–1.6)
Specific phobia	1.6*	(1.4–1.8)	0.9*	(0.8–1.0)	0.9	(0.8–1.1)	1.1	(1.0–1.3)
Disruptive behavior disorders								
Attention-deficit/hyperactivity	1.9*	(1.2–3.0)	1.3	(1.0–1.7)	1.1	(0.9–1.3)	1.0	(0.7–1.5)
Conduct disorder	1.7*	(1.1–2.6)	0.8	(0.6–1.1)	1.2	(0.9–1.5)	1.1	(0.8–1.7)
Intermittent explosive disorder	1.0	(0.8–1.3)	1.0	(0.8–1.3)	1.3*	(1.1–1.5)	1.3	(1.0–1.7)
Oppositional-defiant disorder	1.1	(0.7–1.5)	0.9	(0.7–1.2)	1.0	(0.8–1.2)	1.4	(0.9–2.0)
Substance disorders								
Alcohol abuse[c]	1.0	(0.8–1.3)	0.8*	(0.6–1.0)	0.8	(0.7–1.0)	1.5*	(1.1–2.0)
Alcohol abuse with dependence	1.6*	(1.1–2.3)	0.7	(0.4–1.1)	0.8	(0.6–1.2)	0.6*	(0.4–0.9)
Drug abuse[c]	1.2	(0.9–1.7)	0.9	(0.7–1.3)	1.0	(0.7–1.2)	1.1	(0.7–1.5)
Drug abuse with dependence	0.8	(0.5–1.4)	1.6	(0.9–2.8)	0.9	(0.6–1.4)	1.0	(0.5–2.2)
χ^2_{17} [d]	558.6*		102.0*		103.2*		30.0*	
χ^2_{16} [e]	87.1*		34.3*		58.7*		30.4*	
Part II. Number of disorders[b]								
Exactly 1 disorder	2.1*	(1.9–2.4)	0.8*	(0.8–0.9)	0.9*	(0.8–1.0)	1.1	(1.0–1.3)
Exactly 2 disorders	3.1*	(2.6–3.7)	0.7*	(0.6–0.8)	0.8*	(0.7–0.9)	1.3*	(1.1–1.6)
Exactly 3 disorders	4.4*	(3.5–5.5)	0.7*	(0.5–0.9)	0.7*	(0.6–0.9)	1.4	(1.0–1.8)
Exactly 4 disorders	5.9*	(4.5–7.8)	0.5*	(0.4–0.7)	0.6*	(0.5–0.8)	1.5	(0.9–2.4)
5+ disorders	7.1*	(5.5–9.2)	0.5*	(0.4–0.6)	0.7*	(0.5–0.8)	1.5	(1.0–2.2)
χ^2_5 [d]	466.4*		74.5*		32.9*		16.0*	
(n)	(44,527)		(37,741)		(37,741)		(26,103)	

[a] Based on a multiple logistic regression model with controls for country, sex, level of education, and time since completing education estimated in all countries. Unlike the analyses in Table 9.2, New Zealand and Ukraine were included in the analyses reported in this table. This accounts for the larger total sample size here (n = 44,527) than in Table 9.2 (n = 37,741).
[b] The results in parts I and II are for two different models. The first model has a separate dummy predictor variable for each mental disorder assessed in the surveys. The second model includes a set of dummy predictor variables for the number of disorders the respondent had without distinguishing types of disorders. We also investigated models that included predictors for both type and number of disorders as well as models that included interactions between type and number of disorders, but the less complex models shown here out-performed those other models.
[c] With or without dependence.
[d] Joint significance of the coefficients associated with the disorders assessed in the model.
[e] Significance of differences among the coefficients associated with the disorders assessed in the model.
* Significant at the 0.05 level, two-sided test.

Early-onset mental disorders are associated in quite different ways with the other two components of household income (other household income and probability of spousal employment). The model for other income is complex in that although it is significant overall (Table 9.2: χ^2_{17} = 27.8, p = 0.048), the sign pattern is weak (10 of 17 coefficients negative) and there is only one significant negative coefficient (alcohol abuse) along with two significant positive coefficients (major depression disorder or dysthymia and oppositional-defiant disorder). The model to predict spousal employment is also significant (Table 9.3: $\chi^2_{17} = 30.0$, $p = 0.026$), but distinct from models for all other outcomes in that early-onset mental disorders are associated with a higher, not lower, probability of the outcome.

No single early-onset disorder stands out as accounting for the most components of income. Fifteen of the 17 predictors of disorders or disorder subtypes have at least one significant coefficient across the seven outcomes and none has more than four significant coefficients across these outcomes. The two disorders with the highest number (four) of significant coefficients are major depression disorder or dysthymia and social phobia. The four disorders that have three significant coefficients across outcomes are bipolar disorder, specific phobia, agoraphobia with or without panic disorder, and alcohol abuse. All other significant disorders have only one or two significant coefficients.

Subgroup associations

We replicated the above analyses by sex and country income level. The best-fitting model in most cases was the number-of-disorders model. Based on this model, early-onset mental disorders significantly predict total household income separately among men and women in high-income countries ($\chi^2_5 = 29.9$–41.3, $p < 0.001$), only among women ($\chi^2_5 = 11.6$, $p = 0.041$) in upper-middle-income countries, and among neither men nor women in low/lower-middle-income countries ($\chi^2_5 = 5.5$–6.2, $p = 0.29$–0.36) (Table 9.4). As in the total sample, the sign pattern is largely negative in each significant subsample. High comorbidity is generally associated with the largest drops in income, with household income in the range of 16% (1 – the antilog of the regression coefficient of −0.17) to 33% (1 – the antilog of the regression coefficient −0.40) lower than the national medians among respondents with a history of highly comorbid early-onset disorders.

We also estimated models for income components in the same subsamples (see Appendix Tables 9.6 to 9.9). Considering each of these seven components separately for women and men and for women and men combined resulted in 21 equations for each set of countries. Early-onset mental disorders significantly predict only two of these 21 in low/lower-middle-income countries (other income in the total sample and among men; $\chi^2_5 = 18.0$–22.9, $p = 0.003$ to < 0.001),

7 of 21 in upper-middle-income countries (other income, disability, and spousal employment in the total sample; employed and being married among women and in the total sample; $\chi^2_5 = 11.1$–20.5, $p = 0.001$–0.049), and 20 of 21 in high-income countries (all outcomes except personal earnings among men; $\chi^2_5 = 16.4$–66.3, $p = 0.006$ to < 0.001). These significant subsample associations are consistently stronger than those in the total sample.

Population attributable risk proportions (PARPs)

As noted above, PARPs can be interpreted as the proportional reduction in total income that would be prevented if early-onset mental disorders were eliminated (either prevented or effectively treated), based on the assumption that the regression coefficients represent causal effects. PARP estimates showed that early-onset mental disorders are associated with 1.1% of gross household income (GHI) in the total sample, 0.5% in low/lower-middle-income countries, 1.0% in upper-middle-income countries, and 1.4% in high-income countries (Table 9.5). Percentages are consistently higher among women than men (1.2% vs. 0.8% in all countries combined; 0.6–1.6% vs. 0.4–1.2% in subsets of countries defined by income level). These are non-trivial proportions of GHI. To put them into perspective, we noted that 1% of GHI in the USA is equal to roughly $79 billion, which in turn is roughly equivalent to the entire annual budget of the US Department of Health and Human Services ($78 billion).

Estimates of decomposition percentages were obtained by recalculating the PARPs from Table 9.4 seven times, each time including a control for one of the seven components of total family income in the prediction equation, and comparing the adjusted PARP estimates to the total PARP estimates shown in Table 9.5 to calculate the proportions of total PARP due to the controlled components. (See the footnote to Table 9.6 for a more detailed description.) As these components are interrelated and the decomposition controls separately for each one, the sum of the percentage estimates across components adds up to much more than 100% (Table 9.6). Indeed, percentages of a few components exceed 100% due to sign reversals in residual associations. Data patterns should consequently be interpreted only in general terms. With this in mind, five broad observations can be made about the data patterns in the decomposition.

Table 9.4 Associations of number of early-onset mental disorders predicting total household income by sex and country income level. The WMH surveys.[a]

Country income level	Number of disorders										X^2_5[b]	N
	Exactly 1 disorder		Exactly 2 disorders		Exactly 3 disorders		Exactly 4 disorders		5+ disorders			
	Estimate	(SE)	Estimate	(SE)	Estimate	(SE)	Estimate	(SE)	Estimate	(SE)		
I. All countries												
Female	−0.03	(0.02)	−0.01	(0.03)	−0.06	(0.04)	−0.23*	(0.06)	−0.30*	(0.07)	28.9*	21,177
Male	−0.02	(0.02)	−0.03	(0.03)	−0.10*	(0.04)	−0.11	(0.06)	−0.11*	(0.05)	10.9	16,564
Total	−0.02	(0.02)	−0.02	(0.02)	−0.08*	(0.03)	−0.18*	(0.04)	−0.18*	(0.04)	40.0*	37,741
II. Low/lower-middle												
Female	0.00	(0.04)	0.06	(0.10)	−0.24*	(0.12)	−0.10	(0.12)	−0.20	(0.42)	5.5	6,508
Male	0.02	(0.05)	0.18*	(0.08)	0.04	(0.16)	−0.15	(0.18)	−0.38	(0.41)	6.2	5,654
Total	0.01	(0.03)	0.11	(0.07)	−0.08	(0.12)	−0.13	(0.10)	−0.32	(0.30)	6.9	12,162
III. Upper-middle												
Female	−0.03	(0.15)	0.07	(0.06)	−0.09	(0.09)	−0.04	(0.16)	−0.40*	(0.17)	11.6*	4,745
Male	0.00	(0.06)	0.17*	(0.07)	−0.07	(0.12)	0.17	(0.14)	−0.17	(0.13)	10.2	3,310
Total	−0.02	(0.04)	0.11*	(0.04)	−0.09	(0.07)	−0.10	(0.09)	−0.26*	(0.10)	21.0*	8,055
IV. High												
Female	−0.04	(0.02)	−0.07	(0.04)	−0.03	(0.05)	−0.29*	(0.07)	−0.30*	(0.07)	29.9*	9,924
Male	−0.04	(0.03)	−0.16*	(0.03)	−0.13*	(0.04)	−0.21*	(0.08)	−0.10	(0.05)	41.3*	7,600
Total	−0.04*	(0.02)	−0.11*	(0.03)	−0.08*	(0.03)	−0.25*	(0.04)	−0.17*	(0.04)	57.7*	17,524

[a] Based on GLM multiple regression models with controls for country, level of education, time since completing education, and sex (in the models that combine men and women) estimated in all countries other than New Zealand and Ukraine (where information on earnings was not collected). The equations all use a log link function and Poisson error variance structure. Exponentiated values of the coefficients can be interpreted as the ratio of expected incomes among respondents with versus without the predictor disorder. For example, coefficients of −0.05, −0.10, −0.20, and −0.30 represent mean income ratios of 0.95, 0.90, 0.82, and 0.74 among respondents with versus without the predictor disorder.

[b] Joint significance of the coefficients associated with the disorders assessed in the model.

* Significant at the 0.05 level, two-sided test.

Table 9.5 Population attributable risk proportions (PARPs) of total household income due to early-onset mental disorders by sex and country income level. The WMH surveys.[a]

Country income level	Female	Male	Total
	PARP (%)	PARP (%)	PARP (%)
All countries	1.2	0.8	1.1
Low/lower-middle	0.6	0.4	0.5
Upper-middle	1.1	0.7	1.0
High	1.6	1.2	1.4

[a] The entries in this table are based on simulations using parameters from the models described in footnotes *a–b* of Table 9.2. The outcome is total household income. See the text for a description of the simulation methods.

First, while decomposition percentages do not vary greatly across country income levels, they do differ by sex, with the PARPs among men better explained by personal earnings and the PARPs among women due roughly equally to spousal earnings and personal earnings. Second, consistent with these sex differences, the PARP percentages associated with marriage and spousal employment are consistently higher among women than men, while PARP percentages due to personal disability and employment are consistently higher among men than women. Third, the PARP percentages due to personal earnings are consistently higher than those due to employment. This means that early-onset disorders are associated not only with being employed but also with the amount earned during employment. Fourth, the ratio of PARP percentages associated with the amount earned versus being

Table 9.6 Population attributable risk proportions (PARPs) of each of the seven components of total household income due to early-onset mental disorders by sex and country income level. The WMH surveys.[a]

	Components of total household income							
	Disability	Employment	Marriage	Spouse employment	Personal earnings	Spouse earnings	Other household income	N
I. Female								
All countries	41.2	21.4	28.0	34.2	58.6	60.0	1.3	(21,177)
Low/lower-middle	46.0	24.3	33.0	39.1	76.8	65.8	−8.8	(6,508)
Upper-middle	44.9	22.9	30.4	36.9	65.3	64.8	−2.8	(4,745)
High	39.1	20.4	26.0	31.9	53.2	56.9	5.3	(9,924)
II. Male								
All countries	54.9	78.9	19.2	5.8	119.0	8.7	10.3	(16,564)
Low/lower-middle	63.9	86.4	19.8	0.5	122.3	−0.5	23.2	(5,654)
Upper-middle	58.4	83.7	19.9	3.8	119.0	4.6	18.2	(3,310)
High	51.8	76.0	18.8	7.4	118.3	11.7	6.1	(7,600)
III. Female and male combined								
All countries	45.2	45.5	23.9	14.8	90.0	30.2	4.7	(37,741)
Low/lower-middle	50.8	52.5	26.1	11.8	103.3	26.7	4.7	(12,162)
Upper-middle	48.0	49.0	25.0	13.7	94.9	28.4	6.4	(8,055)
High	43.2	43.0	22.8	15.4	85.7	31.0	4.9	(17,524)

[a] The simulations in Table 9.5 were rerun seven times, each time with a control for one of the seven components of total household income. The entries here are equal to 100% minus the ratio of the simulation, with the additional control over the corresponding simulation from Table 9.5 (i.e., without the additional control). These numbers represent the percent of PARP explained by the additional control. For example, if disorders no longer predicted total household income at all after controlling for a given component, the entry would be 100%, indicating that the control fully accounts for the PARP. If the addition of a control reverses the sign of disorders predicting total household income, the entry in Table 9.6 will be greater than 100%. If the addition of the control makes the association between disorders and household income stronger (i.e., more negative), the entry in Table 9.6 will be negative.

employed is higher for women (2.6–3.2) than for men (1.4–1.6), meaning that the amount earned by the employed is relatively more important than employment among women than men, presumably reflecting the fact that unemployment is more indicative of pre-existing emotional problems among men than women. Fifth, other household income is of very little importance either for women or for men in any country subsample.

Discussion

The above results show that common early-onset mental disorders are strongly associated with low current household income after adjusting for education, but that this association is considerably stronger in high-income than in upper-middle-income countries and not significant at all in low/lower-middle-income countries. In considering these differences, it is important to remember that early onset is defined as onset prior to educational completion. Given that the level of educational attainment is linked to country income level, the average age of onset of early-onset disorders is inversely related to country income level, which means that some part of the cross-national variation in the strength of associations could be due to differences in age of onset. Further analyses in subsamples with a constant level of educational attainment could be carried out to compare effect sizes across countries, but this would also raise the issues of historical-cohort changes in levels of educational attainment within and across countries, and differences in the effects of early-onset disorders across different parts of the life course, neither of which we considered because of the difficulty of examining these complex interactions.

We also found that the association of early-onset mental disorders with current income varies by sex, that a wide variety of early-onset mental disorders are involved in these associations, and that the overall associations are mediated by a number of components. The relative importance of the components differs in men and women, due to stronger associations with personal employment and earnings among men and with spousal employment and spousal earnings among women. In keeping with the fact that no single disorder has a dominant effect in accounting for these associations, significant individual-level coefficients were stronger for high comorbidity than for individual disorders.

We found that PARP estimates are in the range 1.0–1.4% of total GHI in upper-middle-income and high-income countries. These percentages might seem low, but are actually quite high in substantive terms. For example, 1% of GHI is more than twice the amount spent on all federal health research in the USA. Importantly, these are *annual* costs averaged over the entire life course up to age 65 among people who had early-onset mental disorders, with ages of onset typically in childhood or early–middle adolescence.

Results as dramatic as these naturally raise the question as to the extent to which these losses could be averted through child/adolescent interventions to prevent and treat early-onset mental disorders. The answer is that we do not know. No large-scale, long-term intervention programs have ever been carried out that would allow for the evaluation of the long-term effects of broad-based interventions for early-onset mental disorders on adult income and earnings. Various different relevant interventions have been carried out that could be pooled to create long-term follow-up data for an evaluation like this (Barlow & Parsons 2002, Embry 2002, Waddell *et al.* 2007, Bayer *et al.* 2009), but it has never been done. The results presented here might provide a rationale for a pooled study of this sort. However, even in the absence of such a study, our results make a strong inferential case that early-onset mental disorders are, if not important *causal* risk factors, at least important early risk *markers* (Kraemer *et al.* 1997) that should be the subject of greater focus as potentially valuable targets of early intervention to increase societal human capital. Our finding in Chapter 4 that early-onset mental disorders predict low educational attainment is also relevant in this regard.

The results are limited by the fact that the WMH surveys do not assess a number of mental disorders that have been found to be significantly related to income and earnings, including psychosis, alcohol and drug dependence without a history of abuse, and a number of other disorders that could be significant predictors of income and earnings (Marwaha & Johnson 2004). In addition, DSM-IV categories might not capture the full relevant range of psychopathology in all countries studied. An additional measurement limitation is that mental disorders were assessed retrospectively with fully structured interviews. Retrospective recall bias might have distorted prevalence estimates, while the use of fully structured rather than semi-structured clinical interviews might have led to a certain degree of inaccuracy in the estimates. While these measurement errors likely resulted in conservative prevalence estimates, they may have led to exaggerated estimates of the effects of these disorders on adult household income, in that people with low household incomes have a lesser tendency towards downward bias in disorder reporting than other respondents. By ignoring later-onset disorders we also ignored information about the chronicity of disorders. These decisions presumably make the PARP estimates more conservative than they would have otherwise been.

The measures of income and earnings are also limited in two ways. First, item-level missing data rates were high for these questions. Although we used a sophisticated imputation method to address this problem and found that mental disorders were not strongly related to missing income/earnings data, this missing data problem raises concerns about the external validity of our findings. Second, we did not assess either *informal* economic activity (i.e., barter) or production by household members for their own end use (e.g., agricultural subsistence). Although there are conceptual and operational challenges in expanding the assessment of economic activity to include these components, progress has been made in developing international standards for doing so that should be used to expand the outcomes of future studies (Organization for Economic Co-operation and Development 2002). This expansion might be especially important in low/lower-middle-income countries, where our analysis failed to find significant economic effects of early-onset mental disorders.

Another potentially important limitation involving measurement that may have given rise to overestimations in some cases is that unmeasured common causes were not controlled. The only way to definitively correct this problem would be through the analysis of the long-term effects of child/adolescent experimental interventions, adding further support for pooled long-term follow-ups of previously conducted child/adolescent interventions. It would also be valuable to carry out long-term prospective naturalistic studies in countries at different developmental stages and with different cultures, both to confirm our findings longitudinally and to trace out developmental pathways linking early-onset mental disorders with the components of total household income examined here.

Acknowledgments

Portions of this chapter are based on Kawakami, N., Abdulrazaq Abdulghani, E., Alonso, J., *et al.* (2012). Early-life mental disorders and adult household income in the World Mental Health surveys. *Biological Psychiatry* 72, 228–37. © 2012. The Society of Biological Psychiatry. Reproduced with permission.

References

Barlow, J., & Parsons, J. (2002). Group-based parent-training programmes for improving emotional and behavioural adjustment in 0–3 year old children. *Cochrane Database of Systematic Reviews* (4), CD003680.

Bayer, J., Hiscock, H., Scalzo, K., *et al.* (2009). Systematic review of preventive interventions for children's mental health: what would work in Australian contexts? *Australian and New Zealand Journal of Psychiatry* 43, 695–710.

Buntin, M. B., & Zaslavsky, A. M. (2004). Too much ado about two-part models and transformation? Comparing methods of modeling Medicare expenditures. *Journal of Health Economics* 23, 525–42.

Dooley, D., Fielding, J., & Levi, L. (1996). Health and unemployment. *Annual Review of Public Health* 17, 449–65.

Embry, D. D. (2002). The good behavior game: a best practice candidate as a universal behavioral vaccine. *Clinical Child and Family Psychology Review* 5, 273–97.

Fergusson, D. M., Boden, J. M., & Horwood, L. J. (2007). Recurrence of major depression in adolescence and early adulthood, and later mental health, educational and economic outcomes. *British Journal of Psychiatry* 191, 335–42.

Gibb, S. J., Fergusson, D. M., & Horwood, L. J. (2010). Burden of psychiatric disorder in young adulthood and life outcomes at age 30. *British Journal of Psychiatry* 197, 122–7.

Goodman, A., Joyce, R., & Smith, J. P. (2011). The long shadow cast by childhood physical and mental problems on adult life. *Proceedings of the National Academy of Sciences of the United States of America* 108, 6032–7.

Greenberg, P. E., Stiglin, L. E., Finkelstein, S. N., & Berndt, E. R. (1993). The economic burden of depression in 1990. *Journal of Clinical Psychiatry* 54, 405–18.

Henderson, M., Harvey, S. B., Overland, S., Mykletun, A., & Hotopf, M. (2011). Work and common psychiatric disorders. *Journal of the Royal Society of Medicine* 104, 198–207.

Jones, L. (1991). The health consequences of economic recessions. *Journal of Health & Social Policy* 3, 1–14.

Kessler, R. C., Angermeyer, M., Anthony, J. C., *et al.* (2007). Lifetime prevalence and age-of-onset distributions of mental disorders in the World Health Organization's World Mental Health Survey Initiative. *World Psychiatry* 6, 168–76.

Kessler, R. C., Ormel, J., Petukhova, M., *et al.* (2011). Development of lifetime comorbidity in the World Health Organization world mental health surveys. *Archives of General Psychiatry* 68, 90–100.

Kraemer, H. C., Kazdin, A. E., Offord, D. R., *et al.* (1997). Coming to terms with the terms of risk. *Archives of General Psychiatry* **54**, 337–43.

Levinson, D., Lakoma, M. D., Petukhova, M., *et al.* (2010). Associations of serious mental illness with earnings: results from the WHO World Mental Health surveys. *British Journal of Psychiatry* **197**, 114–21.

Lo Sasso, A. T., Rost, K., & Beck, A. (2006). Modeling the impact of enhanced depression treatment on workplace functioning and costs: a cost-benefit approach. *Medical Care* **44** (4): 352–8.

Marwaha, S., & Johnson, S. (2004). Schizophrenia and employment: a review. *Social Psychiatry and Psychiatric Epidemiology* **39**, 337–49.

McCullagh, P., & Nelder, J. A. (1989). *Generalized Linear Models*, 2nd edn. London: Chapman & Hall.

Morgan, J., & David, M. (1963). Education and income. *The Quarterly Journal of Economics* **77**, 423–37.

Northridge, M. E. (1995). Public health methods-attributable risk as a link between causality and public health action. *American Journal of Public Health* **85**, 1202–4.

Organization for Economic Co-operation and Development (2002). *Measuring the Non-Observed Economy: a Handbook*. OECD Statistics Directorate, International Monetary Fund, Bureau of Statistics. Paris: OECD Publication Services.

Sanderson, K., & Andrews, G. (2006). Common mental disorders in the workforce: recent findings from descriptive and social epidemiology. *Canadian Journal of Psychiatry* **51**, 63–75.

SAS Institute Inc. (2008). *SAS/STAT® Software, Version 9.2 for Unix*. Cary, NC: SAS Institute Inc.

Sharac, J., McCrone, P., Clement, S., & Thornicroft, G. (2010). The economic impact of mental health stigma and discrimination: a systematic review. *Epidemiolgia Psichiatria Sociale* **19**, 223–32.

Smith, J. P., & Smith, G. C. (2010). Long-term economic costs of psychological problems during childhood. *Social Science and Medicine* **71**, 110–15.

Tyrer, P. (2007). Personality diatheses: a superior explanation than disorder. *Psychological Medicine* **37**, 1521–5.

Waddell, C., Hua, J. M., Garland, O. M., Peters, R. D., & McEwan, K. (2007). Preventing mental disorders in children: a systematic review to inform policy-making. *Canadian Journal of Public Health* **98**, 166–73.

Wang, P. S., Simon, G. E., Avorn, J., *et al.* (2007). Telephone screening, outreach, and care management for depressed workers and impact on clinical and work productivity outcomes: a randomized controlled trial. *JAMA* **298**, 1401–11.

Wolter, K. M. (1985). *Introduction to Variance Estimation*. New York, NY: Springer-Verlag.

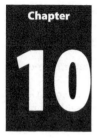
Family burden associated with mental and physical disorders

Maria Carmen Viana, Michael J. Gruber, Victoria Shahly, Peter de Jonge, Yanling He, Hristo Hinkov, and Ronald C. Kessler

Introduction

While most of the chapters in this volume focus on the adverse effects of mental disorders on the people who have these disorders, it is also important to recognize that health problems can affect the family members of ill people. A considerable amount of research has been carried out on these adverse effects of health problems on family members. Family caregivers shoulder the vast majority of long-term care responsibilities worldwide without pay or compensation (Carter 2008). Widespread health trends such as longer life expectancy and prolonged survival with severely disabling conditions (Wiener 2003, Lee 2011) are steadily increasing the demand for informal care at the same time as sociodemographic trends such as delayed childbearing, smaller families, more divorce and remarriage, more female employment and dual-earner households, higher migration and globalization, and less intergenerational co-residency are reducing the supply of family caregivers (Heitmueller & Inglis 2007, Lamura et al. 2008). Changing healthcare policies (e.g., limiting hospital beds for chronic physical conditions, psychiatric deinstitutionalization) and escalating healthcare costs compound the demand for informal caregiving (Dosman & Keating 2005, Awad & Voruganti 2008). While this shift toward community care has enormous positive value from a societal perspective by sparing professional and economic resources, it presumably has negative consequences for the caregivers, including opportunity costs or forgone income, reduced quality of life, and increased stress-related conditions (Jacobzone 2000, Sales 2003, Carter 2008). Indeed, considerable research over the past several decades has documented numerous adverse impacts on caregivers, ranging from financial strain (Hickenbottom et al. 2002, Heitmueller & Inglis 2007) and depression (Pinquart & Sorensen 2003, Opree &

Kalmijn 2012) to excess mortality (Christakis & Allison 2006). Such impacts may importantly undermine the daily functioning of the caregivers themselves, and might also predict worse prognosis and costly institutionalization for care recipients (Lauber et al. 2005).

Given the dual importance of caregiving for both caregivers and care recipients, it is especially important to monitor or benchmark broad patterns in caregiver burden. However, most available research focuses narrowly on particular family conditions such as dementia (Torti et al. 2004, Wimo et al. 2007), stroke (Hickenbottom et al. 2002), or schizophrenia (Awad & Voruganti 2008) in geographically homogeneous samples. Such focused studies are invaluable resources regarding condition-specific and region-specific caregiver burdens, but cannot be used to generate reliable population-level estimates of total burden associated with the fuller range of mental and physical conditions occurring throughout the world population.

In the current chapter we extend prior epidemiologic research on caregiving by describing the prevalence and correlates of family burden associated with a wide range of first-degree-relative mental and physical health problems in the culturally diverse and geographically heterogeneous WMH samples, providing a broader perspective on the total magnitude of caregiver burden than previously available.

Methods

Sample

We analyzed data on caregiver burden collected in 20 of the 25 surveys considered in this volume. The surveys carried out in India–Pondicherry, Israel, PRC–Beijing/Shanghai, New Zealand, and South Africa were excluded

The Burdens of Mental Disorders, ed. Jordi Alonso, Somnath Chatterji, and Yanling He. Published by Cambridge University Press. © World Health Organization 2013.

because they did not assess family caregiver burden. As family burden was not a core focus of the WMH surveys, only a probability subsample of respondents in many of the remaining surveys were administered the family burden question series, as explained in detail in Chapter 2. They were administered to a random 15% of respondents in Portugal, and to random proportions ranging from 25% (in six surveys) to 100% (in five surveys). A total of $n = 43,732$ respondents were assessed for family burden across these countries.

Measures

The design of the WMH surveys did not lend itself to replicating the kinds of studies of family burden that have been implemented in the past, in which a sample of focal respondents with serious health problems is selected for study and the family members of these ill individuals are interviewed. This kind of approach would have required a completely separate design to generate a representative sample of the relatives of the WMH respondents who had serious health problems. As a result, we used a different approach to assessing family burden by treating WMH respondents as a representative sample of family caregivers rather than of the people with health problems. In order to do this, we asked WMH respondents if they had any first-degree relatives with serious mental or physical disorders and then assessed the burdens associated with caring for these family-member disorders in the subsample of respondents who reported having such family members.

Research on caregiving traditionally distinguishes between subjective burden (e.g., distress, embarrassment) and objective burden (most notably, time and money). We follow that custom in the current report (Hudson *et al.* 2010, Idstad *et al.* 2011). Once the conditions experienced by each first-degree relative were recorded, the burden associated with caregiving was assessed by asking respondents with at least one family member with at least one health problem: "Taking into consideration your time, energy, emotions, finances, and daily activities, would you say that (*his/her/their*) health problems affect your life a lot, some, a little, or not at all?" Only respondents who answered "a lot" or "some" were administered further questions about burden. The first two such questions asked about subjective burden: if their relatives' health problems caused them to be psychologically distressed (worried, anxious, or depressed) and if it caused them embarrassment

(response options to both questions were: a lot, some, a little, not at all). Objective burden was then assessed, initially exploring the type of help required (self-care such as washing, dressing, or eating; practical things like paperwork, getting around, housework, or taking medications; spending time keeping them company or giving them emotional support than would otherwise be the case; or spending any time doing other things), and inquiring about the amount of time spent with such help (number of hours spent currently in an average week). Respondents were also asked whether they had any financial burden (either money spent or earnings lost) due to their relatives' health problems and, if so, the average monthly amount spent during the past year. All financial expenses reported were compared to median monthly national household income and expressed as a proportion of median income within the country. This transformation allowed results to be pooled across countries for purposes of cross-national comparisons.

It is important to note that the questions about subjective and objective burden were all asked *in the aggregate*: that is, with regard to all the health problems of all the relatives reported. No attempt was made to have respondents with multiple family members having multiple health problems estimate the amount of distress or time or financial loss associated uniquely with condition X of family member Y. Instead, we asked respondents to report the overall levels of subjective and objective burden associated with providing informal caregiving for all the health problems experienced by all their first-degree relatives. However, as described below, we did carry out statistical analyses aimed at sorting out the relative effects of the different health problems of different family members on these measures of overall burden.

Five dichotomous outcome variables were included in the analysis (any burden, a lot/some psychological distress, a lot/some embarrassment, any time burden, and any financial burden), and two continuous variables (amount of time in hours spent and amount of financial burden as a proportion of median household income in the country).

Respondents were asked how many living parents, spouses, children, and siblings they had and whether each of them suffered from a series of serious mental and physical health problems. The health problems included four broadly defined classes of physical conditions (cancer, serious heart problems, permanent physical disability such as blindness or paralysis, and any other serious chronic physical illness) and eight classes of mental disorders (serious memory problems such as senility or dementia, mental retardation, alcohol- or drug-related problems, depression, anxiety, schizophrenia or psychosis, bipolar disorder, any other serious chronic mental problem). It is important to note that the final entry in each of these two sets asked about "any other serious" illness or problem. The logic here was to use the more concrete examples to help provide a nominal definition of the word "serious" in the final question in each series, while using the final question to obtain data about the great many other types of serious family-member health problems that we could not capture in a condition checklist of reasonable length.

Statistical analysis

Regression analysis was used to sort out the relative importance of different types of health problems experienced by different types of family members in accounting for each outcome in the subsample of respondents who reported having at least one first-degree relative with at least one of the health problems assessed. Predictors included count variables (coded 0–4) for number of types of relatives with each of the 12 health problems (i.e., 12 separate variables, each coded in the range 0–4), three count variables, each coded 0–12, for the number of types of health problems experienced by each of three types of relatives (parents, spouse, children, compared to the contrast category of siblings), and demographic controls (respondent age, sex, marital status, and education). All equations were estimated in all 20 countries combined and then separately in the three World Bank categories of low/lower-middle-income, upper-middle-income, and high-income countries (World Bank 2008).

Logistic regression analysis was used to predict dichotomous outcomes. Coefficients and standard errors were exponentiated to produce odds ratios (OR) with 95% confidence intervals (95% CI). Generalized linear models (GLMs) with a log link function and Poisson error variance structure were used to predict continuous outcomes. As in earlier chapters that used GLM, we explored a number of different model specifications and selected the log link/Poisson model based on standard fit comparisons. Coefficients and standard errors were exponentiated to produce incidence density ratios (IDR) with 95% confidence intervals. IDRs can be interpreted as ratios of expected scores on the continuous outcomes among respondents who differ by one point on the predictors. Population attributable risk proportions (PARPs) of the two continuous outcomes were calculated to characterize proportions of time and financial burden due to particular types of relatives and health problems. PARP can be interpreted as the proportion of burden that would be prevented if a particular subset of health problems were eliminated, based on the assumption that the regression coefficients represent causal effects (Northridge 1995). PARP was calculated with simulation methods described in Chapter 2 (Levinson *et al.* 2010). The design-based Jackknife Repeated Replication method (Wolter 1985) was used to adjust standard errors for the weighting and clustering of WMH data. Statistical significance was consistently evaluated using 0.05-level, two-sided design-based tests.

Results

Prevalence of family caregiving burden

More respondents reported serious health problems affecting their parents (12.8–22.0%) than spouses (1.9–5.7%), children (1.5–5.3%), or siblings (5.3–16.5%). Frequency was higher in more developed countries. Any serious mental or physical problem among first-degree relatives was reported by 18.9–40.3% of respondents across country groups in the total sample (Table 10.1). Mean number of problems among those reporting any was 1.5–1.8 across country income groups, with an overall mean (standard error) of 1.7 (0.02). Family physical conditions were reported by more respondents (15.2–30.6%) than mental health problems (6.3–19.0%) in the total sample. Among those with family health problems, serious physical conditions were reported by 67.7–80.4% and serious mental health problems by 33.1–53.5% of respondents. It is noteworthy that these results do not account for the number of family members a respondent actually had or the number of family members with serious health problems a respondent had at the time of interview. Among respondents who had ill relatives, almost 40% reported any burden in all country income groups. Regarding subjective burden, 23.3–27.1% of respondents with an ill relative experienced psychological distress and 6.0–17.2% reported embarrassment due to their family health problems. Objective burden was reported by 22.0–31.1% who devoted time and 10.6–18.8% who reported financial burden.

Table 10.1 Prevalence and reported burden of family health problems by country income level. The WMH surveys.

	Total sample								Subsample with family health problems							
	Total		Country income level						Total		Country income level					
			Low/lower-middle		Upper-middle		High				Low/lower-middle		Upper-middle		High	
	%	(SE)	%	(SE)	%	(SE)	%	(SE)	%	(SE)	%	(SE)	%	(SE)	%	(SE)
I. Prevalence of relatives with problems																
Parent	17.5	(0.2)	12.8	(0.4)	17.2	(0.4)	22.0	(0.4)	57.7	(0.5)	68.0	(1.1)	55.0	(0.9)	54.5	(0.7)
Spouse	3.9	(0.1)	1.9	(0.2)	4.0	(0.2)	5.7	(0.2)	12.9	(0.4)	10.3	(0.8)	12.7	(0.6)	14.0	(0.6)
Child	3.4	(0.1)	1.5	(0.1)	3.3	(0.2)	5.3	(0.2)	11.4	(0.3)	8.0	(0.6)	10.7	(0.6)	13.1	(0.5)
Sibling	11.6	(0.2)	5.3	(0.3)	12.9	(0.4)	16.5	(0.4)	38.1	(0.5)	28.4	(1.2)	41.2	(1.0)	40.8	(0.7)
II. Prevalence of family health problems																
Any mental	14.0	(0.2)	6.3	(0.3)	16.7	(0.4)	19.0	(0.4)	45.9	(0.5)	33.1	(1.2)	53.5	(1.2)	47.1	(0.7)
Any physical	22.9	(0.3)	15.2	(0.4)	21.1	(0.4)	30.6	(0.5)	74.6	(0.5)	80.4	(1.0)	67.7	(1.0)	75.9	(0.6)
Any mental or physical	30.6	(0.3)	18.9	(0.4)	31.2	(0.5)	40.3	(0.5)	—		—		—		—	
Mean number[a]	0.530	(0.007)	0.280	(0.009)	0.532	(0.009)	0.744	(0.015)	1.730	(0.015)	1.476	(0.020)	1.704	(0.020)	1.845	(0.024)
III. Burden of family health problems																
Any burden	12.1	(0.2)	7.5	(0.3)	12.2	(0.4)	15.9	(0.4)	39.1	(0.5)	39.6	(1.3)	39.0	(1.0)	39.0	(0.7)
Psychological distress[b]	7.7	(0.2)	5.1	(0.3)	8.4	(0.3)	9.5	(0.3)	25.1	(0.5)	27.1	(1.2)	27.0	(0.8)	23.3	(0.6)
Embarrassment[b]	2.9	(0.1)	1.6	(0.2)	5.4	(0.3)	2.4	(0.1)	9.5	(0.3)	8.6	(0.8)	17.2	(0.8)	6.0	(0.3)
Any time burden	8.3	(0.2)	5.9	(0.3)	6.9	(0.3)	11.3	(0.3)	26.8	(0.4)	31.1	(1.2)	22.0	(0.8)	27.6	(0.6)
Any financial burden	4.0	(0.1)	3.6	(0.2)	4.1	(0.2)	4.3	(0.2)	13.0	(0.3)	18.8	(0.9)	13.1	(0.7)	10.6	(0.4)
(n)	43,732		14,979		11,464		17,289		13,899		3,027		3,792		7,080	

[a] Mean number of family health problems out of 48 (12 types of problems for each of four types of family members).
[b] "A lot" or "some" distress or embarrassment reported in response to questions about intensity of these feelings.

Table 10.2 Individual-level and population-level time and financial burdens of family health problems by country income level. The WMH surveys.

	Country income level							
	All countries		Low/lower-middle		Upper-middle		High	
	Estimate	(SE)	Estimate	(SE)	Estimate	(SE)	Estimate	(SE)
I. Time (number of hours per week)								
Individual level (mean)[a]	13.9	(0.6)	12.9	(0.9)	16.5	(1.6)	13.3	(0.7)
Per 100 in the population (total)[b]	118.0	(1.2)	83.7	(2.8)	117.8	(1.6)	147.9	(2.2)
II. Financial (mean percent of median household income)								
Individual level[c]	24.0	(1.1)	44.1	(5.3)	32.2	(2.1)	15.1	(0.9)
Per 100 in the population[d]	1.01	(0.03)	1.81	(0.07)	1.09	(0.04)	0.50	(0.02)
(n_1)[e]		(3,680)		(969)		(820)		(1,891)
(n_2)[e]		(1,738)		(601)		(395)		(742)
(n_3)[e]		(43,732)		(14,979)		(11,464)		(17,289)

[a] Individual-level reports of hours per week spent with or doing things for ill family members.
[b] The population-level estimate was obtained by multiplying the individual-level estimate by the proportion of respondents who reported spending any time.
[c] Individual-level reports of financial burden were converted to percentages of median household income in the country. The means of these transformed scores among respondents who reported any financial burden are reported here. For example, the mean monthly financial impact of family illness (due either to out-of-pocket expenses or foregone income) across countries among respondents who reported such costs was equal to 24.0% of the median monthly household income in the country.
[d] The population-level estimate of financial burden was obtained by multiplying the individual-level estimate by the proportion of respondents who reported such burdens. The resulting estimate can be interpreted as the total financial costs of family health problems as a percentage of total household income in the country.
[e] n_1 = subsample of respondents who devoted any time to family health problems; n_2 = subsample of respondents with any financial burden due to family health problems (Romania was removed from the models for financial burden, as this aspect of burden was not assessed in Romania); n_3 = total sample, including respondents who had no family health problems.

Despite the likely conservative estimates of burden, as only serious health conditions affecting only first-degree relatives were assessed, mean caregiving hours/week among those devoting any time are considerable: 13.9 hours/week across all countries, slightly less in low/lower-middle-income countries (12.9) than in other countries (13.3–16.5) (Table 10.2). Population-level equivalents are 83.7–147.9 hours/week/100 people aged 18+ in the general population (which includes in the denominator those who do not have ill relatives and those with ill relatives who reported that this did not affect their lives). Mean financial burden among those reporting any is also substantial: equivalent to 24.0% of the median within-country family income, with lower estimates in high-income countries (15.1%) than in upper-middle-income countries (32.2%), and up to almost half (44.1%) of the median family income in low/lower-middle-income countries. Population-level equivalents are 0.50–1.81% of total sample-wide median family income among all people aged 18+ in the countries (which again includes in the denominator those who do not have ill relatives and those with ill relatives who reported that this did not affect their lives). The resulting estimates can be interpreted as the total financial costs of first-degree-relative serious health problems imposed on family caregivers as a percentage of total median household income in the country.

Sociodemographic correlates of family caregiving-associated burden

Sociodemographic correlates of family caregiving burden are reported in Table 10.3. Older cohorts (age 50–64) were more likely to spend any time and report any financial burden in caring for ill family members than younger cohorts (age 18–49) or the oldest

Table 10.3 Demographic correlates of family burden among respondents with family health problems by country income level. The WMH surveys.[a]

	Any burden		Psychological distress		Embarrassment		Any time burden		Any financial burden		Amount of time[b]		Amount of financial burden[c]	
	OR	(95% CI)	OR	(95% CI)	OR	(95% CI)	OR	(95% CI)	OR	(95% CI)	OR	(95% CI)	OR	(95% CI)
Age 18–34 (compared to 65+)														
All countries	0.9	(0.8–1.1)	1.0	(0.8–1.2)	1.1	(0.8–1.4)	1.0	(0.8–1.2)	0.9	(0.7–1.3)	0.6	(0.4–0.8)	0.6	(0.2–1.9)
Low/lower-middle-income countries	1.5	(0.9–2.5)	1.8	(1.0–3.4)	1.4	(0.6–3.0)	1.6	(0.9–2.6)	1.7	(0.8–3.4)	0.5*	(0.3–1.0)	0.3	(0.0–1.2)
Upper-middle-income countries	1.0	(0.7–1.3)	1.0	(0.7–1.5)	1.2	(0.8–1.7)	1.4	(1.0–2.0)	0.8	(0.4–1.6)	0.5	(0.2–0.9)	1.9	(0.7–5.2)
High-income countries	0.8	(0.6–1.1)	0.9	(0.6–1.2)	0.9	(0.6–1.4)	0.8	(0.6–1.0)	0.8	(0.5–1.2)	0.7	(0.4–1.0)	1.8*	(1.0–3.4)
Age 35–49 (compared to 65+)														
All countries	1.1	(0.9–1.3)	1.1	(0.9–1.3)	1.1	(0.9–1.4)	1.2	(1.0–1.4)	1.1	(0.8–1.4)	0.6*	(0.5–0.8)	1.1	(0.6–2.2)
Low/lower-middle-income countries	1.4	(0.9–2.2)	1.7	(0.9–3.0)	1.4	(0.7–2.9)	1.5	(0.9–2.6)	1.9*	(1.0–3.6)	0.7	(0.4–1.2)	0.5	(0.2–1.6)
Upper-middle-income countries	1.2	(0.9–1.6)	1.1	(0.8–1.6)	1.2	(0.8–1.7)	1.4	(1.0–2.1)	1.0	(0.6–1.9)	0.6*	(0.4–1.0)	2.2	(0.6–7.5)
High-income countries	1.0	(0.8–1.3)	1.0	(0.8–1.2)	1.0	(0.7–1.6)	1.0	(0.8–1.3)	1.0	(0.7–1.3)	0.6	(0.4–0.9)	1.6	(1.0–2.6)
Age 50–64 (compared to 65+)														
All countries	1.1	(0.9–1.2)	1.1	(0.9–1.3)	1.0	(0.8–1.2)	1.2*	(1.0–1.4)	1.2*	(1.0–1.6)	0.7*	(0.6–0.9)	0.6	(0.4–1.2)
Low/lower-middle-income countries	1.1	(0.7–1.8)	1.4	(0.7–2.5)	1.0	(0.5–2.0)	1.4	(0.9–2.4)	1.7	(0.9–3.0)	0.7	(0.4–1.2)	0.3	(0.1–1.4)
Upper-middle-income countries	1.0	(0.8–1.4)	1.1	(0.7–1.5)	1.1	(0.8–1.4)	1.4*	(1.1–2.0)	1.0	(0.6–1.7)	1.0	(0.7–1.4)	1.0	(0.6–1.6)
High-income countries	1.1	(0.9–1.4)	1.1	(0.9–1.4)	0.9	(0.7–1.3)	1.2	(0.9–1.4)	1.3*	(1.0–1.8)	0.7*	(0.5–1.0)	1.3	(0.8–2.2)
Female (compared to male)														
All countries	1.5*	(1.4–1.6)	1.6*	(1.4–1.8)	1.1	(1.0–1.4)	1.4*	(1.3–1.6)	1.0	(0.9–1.1)	1.4*	(1.2–1.6)	0.8	(0.5–1.2)
Low/lower-middle-income countries	1.2*	(1.0–1.5)	1.2	(1.0–1.6)	0.7	(0.4–1.0)	1.2	(1.0–1.4)	0.7	(0.6–0.9)	1.5*	(1.2–1.9)	0.5	(0.3–1.0)
Upper-middle-income countries	1.8*	(1.4–2.1)	2.0*	(1.6–2.5)	1.6*	(1.2–2.1)	1.8*	(1.4–2.2)	1.4*	(1.0–1.9)	1.2	(0.9–1.6)	1.0	(0.6–1.9)
High-income countries	1.5*	(1.3–1.7)	1.6*	(1.4–1.8)	1.0	(0.8–1.3)	1.4*	(1.2–1.6)	1.0	(0.8–1.3)	1.3*	(1.1–1.6)	1.1	(0.8–1.4)
Never married (compared to married)														
All countries	1.1	(1.0–1.2)	1.1	(1.0–1.3)	1.1	(0.9–1.4)	1.2*	(1.0–1.3)	0.8	(0.7–1.1)	0.9	(0.7–1.2)	1.0	(0.5–1.9)
Low/lower-middle-income countries	1.2	(0.9–1.6)	1.3	(1.0–1.8)	1.7*	(1.1–2.6)	1.3	(1.0–1.7)	0.8	(0.5–1.3)	1.3	(0.9–1.8)	0.7	(0.3–2.0)
Upper-middle-income countries	1.0	(0.8–1.3)	0.9	(0.7–1.2)	0.8	(0.6–1.1)	1.1	(0.9–1.4)	0.8	(0.5–1.2)	0.8	(0.4–1.4)	1.9*	(1.2–3.2)
High-income countries	1.1	(0.9–1.3)	1.1	(0.9–1.4)	1.1	(0.8–1.7)	1.2	(1.0–1.4)	1.0	(0.7–1.3)	0.8	(0.6–1.1)	1.2	(0.7–2.0)

Table 10.3 (cont.)

	Any burden		Psychological distress		Embarrassment		Any time burden		Any financial burden		Amount of time[b]		Amount of financial burden[c]	
	OR	(95% CI)	OR	(95% CI)	OR	(95% CI)	OR	(95% CI)	OR	(95% CI)	OR	(95% CI)	OR	(95% CI)
Previously married (compared to married)														
All countries	0.8	(0.7–0.9)	0.9	(0.7–1.0)	1.0	(0.7–1.3)	0.8*	(0.7–0.9)	0.7	(0.6–0.9)	0.9	(0.7–1.2)	0.8	(0.3–2.1)
Low/lower-middle-income countries	1.4	(0.9–2.0)	1.3	(0.8–2.0)	1.7	(0.8–3.7)	1.2	(0.8–1.9)	0.6	(0.3–1.2)	1.2	(0.6–2.4)	0.6	(0.2–2.5)
Upper-middle-income countries	0.9	(0.7–1.2)	0.9	(0.7–1.3)	0.8	(0.5–1.2)	1.1	(0.8–1.5)	0.7	(0.4–1.1)	0.7	(0.4–1.4)	2.2*	(1.0–4.8)
High-income countries	0.7	(0.6–0.8)	0.8	(0.6–0.9)	1.1	(0.8–1.7)	0.6*	(0.5–0.8)	0.8	(0.6–1.1)	0.9	(0.6–1.2)	0.6	(0.3–1.1)
Education[d]														
All countries	1.0	(1.0–1.0)	1.0	(1.0–1.0)	1.0	(0.9–1.0)	1.0	(1.0–1.1)	1.1*	(1.0–1.1)	1.0	(1.0–1.0)	1.0	(0.9–1.1)
Low/lower-middle-income countries	1.0	(0.9–1.0)	1.0	(0.9–1.0)	0.9	(0.8–1.0)	1.0	(0.9–1.1)	1.0	(0.9–1.1)	1.0	(0.9–1.1)	1.0	(0.8–1.2)
Upper-middle-income countries	1.0	(1.0–1.0)	1.0	(1.0–1.1)	1.0	(0.9–1.0)	1.0	(0.9–1.1)	1.0	(1.0–1.1)	1.0	(0.9–1.0)	1.0	(0.8–1.3)
High-income countries	1.0	(1.0–1.1)	1.0	(1.0–1.1)	0.9	(0.9–1.0)	1.1*	(1.0–1.1)	1.1*	(1.0–1.2)	1.0	(0.9–1.1)	1.1	(0.9–1.3)

[a] Based on multivariate models (logistic for dichotomous outcomes; GLM for continuous outcomes with log link function and Poisson error distribution) with predictors that included a separate count variable (coded 0–4) for the number of types of relatives with each of the 12 health problems, a separate count variable (coded 0–12) for the number of types of health problems experienced by each of three types of relatives (parents, spouse, children, compared to the implicit contrast category of siblings), and demographic controls (respondent age, sex, marital status, and level of educational attainment). All equations were estimated in a pooled dataset across either the entire set of 19 countries or in high-income, upper-middle-income, and low/lower-middle-income countries. Romania was removed from the models for financial burden, as this aspect of burden was not assessed in Romania.
[b] Amount of time among those devoting any time.
[c] Amount of financial burden among those with any.
[d] Coded in the range 1–7 (1 = no education, 7 = college graduate).
* Significant at the 0.05 level, two-sided test.

respondents (65+), but all younger age groups reported spending less time on family health problems than older respondents (65+), with ORs in the range 0.5–0.7. With the exception of amount of financial burden, which showed no differences by sex, women reported significantly more burden than men on all indicators of family burden associated with caregiving, with ORs in the range 1.2–2.0. These differences by sex are relatively consistent across country income groups. The highest female-to-male ORs are related to reporting significantly more distress (OR = 1.6 [95% CI 1.4–1.8] to 2.0 [95% CI 1.6–2.5]), any burden (OR = 1.2 [95% CI 1.0–1.5] to 1.8 [95% CI 1.4–2.1]), and any time (OR = 1.2 [95% CI 1.0–1.4] to 1.8 [95% CI 1.4–2.2]) due to family health conditions. There are no consistent patterns related to marital status predicting burden, although those never married reported more embarrassment (OR = 1.7, 95% CI 1.1–2.6) in low/lower-middle-income countries and higher amount of financial expenditure (OR = 1.9, 95% CI 1.2–3.2) in upper-middle-income countries than married respondents; and those previously married reported less time burden (OR = 0.6, 95% CI 0.5–0.8) in high-income countries and higher amount of financial expenditure (OR = 2.2, 95% CI 1.0–4.8) in upper-middle-income countries compared to married respondents. Education is significantly related to time and financial burden only in high-income countries, but with quite small ORs (1.1).

Variations in burden by type of ill relative and health problem

Total-sample multivariate models show that spouse and child health problems are associated with highest burden, parents' health problems with intermediate burden, and sibling problems with lowest burden across all indicators of burden associated with caregiving (Table 10.4). The only exception is amount of financial expenditure, where type of ill relative is not significant. This pattern is consistent for high-income and upper-middle-income country groups, while for low/lower-middle-income countries, only children's health problems are consistently associated with all burden outcomes.

Significant variation in family burden is also related to type of health problems (Table 10.5). Regarding mental disorders, serious memory problem, mental retardation, depression, and anxiety are associated with increased odds of several burden

outcomes, with ORs in the range of 1.2–1.7. Family alcohol/drug-related problems is the only condition associated with reduced odds of devoting any time (OR = 0.8, 95% CI 0.6–0.9), and reporting financial burden (OR = 0.8, 95% CI 0.7–1.0) and reduced magnitude of time devoted (OR = 0.7, 95% CI 0.6–0.8), but also with elevated odds for reporting embarrassment (OR = 1.7, 95% CI 1.5–2.0). Furthermore, anxiety is associated with significantly lower amounts of time spent among people who devote any time (OR = 0.8, 95% CI 0.6–0.9). Physical conditions, overall, are not related to reporting embarrassment. Cancer and permanent physical disability are the conditions associated with more family burden indicators, with ORs in the range 1.2–2.1. The conditions significantly associated with reporting any burden are cancer (OR = 1.2, 95% CI 1.0–1.3), physical disability (OR = 1.2, 95% CI 1.0–1.4), serious memory problem (OR = 1.5, 95% CI 1.2–1.8), mental retardation (OR = 1.3, 95% CI 1.0–1.6), and depression (OR = 1.2, 95% CI 1.0–1.3). The health conditions associated with devoting any time are cancer (OR = 1.3, 95% CI 1.1–1.5), permanent physical disability (OR = 1.5, 95% CI 1.3–1.7), other serious chronic physical illness (OR = 1.2, 95% CI 1.1–1.4), and serious memory problem (OR = 1.7, 95% CI 1.4–2.0). Having a family member with heart problems is associated with lower embarrassment (OR = 0.8, 95% CI 0.6–0.9).

Population attributable risk proportions (PARPs)

As noted above, PARP can be interpreted as the percentage of all burden of a particular type in the population that can be attributed to a particular condition or set of conditions. PARPS are consistently highest for caring for parent health problems in all country income groups, for both amount of time (26.9–31.4%) and financial resources (31.0–35.2%) devoted (Table 10.6). It is noteworthy that this is true despite the fact that parent health problems were not found to be associated with the highest levels of burden at the individual level. The reason for the discrepancy is that PARP takes into consideration both individual-level strength of associations and distributions of the predictors. Parent health problems have the highest PARPs because they are both commonly occurring, compared to the health problems of other relatives, and impactful.

Table 10.4 Differential burdens of family health problems by type of relative and by country income level. The WMH surveys.[a]

	Total		Low/lower-middle		Upper-middle		High	
	Est[b]	(95% CI)	Est[b]	(95% CI)	Est[b]	(95% CI)	Est[b]	(95% CI)
I. Any burden (compared to siblings)								
Parent	1.4*	(1.3–1.4)	1.2	(1.0–1.5)	1.3*	(1.2–1.5)	1.4*	(1.3–1.5)
Spouse	2.0*	(1.8–2.3)	1.1	(0.8–1.5)	1.9*	(1.5–2.3)	2.4*	(2.1–2.8)
Child	1.9*	(1.7–2.1)	3.6*	(2.3–5.8)	2.0*	(1.5–2.6)	1.8*	(1.6–2.0)
χ^2_3	245.3*		31.2*		57.1*		204.7*	
II. Distress (compared to siblings)								
Parent	1.3*	(1.2–1.4)	1.2*	(1.0–1.4)	1.3*	(1.2–1.5)	1.3*	(1.2–1.4)
Spouse	1.7*	(1.5–2.0)	1.1	(0.8–1.3)	1.8*	(1.4–2.2)	1.9*	(1.6–2.2)
Child	1.9*	(1.7–2.1)	3.8*	(2.5–5.8)	1.9*	(1.5–2.5)	1.8*	(1.6–2.0)
χ^2_3	183.6*		38.1*		55.5*		120.9*	
III. Embarrassment (compared to siblings)								
Parent	1.3*	(1.1–1.4)	1.1	(0.8–1.4)	1.3*	(1.1–1.5)	1.4*	(1.1–1.7)
Spouse	1.6*	(1.4–1.9)	1.0	(0.8–1.3)	1.7*	(1.4–2.2)	1.9*	(1.6–2.4)
Child	1.7*	(1.5–1.9)	1.7*	(1.1–2.6)	1.8*	(1.4–2.3)	1.8*	(1.4–2.1)
χ^2_3	86.7*		6.5		49.3*		54.3*	
IV. Any time burden (compared to siblings)								
Parent	1.4*	(1.3–1.5)	1.2	(1.0–1.5)	1.3*	(1.1–1.5)	1.5*	(1.3–1.6)
Spouse	1.9*	(1.6–2.1)	1.0	(0.8–1.3)	1.8*	(1.4–2.2)	2.3*	(2.0–2.6)
Child	1.7*	(1.5–1.9)	3.0*	(1.8–5.0)	1.6*	(1.2–2.0)	1.6*	(1.4–1.9)
χ^2_3	180.4*		20.1*		38.3*		145.1*	
V. Any financial burden (compared to siblings)								
Parent	1.3*	(1.1–1.4)	1.1	(0.9–1.4)	1.3*	(1.1–1.6)	1.4*	(1.2–1.6)
Spouse	2.3*	(2.0–2.7)	1.0	(0.8–1.3)	2.5*	(1.8–3.4)	2.9*	(2.4–3.4)
Child	2.2*	(1.9–2.5)	3.0*	(1.8–4.9)	2.0*	(1.5–2.6)	2.3*	(1.9–2.7)
χ^2_3	195.8*		19.3*		45.7*		170.7*	
VI. Amount of time (among those devoting any time)								
Parent	1.1*	(1.0–1.2)	1.4*	(1.2–1.7)	1.1	(0.9–1.4)	1.1	(0.9–1.2)
Spouse	1.3*	(1.1–1.5)	1.0	(0.8–1.4)	1.3	(1.0–1.7)	1.4*	(1.1–1.6)
Child	1.4*	(1.2–1.6)	1.6*	(1.2–2.0)	1.2	(1.0–1.5)	1.4*	(1.2–1.7)
F_3	10.7*		9.9*		1.9		12.1*	
VII. Amount of financial burden (among those with any)								
Parent	1.0	(0.7–1.4)	1.0	(0.7–1.5)	0.8	(0.7–1.1)	0.9	(0.8–1.2)
Spouse	0.7*	(0.6–1.0)	0.4*	(0.2–0.7)	1.1	(0.8–1.5)	1.0	(0.8–1.3)
Child	1.0	(0.8–1.2)	1.3	(0.9–2.0)	0.9	(0.7–1.2)	1.1	(0.9–1.4)
F_3	2.1		4.6*		0.7		1.2	
$(n_1)^c$	13,899		3,027		3,792		7,080	
$(n_2)^c$	3,680		969		820		1,891	
$(n_3)^c$	1,738		601		395		742	

[a] Based on multivariate models (logistic for dichotomous outcomes; GLM for continuous outcomes with log link function and Poisson error distribution) with predictors that included a separate count variable (coded 0–4) for the number of types of relatives with each of the 12 health problems, a separate count variable (coded 0–12) for the number of types of health problems experienced by each of three types of relatives (parents, spouse, children, compared to the implicit contrast category of siblings), and demographic controls (respondent age, sex, marital status, and level of educational attainment). All equations were estimated in a pooled dataset across either the entire set of 19 countries or in the high, upper-middle, and low/lower-middle-income countries. Romania was removed from the models for financial burden, as this aspect of burden was not assessed in Romania.
[b] Coefficient estimates (Est) are odds ratios for the first five outcomes (I–V), all of which are dichotomies, and incidence density ratios for the last two outcomes (VI–VII), which are continuous.
[c] n_1 = total subsample of respondents with family health problems; n_2 = subsample of respondents who devoted any time to family health problems; n_3 = subsample of respondents with any financial burden due to family health problems.
* Significant at the 0.05 level, two-sided test.

Table 10.5 Differential burdens of family health problems by type of problem in the total sample (n = 13,899). The WMH surveys.[a]

	Any burden		Psychological distress		Embarrassment		Any time burden		Any financial burden		Amount of time		Amount of financial burden	
	OR	(95% CI)	OR	(95% CI)	OR	(95% CI)	OR	(95% CI)	OR	(95% CI)	IDR[b]	(95% CI)	IDR[b]	(95% CI)
I. Mental disorder														
Serious memory problem	1.5*	(1.2–1.8)	1.3*	(1.1–1.5)	1.4*	(1.0–1.8)	1.7*	(1.4–2.0)	1.2	(0.9–1.5)	1.0	(0.8–1.3)	0.7	(0.4–1.3)
Mental retardation	1.3*	(1.0–1.6)	1.2	(1.0–1.5)	1.1	(0.8–1.5)	1.4*	(1.1–1.7)	1.7*	(1.3–2.2)	1.2	(1.0–1.5)	0.6	(0.4–1.1)
Alcohol/drug problem	1.0	(0.9–1.2)	1.1	(1.0–1.2)	1.7*	(1.5–2.0)	0.8*	(0.6–0.9)	0.8*	(0.7–1.0)	0.7*	(0.6–0.8)	1.2	(0.7–2.0)
Depression	1.2*	(1.0–1.3)	1.2*	(1.0–1.4)	1.4*	(1.1–1.7)	1.2*	(1.0–1.4)	1.0	(0.8–1.3)	1.0	(0.9–1.2)	1.5*	(1.1–2.0)
Anxiety	1.1	(1.0–1.3)	1.2*	(1.1–1.4)	0.9	(0.7–1.2)	1.1	(0.9–1.3)	0.9	(0.7–1.1)	0.8*	(0.6–0.9)	1.5*	(1.0–2.0)
Schizophrenia/psychosis	1.0	(0.7–1.3)	1.0	(0.7–1.3)	1.4	(0.9–2.2)	1.0	(0.7–1.3)	1.1	(0.7–1.7)	1.1	(0.8–1.5)	1.1	(0.4–2.9)
Bipolar disorder	1.0	(0.7–1.3)	0.7	(0.5–1.0)	1.1	(0.7–1.9)	1.0	(0.7–1.4)	1.0	(0.6–1.5)	0.8	(0.6–1.0)	1.1	(0.3–3.6)
Other serious chronic mental problem	1.1	(0.9–1.4)	1.1	(0.8–1.4)	1.1	(0.7–1.6)	1.3	(1.0–1.6)	1.6*	(1.2–2.2)	1.3	(1.0–1.6)	0.8	(0.4–1.5)
χ^2_8/F_3[c]	37.9*		31.9*		58.5*		78.7*		40.5*		3.7*		7.6*	
χ^2_{12}/F_{12}[c]	42.0*		34.1*		111.6*		112.9*		49.5*		3.3*		8.0*	
II. Physical condition														
Cancer	1.2*	(1.0–1.3)	1.2*	(1.1–1.4)	1.0	(0.8–1.2)	1.3*	(1.1–1.5)	1.0	(0.8–1.2)	1.1	(0.9–1.4)	2.1*	(1.2–3.7)
Serious heart problems	1.1	(1.0–1.2)	1.1*	(1.0–1.3)	0.8*	(0.6–0.9)	1.0	(0.9–1.2)	1.0	(0.9–1.2)	1.0	(0.8–1.1)	1.3	(1.0–1.7)
Permanent physical disability	1.2*	(1.0–1.4)	1.2	(1.0–1.3)	1.1	(0.9–1.4)	1.5*	(1.3–1.7)	1.3*	(1.1–1.6)	1.2	(1.0–1.4)	1.1	(0.7–1.8)
Other serious chronic physical illness	1.1	(1.0–1.2)	1.1	(1.0–1.2)	0.8	(0.7–1.0)	1.2*	(1.1–1.4)	1.2*	(1.0–1.4)	0.9	(0.8–1.1)	0.8	(0.5–1.3)
χ^2_4	10.1*		13.0*		13.2*		46.1*		11.7*		2.3		2.9*	

[a] Based on multivariate models (logistic for dichotomous outcomes; GLM for continuous outcomes with log link function and Poisson error distribution) with predictors that included a separate count variable (coded 0–4) for the number of types of relatives with each of the 12 health problems, a separate count variable (coded 0–12) for the number of types of health problems experienced by each of three types of relatives (parents, spouse, children, compared to the implicit contrast category of siblings), and demographic controls (respondent age, sex, marital status, and level of educational attainment). All equations were estimated in a pooled dataset across the entire set of 19 countries. Romania was removed from the models for financial burden, as this aspect of burden was not assessed in Romania. Parallel tables for high-income, upper-middle-income, and low/lower-middle-income countries are not presented but are available on request.

[b] IDR: incidence density ratio.

[c] χ^2 tests were used for the first five (dichotomous) outcomes and F tests for the last two (continuous) outcomes.

* Significant at the 0.05 level, two-sided test.

Table 10.6 Significant population attributable risk proportions (PARPs) of time and financial burdens due to family health problems by country income level. The WMH surveys.

	Country income level							
	Total		Low/lower-middle		Upper-middle		High	
	Time burden	Financial burden	Time burden	Financial burden	Time burden	Financial burden	Time burden	Financial burden
	PARP (%)[a]	PARP (%)[a]	PARP (%)[a]	PARP (%)[a]	PARP (%)[a]	PARP (%)[a]	PARP (%)[a]	PARP (%)[a]
I. Type of relative								
Parent	28.4	31.9	31.4	31.0	26.9	31.6	27.8	35.2
Spouse	17.0	10.4	11.5	9.3	18.6	13.6	18.7	10.3
Child	17.5	14.5	16.9	13.2	17.7	16.7	17.6	15.8
Sibling	2.5	10.2	3.0	10.2	1.8	9.7	2.6	10.6
II. Type of health problem								
Mental[b]	27.7	26.9	22.4	20.7	28.7	36.8	29.6	35.5
Physical[c]	44.5	47.3	46.0	47.8	44.0	45.8	44.1	47.6
(n)		(13,899)		(3,027)		(3,792)		(7,080)

[a] The numbers presented represent the % increase in time/money spent when the given conditions are present (for example, there is a 28.4 increase in time spent when parent burdens are accounted for vs. when they are taken completely out).
[b] All mental conditions include serious memory problems, mental retardation, alcohol/drug, depression, anxiety, schizophrenia or psychosis, bipolar disorder, other serious chronic mental problems (8 total).
[c] All physical conditions include cancer, serious heart problems, permanent physical disability, other serious chronic physical illness (4 total).

Similarly, sibling health problems were associated with smallest PARPs in all country groups, less for time devoted (1.8–3.0%) than for financial burden (9.7–10.6%). This reflects the joint occurrence of low prevalence and low individual-level effects of sibling health problems. In high-income and upper-middle-income countries, PARPs related to time devoted to health problems of spouses (18.6–18.7%) and children (17.6–17.7%) were similar, but were greater for children (15.8–16.7%) than for spouses (10.3–13.6%) where financial burden is concerned. In low/lower-middle-income countries, PARPs associated with both time and financial resources are greater for children (16.9%; 13.2%) compared to spouses (11.5%; 9.3%). Despite these between-relative differences in PARPs, the health problems of parents, spouses, and children all have meaningful PARPs with time and/or financial burden for these sets of relatives, accounting for meaningful components of burden in all three country groups.

Another consistent pattern is that PARPs associated with physical disorders are higher than those associated with mental disorders in all country income groups (44.0–47.8% vs. 20.7–36.8%). However, the comparative importance of mental disorders is much higher than that expected from relative prevalence, which might be explained by the generally higher individual-level associations of mental disorders (especially mental retardation, serious memory problems, and depression) than physical disorders with most burden dimensions. In other words, physical disorders are more important than mental disorders in terms of PARP because of their higher prevalence, not because of higher individual-level effects.

It is noteworthy that the sums of PARP estimates across types of relative are consistently less than 100 (varying from 62.8 to 71.9) and the sums of PARP estimates across types of illness vary from 72.2 to 83.1. This is due to the fact that PARP estimates were calculated one at a time for individual conditions that in many cases overlapped in their occurrence with other conditions. This pattern indicates that the joint effects of compound caregiving on burden are not completely captured in the disorder-specific and relative-specific PARP estimates computed here.

Discussion

The results reported here indicate that the caregiving burdens associated with serious family mental and physical conditions are substantial in the 19 countries considered. Although the magnitude and characteristics of burden are broadly consistent with the previous reports on burden associated with more specific health conditions (Hickenbottom *et al.* 2002, Wimo *et al.* 2007, Awad & Voruganti 2008), our results are unique in providing population-level estimates of subjective and objective burden associated with the full range of health problems affecting first-degree relatives that people considered to be serious. The magnitudes of these population-level estimates are stunning. Concerning financial burden, the 3.6% of people in low/lower-middle-income countries who report financial burden associated with caregiving for ill relatives devote up to 44% of median household income to these activities, and 32% in upper-middle-income countries (among those 4.1% reporting this burden). The population-level equivalent financial burden of informal family caregiving is estimated to be, respectively, 1.8% and 1.1% of total household income in the country. These population-level estimates are helpful in assessing the magnitude of the objective burden associated with informal family caregiving. An earlier analysis of family caregiver burden among older caregivers (50+) assessed within part of the same sampling frame (Shahly *et al.* 2012) found that, on individual-level analyses across country income groups, older family caregivers were more likely to devote time and less likely to spend money, possibly as a result of their age-related condition, i.e., being retired and having grown-up children.

As noted in the introduction, women have traditionally been responsible for caring for ill family members in most cultures (Mendez-Luck *et al.* 2008, Javadpour *et al.* 2009, Wells *et al.* 2009). It is notable in this regard that we found women are more burdened than men with family caregiving demands regarding time, and also experience the greatest subjective burdens associated with caregiving. These findings are consistent with previous, more focused studies of caregivers of relatives with one particular type of condition (Navaie-Waliser *et al.* 2002, Torti *et al.* 2004, Pinquart & Sorensen 2006). It is interesting that we found higher psychological distress related to family caregiving among women than men, with higher ORs than for other dimensions of burden. This means that it is not merely that women devote more time and that the time itself is the key determinant of the distress and other psychological burdens experienced by female caregivers. Instead, we find implicitly that female

caregivers are more likely to experience subjective burden than male caregivers who devote the same amounts of time and money to their ill relatives. The only exception to this pattern is the magnitude of financial expenditure, as, compared to men, women are less likely to be employed and more likely to earn less on the same jobs and raise children alone (Jutting *et al.* 2008, World Bank 2012).

As reported in previous studies, there was evidence that family mental health conditions were associated with higher family burden than were physical conditions *at the individual level* (Hastrup *et al.* 2011, Pinquart & Sorensen 2011); that is, in comparing the likelihood of a given caregiver experiencing burden as a function of whether the relative's illness was a mental disorder or a physical disorder. This finding is especially striking, given that the analysis was biased against finding between-condition differences in burden (since we asked respondents to tell us only about *serious* relative health problems) and we would expect this truncation of the severity distribution to reduce evidence of between-condition differences in burden. The results were different at the societal level, however, where we found that physical health problems were more important than mental health problems in the aggregate, due to the much higher prevalence of the former than the latter.

In a similar way, although we found, consistent with previous research (Chumbler *et al.* 2003, Pinquart & Sorensen 2011), that the individual-level burden of the health conditions of spouses and children was higher than that of the health conditions of parents or siblings, the societal-level burden was most strongly associated with the conditions of parents. This higher importance of parents at the population level reflects the fact that parent illnesses requiring assistance are more common than those of other first-degree relatives. It is worth emphasizing that family alcohol- and drug-related problems were the only conditions associated with reduced objective burden and with higher embarrassment, possibly reflecting the common view of substance abuse as a stigmatized social problem, rather than as a health-related condition.

The results must be interpreted in the context of several study limitations. People with the greatest caregiver burden might have been less likely than others to participate in the survey because of the demands on their time, in which case our estimates of caregiver burden would be conservative. As respondents were asked to report only on self-defined *serious* family health problems that occurred only to first-degree relatives, some unknown proportion of overall caregiver burden was excluded from analysis. Finally, the broader focus of this study design did not allow in-depth explorations of other important aspects of family caregiving and associated burden, such as the impact on the caregiver's quality of life, physical health, or stress-buffering supports that have been the focus of other studies (Pinquart & Sorensen 2003, Torti *et al.* 2004, Knight & Sayegh 2010, Opree & Kalmijn 2012). Finally, the WMH surveys did not collect data on the number of family members a respondent had and/or lived with, the extent of relatives that were encompassed within the core family in different countries, or the number of family members of a given type with a particular type of illness, imposing restrictions on the extent to which we could carry out fine-grained analyses of complex caregiving situations.

Notwithstanding the foregoing limitations, this study provides robust evidence for the existence of substantial burden across a wide range of countries associated with informal family caregivers of first-degree relatives having serious health problems. Such uncompensated family caregiving has tremendous value from a public health perspective by way of offsetting the costs and services of expensive and critically shorthanded healthcare professionals. It is consequently vital from a societal perspective to maintain the functional integrity of the informal family caregiving system. But results such as those presented here, documenting as they do high and perhaps ultimately unsustainable levels of caregiver burden, should raise serious concerns among policy makers. This is all the more true given widespread demographic trends persistently moving in a direction predictive of increased demands on the world's informal family caregivers. It is therefore crucial that we continue to refine our understanding of the correlations and magnitude of caregiver burden, and develop, implement, evaluate, and sustain effective interventions to reduce these burdens in an effort to guarantee the continued integrity of the informal family caregiving system.

Acknowledgments

Portions of this chapter are based on Viana, M. C., Gruber, M. J., Shahly, V., *et al.* (in press). Family burden related to mental and physical illness in the world: results from the WHO World Mental Health Surveys. *Revista Brasileira de Psiquiatria.* © 2012. Reproduced with permission.

References

Awad, A. G., & Voruganti, L. N. (2008). The burden of schizophrenia on caregivers: a review. *Pharmacoeconomics* **26**, 149–62.

Carter, R. (2008). Addressing the caregiving crisis. *Preventing Chronic Disease* **5** (1), A02.

Christakis, N. A., & Allison, P. D. (2006). Mortality after the hospitalization of a spouse. *New England Journal of Medicine* **354**, 719–30.

Chumbler, N. R., Grimm, J. W., Cody, M., & Beck, C. (2003). Gender, kinship and caregiver burden: the case of community-dwelling memory impaired seniors. *International Journal of Geriatric Psychiatry* **18**, 722–32.

Dosman, D., & Keating, N. (2005). Cheaper for whom? Costs experienced by formal caregivers in adult family living programs. *Journal of Aging and Social Policy* **17**, 67–83.

Hastrup, L. H., Van Den, B. B., & Gyrd-Hansen, D. (2011). Do informal caregivers in mental illness feel more burdened? A comparative study of mental versus somatic illnesses. *Scandinavian Journal of Public Health* **39**, 598–607.

Heitmueller, A., & Inglis, K. (2007). The earnings of informal carers: wage differentials and opportunity costs. *Journal of Health Economics* **26**, 821–41.

Hickenbottom, S. L., Fendrick, A. M., Kutcher, J. S., *et al.* (2002). A national study of the quantity and cost of informal caregiving for the elderly with stroke. *Neurology* **58**, 1754–9.

Hudson, P. L., Trauer, T., Graham, S., *et al.* (2010). A systematic review of instruments related to family caregivers of palliative care patients. *Palliative Medicine* **24**, 656–68.

Idstad, M., Roysamb, E., & Tambs, K. (2011). The effect of change in mental disorder status on change in spousal mental health: the HUNT study. *Social Science and Medicine* **73**, 1408–15.

Jacobzone, S. (2000). Coping with aging: international challenges. *Health Affairs (Project Hope)* **19**, 213–25.

Javadpour, A., Ahmadzadeh, L., & Bahredar, M. J. (2009). An educative support group for female family caregivers: impact on caregivers psychological distress and patient's neuropsychiatry symptoms. *International Journal of Geriatric Psychiatry* **24**, 469–71.

Jutting, J. P., Morrisson, C., Dayton-Johnson, J., & Drechsler, D. (2008). Measuring gender (in)equality: the OECD Gender, Institutions and Development Data Base. *Journal of Human Development* **9**, 65–86.

Knight, B. G., & Sayegh, P. (2010). Cultural values and caregiving: the updated sociocultural stress and coping model. *Journals of Gerontology Series B* **65B**, 5–13.

Lamura, G., Mnich, E., Nolan, M., *et al.* (2008). Family carers' experiences using support services in Europe: empirical evidence from the EUROFAMCARE study. *The Gerontologist* **48**, 752–71.

Lauber, C., Keller, C., Eichenberger, A., & Rössler, W. (2005). Family burden during exacerbation of schizophrenia: quantification and determinants of additional costs. *International Journal of Social Psychiatry* **51**, 259–64.

Lee, R. (2011). The outlook for population growth. *Science* **333**, 569–73.

Levinson, D., Lakoma, M. D., Petukhova, M., *et al.* (2010). Associations of serious mental illness with earnings: results from the WHO World Mental Health surveys. *British Journal of Psychiatry* **197**, 114–21.

Mendez-Luck, C. A., Kennedy, D. P., & Wallace, S. P. (2008). Concepts of burden in giving care to older relatives: a study of female caregivers in a Mexico City neighborhood. *Journal of Cross Cultural Gerontology* **23**, 265–82.

Navaie-Waliser, M., Spriggs, A., & Feldman, P. H. (2002). Informal caregiving: differential experiences by gender. *Medical Care* **40**, 1249–59.

Northridge, M. E. (1995). Public health methods: attributable risk as a link between causality and public health action. *American Journal of Public Health* **85**, 1202–4.

Opree, S. J., & Kalmijn, M. (2012). Exploring causal effects of combining work and care responsibilities on depressive symptoms among middle-aged women. *Ageing and Society*, **32**, 146.

Pinquart, M., & Sorensen, S. (2003). Differences between caregivers and noncaregivers in psychological health and physical health: a meta-analysis. *Psychology of Aging* **18**, 250–67.

Pinquart, M., & Sorensen, S. (2006). Gender differences in caregiver stressors, social resources, and health: an updated meta-analysis. *Journal of Gerontology Series B Psychology* **61**, 33–45.

Pinquart, M., & Sorensen, S. (2011). Spouses, adult children, and children-in-law as caregivers of older adults: a meta-analytic comparison. *Psychology and Aging* **26**, 1–14.

Sales, E. (2003). Family burden and quality of life. *Quality of Life Research* **12** (Suppl 1), 33–41.

Shahly, V., Chatterji, S., Gruber, M. J., *et al.* (2012) Cross-national differences in the prevalence and correlates of burden among older family caregivers in the World Health Organization World Mental Health (WMH) Surveys. *Psychological Medicine* Aug 9, 1–15. [Epub ahead of print].

Torti, F. M., Gwyther, L. P., Reed, S. D., Friedman, J. Y., & Schulman, K. A. (2004). A multinational review of recent trends and reports in dementia caregiver burden. *Alzheimer Disease and Associated Disorders* **18**, 99–109.

Wells, J. N., Cagle, C. S., Marshall, D., & Hollen, M. L. (2009). Perceived mood, health, and burden in female Mexican American family cancer caregivers. *Health Care for Women International* **30**, 629–54.

Wiener, J. (2003). The role of informal support in long-term care. In J. Brodsky, J. Habib, & M. Hirschfeld, eds., *Key Policy Issues in Long-Term Care*. Geneva: World Health Organization, pp. 3–24. http://whqlibdoc.who.int/publications/2003/9241562250.pdf. Accessed November 2012.

Wimo, A., Winblad, B., & Jonsson, L. (2007). An estimate of the total worldwide societal costs of dementia in 2005. *Alzheimers and Dementia* **3**, 81–91.

Wolter, K. (1985). *Introduction to Variance Estimation*. New York, NY: Springer-Verlag.

World Bank (2008). Data and statistics. http://go.worldbank.org/D7SN0B8YU0. Accessed May 12, 2009.

World Bank (2012). Genderstats: gender equality data and statistics. Electronic database. http://datatopics.worldbank.org/gender. Accessed November 2012.

Days totally out of role associated with common mental and physical disorders

Jordi Alonso, Maria V. Petukhova, Gemma Vilagut, Evelyn J. Bromet, Hristo Hinkov, Elie G. Karam, Viviane Kovess-Masféty, Kate M. Scott, and Dan J. Stein

Introduction

A growing body of research has aimed to quantify the societal impacts of mental and physical disorders on functioning in order to influence social policy decisions on healthcare investments (Davis *et al.* 2005, Suhrcke *et al.* 2008, American College of Occupational and Environmental Medicine 2009, Loeppke *et al.* 2009). One important component of this research examines the effects of health problems on days out of role. In the USA, for example, these studies have estimated an annual 3.6 billion health-related days out of role attributable to common mental and physical disorders (Merikangas *et al.* 2007). A recent study in Europe estimated that the annual human capital costs of health-related days out of role due to mental and neurological (i.e., brain) disorders exceeded 798 billion euros in 2010 (Gustavsson *et al.* 2011). It is also important to quantify the relative importance of specific disorders in accounting for these disability effects, and to evaluate the extent to which expanded outreach and best-practice treatment of the disorders associated with the largest losses can reduce these effects.

The first step in a research program such as this should be to distinguish between the relative disability effects of specific disorders: that is, the disability that might be accounted for by the presence of a particular disorder. This requires epidemiological data on a broad range of disorders in order to adjust for the high rates of comorbidity within and between mental and physical disorders (Stang *et al.* 2006, Von Korff 2009). While some studies of this sort have been carried out in the USA (Stang *et al.* 2006, Merikangas *et al.* 2007), at the time of our analyses comparable data on the impact of common mental and physical disorders on days out of role were not available for numerous countries in the world.

In this chapter we examine the variation in the average numbers of days out of role in the month prior to the interview associated with a wide range of mental and physical disorders. We specifically estimate the number of days that individuals report to be totally out of role. By focusing on the extreme end of the disability continuum, this chapter aims to maximize the substantive relevance of the associations assessed. Obviously, this approach results in an underestimation of the degree of disability attributable to the various disorders studied; therefore, a parallel assessment of partial days out of role is presented in Chapter 12. It is important to keep in mind that the WMH surveys are based on the general adult population, including working and non-working individuals. Therefore, the WMH surveys expand upon the large body of knowledge presented in the literature dealing with the association between common disorders and absenteeism among the employed population.

Methods

Sample

The analysis is based on all 25 WMH surveys considered in this volume. Specifically, this chapter focuses on part 2 of the interview, which had a total number of respondents across surveys of $n = 63{,}678$. However, 429 respondents in Lebanon and 278 in Northern Ireland were not included in the analysis because their chronic conditions were not assessed, leading to a final sample of $n = 62{,}971$ respondents (see Appendix Table 2.1).

The Burdens of Mental Disorders, ed. Jordi Alonso, Somnath Chatterji, and Yanling He. Published by
Cambridge University Press. © World Health Organization 2013.

Measures

Days totally out of role were assessed with a modified version (Von Korff *et al.* 2008) of the World Health Organization Disability Assessment Schedule 2.0 (WHODAS 2) (Üstün *et al.* 2010). Respondents were asked to provide the number of days in the 30 days prior to the interview (that is, beginning yesterday and going back 30 days) in which they were totally unable to work or carry out their normal activities because of problems with their mental health, their use of alcohol or drugs, or their physical health. Scores were recorded in the range 0–30. Good concordance of such reports has been documented both with payroll records of employed people (Revicki *et al.* 1994, Kessler *et al.* 2003) and with prospective daily diary reports (Kessler *et al.* 2004).

Nine mental disorders were considered, including alcohol abuse with or without dependence, bipolar disorder (i.e., bipolar I disorder, bipolar II disorder, and subthreshold bipolar disorder combined into a single variable), drug abuse with or without dependence, generalized anxiety disorder (GAD), major depressive disorder (MDD), panic disorder and/or agoraphobia, post-traumatic stress disorder (PTSD), social phobia, and specific phobia. The focus was on mental disorders that were present at some time in the 12 months prior to the interview. Ten chronic physical conditions were also included: arthritis, cancer, cardiovascular disorders (heart attack, heart disease, hypertension, and stroke), chronic pain (chronic back or neck pain and other chronic pain), diabetes, digestive disorders (stomach or intestinal ulcer or irritable bowel disorder), frequent or severe headache or migraine, insomnia, neurological disorders (multiple sclerosis, Parkinson's disease, and epilepsy or seizures), and respiratory disorders (seasonal allergies such as hay fever, asthma, and chronic obstructive pulmonary disease [COPD] or emphysema). As detailed in Chapter 2, these conditions were assessed using a checklist adapted from the US National Health Interview Survey. Methodological studies have documented moderate to good concordance between reports based on such checklists and medical records (Baker *et al.* 2001, Knight *et al.* 2001, Schoenborn *et al.* 2003). The *silent conditions* (i.e., conditions that cannot be detected by sufferers based on signs or symptoms, but must be detected based on medical tests, such as cancer or heart disease) were ascertained by asking respondents whether a doctor or other health professional had ever told them that

they had the condition, while the *symptom-based conditions* (i.e., conditions that sufferers can detect without medical diagnoses, such as chronic headaches or chronic back pain) were assessed by asking respondents whether they had ever had the condition. As with the mental disorders, only physical conditions present in the 12 months prior to the interview were considered.

Statistical analysis

Multiple regression analysis was used to examine the multivariate associations of the mental and physical disorders with the number of days totally out of role. However, as the distribution of the 0–30 days out of role measure was highly skewed – there was a considerable proportion of respondents with no disability – we used special modeling procedures to address the fact that standard ordinary least squares (OLS) regression methods often yield biased and inefficient results when predicting these kinds of outcomes. As detailed in Chapter 2, both two-part models (i.e., a logistic model to predict having at least one day out of role in the total sample and a linear regression model to predict the number of days out of role among respondents reporting at least one) and one-part generalized linear models (GLMs) with non-linear link functions and complex error structures were used to predict skewed outcomes. We explored the use of both of these approaches, as shown in Appendix Table 11.1, and found that a GLM with a log link function and constant error variance was the best-fitting specification to predict days out of role in the WMH survey data. The log link function and constant variance show the lowest mean squared error (MSE) value among every set of six models; only square root link function and constant variance mean absolute percentage error (MAPE) values are slightly lower than log link function and constant variance values for upper-middle-income and high-income countries (Appendix Table 11.1). All the results reported in this chapter are consequently based on models that use this link function (link) and error structure (constant).

A major problem with previous studies examining days out of role is that they generally do not convincingly address the presence of a great deal of comorbidity between different types of mental disorders and between mental and physical disorders (Gureje 2009). A simplistic way to deal with comorbidity is to create a conventional additive

Table 11.1 Distribution of days out of role by country income level. The WMH surveys.

	All countries		Low/lower-middle		Upper-middle		High		Tests	
	%	(SE)	%	(SE)	%	(SE)	%	(SE)	χ^2	DF
Percentage of respondents who reported any days out of role	12.8	(0.2)	14.6	(0.4)	10.4	(0.4)	13.1	(0.3)	29.8**	2
1 day[a]	15.6	(0.6)	13.5	(0.9)	12.5	(1.2)	17.8	(0.9)		
2 days[a]	16.8	(0.5)	18.4	(1.0)	17.0	(1.2)	15.8	(0.7)		
3–5 days[a]	25.7	(0.7)	29.4	(1.2)	29.6	(1.6)	22.2	(0.9)		
6–10 days[a]	14.5	(0.5)	17.1	(1.1)	14.3	(1.0)	13.2	(0.7)		
11–20 days[a]	9.1	(0.4)	8.1	(0.8)	10.6	(0.9)	9.1	(0.5)		
21–30 days[a]	18.3	(0.6)	13.5	(1.0)	16.1	(1.2)	21.9	(0.8)	81.2**	10
	Mean	(SE)	Mean	(SE)	Mean	(SE)	Mean	(SE)	χ^2	DF
Mean days out of role per month (all respondents)	1.2	(0.0)	1.2	(0.1)	1.0	(0.1)	1.4	(0.0)	35.1**	2
Mean days out of role per month (respondents with any day out of role)	9.6	(0.2)	8.3	(0.3)	9.3	(0.3)	10.3	(0.2)	29.7**	2
Median days out of role per month (respondents with any day out of role)	4.2	(0.0)	4.0	(0.2)	4.3	(0.1)	4.3	(0.0)		

[a] Days per month: percentage of respondents with any day out of role.
** Significant at the 0.001 level.

multivariate model in which all the disorders under consideration are included as predictors in the same model. As discussed in Chapter 2, this approach adjusts for simple additive associations, but it fails to consider the possibility of synergy: that is, the possibility that the effect of a given disorder on days out of role varies depending on the presence or absence of other disorders. We have already seen evidence for such synergy in the joint effects of mental disorders earlier in this volume (e.g., in the analysis of marriage and divorce in Chapter 5). It is not possible to include terms to capture the effects of every logically possible profile of comorbidity, given that the number of possible combinations of comorbid disorders in the data (2^{19} − 20 = 524,268) far exceeds the number of respondents. We therefore needed to make some simplifying assumptions about the effects of comorbidity.

One solution to this problem was to create a hierarchy of models that began with an additive model (model 1). Model 2 then included instead a series of dummy predictor variables for number of disorders (e.g., a dummy variable for respondents who had exactly one disorder, another for respondents with exactly two disorders, etc.) without information about types of disorders. The assumption in model 2 was that the disorder is unimportant once the number of disorders is known. Model 3 then combined the 19 predictors for each disorder from model 1 with the dummy predictors for the number of disorders (starting with 2) from model 2. Model 4 was similar to model 3 but allowed for the effects of each disorder to be a linear function of the number of other disorders by including the interaction terms of disorder with the number of other mental or physical disorders. Model 5, finally, expanded on model 4 by weighting the interactions of type with number by the importance of the disorders. This complex statistical model included a term equal to the sum of the regression coefficients for each of the respondents' disorders, as well as the interaction of this term with each disorder. For each disorder, this term is called the "importance score," and it is only positive for respondents with at least two comorbid disorders. Iterative procedures were required to estimate this last model (Seber & Wild 1989) because each interaction term was constructed from coefficients estimated in the previous iteration of the model. This iterative approach was continued until the coefficients converged. All models controlled for age, sex, employment status, and country. Model 5 was found to provide the best fit for the data.

We estimated both the individual-level and the societal-level effects of mental and physical disorders on days totally out of role. Societal-level effects were estimated using population attributable risk proportions (PARPs). As noted in Chapter 2, a PARP can be interpreted as the proportion of all days out of role in the general population that would be prevented if the effects of a given disorder on days totally out of role were eliminated. See Chapter 2 for a discussion of individual-level effects and PARPs. Standard errors of prevalence estimates were obtained using the Taylor Series Linearization (TSL) method, while standard errors of individual- and societal-level coefficients were estimated using SAS macros for the Jackknife Repeated Replication (JRR) method to account for the complex sample design (Wolter 1985). As in all other chapters in this volume, statistical significance was consistently evaluated using 0.05-level, two-sided design-based tests.

Results

As shown in Appendix Table 2.1, the mean age of respondents was 42, about 52% were female, just over a third of the overall sample of individuals were not married, more than half reported having completed high school or a more advanced educational level, and 42% were unemployed.

Distribution of days totally out of role

The mean number of health-related days totally out of role reported in the month prior to the interview was 1.2 in the total sample, with a range of 1.0–1.4 across countries in the three income levels (Table 11.1). The overall mean can be broken down to show that 12.8% of respondents reported at least one day out of role (14.6% in low/lower-middle-income countries, 10.4% in upper-middle-income countries, and 13.1% in high-income countries), and the mean number of days for respondents reporting at least one day out of role within the previous month was 9.6 (8.3 in low/lower-middle-income countries, 9.3 in upper-middle-income

countries, and 10.3 in high-income countries). The distribution is skewed to the right, as indicated by the fact that the median number of respondents reporting any days out of role, 4.2 in the total sample (4.0 in low/lower-middle-income countries, 4.3 in upper-middle-income countries, and 4.3 in high-income countries) is lower than the mean.

Prevalence of disorders

More than half (58.0%) of respondents across countries reported having one or more disorder (Table 11.2). The proportion of those reporting at least one chronic physical condition (53.2%) is considerably higher than the proportion of those reporting at least one mental disorder (15.4%). The prevalence of having any chronic physical condition and any mental disorder both increase monotonically with country income level: from 45.6% in low/lower-middle-income to 52.2% in upper-middle-income and 57.4% in high-income countries for any chronic physical condition; and from 12.1% to 15.4% and 17.0%, respectively, for any mental disorder.

This monotonic increase is seen in 11 of the 19 individual disorders, with five others either having their lowest prevalence in low/lower-middle-income countries or having their highest prevalence in high-income countries. The three exceptions are frequent or severe headaches or migraines and chronic pain conditions, both of which have their highest prevalence in upper-middle-income countries, and digestive disorders, with the highest prevalence in low/lower-middle-income countries. The rank order of prevalence estimates across disorders is very similar in the three groups of countries, with rank-order correlations across groups in the range of 0.87–0.97. Chronic pain conditions are among the two most commonly reported disorders in all three groups of countries (21.6–23.7%), headaches among the top two in low/lower-middle-income and upper-middle-income countries (14.5–19.4%), and cardiovascular disorders among the top three in upper-middle-income and high-income countries (18.2–18.8%). Major depressive disorder is the most commonly reported mental disorder in all three groups of countries (4.9–6.2%), followed by specific phobia (4.2–6.0%). Other highly prevalent conditions in all groups of countries are arthritis (12.5–16.6%) and respiratory disorders (11.9–21.9%).

Table 11.2 Prevalence of the disorder and mean number of days out of role (DOR) per year, by country income level. The WMH surveys.

Disorder	Country income level															
	All countries				Low/lower-middle				Upper-middle				High			
	Prevalence (%)	(SE)	Mean yearly DOR	(SE)	Prevalence (%)	(SE)	Mean yearly DOR	(SE)	Prevalence (%)	(SE)	Mean yearly DOR	(SE)	Prevalence (%)	(SE)	Mean Yearly DOR	(SE)
Alcohol abuse	2.1	(0.1)	30.6	(0.7)	1.8	(0.1)	29.0	(1.4)	2.8	(0.2)	27.9	(1.2)	1.9	(0.1)	33.1	(1.0)
Bipolar	0.8	(0.0)	41.2	(1.1)	0.4	(0.1)	30.8	(2.5)	0.6	(0.1)	42.4	(2.5)	1.1	(0.1)	42.6	(1.4)
Drug abuse	0.6	(0.0)	36.6	(1.3)	0.2	(0.0)	40.8	(4.8)	0.7	(0.1)	32.1	(1.9)	0.7	(0.1)	37.8	(1.6)
Generalized anxiety	1.4	(0.1)	39.8	(0.8)	1.1	(0.1)	38.1	(1.9)	1.1	(0.1)	41.4	(1.9)	1.7	(0.1)	39.9	(1.0)
Major depressive disorder	5.7	(0.1)	34.4	(0.4)	4.9	(0.2)	35.8	(0.9)	5.4	(0.2)	34.8	(0.9)	6.2	(0.1)	33.7	(0.6)
Panic and/or agoraphobia	1.9	(0.1)	42.9	(0.8)	1.1	(0.1)	39.6	(1.9)	2.7	(0.1)	39.7	(1.3)	2.0	(0.1)	45.6	(1.1)
Post-traumatic stress	1.6	(0.1)	42.7	(0.9)	0.7	(0.1)	44.9	(2.1)	1.0	(0.1)	40.9	(2.3)	2.2	(0.1)	42.7	(1.1)
Social phobia	2.4	(0.1)	39.3	(0.7)	1.1	(0.1)	33.3	(1.8)	2.0	(0.1)	41.3	(1.8)	3.3	(0.1)	39.7	(0.8)
Specific phobia	5.2	(0.1)	33.8	(0.5)	4.2	(0.2)	28.9	(1.2)	4.6	(0.2)	35.2	(1.1)	6.0	(0.2)	34.8	(0.6)
Arthritis	14.8	(0.2)	29.5	(0.3)	13.1	(0.4)	28.7	(0.5)	12.5	(0.3)	30.2	(0.6)	16.6	(0.3)	29.6	(0.3)
Cancer	2.2	(0.1)	31.9	(0.7)	0.4	(0.1)	30.4	(2.6)	0.8	(0.1)	37.2	(3.4)	3.7	(0.2)	31.5	(0.8)
Cardiovascular	16.9	(0.2)	28.7	(0.3)	11.9	(0.4)	29.8	(0.6)	18.2	(0.4)	29.6	(0.5)	18.8	(0.3)	27.9	(0.4)
Chronic pain	22.2	(0.3)	28.3	(0.2)	21.9	(0.6)	26.8	(0.4)	23.7	(0.5)	28.5	(0.4)	21.6	(0.3)	28.9	(0.3)
Diabetes	4.2	(0.1)	30.3	(0.5)	2.5	(0.2)	29.4	(1.1)	4.4	(0.2)	32.1	(0.9)	4.9	(0.2)	29.8	(0.8)
Digestive	3.3	(0.1)	34.9	(0.6)	4.5	(0.2)	29.4	(0.9)	3.9	(0.2)	37.2	(1.1)	2.5	(0.1)	37.7	(1.0)
Headache/migraine	13.9	(0.2)	30.7	(0.3)	14.5	(0.4)	29.8	(0.5)	19.4	(0.5)	29.3	(0.5)	11.1	(0.2)	32.3	(0.4)
Insomnia	5.0	(0.1)	36.7	(0.5)	4.3	(0.2)	37.8	(1.1)	4.1	(0.2)	36.0	(1.1)	5.7	(0.2)	36.5	(0.6)
Neurological	1.1	(0.1)	37.2	(1.1)	0.8	(0.1)	37.8	(2.4)	1.4	(0.1)	39.8	(2.2)	1.2	(0.1)	35.5	(1.4)
Respiratory	17.3	(0.3)	28.4	(0.3)	11.9	(0.4)	26.2	(0.6)	13.1	(0.4)	30.7	(0.6)	21.9	(0.4)	28.2	(0.4)
Any mental disorder	15.4	(0.2)	31.3	(0.3)	12.1	(0.3)	30.5	(0.6)	15.4	(0.4)	32.0	(0.4)	17.0	(0.3)	31.2	(0.4)

Table 11.2 (cont.)

Disorder	Country income level															
	All countries				Low/lower-middle				Upper-middle				High			
	Prevalence (%)	(SE)	Mean yearly DOR	(SE)	Prevalence (%)	(SE)	Mean yearly DOR	(SE)	Prevalence (%)	(SE)	Mean yearly DOR	(SE)	Prevalence (%)	(SE)	Mean Yearly DOR	(SE)
Any physical disorder	53.2	(0.3)	24.5	(0.1)	45.6	(0.6)	23.7	(0.6)	52.2	(0.7)	24.8	(0.3)	57.4	(0.5)	24.7	(0.2)
Any disorder	58.0	(0.3)	24.2	(0.1)	49.8	(0.6)	23.5	(0.6)	56.8	(0.6)	24.5	(0.3)	62.5	(0.5)	24.4	(0.2)
Respondents with positive days out of role			116.2	(1.9)			101.3	(3.5)			113.6	(3.8)			125.4	(2.8)
All respondents			15.0	(0.4)			14.8	(0.6)			11.8	(0.6)			16.4	(0.5)

Days totally out of role by type of disorder

The mean number of days totally out of role per year was found to vary by disorder. Individuals with panic disorder (42.9), PTSD (42.7), and bipolar disorder (41.2) had the highest mean numbers of days out of role. Trends were similar across types of countries. The correlations between mean days totally out of role across conditions were high in each of the three country income groups (Spearman rank-order correlations in the range 0.62–0.77). PTSD, panic disorder, and GAD were among the top six conditions with the highest mean days totally out of role in all three income groups. Individuals with at least one disorder reported an average of 24.2 more days totally out of role in a year (31.3 days those with any mental disorder, 24.5 those with any physical condition) than those with no conditions.

Respondents who reported having at least one disorder had an average of 2.1 disorders. Comorbidity is the norm, with 55.9% of respondents with a disorder reporting at least two. Odds ratios (ORs) between pairs of disorders were largely positive (94.1% of all the 19*18/2 = 171 ORs between pairs of disorders) and statistically significant (90.0% of all ORs). The ORs were found to be higher (median and interquartile range) among pairs of chronic physical conditions (2.5, 1.9–3.0) and mental disorders (7.2, 4.0–8.7) than between physical–mental pairs (2.0, 1.4–2.6) (Appendix Table 11.2). Similar patterns were revealed for each of the three groups of countries.

Individual and societal effects of disorders on days totally out of role

Table 11.3 shows the additional number of days totally out of role in a year among respondents with a disorder (individual-level effect), adjusting for age, sex, marital status, and employment, as well as the number and type of comorbid disorders. The most disabling disorders were bipolar disorder (36.5 additional days), neurological disorders (33.7), and panic disorder (24.3) in low/lower-middle-income countries, GAD (24.6 additional days), bipolar disorder (23.2), neurological disorder (18.6), and panic disorder (17.7) in upper-middle-income countries, and chronic pain conditions (19.6 additional days), digestive disorders (16.6), and PTSD (16.2) in high-income countries. Rank correlations of the individual effects of the conditions were very low across country type (from 0.12 to 0.26).

Interactions were found to be sub-additive for most disorders in all three country income groups: the incremental increase in days totally out of role was lower when a disorder occurred comorbidly compared to when the same disorder occurred in isolation (Appendix Table 11.3). Table 11.3 also shows the PARPs of days totally out of role for each condition. Chronic pain conditions accounted for the highest proportion of days out of role (21.5% on average), followed by frequent or severe headaches or migraines (6.9%), cardiovascular disorders (6.3%), and major depressive disorder (5.1%). For each condition, the PARPs tend to be fairly similar across country types, especially between low/lower-middle-income and upper-middle-income countries (Spearman correlations 0.32). The individual effects and PARPs for all countries combined are presented in Figure 11.1. The figure clearly shows that the disorders with the highest impacts in terms of their individual-level effects – most notably neurological disorders, bipolar disorder, and chronic pain conditions (Figure 11.1a) – are quite different from those that have the most impact at the societal level – chronic pain conditions, cardiovascular disorders, and major depressive disorder (Figure 11.1b).

Discussion

A number of limitations must be considered before interpreting the estimated effects of common mental and physical disorders on the days totally out of role presented above. First, only a restricted set of the most common disorders was included in the analysis, and some were pooled to form larger disorder groups. Some burdensome disorders, such as dementia and psychosis, were not included. While the disorders we did consider are among those most commonly reported in previous population studies (Merikangas *et al.* 2007), an expansion and disaggregation of these disorders is clearly needed in future studies. Secondly, diagnoses of chronic physical conditions were based on self-reports. Prior research has demonstrated reasonable correspondence between self-reported chronic conditions, such as diabetes, heart disease, and asthma, and general practitioner records (Kriegsman *et al.* 1996), but some bias might account for the generally higher prevalence estimates of these conditions in developed countries than in developing countries. Higher rates of medical treatment and detection in developed countries likely artificially inflate differences in prevalence by country. Thirdly, we only considered the days out of role that the

Table 11.3 Additional days out of role per year ("individual effects") and population attributable risk proportions (PARPs) of days out of role due to each condition considered, by country income level. The WMH surveys.

Disorder	All countries				Low/lower-middle				Upper-middle				High			
	Additional days		PARP		Additional days		PARP		Additional days		PARP		Additional days		PARP	
	Mean	(SE)	%	(SE)	Mean	(SE)	%	(SE)	Mean	(SE)	%	(SE)	Mean	(SE)	%	(SE)
Alcohol abuse	1.9	(3.2)	0.3	(0.5)	−2.8	(7.2)	−0.5	(1.3)	8.2	(5.0)	1.9	(1.2)	−0.3	(4.5)	0.0	(0.6)
Bipolar disorder	17.3	(4.9)	1.4	(0.4)	36.5	(15.0)	1.6	(0.7)	23.2	(9.6)	1.7	(0.7)	9.6	(5.8)	1.0	(0.6)
Drug abuse	2.5	(4.0)	0.1	(0.2)	14.7	(13.9)	0.3	(0.3)	3.9	(12.2)	0.2	(0.6)	1.2	(5.5)	0.1	(0.3)
Generalized anxiety	7.7	(3.6)	1.0	(0.5)	13.5	(9.1)	1.4	(1.0)	24.6	(8.4)	3.4	(1.1)	7.6	(4.9)	1.2	(0.7)
Major depressive disorder	9.0	(2.5)	5.1	(1.4)	13.1	(5.0)	8.1	(3.1)	14.7	(4.1)	9.7	(2.5)	4.1	(3.2)	2.2	(1.7)
Panic and/or agoraphobia	14.3	(3.5)	2.6	(0.6)	24.3	(12.9)	3.3	(1.8)	17.7	(5.5)	4.9	(1.4)	11.7	(4.1)	2.2	(0.8)
Post-traumatic stress	15.2	(3.5)	2.2	(0.5)	15.3	(11.3)	1.2	(0.9)	−1.1	(9.5)	−0.1	(1.0)	16.2	(4.0)	3.1	(0.8)
Social phobia	7.3	(2.8)	1.7	(0.6)	5.7	(10.0)	0.6	(1.1)	9.0	(8.4)	1.9	(1.9)	7.5	(2.9)	2.2	(0.9)
Specific phobia	3.9	(2.5)	1.8	(1.2)	−6.6	(5.2)	−2.6	(2.1)	4.2	(4.7)	2.2	(2.3)	6.7	(3.3)	3.4	(1.6)
Arthritis	2.7	(1.8)	2.7	(1.8)	6.1	(4.4)	6.5	(5.0)	0.8	(5.0)	0.9	(5.6)	1.8	(2.4)	1.7	(2.3)
Cancer	5.5	(3.5)	0.7	(0.5)	19.4	(17.9)	0.7	(0.7)	−4.2	(12.9)	−0.3	(0.9)	6.9	(3.6)	1.4	(0.7)
Cardiovascular	5.7	(2.1)	6.3	(2.3)	2.7	(6.7)	2.5	(6.2)	1.0	(3.6)	1.7	(6.0)	7.3	(2.7)	7.6	(2.8)
Chronic pain	14.3	(1.5)	21.5	(2.3)	0.9	(3.1)	1.6	(5.5)	11.0	(2.5)	21.8	(5.2)	19.6	(2.1)	25.7	(2.9)
Diabetes	8.6	(2.8)	2.3	(0.7)	4.0	(6.4)	0.8	(1.2)	0.5	(5.6)	0.2	(2.2)	9.6	(3.8)	2.6	(1.0)
Digestive	7.6	(3.0)	1.8	(0.7)	−4.3	(4.8)	−1.5	(1.8)	−0.4	(4.0)	−0.2	(1.5)	16.6	(4.8)	2.6	(0.7)
Headache/ migraine	7.1	(1.5)	6.9	(1.5)	10.4	(3.6)	11.7	(3.8)	6.5	(3.3)	10.7	(5.5)	4.5	(2.1)	3.3	(1.5)
Insomnia	7.9	(2.7)	3.0	(1.0)	5.7	(5.3)	2.2	(2.1)	4.6	(5.4)	2.0	(2.2)	9.4	(3.2)	3.5	(1.2)
Neurological	17.4	(5.8)	1.5	(0.5)	33.7	(23.0)	2.5	(1.6)	18.6	(7.0)	2.4	(0.9)	15.3	(7.4)	1.2	(0.6)
Respiratory	2.6	(1.3)	2.9	(1.4)	10.7	(3.0)	9.2	(2.9)	−1.1	(2.6)	−1.2	(2.7)	0.9	(1.4)	1.1	(1.7)
All mental disorders	11.9	(1.4)	16.5	(1.8)	10.5	(3.1)	13.7	(4.3)	12.8	(2.3)	20.7	(3.1)	11.3	(1.7)	16.0	(2.2)
All physical disorders	14.1	(0.8)	47.6	(2.7)	12.6	(3.1)	42.7	(8.3)	9.3	(1.9)	39.9	(7.9)	16.3	(1.0)	52.7	(3.4)
All disorders	16.5	(0.7)	62.2	(2.1)	15.3	(1.9)	58.1	(5.7)	12.5	(1.7)	59.2	(7.2)	18.4	(0.8)	66.6	(2.6)

Country income level

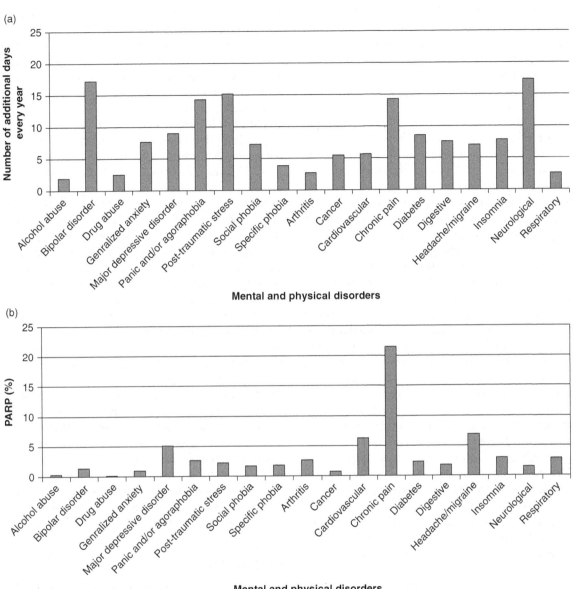

Figure 11.1 Yearly days totally out of role associated with common mental and physical disorders. The WMH surveys.
(a) Additional days totally out of role among those suffering the disorder ("individual effect").
(b) Population attributable risk proportions (PARPs) of days totally out of role ("societal effect").

respondents reported that they were *totally* unable to do their work or usual activities. It is not uncommon for individuals to perform their role activities despite health issues, albeit to a lesser or worse degree than expected (e.g., presenteeism) (Sanderson & Andrews 2006), and therefore information about days out of role underestimates total productivity loss. This limitation is, however, overcome in Chapter 12, which applies the same

analytical approach presented here to "partial" disability, that is, role limitations that do not incur days totally out of role. Finally, to increase the validity of the self-reports, we limited the reporting of restriction of activity to 30 days prior to the interview and then projected the numbers in this recall interval to the whole year to improve comparability with data in the published literature (Merikangas *et al.* 2007). However, there may be some mismatch between disease severity and prevalence: for more episodic conditions this recall period might have missed a severe exacerbation present in the previous year but not in the month before the interview. Due to the relatively large number of events assessed, we expect this to cancel out the opposite situation and overall not to affect our estimates.

Within the context of these limitations, a number of disorders that cause a great deal of disability have been identified. For the overall sample (Table 11.3), sufferers of bipolar disorder, PTSD, and panic disorder have the highest degree of disability, followed closely by those with GAD and social phobia. These results show that mental disorders are among the conditions most strongly associated with productivity loss. This finding is broadly consistent with previous studies (Goetzel *et al.* 2003, Polder & Achterberg 2004, Bowden 2005, Kessler *et al.* 2006). Nevertheless, as comorbidity is so common, especially between mental disorders, the associations found in previous studies, which failed to adjust adequately for comorbidity, could have been due not to the particular conditions themselves but rather to their high comorbidity. This possibility was addressed in the analysis reported here by controlling for comorbidity. Table 11.3 (individual effects) shows that the rank ordering of disorders in terms of relative impacts on days totally out of role changes when adjusted for comorbidity. Therefore, it is important to consider comorbidity in assessing the relative effects of particular disorders on days out of role.

Results presented here show that the 19 common disorders considered account for almost two-thirds of all days totally out of role in the general populations of the countries studied (PARP = 62.2%). Chronic physical conditions accounted for 47.6% and mental disorders for 16.5% of days out of role. It should be noted that the chronic physical conditions include neurological disorders (epilepsy, multiple sclerosis, and stroke), pain conditions (including frequent or severe headaches or migraines), and insomnia. If insomnia were considered a mental disorder instead of a chronic physical condition, mental disorders would account for up to 20.3% of days out of role. Pain conditions are disabling and highly prevalent and they are, by far, the most important contributor to days totally out of role in the population. Cardiovascular disorders, depression, and migraine are also major contributors to population-level days totally out of role. As a consequence, attempts at improving the productivity of our societies should seriously consider addressing

these disorders. Nonetheless, while PARPs indicate the theoretical proportion of outcome events that could be avoided if the exposure (i.e., the disorders in our study) was completely eliminated, and are useful for identifying burdensome targets for population-wide intervention, it should be borne in mind that disability days avoided by eliminating one disorder might limit the opportunity for preventing the same days lost by eliminating another condition (Steenland & Armstrong 2006).

With some exceptions, the results presented here are similar across the types of countries studied. We had anticipated that cultural, social, and economic differences might modulate the association of disorders with days totally out of role. First, we found relatively small differences across types of countries in the average proportion of individuals reporting days totally unable to carry out normal activities. There is little variation in the mean number of yearly days totally out of role among those with at least one day out of role. Specifically, individuals reporting at least one day totally out of role in high-income countries reported two more days than those in the low/lower middle-income countries and one more day than those in upper-middle-income countries. These differences might be due to the higher severity of the disorders in those countries or to a more developed welfare system. When comparing the number of days out of role associated with specific disorders across country income levels, no systematic differences were found in either the bivariate or the multivariate analyses. Nevertheless, country differences in disability attributable to common mental and physical disorders deserve further research.

Implications

A first implication of the results presented in this chapter is the identification of the relative contribution of different common disorders to the loss of productivity in a population. Lowering the impact of common and disabling disorders such as pain and migraine, as well as cardiovascular disease and depression, would give rise to major productivity returns. Considering that indirect costs are usually higher than direct medical and social services costs to treat disorders (Rice & Miller 1998, Smit *et al.* 2006), the prevention and treatment of these disorders should be cost-effective.

Another implication is that interactions were found to be sub-additive in the best-fitting model.

This does not mean that comorbidity is not highly disabling. On the contrary, there is clear evidence of its high burden (Turner *et al.* 2008). But it does mean that, in the presence of comorbidity, disability increases less than the sum of the coefficients associated with each comorbid disorder. This finding might have an important implication for the prevention of disability: addressing only one disorder (treatment or prevention) when it coexists with other disorders might render a less effective outcome than addressing all coexisting conditions (Kessler *et al.* 2012).

Acknowledgments

Portions of this chapter are based on Alonso, J., Petukhova, M., Vilagut, G., *et al.* (2011). Days out of role due to common physical and mental conditions: results from the WHO World Mental Health surveys. *Molecular Psychiatry* **16**, 1234–46. © 2011. Nature Publishing Group. Reproduced with permission.

References

American College of Occupational and Environmental Medicine (2009). Healthy workforce/healthy economy: the role of health, productivity, and disability management in addressing the nation's health care crisis: why an emphasis on the health of the workforce is vital to the health of the economy. *Journal of Occupational and Environmental Medicine* **51**, 114–19.

Baker, M., Stabile, M., & Deri, C. (2001). *What Do Self-reported, Objective Measures of Health Measure?* NBER Working Paper Series 8419. Cambridge, MA: National Bureau of Economic Research.

Bowden, C. L. (2005). Bipolar disorder and work loss. *American Journal of Managed Care* **11** (3 Suppl), S91–4.

Davis, K., Collins, S. R., Doty, M. M., Ho, A., & Holmgren, A. (2005). Health and productivity among U.S. workers. *Issue Brief (Commonwealth Fund)* **856**, 1–10.

Goetzel, R. Z., Hawkins, K., Ozminkowski, R. J., & Wang, S. (2003). The health and productivity cost burden of the "top 10" physical and mental health conditions affecting six large U.S. employers in 1999. *Journal of Occupational and Environmental Medicine* **45**, 5–14.

Gureje, O. (2009). The pattern and nature of mental–physical comorbidity: specific or general? In M. R. Von Korff, K. M. Scott, & O. Gureje, eds., *Global Perspectives on Mental–Physical Comorbidity in the WHO World Mental Health Surveys*. New York, NY: Cambridge University Press, pp. 51–83.

Gustavsson, A., Svensson, M., Jacobi, F., *et al.* (2011). Cost of disorders of the brain in Europe 2010. *European Neuropsychopharmacology* **21**, 718–79.

Kessler, R. C., Ormel, J., Demler, O., & Stang, P. E. (2003). Comorbid mental disorders account for the role impairment of commonly occurring chronic physical disorders: results from the National Comorbidity Survey. *Journal of Occupational and Environmental Medicine* **45**, 1257–66.

Kessler, R. C., Ames, M., Hymel, P. A., *et al.* (2004). Using the World Health Organization Health and Work Performance Questionnaire (HPQ) to evaluate the indirect workplace costs of illness. *Journal of Occupational and Environmental Medicine* **46** (6 Suppl), S23–37.

Kessler, R. C., Akiskal, H. S., Ames, M., *et al.* (2006). Prevalence and effects of mood disorders on work performance in a nationally representative sample of U.S. workers. *American Journal of Psychiatry* **163**, 1561–8.

Kessler, R. C., Avenevoli, S., Costello, E. J., *et al.* (2012). Severity of 12-month DSM-IV disorders in the NCS-R Adolescent Supplement (NCS-A). *Archives of General Psychiatry* **69**, 381–9.

Knight, M., Stewart-Brown, S., & Fletcher, L. (2001). Estimating health needs: the impact of a checklist of conditions and quality of life measurement on health information derived from community surveys. *Journal of Public Health Medicine* **23**, 179–86.

Kriegsman, D. M., Penninx, B. W., van Eijk, J. T., Boeke, A. J. P., & Deeg, D. J. H. (1996). Self-reports and general practitioner information on the presence of chronic diseases in community dwelling elderly: a study on the accuracy of patients' self-reports and on determinants of inaccuracy. *Journal of Clinical Epidemiology* **49**, 1407–17.

Loeppke, R., Taitel, M., Haufle, V., *et al.* (2009). Health and productivity as a business strategy: a multiemployer study. *Journal of Occupational and Environmental Medicine* **51**, 411–28.

Merikangas, K. R., Ames, M., Cui, L., *et al.* (2007). The impact of comorbidity of mental and physical conditions on role disability in the US adult household population. *Archives of General Psychiatry* **64**, 1180–8.

Polder, J. J., & Achterberg, P. W. (2004). *Cost of Illness in the Netherlands*. Bilthoven, the Netherlands: National Institute for Public Health and the Environment.

Revicki, D. A., Irwin, D., Reblando, J., & Simon, G. E. (1994). The accuracy of self-reported disability days. *Medical Care* **32**, 401–4.

Rice, D. P., & Miller, L. S. (1998). Health economics and cost implications of anxiety and other mental disorders in the United States. *British Journal of Psychiatry Supplement* **34**, 4–9.

Sanderson, K., & Andrews, G. (2006). Common mental disorders in the workforce: recent findings from descriptive and social epidemiology. *Canadian Journal of Psychiatry* **51**, 63–75.

Schoenborn, C. A., Adams, P. F., & Schiller, J. S. (2003). Summary health statistics for the U.S. population: National Health Interview Survey, 2000. *Vital Health Statistics* 10 (214), 1–83.

Seber, G. A. F. & Wild, C. L. (1989). *Nonlinear Regression*. New York, NY: Wiley.

Smit, F., Cuijpers, P., Oostenbrink, J., *et al.* (2006). Costs of nine common mental disorders: implications for curative and preventive psychiatry. *Journal of Mental Health Policy and Economics* 9, 193–200.

Stang, P. E., Brandenburg, N. A., Lane, M. C., *et al.* (2006). Mental and physical comorbid conditions and days in role among persons with arthritis. *Psychosomatic Medicine* 68, 152–8.

Steenland, K., & Armstrong, B. (2006). An overview of methods for calculating the burden of disease due to specific risk factors. *Epidemiology* 17, 512–19.

Suhrcke, M., Arce, R. A., McKee, M., & Rocco, L. (2008). *Economic Costs of Ill Health in the European Region*. Copenhagen: European Observatory on Health Systems and Policies, World Health Organization.

Turner, B. J., Hollenbeak, C. S., Weiner, M., Ten Have, T., & Tang, S. S. (2008). Effect of unrelated comorbid conditions on hypertension management. *Annals of Internal Medicine* 148, 578–86.

Üstün, T. B., Kostanjsek, N., Chatterji, S., & Rehm, J. (2010). *Measuring Health and Disability: Manual for WHO Disability Assessment Schedule (WHODAS 2.0)* Geneva: World Health Organization.

Von Korff, M., Crane, P. K., Alonso, J., *et al.* (2008). Modified WHODAS-II provides valid measure of global disability but filter items increased skewness. *Journal of Clinical Epidemiology* 61, 1132–43.

Von Korff, M. R. (2009). Global perspectives on mental–physical comorbidity. In M. R. Von Korff, K. M. Scott, & O. Gureje, eds., *Global Perspectives on Mental–Physical Comorbidity in the WHO World Mental Health Surveys*. New York, NY: Cambridge University Press, pp. 1–11.

Wolter, K. M. (1985). *Introduction to Variance Estimation*. New York, NY: Springer-Verlag.

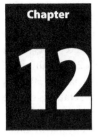

Chapter

12

Partial disability associated with common mental and physical disorders

Ronny Bruffaerts, Gemma Vilagut, Ali Obaid Al-Hamzawi, Brendan Bunting, Koen Demyttenaere, Yanling He, Silvia Florescu, Chiyi Hu, J. Elisabeth Wells, and Miguel Xavier

Introduction

Epidemiological research clearly shows that both mental and physical disorders are quite common among home-dwelling adults all over the world, and the published estimates of the prevalence of some of these conditions are relatively consistent. For example, between 10% and 25% of the adult general population in Western countries meet the criteria for a DSM-IV mental disorder in any given year (Demyttenaere *et al.* 2004), while about 40% report having chronic pain (Breivik *et al.* 2006, Tsang & Lee 2009). Furthermore, both mental and physical disorders have consistently been found to place a considerable burden on the daily lives of those who suffer from them. Although burden has traditionally been defined in terms of condition-specific rates of morbidity and mortality (Goetzel *et al.* 2004), research is increasingly moving beyond these actuarial data to consider additional information about the impairments associated with different mental and physical disorders, such as the comparative effects of different conditions on role functioning. Systematic studies using these definitions of burden have consistently shown that mental disorders imply substantial burdens in terms of role impairments (e.g., Von Korff *et al.* 2005, Demyttenaere *et al.* 2006, 2008, Merikangas *et al.* 2007, Bruffaerts *et al.* 2008). Comparable burdens have been found to be associated with commonly occurring chronic physical conditions (Alonso *et al.* 2004).

However, a shortcoming of these studies is that most of them focus on the extent to which disorders are associated with being *totally* out of role: that is, the number of days in which individuals are *not at all able* to perform as usual. According to data presented in Chapter 11, approximately 13% of the general population samples in the WMH surveys reported at least one day of being totally out of role due to a health problem in the month prior to the interview. Among those reporting any number of days at all in which they were totally out of role, the median number of days out of role was about four in the past month, with the highest numbers for panic disorder, post-traumatic stress disorder, and bipolar disorder (Alonso *et al.* 2011). But there is growing evidence that health disorders are also associated with *partial* disability: that is, days in which some people are *partially unable* to perform as usual (World Health Organization 2011). Partial-disability days have for the most part been studied among working populations (e.g., Kessler *et al.* 1997, Dewa *et al.* 2007). In these studies, mental and physical disorders have both been shown to be associated with significant losses of work productivity due to reduced performance. Up to one-third of working adults report that they have gone to work at least once in the past month despite feeling that they should have stayed home because of health problems, and that their work performance suffered because of those health problems (Aronsson *et al.* 2000). The aggregate loss in productive functioning associated with this partial disability is very substantial. Moreover, current partial disability may predict full disability later. In an interesting prospective study by Bergström and colleagues (2009) among public- and private-sector employees (*n* = 6,242), the number of days a worker went to work feeling unwell was significantly associated with an 11–40% increase in the odds of being absent for more than 30 days 2–3 years after the baseline assessment.

Based on these results, the study of partial disability seems to be an important undertaking, especially in light of the emphasis of public health research on the identification of major high-burden disorders (Merikangas *et al.* 2007). Ever-increasing healthcare costs may strain the capability of a society to provide health care for everyone with chronic conditions (Kessler *et al.* 2001). Resources for providing health care are by definition scarce and insufficient (Drummond 1987) and, therefore, the question arises whether it would be possible to identify specific burdensome disorders in order to prioritize healthcare needs and the (re)allocation of resources. After all, an optimal allocation of healthcare resources implies that planners and administrators are aware of comparable estimates of disease burdens worldwide.

There are three important limitations to the previous research on partial disability. First, no cross-national analyses have been conducted on the comparative effects of mental and physical disorders on partial disability. Second, as noted above, most previous studies estimated the effects of disorders on partial disability in the workplace rather than studying more general role impairments. Third, most previous studies examined only individual-level effects: that is, the effects of disorders on the daily lives of those who have a disorder. However, from a public health perspective it is also of considerable importance to estimate the societal-level burden. All of these limitations are addressed in this chapter, which examines partial-disability days in the month prior to the interview as a function of mental and physical disorders at both individual and societal levels. We also examine the extent to which these estimates vary by country income level.

Methods

Sample

We based our analysis on all 25 of the WMH surveys considered in this volume. Because partial disability was assessed in part 2 of the interview, that part was taken as the focus of the analysis. As noted in Chapter 2, the total number of respondents in this part of the interview was $n = 63,678$. However, the sample size for the analysis conducted in this chapter is $n = 61,259$ (Appendix Table 2.1), as 429 respondents in Lebanon and 278 in Northern Ireland were excluded because their chronic conditions were not assessed. Respondents that reported full disability were also excluded ($n = 1,712$).

Measures

Partial disability was assessed using a modified version (Von Korff *et al.* 2008) of the WHO Disability Assessment Schedule 2.0 (WHODAS 2) (Üstün *et al.* 2010). The time frame of WHODAS is the 30 days prior to the assessment. The interpretation of the number of partial-disability days goes beyond job productivity to focus on the number of days with functional limitations in daily activities without being fully out of role. Specifically, a partial-disability day was defined as a day in which respondents had: (a) *to cut down on what they did* (hereafter referred to as "quantity cut-down days" and assessed by the question, "How many days out of the past 30 were you able to work and carry out your normal activities, but had to cut down on what you did or not get as much done as usual because problems with either your physical health, your mental health, or your use of alcohol or drugs?"); or (b) *to cut back on the quality of what they did* (hereafter referred to as "quality cut-back days" and assessed by the question, "How many days out of the past 30 did you cut back on the quality of your work or how carefully you worked because of problems with either your physical health, your mental health, or your use of alcohol or drugs?"); or (c) *to make an extreme effort to perform as usual* (hereafter referred to as "extreme-effort days" and assessed by the question, "How many days out of the past 30 did it take an extreme effort to perform up to your usual level at work or at your other normal daily activities because of problems with either your physical health, your mental health, or your use of alcohol or drugs?"). Good concordance of reported disability days has been documented both with payroll records of employed people and with prospective daily diary reports (Kessler *et al.* 2004). Responses to the quantity cut-down, quality cut-back, and extreme-effort days were added together to calculate an aggregate measure of partial disability, with weighted items (Von Korff *et al.* 2008) of ([0.50]*quantity cut-down days) + ([0.50]*quality cut-back days) + ([0.25]*extreme-effort days). If this sum exceeded 30, it was recoded to equal 30, resulting in a sum ranging from 0 to 30. These four measures (i.e., the number of quantity cut-down, quality cut-back, extreme-effort, and aggregate partial-disability days) are considered as the four dependent variables in this chapter.

The 10 chronic physical conditions considered in our analysis were arthritis, cancer, cardiovascular disorders (heart attack, heart disease, hypertension, and stroke), chronic pain (chronic back or neck pain and other chronic pain), diabetes, digestive disorders (stomach or intestine ulcer and irritable bowel disorder), frequent or severe headache or migraine, insomnia, neurological disorders (multiple sclerosis, Parkinson's disease, and epilepsy or seizures), and respiratory disorders (seasonal allergies such as hay fever, asthma, and chronic obstructive pulmonary disease [COPD] or emphysema). As described in Chapter 2, these conditions were assessed using a checklist adapted from the US National Health Interview Survey (National Center for Health Statistics 1994). Methodological studies have documented moderate to good concordance between reports based on such checklists and medical records (Baker *et al.* 2001, Knight *et al.* 2001, Schoenborn *et al.* 2003). The *silent conditions* (i.e., conditions that cannot be detected by sufferers based on signs or symptoms, but must be detected based on medical tests, such as cancer or heart disease) were ascertained by asking respondents whether a doctor or other health professional ever told them that they had the condition, while the *symptom-based conditions* (i.e., conditions that sufferers can detect without medical diagnoses, such as chronic headaches or chronic back pain) were assessed by asking respondents whether they had ever had the condition. For the purposes of this study, our focus is on the conditions that were present at some time in the 12 months prior to the interview. In order to construct a comparison set of mental disorders roughly equal in number to the chronic physical conditions, we considered only nine mental disorders: alcohol abuse with or without dependence, bipolar disorder (i.e., bipolar I disorder, bipolar II disorder, and subthreshold bipolar disorder), drug abuse with and without dependence, generalized anxiety disorder (GAD), major depressive disorder (MDD), panic disorder and/or agoraphobia, post-traumatic stress disorder (PTSD), social phobia, and specific phobia. As with the chronic physical conditions, only mental disorders present in the 12 months before the interview were considered.

Statistical analysis

We examined the individual-level and societal-level associations of mental and physical disorders with the three partial-disability outcomes and the aggregate measure using generalized linear models (GLMs) to examine joint associations, controlling for age, sex, employment status, and country. As noted in Chapter 2, GLMs were used here to adjust for the fact that the four outcomes are highly skewed, making estimates of predictive associations based on ordinary least squares (OLS) regression analysis both biased and inefficient. As in the earlier chapters that used this analysis approach, we began by examining a number of two-part models as well as a number of standard GLM specifications and selected the best specification using standard empirical model comparison procedures (Buntin & Zaslavsky 2004). As the sample size was too small to allow each of the 524,268 (2^{19} − 20) logically possible combinations of comorbid disorders to be treated as separate predictors of partial disability, the GLM models necessarily made a number of simplifying assumptions about the effects of comorbidity, and we ultimately focused on five statistical models to investigate the association between mental and physical disorders and partial disability. Model 1 assumed additivity: that is, we included a separate predictor variable for sex, age, country, and for each of the 19 disorders without additional terms for comorbidities. This implied that the effects of comorbid disorders equaled the sum of their individual effects. Model 2 included, besides age, sex, and country, a series of dummy predictor variables for number of disorders (e.g., one such variable for respondents who had exactly one condition, another for respondents with exactly two disorders, etc.) without information about types of disorders. The assumption in model 2 was that the type of condition is unimportant once the number of disorders is known. Model 3 included, apart from age, sex, and country, 19 predictors for type and dummy predictors for number of disorders (starting with 2). Model 4 was built on model 3 but allowed the effects of type to be a linear function of number of other disorders by including interaction terms of type of disorder with number of other mental or physical disorders. Finally, a more complex statistical model (model 5) allowed for interactions of type with number using weighted counts based on type coefficients. Based on the Bayesian information criterion (BIC), model 3 was found to provide the best fit for each of the dependent variables (Appendix Table 12.1). Therefore, we focused on the coefficients from that model.

We calculated both the individual and the societal effects of disorders on partial disability. Individual-level effects refer to the difference in partial disability for those with and without mental or physical disorders or the *additional* number of days of partial disability for a respondent with a specific mental or physical disorder. Societal-level effects were estimated using population attributable risk proportions (PARPs). From a public health perspective, such an approach may help in identifying which disorders will have the most impact when it comes to making decisions about the (re)allocation of scarce resources in the general population. A PARP is to be interpreted as the proportion by which the number of partial-disability days in the general population could be reduced if a specific disorder were eliminated. See Chapter 2 for a discussion of individual-level effects and PARPs. Standard errors of prevalence estimates were calculated using the Taylor Series Linearization (TSL) method to account for the complex sample design (Wolter 1985). Standard errors of individual and societal-level coefficients were estimated using SAS macros for the Jackknife Repeated Replication method (JRR) for complex sample data (SAS Institute Inc. 2002). The macros written for this purpose were used to obtain standard errors of the simulated estimates of individual-level and societal-level disorder effects. Significance tests were consistently evaluated using 0.05-level, two-sided design-based tests.

Results

The prevalence of mental and physical disorders by country income level is shown in Table 11.2 (Chapter 11).

Distribution of partial-disability days

The mean number of partial-disability days was found to be 1.6 per month (Table 12.1), with ranges between 1.2 (in low/lower-middle-income countries) and 1.9 (in high-income countries). Interestingly, most partial-disability days were found in countries with higher incomes. About one in five (i.e., 21.6%) of respondents in the WMH sample reported experiencing at least one partial-disability day. Again, we found that respondents from high-income countries were more likely to report partial-disability days (25.4%) than those from upper-middle-income (15.4%) or low/lower-middle-income countries (19.7%). Among those claiming at least one partial-disability day, the average number of such days was approximately 7.3/month for the entire sample, with ranges between 6.2 per month (for respondents from low/lower-middle-income countries) and 8.2 per month (for those from upper-middle-income countries). A similar country

income level trend is found of all the specific component indicators of partial disability.

Partial disability among respondents with mental and physical disorders

The average number of partial-disability days reported varied considerably by type of disorder, but all were in the 2.4–4.6 range for individuals with chronic physical conditions (median = 3.3 days per month) and in the 2.4–5.8 range for mental disorders (median = 4.4 days per month). Interestingly, we found that although mental disorders are 3–4 times less common than chronic physical conditions (Table 11.2), mental disorders are associated with more overall partial-disability days (Table 12.2). More precisely, PTSD (5.8 days per month), GAD (5.0 days), and bipolar disorder (4.6 days) were related to the highest number of partial-disability days. Respondents with mental disorders systematically reported 15–28% more partial-disability days than respondents with chronic physical conditions. Among the chronic physical conditions, insomnia and neurological disorders were especially associated with partial disability (4.6 and 4.3 partial-disability days per month, respectively). When we broke down partial-disability days into the three subdomains, all disorders had a comparable impact. More information on the mean number of partial-disability days by country income level is shown in Appendix Table 12.2.

Individual-level effects of mental and physical disorders on partial-disability days

Table 12.3 shows the *additional* days per month with partial disability for respondents with mental and physical disorders, in comparison to those respondents with no disorders. The presence of any disorder is associated with an additional 1.6 partial-disability days per month (corresponding to about 19 days per year). Mental disorders take an especially high toll of partial disability, with 1.9 additional days per month for PTSD, 1.7 for MDD, and 1.7 for bipolar disorder. For chronic physical conditions, the additional days per month with partial disability are highest for insomnia (1.5), chronic pain conditions (1.5), and neurological disorders (1.2). Overall, the number of additional partial-disability days is similar for mental disorders and physical conditions: an average of 1.5 for the former and 1.4 for the latter, corresponding to 18

Table 12.1 Distribution of partial-disability days per month by country income level. The WMH surveys.

	All countries		Low/lower-middle		Upper-middle		High	
	%	(SE)	%	(SE)	%	(SE)	%	(SE)
Any days had to cut down quantity	16.8	(0.2)	16.2	(0.4)	13.0	(0.4)	19.0	(0.3)
1 day[a]	12.4	(0.4)	12.9	(0.9)	10.5	(0.9)	12.8	(0.5)
2 days[a]	18.0	(0.5)	22.3	(1.2)	16.0	(1.1)	16.8	(0.6)
3–5 days[a]	25.8	(0.5)	27.5	(1.1)	24.2	(1.1)	25.5	(0.7)
6–10 days[a]	15.8	(0.5)	18.8	(1.2)	15.2	(1.0)	14.7	(0.6)
11–20 days[a]	11.7	(0.4)	10.1	(0.8)	11.9	(0.9)	12.2	(0.5)
21–30 days[a]	16.4	(0.5)	8.5	(0.8)	22.1	(1.2)	17.9	(0.7)
	Mean	(SE)	Mean	(SE)	Mean	(SE)	Mean	(SE)
Mean number of quantity cut-down days	1.6	(0.03)	1.2	(0.05)	1.4	(0.06)	1.9	(0.05)
Mean number of quantity cut-down days, among those with any quantity cut-down days	9.5	(0.1)	7.3	(0.2)	11.1	(0.3)	9.9	(0.2)
Any days had to cut back quality	13.0	(0.2)	13.1	(0.4)	9.2	(0.3)	14.7	(0.3)
1 day[b]	12.3	(0.5)	12.4	(1.1)	11.7	(1.0)	12.3	(0.6)
2 days[b]	18.9	(0.6)	21.3	(1.4)	16.8	(1.2)	18.5	(0.7)
3–5 days[b]	30.5	(0.6)	31.2	(1.4)	31.4	(1.5)	29.9	(0.8)
6–10 days[b]	16.4	(0.5)	19.3	(1.3)	17.0	(1.4)	14.9	(0.6)
11–20 days[b]	11.3	(0.5)	10.0	(0.9)	12.5	(1.0)	11.6	(0.6)
21–30 days[b]	10.6	(0.4)	5.7	(0.7)	10.7	(0.9)	12.7	(0.6)
	Mean	(SE)	Mean	(SE)	Mean	(SE)	Mean	(SE)
Mean number of quality cut-back days	1.0	(0.02)	0.9	(0.03)	0.8	(0.04)	1.2	(0.03)
Mean number of quality cut-back days, among those with any quality cut-back days	8.0	(0.1)	6.7	(0.2)	8.3	(0.3)	8.5	(0.2)
Any days took extreme effort	13.5	(0.2)	11.8	(0.3)	9.4	(0.3)	16.3	(0.3)
1 day[c]	12.1	(0.5)	11.2	(1.1)	11.8	(1.4)	12.4	(0.6)
2 days[c]	17.1	(0.5)	17.2	(1.2)	15.9	(1.2)	17.5	(0.6)
3–5 days[c]	28.5	(0.6)	31.3	(1.5)	29.7	(1.6)	27.2	(0.7)
6–10 days[c]	17.9	(0.5)	21.5	(1.3)	18.2	(1.4)	16.6	(0.7)
11–20 days[c]	11.0	(0.4)	10.0	(0.8)	11.2	(0.9)	11.3	(0.6)
21–30 days[c]	13.4	(0.5)	8.8	(0.9)	13.2	(1.0)	15.1	(0.6)
	Mean	(SE)	Mean	(SE)	Mean	(SE)	Mean	(SE)
Mean number of extreme-effort days	1.2	(0.02)	0.9	(0.04)	0.8	(0.04)	1.5	(0.04)
Mean number of extreme-effort days, among those with any extreme-effort days	8.7	(0.1)	7.7	(0.3)	8.8	(0.3)	9.1	(0.2)
Any days with partial disability	21.6	(0.2)	19.7	(0.4)	15.4	(0.5)	25.4	(0.4)
1 day[d]	18.9	(0.4)	20.3	(1.0)	15.6	(0.9)	19.2	(0.5)
2 days[d]	15.7	(0.4)	15.7	(0.9)	14.5	(0.9)	16.0	(0.6)
3–5 days[d]	24.0	(0.5)	26.5	(1.2)	21.8	(1.1)	23.7	(0.5)
6–10 days[d]	15.1	(0.4)	16.9	(0.9)	15.1	(0.8)	14.4	(0.5)
11–20 days[d]	17.6	(0.4)	15.2	(0.7)	23.9	(1.1)	16.8	(0.5)
21–30 days[d]	8.7	(0.3)	5.4	(0.6)	9.2	(0.7)	9.9	(0.4)
	Mean	(SE)	Mean	(SE)	Mean	(SE)	Mean	(SE)
Mean number of partial-disability days	1.6	(0.03)	1.2	(0.04)	1.3	(0.05)	1.9	(0.04)
Mean number of partial-disability days, among those with any	7.3	(0.1)	6.2	(0.2)	8.2	(0.2)	7.4	(0.1)

[a] Percentage of respondents with any quantity cut-down day.
[b] Percentage of respondents with any quality cut-back day.
[c] Percentage of respondents with any extreme-effort day.
[d] Percentage of respondents with any partial-disability day.

Table 12.2 Mean number of partial-disability days per month associated with different mental disorders and physical conditions. The WMH surveys.

Disorder	Quantity cut-down days		Quality cut-back days		Extreme-effort days		Partial-disability days	
	Mean	(SE)	Mean	(SE)	Mean	(SE)	Mean	(SE)
Alcohol abuse	2.2	(0.2)	1.7	(0.1)	1.9	(0.1)	2.4	(0.2)
Bipolar	3.9	(0.3)	3.6	(0.3)	3.8	(0.3)	4.6	(0.3)
Drug abuse	2.9	(0.3)	2.6	(0.3)	2.8	(0.3)	3.4	(0.4)
Generalized anxiety	4.6	(0.3)	3.6	(0.3)	4.1	(0.3)	5.0	(0.3)
Major depressive disorder	3.9	(0.1)	3.2	(0.1)	3.8	(0.1)	4.4	(0.1)
Panic and/or agoraphobia	4.1	(0.3)	3.3	(0.2)	3.9	(0.2)	4.6	(0.2)
Post-traumatic stress	5.2	(0.3)	4.4	(0.3)	5.0	(0.3)	5.8	(0.3)
Social phobia	3.6	(0.2)	2.9	(0.2)	3.5	(0.2)	4.0	(0.2)
Specific phobia	2.8	(0.1)	2.3	(0.1)	2.8	(0.2)	3.1	(0.1)
Arthritis	3.2	(0.1)	2.3	(0.1)	2.7	(0.1)	3.3	(0.1)
Cancer	3.6	(0.3)	2.6	(0.2)	3.2	(0.2)	3.8	(0.3)
Cardiovascular	3.0	(0.1)	2.1	(0.1)	2.4	(0.1)	3.1	(0.1)
Chronic pain	3.2	(0.1)	2.3	(0.1)	2.8	(0.1)	3.4	(0.1)
Diabetes	3.0	(0.2)	2.3	(0.2)	2.7	(0.2)	3.2	(0.2)
Digestive	3.2	(0.2)	2.5	(0.2)	2.9	(0.2)	3.4	(0.2)
Headache/migraine	2.9	(0.1)	2.2	(0.1)	2.5	(0.2)	3.1	(0.1)
Insomnia	4.1	(0.2)	3.4	(0.1)	4.0	(0.2)	4.6	(0.2)
Neurological	4.0	(0.4)	3.1	(0.3)	3.6	(0.4)	4.3	(0.3)
Respiratory	2.3	(0.1)	1.7	(0.1)	1.9	(0.1)	2.4	(0.1)
Any mental	3.1	(0.1)	2.5	(0.1)	2.9	(0.1)	3.4	(0.1)
Any physical	2.3	(0.1)	1.6	(0.0)	1.8	(0.0)	2.3	(0.0)
Any disorder	2.2	(0.1)	1.6	(0.0)	1.8	(0.0)	2.3	(0.0)

and 17 additional days of partial disability per year, respectively.

After disaggregation by country income level (Table 12.4), the impact of disorders on the number of additional disability days was strongest in high-income countries, where 1.9 additional partial-disability days were reported per month, compared to 1.1 in upper-middle-income countries and 1.2 in low/lower-middle-income countries. No considerable difference between the impact of mental disorders and the impact of chronic physical conditions was found in low/lower-middle-income and high-income countries; the number of additional disability days in low/lower-middle-income countries was 1.0–1.1 (or about 12–13 days per year), while comparable figures for high-income

countries approached 1.7 for both mental and physical disorders (or about 20–21 days per year). This was not the case for upper-middle-income countries, in which there was a difference in the impact of mental and physical disorders on partial disability. As shown in Table 12.4, mental disorders have an 80% higher impact on partial disability than chronic physical conditions (1.6 and 0.9 additional partial days, respectively). At the level of individual disorders, the disorders with the highest impact are PTSD, insomnia, and GAD (all in the 2.2–3.0 range of additional days of partial disability per month, or 26–36 days per year) in low/lower-middle-income countries. PTSD, panic disorder, and MDD (all in the 1.6–2.0 range of additional partial-disability days per month, or 20–24 days per year) have the

Table 12.3 Additional partial-disability days per month (individual effects) associated with mental disorders and physical conditions in the overall sample. The WMH surveys.

Disorder	Additional quantity cut-down days			Additional quality cut-back days			Additional extreme-effort days			Any additional partial-disability days		
	Est[a]	SE	Rank	Est[a]	SE	Rank	Est[a]	SE	Rank	Est[a]	SE	Rank
Alcohol abuse	0.4	(0.2)	18	0.3	(0.2)	18	0.2	(0.2)	19	0.4	(0.2)	18
Bipolar	1.5	(0.4)	2	1.3	(0.3)	3	1.1	(0.4)	6	1.7	(0.5)	2
Drug abuse	0.4	(0.4)	16	0.7	(0.4)	12	0.8	(0.4)	12	0.8	(0.5)	13
Generalized anxiety	1.4	(0.3)	3	1.0	(0.3)	7	1.0	(0.3)	9	1.4	(0.4)	6
Major depressive disorder	1.3	(0.2)	5	1.3	(0.2)	2	1.6	(0.2)	2	1.7	(0.2)	3
Panic and/or agoraphobia	1.1	(0.3)	8	1.0	(0.2)	8	1.2	(0.2)	5	1.3	(0.2)	7
Post-traumatic stress	1.6	(0.3)	1	1.6	(0.3)	1	1.7	(0.3)	1	1.9	(0.4)	1
Social phobia	0.8	(0.2)	11	0.8	(0.2)	9	0.9	(0.2)	11	1.0	(0.2)	10
Specific phobia	0.4	(0.1)	17	0.6	(0.2)	13	0.7	(0.2)	13	0.7	(0.2)	15
Arthritis	0.8	(0.1)	10	0.5	(0.1)	16	0.7	(0.1)	14	0.8	(0.2)	12
Cancer	1.0	(0.3)	9	0.8	(0.2)	10	1.0	(0.3)	8	1.0	(0.3)	9
Cardiovascular	0.6	(0.1)	13	0.6	(0.1)	15	0.5	(0.1)	17	0.7	(0.2)	16
Chronic pain	1.3	(0.1)	6	1.1	(0.1)	5	1.4	(0.1)	3	1.5	(0.3)	5
Diabetes	0.6	(0.2)	14	0.6	(0.2)	14	0.7	(0.2)	15	0.7	(0.2)	14
Digestive	0.8	(0.2)	12	0.7	(0.2)	11	0.9	(0.2)	10	0.9	(0.3)	11
Headache/ migraine	0.5	(0.1)	15	0.5	(0.1)	17	0.6	(0.1)	16	0.7	(0.2)	17
Insomnia	1.4	(0.2)	4	1.1	(0.2)	4	1.4	(0.2)	4	1.5	(0.2)	4
Neurological	1.2	(0.4)	7	1.0	(0.3)	6	1.1	(0.4)	7	1.2	(0.5)	8
Respiratory	0.3	(0.1)	19	0.3	(0.1)	19	0.3	(0.1)	18	0.3	(0.1)	19
Any physical	1.3	(0.1)	–	1.1	(0.0)	–	1.2	(0.1)	–	1.4	(0.3)	–
Any mental	1.2	(0.1)	–	1.2	(0.1)	–	1.4	(0.1)	–	1.5	(0.1)	–
Any disorder	1.4	(0.1)	–	1.2	(0.0)	–	1.4	(0.1)	–	1.6	(0.2)	–

[a] Individual-effect estimate.

highest impact in upper-middle-income countries, and chronic pain conditions, digestive disorders, and bipolar disorder (all around 2.0 additional days per month, or 23–24 days per year) have the highest influence in high-income countries. Interestingly, these figures suggest that, although the overall impact of mental and physical disorders in low/lower-middle-income countries is generally lower than in high-income countries, the impact of specific disorders is considerably higher.

If the partial-disability measure is disaggregated by income category and the separate components of the aggregate measure (Table 12.4; Figure 12.1), it becomes clear that the impact of mental disorders on quantity cut-down, quality cut-back, and extreme-effort days is comparable (Figure 12.1A). Moreover, this impact seems quite similar in high- and upper-middle-income countries, as opposed to low/lower-middle-income countries. When comparing the impact of chronic physical conditions across income categories (Figure 12.1B), a different picture emerges. Indeed, the impact of chronic physical conditions on additional partial disability is the highest in high-

Table 12.4 Individual effects of mental and physical disorders on partial-disability days per month by country income level. The WMH surveys.

Disorder	Quantity cut-down days						Quality cut-back days						Extreme-effort days						Partial-disability days					
	Country income level						Country income level						Country income level						Country income level					
	Low/lower-middle		Upper-middle		High		Low/lower-middle		Upper-middle		High		Low/lower-middle		Upper-middle		High		Low/lower-middle		Upper-middle		High	
	Est[a]	SE	Est[a]	SE	Est[a]	SE	Est[a]	SE	Est[a]	SE	Est[a]	SE	Est[a]	SE	Est[a]	SE	Est[a]	SE	Est[a]	SE	Est[a]	SE	Est[a]	SE
Alcohol Abuse	0.6	(0.2)	0.5	(0.4)	0.3	(0.3)	0.4	(0.4)	0.1	(0.3)	0.5	(0.3)	0.2	(0.4)	0.4	(0.3)	0.3	(0.3)	0.5	(0.4)	0.4	(0.3)	0.5	(0.3)
Bipolar	0.3	(0.6)	1.0	(0.8)	1.8	(0.4)	0.6	(0.7)	1.2	(0.8)	1.4	(0.4)	1.1	(0.9)	0.7	(2.1)	1.3	(0.5)	0.8	(0.5)	1.5	(0.9)	2.0	(0.4)
Drug Abuse	1.1	(0.8)	0.2	(0.9)	0.4	(0.5)	2.6	(1.1)	0.1	(0.5)	0.6	(0.5)	0.5	(1.1)	-0.2	(4.4)	1.2	(0.6)	2.0	(0.7)	0.0	(0.7)	0.8	(0.5)
Generalized anxiety	2.6	(0.9)	1.2	(0.7)	0.9	(0.4)	1.7	(1.0)	0.9	(0.6)	0.7	(0.4)	0.9	(0.7)	1.1	(0.6)	1.0	(0.4)	2.2	(0.8)	1.3	(0.6)	1.0	(0.4)
Major depressive disorder	0.5	(0.4)	1.8	(0.4)	1.4	(0.2)	0.8	(0.3)	1.6	(0.3)	1.4	(0.2)	1.1	(0.4)	1.6	(0.6)	1.7	(0.2)	0.9	(0.3)	2.0	(0.4)	1.8	(0.2)
Panic and/or agoraphobia	1.1	(1.0)	1.5	(0.5)	0.9	(0.3)	0.1	(0.5)	1.0	(0.4)	1.2	(0.3)	0.3	(0.6)	1.9	(1.2)	1.2	(0.3)	0.8	(0.7)	1.6	(0.4)	1.2	(0.3)
Post-traumatic stress	2.5	(0.9)	1.1	(0.8)	1.5	(0.4)	2.4	(0.8)	1.9	(0.7)	1.3	(0.4)	2.7	(0.9)	2.0	(0.8)	1.4	(0.4)	3.0	(0.8)	1.8	(0.7)	1.7	(0.4)
Social phobia	0.4	(0.9)	1.1	(0.6)	0.8	(0.2)	-0.0	(0.3)	1.2	(0.5)	0.8	(0.2)	0.2	(0.4)	1.3	(0.6)	0.9	(0.2)	0.3	(0.6)	1.3	(0.6)	1.0	(0.2)
Specific phobia	0.1	(0.3)	0.4	(0.3)	0.5	(0.2)	0.3	(0.3)	0.7	(0.3)	0.7	(0.3)	0.3	(0.3)	0.8	(0.5)	0.9	(0.3)	0.3	(0.3)	0.8	(0.3)	0.8	(0.2)
Arthritis	0.3	(0.2)	0.6	(0.3)	1.2	(0.2)	0.4	(0.3)	0.2	(0.2)	0.7	(0.1)	0.6	(0.3)	0.2	(0.2)	1.0	(0.2)	0.5	(0.2)	0.4	(0.2)	1.1	(0.2)
Cancer	0.9	(0.9)	0.8	(0.7)	1.0	(0.4)	1.8	(1.2)	0.4	(0.8)	0.7	(0.2)	1.2	(1.0)	1.1	(2.3)	0.9	(0.3)	1.4	(1.0)	0.9	(0.8)	1.0	(0.3)
Cardiovascular	0.3	(0.3)	0.6	(0.3)	0.9	(0.2)	0.3	(0.2)	0.5	(0.2)	0.7	(0.1)	0.0	(0.4)	0.2	(1.0)	0.8	(0.1)	0.3	(0.3)	0.6	(0.2)	0.9	(0.1)
Chronic pain	0.7	(0.2)	0.5	(0.2)	1.8	(0.2)	0.4	(0.2)	0.8	(0.1)	1.5	(0.1)	0.6	(0.2)	1.0	(0.6)	1.8	(0.2)	0.7	(0.2)	0.9	(0.2)	2.0	(0.1)
Diabetes	0.9	(0.4)	0.5	(0.4)	0.5	(0.3)	0.8	(0.4)	0.2	(0.3)	0.7	(0.2)	0.9	(0.6)	0.6	(0.3)	0.7	(0.3)	1.0	(0.4)	0.5	(0.3)	0.7	(0.3)
Digestive	0.4	(0.3)	-0.2	(0.4)	1.8	(0.4)	0.2	(0.3)	0.3	(0.2)	1.5	(0.4)	0.2	(0.3)	0.1	(0.4)	2.1	(0.4)	0.3	(0.3)	0.0	(0.3)	2.0	(0.4)
Headache/migraine	0.6	(0.2)	0.3	(0.2)	0.7	(0.2)	0.7	(0.2)	0.5	(0.2)	0.5	(0.2)	0.6	(0.2)	0.2	(0.3)	0.7	(0.2)	0.8	(0.2)	0.4	(0.2)	0.8	(0.2)
Insomnia	2.3	(0.6)	0.9	(0.3)	1.1	(0.3)	1.7	(0.5)	0.5	(0.3)	1.1	(0.2)	2.0	(0.6)	1.1	(0.5)	1.2	(0.2)	2.4	(0.5)	1.0	(0.3)	1.4	(0.2)
Neurological	0.5	(0.9)	1.6	(0.7)	1.2	(0.5)	0.4	(0.8)	1.3	(0.5)	1.2	(0.5)	0.7	(0.9)	1.2	(1.3)	1.3	(0.6)	0.8	(0.8)	1.7	(0.6)	1.3	(0.5)
Respiratory	0.4	(0.2)	-0.3	(0.2)	0.4	(0.1)	0.3	(0.2)	-0.2	(0.2)	0.4	(0.1)	0.5	(0.3)	-0.2	(0.8)	0.3	(0.1)	0.5	(0.2)	-0.3	(0.2)	0.4	(0.1)
Any mental	0.8	(0.2)	1.3	(0.2)	1.3	(0.1)	0.8	(0.2)	1.2	(0.2)	1.3	(0.1)	0.9	(0.2)	1.4	(0.3)	1.5	(0.1)	1.0	(0.2)	1.6	(0.2)	1.7	(0.1)
Any physical	1.0	(0.1)	0.7	(0.1)	1.6	(0.1)	0.8	(0.2)	0.7	(0.1)	1.3	(0.1)	0.9	(0.2)	0.8	(0.6)	1.6	(0.1)	1.1	(0.1)	0.9	(0.1)	1.7	(0.1)
Any disorder	1.0	(0.1)	1.0	(0.1)	1.7	(0.1)	0.8	(0.2)	0.9	(0.1)	1.4	(0.1)	1.0	(0.2)	1.0	(0.5)	1.7	(0.1)	1.2	(0.1)	1.1	(0.1)	1.9	(0.1)

[a]Est, estimate of the individual effect.

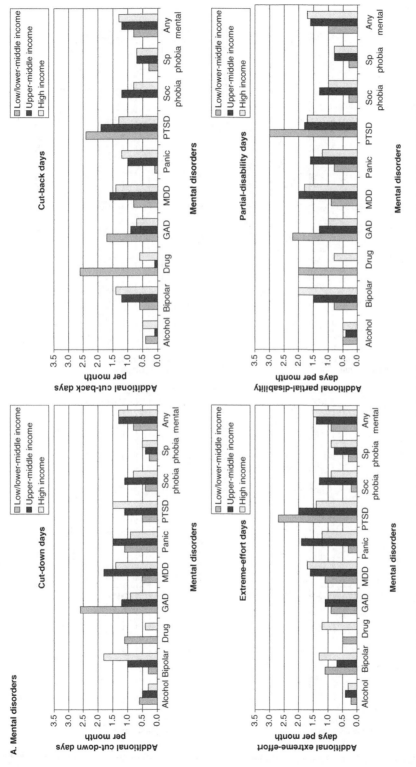

Figure 12.1 Additional partial-disability days per month associated with mental and physical disorders by country income level ("individual effects"). The WMH surveys.
(A) Mental disorders.
(B) Chronic physical conditions.

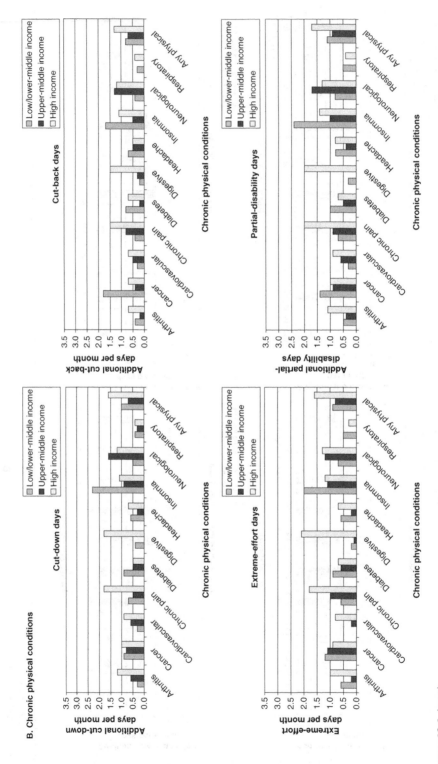

Figure 12.1 (cont.)

income countries, compared to upper-middle- and low/lower-middle-income countries, but their impact on quantity cut-down, quality cut-back, and extreme-effort days remains comparable.

The multivariate interactive regression model shown in Table 12.5 reveals that all the disorders under consideration are significantly associated with additional partial-disability days, even when data are broken down for the three subdomains of partial disability. In both bivariate and multivariate approaches, MDD, bipolar disorder, and chronic pain conditions are the most predictive in this multivariate model. In general, mental disorders have higher regression coefficients than chronic physical conditions in predicting partial disability. When the regression coefficients are broken down for the separate components of partial disability (Table 12.5), it is clear that chronic pain is systematically highly predictive of additional partial disability, and the same holds true for MDD, although to a lesser extent. PTSD also appears to be highly predictive of quality cut-back days, and panic disorder and/or agoraphobia is highly predictive of extreme-effort days.

Interestingly, the regression coefficients associated with the number of mental and chronic physical conditions do not change considerably with an increasing number of disorders. In fact, of the 15 coefficients studied (five groups of dummies for number of disorders by three partial disability subdomains – see bottom of Table 12.5), only five are significant. This particular finding suggests that there are additive interactions among the various disorders, and we interpret this to mean that the joint effects of multiple disorders are additive to those associated with individual disorders.

Societal-level effects of mental and physical disorders on partial-disability days

Table 12.6 shows the population attributable risk proportions (PARPs) of partial-disability days caused by mental and physical disorders. The use of PARPs allowed us to estimate the proportion by which the number of partial-disability days in the general population could (theoretically) be reduced if a specific disorder were eliminated. In general, estimated PARPs are around 59% when all disorders are considered at once, with higher PARPs for physical than for mental disorders (49% vs. 15%). This could be interpreted as meaning that within the theoretical

assumption that all disorders could be prevented, partial disability could be reduced by about 59%. Similarly, in the assumption that all mental or physical disorders could be prevented, the number of partial-disability days could theoretically be reduced by 15% and 49% respectively. When focusing on individual disorders, we find that chronic pain conditions (PARP = 21.0%), arthritis (PARP = 7.8%), and cardiovascular disorders (PARP = 7.2%) yield the highest attributable risk (Table 12.6). Disaggregating the partial disability measure into its three components shows that the highest PARPs correspond to extreme-effort days (PARP = 70.0%), followed by quality cut-back days (PARP = 66.1%), and quantity cut-down days (PARP = 50.5%). This suggests that if these disorders were eliminated, the highest level of performance would be achieved on the extreme-effort days, and not as much on the quantity cut-down or quality cut-back days. Moreover, when individual disorders are taken into account, chronic pain conditions have one of the highest degrees of impact on each of the three domains, with all PARPs in the 17–26% range. Although to a lesser extent, arthritis (especially when it comes to extreme-effort days), cardiovascular disorders (especially in relation to quality cut-back days), depression (especially with regard to extreme-effort and quality cut-back days), and frequent or severe headaches or migraines (especially in relation to quality cut-back and extreme-effort days) also have high PARPs. A summary of PARP estimates is shown in Figure 12.2.

Table 12.7 presents a profile of the societal effects of mental and physical disorders on partial disability across the three country income categories, disaggregated by the different components of partial disability. Based on these analyses, four interesting findings stand out. First, we found a gradient between the PARP estimates for the aggregated partial-disability measure and income category: although the overall PARP for any disorder was around 59%, the highest PARPs were obtained in high-income countries (around 65%), followed by upper-middle-income (around 52%), and low/lower-middle-income countries (around 49%). Second, chronic physical conditions consistently had higher PARPs than mental disorders, but this effect is more pronounced in low/lower-middle-income and in high-income countries than in upper-middle-income countries. Indeed, the PARPs of mental disorders in upper-middle-income countries were approximately 20%, suggesting that partial disability in these

Table 12.5 Multivariate associations between type and number of mental disorders and physical conditions with additional partial-disability days. The WMH surveys.

Disorder	Quantity cut-down days				Quality cut-back days				Extreme-effort days				Partial-disability days			
	Bivariate model		Multivariate additive model		Bivariate model		Multivariate additive model		Bivariate model		Multivariate additive model		Bivariate model		Multivariate additive model	
	Coeff[a]	(SE)	Coeff[a]	(SE)	Coeff[a]	(SE)	Coeff[a]	(SE)	Coeff[a]	(SE)	Coeff[a]	(SE)	Coeff[a]	(SE)	Coeff[a]	(SE)
Alcohol abuse	0.14*	(0.055)	0.15*	(0.058)	0.17*	(0.048)	0.20*	(0.051)	0.10	(0.053)	0.13*	(0.056)	0.16*	(0.046)	0.18*	(0.049)
Bipolar	0.42*	(0.067)	0.46*	(0.068)	0.42*	(0.055)	0.47*	(0.057)	0.33*	(0.060)	0.39*	(0.061)	0.46*	(0.054)	0.52*	(0.055)
Drug abuse	0.14	(0.087)	0.16	(0.089)	0.26*	(0.072)	0.31*	(0.074)	0.31*	(0.075)	0.35*	(0.076)	0.25*	(0.070)	0.29*	(0.071)
Generalized anxiety	0.36*	(0.046)	0.38*	(0.050)	0.30*	(0.039)	0.34*	(0.043)	0.27*	(0.041)	0.32*	(0.045)	0.34*	(0.038)	0.38*	(0.041)
Major depressive disorder	0.40*	(0.027)	0.40*	(0.034)	0.46*	(0.023)	0.49*	(0.030)	0.52*	(0.024)	0.54*	(0.031)	0.49*	(0.022)	0.51*	(0.028)
Post-traumatic stress	0.39*	(0.042)	0.42*	(0.047)	0.45*	(0.035)	0.50*	(0.040)	0.42*	(0.037)	0.48*	(0.042)	0.44*	(0.034)	0.49*	(0.039)
Panic and/or agoraphobia	0.28*	(0.042)	0.31*	(0.046)	0.31*	(0.036)	0.37*	(0.040)	0.36*	(0.037)	0.42*	(0.041)	0.33*	(0.035)	0.38*	(0.038)
Social phobia	0.22*	(0.041)	0.24*	(0.046)	0.27*	(0.035)	0.31*	(0.039)	0.29*	(0.036)	0.33*	(0.041)	0.26*	(0.034)	0.31*	(0.038)
Specific phobia	0.14*	(0.032)	0.15*	(0.037)	0.26*	(0.028)	0.29*	(0.033)	0.28*	(0.028)	0.30*	(0.034)	0.24*	(0.026)	0.26*	(0.031)
Arthtis	0.27*	(0.021)	0.26*	(0.030)	0.21*	(0.019)	0.23*	(0.028)	0.26*	(0.020)	0.27*	(0.029)	0.27*	(0.018)	0.27*	(0.026)
Cancer	0.28*	(0.040)	0.29*	(0.045)	0.26*	(0.035)	0.30*	(0.039)	0.30*	(0.035)	0.32*	(0.040)	0.29*	(0.033)	0.31*	(0.038)
Cardiovascular	0.21*	(0.021)	0.19*	(0.029)	0.23*	(0.019)	0.24*	(0.027)	0.19*	(0.020)	0.19*	(0.028)	0.22*	(0.018)	0.22*	(0.025)
Chronic pain	0.44*	(0.019)	0.42*	(0.028)	0.50*	(0.018)	0.50*	(0.026)	0.58*	(0.019)	0.56*	(0.027)	0.52*	(0.016)	0.51*	(0.024)
Diabetes	0.19*	(0.032)	0.18*	(0.037)	0.24*	(0.028)	0.26*	(0.033)	0.26*	(0.029)	0.27*	(0.034)	0.23*	(0.027)	0.24*	(0.032)
Digestive	0.24*	(0.035)	0.25*	(0.040)	0.28*	(0.030)	0.31*	(0.035)	0.34*	(0.031)	0.37*	(0.036)	0.27*	(0.029)	0.31*	(0.033)
Headache/migraine	0.18*	(0.022)	0.17*	(0.029)	0.22*	(0.020)	0.24*	(0.027)	0.22*	(0.020)	0.23*	(0.029)	0.22*	(0.018)	0.23*	(0.025)
Insomnia	0.40*	(0.028)	0.40*	(0.035)	0.38*	(0.024)	0.41*	(0.030)	0.41*	(0.024)	0.43*	(0.031)	0.42*	(0.023)	0.44*	(0.029)
Neurological	0.31*	(0.052)	0.34*	(0.055)	0.34*	(0.045)	0.38*	(0.048)	0.33*	(0.047)	0.38*	(0.050)	0.33*	(0.043)	0.37*	(0.047)
Respiratory	0.09*	(0.021)	0.08*	(0.028)	0.11*	(0.019)	0.13*	(0.026)	0.11*	(0.019)	0.11*	(0.028)	0.11*	(0.017)	0.12*	(0.025)
2 disorders			0.03	(0.038)			0.03	(0.036)			0.12*	(0.038)			0.04	(0.033)
3 disorders			0.07	(0.057)			−0.04	(0.053)			0.07	(0.056)			0.02	(0.049)
4/5 disorders			0.14	(0.082)			0.07	(0.077)			0.17*	(0.082)			0.11	(0.071)
6/7 disorders			−0.08	(0.126)			−0.27*	(0.116)			−0.15	(0.125)			−0.20	(0.109)
8 disorders			−0.29	(0.183)			−0.34*	(0.165)			−0.33	(0.178)			−0.37*	(0.156)

[a] Coefficients from the GLM model.
* Significant at the 0.05 level, two-sided test.

Table 12.6 Population attributable risk proportions (PARPs) of partial-disability days due to mental and physical disorders. The WMH surveys.

Disorder	Additional quantity cut-down days			Additional quality cut-back days			Additional extreme-effort days			Additional partial-disability days		
	PARP (%)	(SE)	Rank	PARP (%)	(SE)	Rank	PARP (%)	(SE)	Rank	PARP (%)	(SE)	Rank
Alcohol abuse	0.5	(0.2)	18	0.7	(0.3)	18	0.4	(0.3)	19	0.6	(0.3)	18
Bipolar	0.7	(0.2)	17	0.9	(0.3)	17	0.8	(0.2)	17	0.8	(0.4)	17
Drug abuse	0.2	(0.1)	19	0.4	(0.2)	19	0.4	(0.2)	18	0.3	(0.2)	19
Generalized anxiety	1.1	(0.3)	15	1.3	(0.4)	15	1.2	(0.4)	15	1.2	(0.5)	15
Major depressive disorder	4.5	(0.6)	5	6.9	(0.8)	5	7.6	(0.8)	3	5.9	(1.2)	5
Panic and/or agoraphobia	1.2	(0.3)	13	1.8	(0.4)	13	2.0	(0.4)	12	1.5	(0.5)	12
Post-traumatic stress	1.4	(0.3)	10	2.2	(0.4)	10	2.1	(0.4)	11	1.8	(0.7)	11
Social phobia	1.1	(0.3)	14	1.8	(0.4)	12	2.0	(0.4)	13	1.5	(0.6)	13
Specific phobia	1.3	(0.5)	12	3.1	(0.8)	8	3.4	(0.8)	8	2.3	(0.7)	8
Arthritis	7.7	(1.2)	2	7.7	(1.5)	3	9.4	(1.3)	2	7.8	(1.3)	2
Cancer	1.4	(0.4)	11	1.6	(0.5)	14	1.9	(0.5)	14	1.4	(0.7)	14
Cardiovascular	6.6	(1.4)	3	9.0	(1.6)	2	7.5	(1.5)	4	7.2	(1.3)	3
Chronic pain	17.2	(1.6)	1	24.0	(2.0)	1	26.7	(1.9)	1	21.0	(2.4)	1
Diabetes	1.5	(0.5)	9	2.4	(0.7)	9	2.6	(0.7)	10	1.9	(0.8)	9
Digestive	1.5	(0.4)	8	2.2	(0.7)	11	2.7	(0.6)	9	1.8	(0.8)	10
Headache/migraine	4.6	(1.0)	4	7.1	(1.4)	4	6.9	(1.3)	5	6.0	(1.0)	4
Insomnia	4.1	(0.6)	6	5.3	(0.8)	6	5.7	(0.8)	6	4.7	(0.9)	6
Neurological	0.8	(0.2)	16	1.1	(0.3)	16	1.1	(0.4)	16	0.9	(0.5)	16
Respiratory	2.8	(1.1)	7	4.4	(1.5)	7	4.0	(1.4)	7	3.5	(1.1)	7
Any mental	11.5	(0.8)	–	17.5	(1.1)	–	18.3	(1.0)	–	14.7	(4.0)	–
Any physical	42.2	(2.2)	–	54.9	(2.3)	–	58.5	(2.0)	–	49.2	(4.9)	–
Any disorder	50.5	(2.6)	–	66.1	(2.5)	–	70.0	(2.3)	–	59.4	(6.8)	–

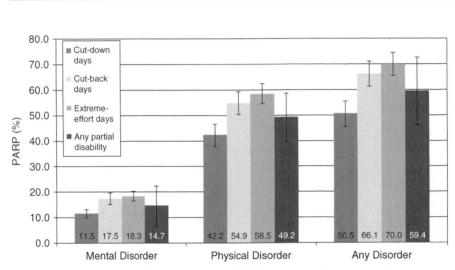

Figure 12.2 Population attributable risk proportions (PARPs) associated with mental and physical disorders. The WMH surveys.

countries could be reduced by 20% if all mental disorders could be eliminated. Comparable figures for the other two groups of countries are considerably lower. Among the individual disorders, chronic pain has the strongest association (in terms of PARPs) with partial disability across all three country income categories. Although the PARPs vary considerably across country income category, they are still between 12.5% and 23.1% for this individual condition. Arthritis and MDD, with moderate to high PARPs, are the next most significant classes of disorders in terms of their impact on daily life functioning.

Third, considering the separate components of partial disability (Table 12.7) shows that, overall, the highest PARPs for chronic physical conditions are obtained in high-income countries (almost 62% for both quality cut-back days and extreme-effort days). This is not the case for mental disorders, in which the highest PARPs are found in upper-middle-income countries for quantity cut-down, quality cut-back, and extreme-effort days. Fourth, on the level of individual disorders, there is one disorder that consistently stands out; a disorder that has a pervasive effect on partial disability across the board at the societal level: chronic pain conditions. The median PARP is about 20% in relation to the societal impact across income and across separate partial disability measures, suggesting that around the world, partial disability could be reduced by about 20% (with ranges between 9% and 27%) if chronic pain conditions were eliminated. Frequent or severe headaches or migraines, cardiovascular disease, arthritis, depression, and insomnia also

have effects at the society level but their influence is far less pervasive than the societal impact of chronic pain conditions.

Discussion

This first worldwide population-based approach has revealed that both mental and physical disorders are associated with considerable partial disability in cross-culturally and cross-economically varied general populations. The general population data from 25 samples around the world shows that people with PTSD, GAD, insomnia, bipolar disorder, or panic disorder report up to 50 days of partial disability per year. On the individual level, mental and physical disorders are associated with about 19 *additional* partial-disability days per year. This is more pronounced in high-income countries (23 additional days) than in upper-middle-income and low/lower-middle-income countries (about 14 additional days). Among the individual disorders, PTSD, depression, and bipolar disorder (all about 20–23 additional partial-disability days per year) were found to have the highest impact on daily life. A different picture emerged when we looked at the impact of disorders at the societal level using population attributable risk proportions (PARPs). We found that all of the disorders together accounted for about 59% of all partial-disability days (65% in high-income, 52% in upper-middle-income, and 49% in low/lower-middle-income countries), with chronic physical conditions having the highest impact at the society level. These accounted for 49% of

Table 12.7 Population attributable risk proportions (PARPs) of partial-disability days due to mental and physical disorders by country income level. The WMH surveys.

Disorder	Quantity cut-down days						Quality cut-back days						Extreme-effort days						Partial-disability days					
	Country income level						Country income level						Country income level						Country income level					
	Low/lower-middle		Upper-middle		High		Low/lower-middle		Upper-middle		High		Low/lower-middle		Upper-middle		High		Low/lower-middle		Upper-middle		High	
	PARP (%)	(SE)	PARP (%)	(SE)	PARP (%)	(SE)	PARP (%)	(SE)	PARP (%)	(SE)	PARP (%)	(SE)	PARP (%)	(SE)	PARP (%)	(SE)	PARP (%)	(SE)	PARP (%)	(SE)	PARP (%)	(SE)	PARP (%)	(SE)
Alcohol abuse	0.9	(0.5)	0.9	(0.8)	0.3	(0.3)	0.9	(0.8)	0.3	(1.0)	0.8	(0.5)	0.5	(0.9)	1.2	(1.2)	0.4	(0.4)	0.8	(0.5)	1.0	(0.7)	0.5	(0.3)
Bipolar	0.1	(0.2)	0.4	(0.3)	1.0	(0.3)	0.3	(0.3)	0.9	(0.6)	1.2	(0.4)	0.5	(0.4)	0.4	(1.5)	0.9	(0.3)	0.2	(0.2)	0.7	(0.4)	1.1	(0.3)
Drug abuse	0.2	(0.1)	0.1	(0.4)	0.2	(0.2)	0.6	(0.3)	0.1	(0.5)	0.4	(0.3)	0.1	(0.2)	-0.1	(3.2)	0.6	(0.3)	0.4	(0.1)	0.0	(0.4)	0.3	(0.2)
Generalized anxiety	2.2	(0.8)	0.8	(0.5)	0.8	(0.3)	1.9	(1.2)	1.3	(0.8)	1.0	(0.5)	1.0	(0.8)	1.3	(1.1)	1.1	(0.5)	1.8	(0.7)	1.1	(0.5)	0.9	(0.3)
Major depressive disorder	2.2	(1.5)	6.5	(1.2)	4.6	(0.7)	4.2	(1.8)	11.1	(2.1)	7.1	(1.1)	6.1	(2.6)	9.0	(8.3)	7.1	(0.9)	3.7	(1.4)	8.6	(1.4)	5.8	(0.7)
Panic disorder	1.0	(0.9)	2.7	(1.0)	0.8	(0.3)	0.2	(0.7)	3.7	(1.3)	1.8	(0.5)	0.4	(0.8)	5.2	(2.6)	1.5	(0.4)	0.7	(0.6)	3.5	(0.9)	1.2	(0.3)
Post-traumatic stress	1.5	(0.6)	0.7	(0.6)	1.6	(0.4)	1.9	(0.7)	2.5	(0.9)	2.2	(0.6)	2.1	(0.8)	2.0	(1.7)	1.9	(0.5)	1.7	(0.6)	1.4	(0.6)	1.8	(0.4)
Social phobia	0.4	(0.9)	1.5	(0.9)	1.3	(0.4)	0.0	(0.4)	3.2	(1.4)	2.2	(0.6)	0.3	(0.6)	2.8	(2.1)	2.1	(0.5)	0.2	(0.5)	2.1	(0.9)	1.7	(0.4)
Specific phobia	0.3	(1.1)	1.4	(1.0)	1.5	(0.6)	1.5	(1.5)	4.3	(1.7)	3.3	(1.2)	1.2	(1.6)	3.9	(3.2)	3.5	(1.0)	1.1	(1.2)	2.9	(1.2)	2.5	(0.7)
Arthritis	3.1	(2.6)	5.1	(2.2)	10.1	(1.7)	6.4	(4.0)	3.1	(3.0)	9.5	(2.0)	9.0	(4.2)	2.9	(3.7)	10.8	(1.7)	5.5	(2.5)	3.8	(1.9)	9.9	(1.3)
Cancer	0.3	(0.3)	0.4	(0.4)	2.0	(0.7)	0.8	(0.5)	0.5	(0.8)	2.3	(0.7)	0.5	(0.5)	0.9	(2.5)	2.3	(0.7)	0.4	(0.3)	0.6	(0.5)	2.0	(0.5)
Cardiovascular	2.6	(2.6)	7.1	(3.6)	8.4	(1.7)	4.0	(3.5)	11.3	(4.5)	11.2	(2.1)	0.2	(5.0)	3.8	(21.6)	10.0	(1.8)	2.8	(2.5)	8.1	(3.1)	9.1	(1.4)
Chronic pain	13.2	(4.2)	8.6	(3.1)	19.8	(1.9)	10.8	(5.1)	25.9	(4.1)	26.7	(2.3)	14.0	(6.0)	25.0	(27.8)	26.8	(2.1)	12.5	(3.5)	16.2	(2.8)	23.1	(1.6)
Diabetes	1.9	(0.8)	1.4	(1.1)	1.3	(0.7)	2.1	(1.2)	1.3	(1.7)	2.7	(0.9)	2.6	(1.8)	2.8	(2.5)	2.3	(0.8)	2.0	(0.8)	1.7	(1.1)	1.9	(0.6)
Digestive	1.5	(1.3)	-0.4	(1.1)	2.2	(0.5)	1.0	(1.6)	1.6	(1.4)	2.8	(0.8)	0.9	(1.5)	0.6	(1.6)	3.3	(0.7)	1.2	(1.2)	0.1	(0.9)	2.4	(0.5)
Headache/migraine	7.2	(2.8)	4.2	(2.3)	3.8	(1.1)	11.8	(3.8)	11.9	(4.2)	4.5	(1.5)	10.5	(4.1)	4.9	(8.4)	5.4	(1.4)	9.4	(2.4)	6.8	(2.6)	4.5	(1.0)

Table 12.7 (cont.)

Disorder	Quantity cut-down days						Quality cut-back days						Extreme-effort days						Partial-disability days					
	Country income level						Country income level						Country income level						Country income level					
	Low/lower-middle		Upper-middle		High		Low/lower-middle		Upper-middle		High		Low/lower-middle		Upper-middle		High		Low/lower-middle		Upper-middle		High	
	PARP (%)	(SE)	PARP (%)	(SE)	PARP (%)	(SE)	PARP (%)	(SE)	PARP (%)	(SE)	PARP (%)	(SE)	PARP (%)	(SE)	PARP (%)	(SE)	PARP (%)	(SE)	PARP (%)	(SE)	PARP (%)	(SE)	PARP (%)	(SE)
Insomnia	8.2	(2.1)	2.6	(1.0)	3.3	(0.7)	7.8	(2.2)	3.0	(1.6)	5.0	(1.0)	9.7	(3.1)	4.8	(4.9)	4.6	(0.9)	8.2	(1.9)	3.3	(1.0)	4.0	(0.7)
Neurological	0.3	(0.6)	1.6	(0.7)	0.7	(0.3)	0.4	(0.7)	2.5	(1.0)	1.1	(0.4)	0.6	(0.7)	1.7	(2.9)	1.0	(0.5)	0.5	(0.6)	1.8	(0.6)	0.8	(0.3)
Respiratory	4.6	(2.6)	-3.1	(2.1)	4.2	(1.4)	4.5	(3.1)	-3.6	(3.1)	6.8	(2.1)	6.6	(3.6)	-2.1	(12.4)	5.0	(1.7)	4.9	(2.4)	-2.6	(2.2)	5.0	(1.3)
Any mental	8.7	(1.9)	14.1	(2.0)	11.5	(1.1)	11.2	(3.2)	24.9	(2.6)	18.2	(1.5)	12.1	(3.7)	23.2	(18.5)	17.7	(1.2)	10.4	(1.8)	19.6	(2.0)	14.9	(1.0)
Any physical	39.1	(4.4)	26.2	(4.6)	48.2	(3.0)	42.1	(8.8)	52.5	(5.8)	61.5	(2.8)	48.7	(13.9)	41.9	(54.6)	61.8	(2.7)	42.2	(3.6)	37.2	(4.4)	54.4	(2.2)
Any disorder	45.3	(5.8)	37.7	(5.1)	56.2	(3.5)	48.3	(11.2)	68.8	(6.1)	73.8	(3.0)	55.2	(16.0)	57.7	(58.0)	73.6	(3.2)	48.9	(4.7)	52.0	(4.7)	64.9	(2.6)

observed partial disability, compared to only 15% accounted for by mental disorders. Chronic pain conditions systematically yielded the highest PARP.

These results should be interpreted in the light of the following limitations. **First**, the set of disorders included in the WMH surveys was not exhaustive. Indeed, a restricted set of common mental and physical disorders was included in the analyses and some of these were pooled to form larger disorder groups. A number of disorders known to be burdensome, such as psychosis, dementia, and chronic fatigue, were not included. Prior research has suggested that disability associated with psychosis is at least similar to disability associated with other mental disorders (Gureje *et al.* 2002). The British National Survey of Psychiatric Morbidity showed that chronic fatigue is not only a chronic prevalent condition (with prevalence estimates of around 15%), but is also significantly associated with increased psychiatric morbidity (Watanabe *et al.* 2008) and impaired daily functioning (Merrill & Verbrugge 1999). Nonetheless, the disorders we did consider included many of those most commonly reported in previous population studies (Alonso *et al.* 2004). Further research should more thoroughly study these possibly high-impact disorders which were not included in this study.

A **second** limitation pertains to the self-report method we used to assess chronic physical conditions. As the WMH surveys were conducted among many different population samples around the world, it was not feasible to include a more comprehensive assessment of chronic physical conditions. Although some prior research has demonstrated a reasonable correspondence between self-reported chronic disorders such as diabetes, heart disease, and asthma and general practitioners' records (Kriegsman *et al.* 1996), other studies have suggested that self-report measures may be more susceptible to under-reporting bias than behavioral measures or physical examinations. They may be biased by cultural norms or demographic factors as well (e.g., lower level of education or poor health literacy) (Harrison 1991, Solomon 2001). There is even some evidence that somatic disorders tend to be forgotten in self-reports (Biering-Sorensen & Hilden 1984, Jamison *et al.* 2006). This suggests that we may have underestimated the contribution of chronic physical conditions to partial disability.

Third, since the WMH surveys are actually cross-sectional in nature, the data obtained from them have no implications whatsoever for causal relationships

between mental and physical disorders on the one hand and partial disability on the other. Whether the disorders cause, follow, or simply co-occur with partial disability is a question for future research in which a focus on the ages of onset of the disorders studied might provide more insight into the course of associated and observed partial disability. Even in the use of PARPs, any inference with regard to causality should be avoided. After all, a PARP is a theoretical measure used to depict the strength of an association in the assumption of causality.

Fourth, a further limitation is that we did not analyze the severity or seriousness of the disorders under consideration. A **fifth** and final limitation is that the time frame we used to assess partial disability was limited to the 30 days previous to the interview. We did this in order to increase the validity of the self-reported data. However, for more episodic disorders or disorders with frequent relapses, the recall period might have missed a severe exacerbation present in the previous year, but not in the month before the actual interview.

Notwithstanding these limitations, several findings yielded by this study expand upon the existing body of knowledge on partial disability in the literature. For individuals, mental disorders are associated with a significant *additional* increase in partial-disability days, even after rigorously controlling for a broad set of sociodemographic variables and comorbidity. These findings expand upon earlier work (Kessler *et al.* 2003, Alonso *et al.* 2004, Polder & Achterberg 2004, Buist-Bouwman *et al.* 2005) by showing that mental disorders are associated with partial disability, above and beyond full disability. Indeed, as shown in the analysis of disability days in Chapter 11, panic disorder, bipolar disorder, and PTSD are associated with about 41–43 days per year on which respondents are totally unable to perform their daily role. In addition to this finding, data from this chapter show that all three of these disorders are also associated with 55–70 days of partial disability per year. But an even closer look at the data illustrates that not only these three but rather a broad range of mental disorders are associated with both days *totally* and days *partially* out of role. Our findings also suggest that, across country income categories and different cultures, mental disorders are systematically associated with an approximate 33% increase in partial-disability days per year compared to chronic physical conditions. Interestingly, this particular finding is in line with the study of total-disability days, in which mental disorders were systematically associated with 22% more total-disability days per year compared to chronic physical conditions.

To the best of our knowledge, our approach is the first cross-national study comparing the relative impact of disorders in respondents who indicate that they are not fully out of role in their daily functioning. Some of our results differ from those yielded by previous studies (Heffler *et al.* 2002). This could be due to methodological differences between this study and previous ones. In general, our estimates may differ from previous studies for three main reasons. First, previous studies often did not adjust disability for comorbidity patterns of disorders. As shown by Merikangas *et al.* (2007) and Alonso *et al.* (2011), accounting for the effects of comorbidity significantly decreases almost all disorder-specific effects and thus allows for more accurate estimates of the precise effects of disorders on either total or partial disability. A second reason why our data differ from those of previous studies is that many studies have focused on disability without clearly differentiating between being *totally* and being *partially* unable to perform as usual (e.g., Stein *et al.* 2006). Third, data obtained in this study also expand upon previous findings by investigating decreases in day-to-day functioning that go beyond mere job productivity (Dewa *et al.* 2000, Lim *et al.* 2000, Cornwell *et al.* 2009) and focus instead on a broader understanding of functioning.

For a given respondent, the type of partial disability caused by a particular disorder is quite similar: mental disorders are associated with an additional 14–16 partial-disability days per year, comparable with the figures for chronic physical conditions of 13–15 days. Interestingly, we were not able to confirm that mental disorders (compared to chronic physical conditions) were more likely associated with an increase in both the number of partial- and total-disability days, as suggested in previous research. Indeed, Dewa and colleagues (2004) found that mental disorders yielded 23 times more *total-disability* days than *partial-disability* days. Comparing the results in this chapter with those discussed in Chapter 11, which examined the associations between mental and physical disorders and the number of days in which respondents were totally out of role, it is striking that mental disorders and chronic physical conditions have a similar impact in both cases. Furthermore, it has been suggested that mental and physical disorders

are similar in their impact on cost of illness (Smit *et al.* 2006).

The impact of disorders on partial disability was most pronounced in high-income countries. In low/lower-middle-income countries, estimates of both individual and societal effects of mental disorders on partial disability were systematically 33–50% lower than those of upper-middle-income or high-income countries. We found the same pattern for chronic physical conditions, although to a lesser extent: estimates of individual and societal effects were on average 15–46% lower in low/lower-middle-income countries. The impact of disorders on partial disability was consistently lower in low/lower-middle-income countries, in contrast to the effect disorders have on days totally out of role. As this is the first study to examine cross-income effects, further research should be undertaken to determine whether these effects can be confirmed.

Our findings also indicate cross-national variability in the prevalence of mental (12-month prevalence estimates between 12% and 16%) and physical disorders (12-month prevalence estimates between 45% and 57%). Moreover, the associations between disorders and partial disability are stronger in some countries than in others. It could be that the phenotype of some disorders (e.g., chronic pain conditions, anxiety disorders, depression, or insomnia) varies due to cultural factors (Kleinman 1995, Waza *et al.* 1999) or societal values (Maercker 2001). For instance, it has been hypothesized that pain may be a cultural equivalent of depression and that somatization, in turn, is more common in non-industrialized countries (Kirmayer *et al.* 1984). However, this hypothesis has been refuted in more recent research (Gureje *et al.* 1997, 1998, Patel 2001). Our research did not reveal a clear pattern with regard to the cross-national variation in the prevalence of disorders, or to the association of disorders with partial disability, making it difficult to draw meaningful conclusions with regard to this variation.

The set of mental and physical disorders included in this study accounted for more than half of all partial-disability days. With a view toward establishing priorities for the allocation of resources amidst ever-increasing healthcare costs, the identification of high-burden disorders is a crucial first step. This requires the evaluation of three criteria: the prevalence of individual disorders, the disorder-specific effects on individual-level estimates of partial disability, and the disorder-specific effects on societal-level estimates of partial disability. Therefore, depression is of particular interest because of its relatively high 12-month prevalence (between 4.7% and 5.9%), its considerable effect on partial disability (on average 20 additional days per year compared to those without a disorder, range 11–24 days), and its relatively high PARP (about 6% on average, range 4–9%). By comparison, among the chronic physical conditions, chronic pain conditions are of great interest because of their high prevalence (with estimates of around 22%, range 21–23%), giving rise on average to 18 additional partial-disability days per year for those with compared to those without the condition (range 8–24 additional days). Furthermore, approximately one-fifth of all partial disability was attributable to these conditions (range 12–23%). It is interesting that prior studies, although often using different methodological approaches, also ranked chronic pain conditions and depression among the disorders with the highest impact at both the individual and the societal level (Knight *et al.* 2001, Smit *et al.* 2006). From a worldwide public health perspective, depression and chronic pain conditions can therefore be classified as high-impact disorders when it comes to partial disability, and thus may be a focus for prioritization with regard to resource allocation.

We could not confirm the findings of prior research that identified cancer as the chronic physical condition that merits the most attention when it comes to identifying high-burden disorders. Using data from the MIDUS study, Kessler and colleagues (2001) found that, although the prevalence of cancer was rather low, this chronic condition had the most powerful effect on disability, at least in the working population. Respondents with cancer reported up to 132 days per year with significant impairment. Findings from the WMH surveys estimate the prevalence of cancer between 0.4% and 3.6%, figures in keeping with previous reports (Broemeling *et al.* 2008), but the associated individual and societal effects were found to be much lower than previous estimates. Respondents with cancer reported approximately 45 partial- and 32 total-disability days per year. Despite the worldwide attention this condition receives (Sullivan *et al.* 2011), it does not fall among the conditions with the most impact on disability as concluded in this study. This is obviously not to suggest that cancer is not strongly associated with daily disability, but it does raise the issue of whether other measures of impact may be more suitable for studying this condition (Elwood & Sutcliffe 2010). The same is true for alcohol and substance use. Although substance use disorders have been identified as highly prevalent and having dramatic effects on both the individual and the societal level of burden (Degenhardt & Wall 2012), our study does not provide sufficient evidence to allow for comparable conclusions. Not only is the prevalence rather low (estimates of 1.8–2.8% for alcohol and 0.2–0.7% for drug abuse disorders), but the individual-level and societal-level effects of these disorders on partial disability are also limited.

Implications

The results obtained in this study may have some important implications. The fact that mental and physical disorders were found to have a similar impact on partial disability emphasizes the importance of prioritizing public health needs. To the extent that partial disability may be a predictor of full disability (Bergström *et al.* 2009), our data underscore the importance of considering partial disability when evaluating functional impairment. Our data indicate that alleviating depression and chronic pain conditions should be considered public health priorities in light of the knowledge that these disorders: (a) have a high impact at both the individual and the societal level; (b) give rise to both full-disability and partial-disability days; and (c) have considerable comorbidity in both clinical and general population settings (Bair *et al.* 2003). How exactly this can be done at the country level remains an open question, although prevention, integrated treatment, and supportive services have been suggested (Katschnig *et al.* 1997). Some recent (health economic) contributions have shown that the treatment of depression mitigates depressive symptoms and reduces the depressive burden, but this effect was only found in the working population and not in the general population (Schoenbaum *et al.* 2001, Hilton *et al.* 2010). At any rate, easing this substantial ill-health burden, in both personal and economic terms, remains a significant challenge.

Acknowledgments

Portions of this chapter are based on Bruffaerts, R., Vilagut, G., Demyttenaere, K., *et al.* (2012). Role of common mental and physical disorders in partial disability around the world. *British Journal of Psychiatry* **200**, 454–61. © 2012. The Royal College of Psychiatrists. Reproduced with permission.

References

Alonso, J., Angermeyer, M., Bernert, S., et al. (2004). Disability and quality of life impact of mental disorders in Europe: results from the European Study on Epidemiology of Mental Disorders (ESEMeD) Project. *Acta Psychiatrica Scandinavica* **109** (Suppl 420), 38–46.

Alonso, J., Petukhova, M., Vilagut, G., et al. (2011). Days out of role due to common physical and mental conditions: results from the WHO World Mental Health surveys. *Molecular Psychiatry* **16**, 1234–46.

Aronsson, G., Gustafsson, K., & Dallner, M. (2000). Sick but yet at work: an empirical study of sickness presenteeism. *Journal of Epidemiology and Community Health* **54**, 502–9.

Bair, M. J., Robinson, R. L., Katon, W., & Kroenke, K. (2003). Depression and pain comorbidity. *Archives of Internal Medicine* **163**, 2433–45.

Baker, M., Stabile, M., & Deri, C. (2001). *What Do Self-reported, Objective Measures of Health Measure?* NBER Working Paper Series 8419. Cambridge, MA: National Bureau of Economic Research.

Bergström, G., Bodin, L., Hagberg, J., Aronsson, G., & Josephson, M. (2009). Sickness presenteeism today, sickness absenteeism tomorrow? A prospective study on sickness presenteeism and future sickness absenteeism. *Journal of Occupational and Environmental Medicine* **51**, 629–38.

Biering-Sorensen, F. & Hilden, J. (1984). Reproductivity of the history of low back trouble. *Spine* **9**, 280–6.

Breivik, H., Collett, B., Ventafridda, V., Cohen, R., & Gallacher, D. (2006). Survey of chronic pain in Europe: prevalence, impact on daily life, and treatment. *European Journal of Pain* **10**, 287–333.

Broemeling, A. M., Watson, D. E., & Prebtani, F. (2008). Population patterns of chronic health conditions, co-morbidity and healthcare use in Canada: implications for policy and practice. *Healthcare Quarterly* **11**, 70–6.

Bruffaerts, R., Demyttenaere, K., Vilagut, G., et al. (2008). The relationship between Body Mass Index, mental health, and functional disability. A European population perspective. *Canadian Journal of Psychiatry* **53**, 37–46.

Buist-Bouwman, M. A., de Graaf, R., Vollebergh, W. A., & Ormel, J. (2005). Comorbidity of physical and mental disorders and the effect on work-loss days. *Acta Psychiatrica Scandinavica* **111**, 436–43.

Buntin, M. B., & Zaslavsky, A. M. (2004). Too much ado about two-part models and transformation? Comparing methods of modeling Medicare expenditures. *Journal of Health Economics* **23**, 525–42.

Cornwell, K., Forbes, C., Inder, B., & Meadows, G. (2009). Mental illness and its effects on labour market outcomes. *Journal of Mental Health Policy and Economics* **12**, 107–18.

Degenhardt, L., & Hall, W. (2012). Extent of illicit drug use and dependence, and their contribution to the global burden of disease. *Lancet* **379**, 55–70.

Demyttenaere, K., Bruffaerts, R., Posada-Villa, J., et al. (2004). Prevalence, severity and unmet need for treatment of mental disorders in the World Health Organization World Mental Health (WMH) surveys. *JAMA* **291**, 2581–90.

Demyttenaere, K., Bonnewyn, A., Bruffaerts, R., et al. (2006). Comorbid painful physical symptoms and depression: prevalence, work loss, and help seeking. *Journal of Affective Disorders* **92**, 185–93.

Demyttenaere, K., Bonnewyn, A., Bruffaerts, R., et al. (2008). Comorbid painful physical symptoms and anxiety disorders: prevalence, work loss, and help seeking. *Journal of Affective Disorders* **109**, 264–74.

Dewa, C., & Lin, E. (2000). Chronic physical illness, psychiatric disorder and disability in the workplace. *Social Science and Medicine* **51**, 41–50.

Dewa, C. S., Lesage, A., Goering, P., & Caveen, M. (2004). Nature and prevalence of mental illness in the workplace. *Healthcare Papers* **5**, 12–25.

Dewa, C. S., Lin, E., Koehoorn, M., & Goldner, E. (2007). Association of chronic work stress, psychiatric disorders, and chronic physical conditions with disability among workers. *Psychiatric Services* **58**, 652–8.

Drummond, M. F. (1987). Resource allocation in health care: a role of quality of life assessments? *Journal of Chronic Disease* **40**, 605–19.

Elwood, M., & Sutcliffe, S. (2010). Cancer control and the burden of cancer. In J. M. Elwood & S. B. Sutcliffe, *Cancer Control*. New York, NY: Oxford University Press, pp. 3–22.

Goetzel, R. Z., Log, S. R., Ozminkowski, R. J., et al. (2004). Health, absence, disability, and presenteeism cost estimates of certain physical and mental health conditions affecting US employers. *Journal of Occupational and Environmental Medicine* **46**, 253–64.

Gureje, O., Simon, G. E., Üstün, T. B., & Goldberg, D. P. (1997). Somatization in cross-cultural perspective: a World Health Organization study in primary care. *American Journal of Psychiatry* **154**, 989–95.

Gureje, O., Von Korff, M., Simon, G. E., & Gater, R. (1998). Persistent pain and well-being. A World Health Organization Study in Primary Care. *JAMA* **280**, 147–51.

Gureje, O., Hermann, H., Harvey, C., Morgen, V., & Jablensky, A. (2002). The Australian National Survey of Psychotic Disorders: profile of psychosocial disability and its risk factors. *Psychological Medicine* **32**, 639–47.

Harrison A (1991). Assessing patients' pain: identifying reasons for error. *Journal of Advanced Nursing* **16**, 1018–25.

Heffler, S., Smith, S., Won, G., et al. (2002). Health spending projections for 2001–2011: the latest outlook. *Health Affairs (Millwood)* **21**, 207–18.

Hilton, M. F. (2010). Using the interaction of mental health symptoms and treatment status to estimate lost employee productivity. *Australia and New Zealand Journal of Psychiatry* **44**, 151–61.

Jamison, R. N., Raymond, S. A., Slawsby, E. A., McHugo, G. J., & Baird, J. C. (2006). Pain assessment in patients with low back pain: comparison of weekly recall and momentary electronic data. *Journal of Pain* 7, 192–9.

Katschnig, H., Freeman, H., & Sartorius, N., eds. (1997). *Quality of Life in Mental Disorders*. New York, NY: Wiley.

Kessler, R. C., & Frank, R. G. (1997). The impact of psychiatric disorders on work loss days. *Psychological Medicine* 27, 861–73.

Kessler, R. C., & Üstün, T. B. (2004). The World Mental Health (WMH) Survey Initiative version of the World Health Organization (WHO) Composite International Diagnostic Interview (CIDI). *International Journal of Methods in Psychiatric Research* 13, 93–121.

Kessler, R. C., Greenberg, P. E., Mickelson, K. D., Meneades, L. M., & Wang, P. S. (2001). The effects of chronic medical conditions on work loss and work cutback. *Journal of Occupational and Environmental Medicine* 43, 218–25.

Kessler, R. C., Ormel, J., Demler, O., & Stang, P. E. (2003). Comorbid mental disorders account for the role impairment of commonly occurring chronic physical conditions: results from the National Comorbidity Survey. *Journal of Occupational and Environmental Medicine* 45, 1257–66.

Kirmayer, L. (1984). Culture, affect and somatization, II. *Transcultural Psychiatric Research Review* 21, 237–62.

Kleinman, A. (1995). Do psychiatric disorders differ in different cultures? The methodological questions. In N. R. Goldberger & J. B. Veroff, eds., *The Culture and Psychology Reader*. New York, NY: New York University Press, pp. 631–51.

Knight, M., Stewart-Brown, S., & Fletcher, L. (2001). Estimating health needs: the impact of a checklist of conditions and quality of life measurement on health information derived from community surveys. *Journal of Public Health Medicine* 23, 179–86.

Kriegsman, D. M., Penninx, B. W., van Eijk, J. T., Boeke, A. J. P., & Deeg, D. J. H. (1996). Self-reports and general practitioner information on the presence of chronic diseases in community dwelling elderly: a study on the accuracy of patients' self- reports and on determinants of inaccuracy. *Journal of Clinical Epidemiology* 49, 1407–17.

Lim, D., Sanderson, K., & Andrews, G. (2000). Lost productivity among full-time workers with mental disorders. *Journal of Mental Health Policy and Economics* 1, 139–46.

Maercker, A. (2001). Association of cross-cultural differences in psychiatric morbidity with cultural values: a secondary data analysis. *German Journal of Psychiatry* 4, 17–23.

Merikangas, K. R., Ames, M., Cui, L., *et al.* (2007). The impact of comorbidity of mental and physical conditions on role disability in the US adult household population. *Archives of General Psychiatry* 64, 1180–8.

Merrill, S. S., & Verbrugge, L. M. (1999). Health and disease in midlife. In S. L. Willis & J. D. Reid, eds., *Life in the Middle: Psychological and Social Development in Middle Age*. San Diego, CA: Academic Press, pp. 78–104.

National Center for Health Statistics (1994). Evaluation of National Health Interview Survey diagnostic reporting. *Vital Health Statistics* 120, 1–116.

Patel, V. (2001). Cultural factors and international epidemiology. *British Medical Bulletin* 57, 33–45.

Polder, J. J., & Achterberg, P. W. (2004). *Cost of Illness in the Netherlands*. Bilthoven, the Netherlands: National Institute for Public Health and the Environment.

SAS Institute Inc. (2002). *SAS/STAT® Software, Version 9.1 for Windows*. Cary, NC: SAS Institute Inc.

Schoenbaum, M., Unutzer, J., Sherbourne, C., *et al.* (2001). Cost-effectiveness of practice-initiated quality improvement for depression: results of a randomized controlled trial. *JAMA* 286, 1325–30.

Schoenborn, C. A., Adams, P. F., & Schiller, J. S. (2003). Summary health statistics for the U.S. population: National Health Interview Survey, 2000. *Vital Health Statistics* 10 (214), 1–83.

Smit, F., Cuijpers, P., Oostenbrink, J., *et al.* (2006). Costs of nine common mental disorders: implications for curative and preventive psychiatry. *Journal of Mental Health Policy and Economics* 9, 193–200.

Solomon, P. (2001). Congruence between health professionals' and patients' pain ratings: a review of the literature. *Scandinavian Journal of Caring Sciences* 15, 174–80.

Stein, M. B., Cox, B. J., Afifi, T. O., Belik, S. H., & Sareen, J. (2006). Does co-morbid depressive illness magnify the impact of chronic physical illness? A population-based perspective. *Psychological Medicine* 36, 587–96.

Sullivan, R., Peppercorn, J., Sikora, K., *et al.* (2011). Delivering affordable cancer care in high-income countries. *Lancet Oncology* 12, 933–80.

Tsang, A., & Lee, S. (2009). The global burden of chronic pain. In M. R. Von Korff, K. M. Scott, & O. Gureje, eds., *Global Perspectives on Mental–Physical Comorbidity in the WHO World Mental Health Surveys*. New York, NY: Cambridge University Press, pp. 22–28.

Üstün, T. B., Kostanjsek, N., Chatterji, S., & Rehm, J. (2010). *Measuring Health and Disability: Manual for WHO Disability Assessment Schedule (WHODAS 2.0)*. Geneva: World Health Organization.

Von Korff, M., Crane, P., Lane, M., *et al.* (2005). Chronic spinal pain and physical–mental comorbidity in the United States: results from the National Comorbidity Survey Replication. *Pain* 113, 331–9.

Von Korff, M., Crane, P. K., Alonso, J., *et al.* (2008). Modified WHODAS-II provides valid measure of global disability but filter items increased skewness. *Journal of Clinical Epidemiology* 61, 1132–43.

Watanabe, N., Stewart, R., Jenkins, R., Bhugra, D., & Furukawa, T. A. (2008). The epidemiology of chronic fatigue, physical illness, and symptoms of common mental disorders: a cross-sectional survey from the second British National Survey of Psychiatric Morbidity. *Journal of Psychosomatic Research* **64**, 357–62.

Waza, K., Graham, A. V., Zyzanski, S. J., & Inoue, K. (1999). Comparison of symptoms in Japanese and American

depressed primary care patients. *Family Practice* **16**, 528–33.

Wolter, K. M. (1985). *Introduction to Variance Estimation.* New York, NY: Springer-Verlag.

World Health Organization (2011). *World Report on Disability.* Geneva: WHO Press.

Disorder-specific disability and treatment of common mental and physical disorders

Johan Ormel, Maria V. Petukhova, Somnath Chatterji, Huibert Burger, Josep Maria Haro, Norito Kawakami, Matthew K. Nock, and T. Bedirhan Üstün

Introduction

As noted in the previous two chapters, increasing healthcare costs will almost certainly require healthcare resource allocation decisions in the years ahead to be based increasingly on information about the prevalence, severity, and chronicity of disorders and the cost-effectiveness of interventions (World Health Organization 2006). This will mean that the attention paid to specific disorders will have to be based not only on information about prevalence and mortality, but also on disability (Ware *et al.* 1986, Wells *et al.* 1989, Verbrugge & Patrick 1995, Murray & López 1996, Katschnig *et al.* 1997, Sprangers *et al.* 2000, Goetzel *et al.* 2003).

Studies from high-income countries have documented significant impairment and loss of quality of life in patients who have been treated by specialty mental health providers, in patients treated in primary care settings, and in people whose mental health disorders have gone untreated (Ormel *et al.* 1994, Kessler & Frank 1997, Bijl & Ravelli 2000, Andrews *et al.* 2001, Buist-Bouwman *et al.* 2006). In all of these studies, people with one or more mental disorders report higher levels of disability compared to people without mental illness. At the population level as a whole, as well, the burden of mental disorders is substantial. The World Bank's Global Burden of Disease (GBD) estimates suggest that common mental disorders account for at least a fifth of all disability-adjusted life years (DALYs) in individuals aged 15–44 worldwide (Murray & López 1996). The high population burden of common mental disorders is due to the combination of a significant impact at the individual level, a high rate of prevalence, the early age of onset compared to most chronic physical conditions, and

the recurrent-chronic course of many mental disorders.

For cross-national comparative purposes, most studies into disability are fraught with considerable limitations. First, most studies use country-specific methods or, if cross-national, target only one or a few common mental disorders (Tylee *et al.* 1999). An exception, to some extent, was the collaborative WHO study on Psychological Problems in Primary Health Care (PPGHC) (Üstün & Sartorius 1995), which used identical methods in each participating country. In that study, patients with one or more mental disorders (regardless of whether or not they had been diagnosed with a mental disorder by a medical professional) showed higher levels of disability compared to patients treated for other ailments without mental health problems (Ormel *et al.* 1994). These findings were consistent across the 15 participating countries, despite huge cross-national differences in the prevalence of mental disorders and disability. The WHO-PPGHC study, however, was limited to patients treated in primary care settings and thus was not population-based. The possibility that the association found was due to patient selection effects can therefore not be ruled out.

A second major limitation is that few studies have assessed the condition-specific disability of a broad range of mental and physical disorders. In a condition-specific approach, respondents are asked to rate the interference in role functioning caused by a particular disorder rather than the interference caused by all their health problems. Most studies assess overall disability, which makes it difficult to compare condition-specific disabilities in the event of comorbidity. Nearly all studies that have used condition-specific approaches to estimate the effects of specific disorders on disability

The Burdens of Mental Disorders, ed. Jordi Alonso, Somnath Chatterji, and Yanling He. Published by Cambridge University Press. © World Health Organization 2013.

have been conducted in high-income countries (Berto *et al.* 2000, Maetzel & Li 2002, Reed *et al.* 2004), and comparable broad-based studies are rare in low/lower-middle-income and upper-middle-income countries (Moussavi *et al.* 2007). Therefore, to date, the available data on the burden of mental disorders in the world are incomplete and have limited comparability.

A third limitation is that few studies assess both mental and physical disorders (Kessler *et al.* 2003, Buist-Bouwman *et al.* 2005). This is a critical issue, given that governments and insurance agencies can introduce disorder-specific co-payment policies. Recently, the Dutch government introduced co-payment for outpatient mental health treatment but spared outpatient physical health treatment. Information on potential differences in associated disability between physical and mental disorders will help to qualify such healthcare policies as reasonable or outright discriminatory for sufferers of mental health disorders.

The aim of this chapter is to compare the condition-specific disability assessments of mental disorders and the disorder-specific disability of physical disorders assessed in the WMH surveys.

Methods

Sample

Chapter 2 described the methods employed in conducting the WMH surveys, including sampling procedures, sample characteristics (Table 2.1), and the classification of countries by income level. The analysis discussed in this chapter is based on 23 of the 25 surveys considered in this volume. The surveys from Iraq and PRC–Shenzhen were excluded, as neither of them included assessments of disorder-specific disability for chronic physical conditions. In addition, 429 respondents in Lebanon and 278 in Northern Ireland were excluded because their chronic physical conditions were not assessed due to skip errors. The resulting sample size is $n = 56,164$ respondents across 23 countries (see Appendix Table 2.1). An earlier report based on 15 WMH surveys found that the mental disorders considered here are associated with more disability than the commonly occurring chronic physical conditions assessed in the WMH surveys (Ormel *et al.* 2008). The results reported in this chapter use the same measures and analysis methods as in that earlier report but expand the sample to evaluate the extent to which the initial results generalize to the

broader set of countries subsequently included in the WMH series.

Measures

Disability was assessed with the Sheehan Disability Scales (SDS), a widely used self-report measure of condition-specific disability that, although to date it has only been used in the assessment of mental disorders, can just as well be used to assess disability caused by physical disorders. The SDS consists of four questions, each asking the respondent to rate on a scale of 0 to 10 the extent to which a particular disorder "interfered with" activities in one of four role domains during the month in the past year when the disorder was most severe. The four domains are: (1) "your home management, like cleaning, shopping, and taking care of the (house/apartment)" (*home*); (2) "your ability to work" (*work*); (3) "your social life" (*social*); and (4) "your ability to form and maintain close relationships with other people" (*close relationships*). The 0–10 response options were presented in a visual analogue format with labels for the response options of none (0), mild (1–3), moderate (4–6), severe (7–9), and very severe (10). A global SDS disability score was also created by assigning each respondent the highest SDS domain score reported across the four domains.

Previous methodological studies have documented good internal consistency reliability across the SDS domains (Leon *et al.* 1997, Hambrick *et al.* 2004), a result that we replicated in the WMH data by finding Cronbach's alpha (a measure of internal consistency reliability) in the range of 0.82–0.97 across countries. Importantly, reliability was consistently high in low/lower-middle-income (0.91), upper-middle-income (0.91), and high-income countries (0.88) (Appendix Table 13.1). Previous methodological studies have also documented good discrimination between role functioning of cases and controls based on SDS scores in studies of social phobia (Hambrick *et al.* 2004), posttraumatic stress disorder (PTSD) (Connor & Davidson 2001), panic disorder (Leon *et al.* 1997), and substance abuse (Pallanti *et al.* 2006). Similar results were found in the WMH surveys, based on responses to a question asked subsequently to the SDS questions: "How many days out of 365 in the past year were you totally unable to work or carry out your normal activities because of (the illness)?" We examined the strength of the SDS scores to predict variation in this relatively objective measure of disability. If the SDS measures genuine disability, we would expect correlations to be significant and comparable for physical and mental disorders. This is, in fact, what we found, although the correlations varied across national income level. In high-income countries, the multiple correlations of the four SDS domain scores predicting days out of role were 0.56 for mental disorders and 0.50 for physical conditions, while the comparable correlations in upper-middle-income countries were 0.42 for mental disorders and 0.37 for physical conditions, and in low/lower-middle-income countries they were 0.38 for mental disorders and 0.34 for physical conditions (Appendix Table 13.2).

It is important to recognize that the SDS scales are *condition-specific*: that is, respondents were asked to rate the interference in role functioning caused by a particular disorder rather than the interference caused by all their health problems. This focused approach to questioning allows SDS scores to be compared across disorders without adjusting for comorbidity. However, this requires respondents with multiple health problems to sort out the relative effects of their various conditions on their overall functioning. An indication that respondents are able to do this comes from controlled treatment studies that have documented significant improvements in SDS measures of condition-specific role functioning with treatment for generalized anxiety disorder (GAD) (Davidson *et al.* 2004), panic disorder (Bertani *et al.* 2004), and major depression (Hudson *et al.* 2007).

Because they are condition-specific, the SDS scales were administered separately for each of the 10 mental disorders considered in this chapter. In the case of the physical conditions, which were only of secondary interest in the WMH surveys, the SDS scales were administered only for one physical disorder per respondent. This one disorder was selected randomly from all the physical conditions that the respondent reported experiencing in the 12 months prior to the interview. This method of selection under-represents comorbid physical conditions, which may be more severe than pure disorders, as a function of the number of such disorders. In order to correct this bias, a weight was applied to each case equal to the number of physical conditions reported by the respondent.

The disorders considered here are somewhat different from those described in Chapters 11 and 12, because we wanted to use the same disorders in this chapter as in our earlier report on disorder-specific disability (Ormel *et al.* 2008). Likewise, the 10 mental disorders considered here are somewhat different from the nine included in Chapters 11 and 12 in that here we consider three disruptive behavior disorders not addressed in the earlier chapters: adult attention-deficit/hyperactivity disorder (ADHD), intermittent explosive disorder (IED), and oppositional-defiant disorder (ODD). Furthermore, the two substance use disorders that we considered in earlier chapters (alcohol abuse with or without dependence, drug abuse with and without dependence) are excluded from this analysis.

As in Chapters 11 and 12, 10 chronic physical conditions are considered in this chapter, although only four coincide with those addressed in those earlier chapters: arthritis, cancer, diabetes, and frequent/severe headaches or migraine. The other six conditions considered here, although included in Chapters 11 and 12, were part of larger summary measures in those chapters, but in this chapter are treated separately. One of these is asthma, which was included as part of a larger category of respiratory disorders (including seasonal allergies, chronic obstructive pulmonary disease [COPD], and emphysema) in the earlier chapters. Two others are chronic back or neck pain and other chronic pain conditions, which were combined into a single category of pain conditions in Chapters 11 and 12. Another is stomach or intestinal ulcer, which was combined with irritable bowel disorder to define a larger category of digestive disorders in Chapters 11 and 12. Finally, heart disease and hypertension are treated as separate categories here, whereas in Chapters 11 and 12 they were combined with heart attack and stroke to define a larger category of cardiovascular disorders. See Chapters 11 and 12 for discussions about how these conditions were measured. As in the earlier chapters, we consider only physical conditions and mental disorders present in the 12 months prior to the interview.

We also consider treatment in this chapter. Treatment of chronic physical conditions was assessed by asking respondents if they had seen a medical doctor or other health professional in the past 12 months for each disorder reported. For mental disorders, disorder-specific treatment was assessed by asking each respondent if "you ever in your life talked to a medical doctor or other professional about (the disorder)" and, if so, if "you receive(d) professional treatment for (the disorder) at any time in the past 12 months." Treatment of mental disorders was also assessed in a series of more general questions that asked respondents whether, in the past 12 months, they had gone to any of a long list of types of professionals (the list varied across countries depending on the types of professionals available in the country) "for problems with your emotions, nerves, or your use of alcohol or drugs." Self-reports about treatment have been shown in previous methodological studies to have generally good concordance with healthcare records (Reijneveld & Stronks 2001), although research verifying this concordance has been carried out exclusively in high-income countries.

Statistical analysis

A separate observational record was created for each 12-month physical condition for which SDS ratings were obtained (i.e., one for each respondent who reported one or more disorders) as well as for each 12-month mental disorder reported by each respondent. So, for example, an otherwise average respondent who met criteria for five 12-month mental disorders and three physical conditions would be represented by six records that had a sum of weights of 8.0: one record for each of the five mental disorders (each with a condition weight of 1.0) and a sixth record for a randomly selected physical condition (with a condition weight of 3.0).

Standard WMH respondent weights were also applied to each observational record. As noted in Chapter 2, these weights adjusted for the differential sampling of respondents in part 1 of the survey as a function of household size and in part 2 of the survey as a function of whether or not core disorders were reported in part 1. These weighted records, which are representative of the conditions present in each population, were pooled across samples for comparative analysis. Domain-specific and global SDS means, proportions rated severe or very severe (hereafter referred to as severe), and the standard errors of these estimates were then calculated separately for each condition in each country and in more aggregated form for all low/lower-middle-income, upper-middle-income, and high-income countries.

Significance tests were used to test the statistical significance of pair-wise differences in SDS scores across all pairs of conditions. Within-disorder comparisons were also made to determine whether disability ratings differed across country income levels. Between-disorder comparisons were made to determine whether disability ratings were more systematically different for

physical than for mental disorders within countries. All of these analyses were then replicated using only the subsample of respondents with treated physical conditions. Finally, all pair-wise comparisons were repeated on a within-person basis: that is, by comparing SDS scores for specific pairs of conditions for the same individual (e.g., a single person who had both depression and cancer who provided separate SDS ratings for these conditions). As in other chapters in this volume, these significance tests adjusted for the clustering and weighting of observations using the Jackknife Repeated Replication (JRR) pseudo-replication simulation method (Kish & Frankel 1974). Significance was consistently evaluated at the 0.05 level with two-sided tests.

Results

Self-reported disorder prevalence and treatment

The broad rank ordering of mental disorder prevalence estimates was found to be fairly similar across country income groups despite the fact that, unlike physical conditions, most mental disorders were estimated to be significantly more prevalent in high-income than in low/lower-middle-income countries. Major depressive disorder (MDD) or dysthymia, specific phobia, social phobia, and IED were estimated to be the most prevalent disorders in each income subsample, while ODD, ADHD, and bipolar disorder were estimated to be the least common. The percentage of respondents who reported being in treatment for the focal disorder at the time of the interview was consistently higher in high-income than in low/lower-middle-income countries.

Although most prevalence estimates of self-reported chronic physical conditions differed significantly and substantially between low/lower-middle-income, upper-middle-income, and high-income countries, the broad pattern of prevalence estimates was also quite similar in the three subsamples (Table 13.1). Chronic back or neck pain, arthritis, chronic headaches, and hypertension were estimated to be the four most common conditions in each income subsample. Cancer, diabetes, and ulcer were among the least common. The percentage of respondents who reported being in treatment for the focal conditions at the time of the interview was generally somewhat to a good deal higher, however, in high-income countries than in lower-income countries. The

Table 13.1 12-month prevalence of disorders and treatment by country income level. The WMH surveys.

Disorders	Prevalence of mental and physical disorders — Country income level												% in treatment among those with conditions — Country income level												
	Low/lower-middle			Upper-middle			High			Test for difference between income groups		Low/lower-middle			Upper-middle			High			Test for difference between income groups
	N^a	%	SE	N^a	%	SE	N^a	%	SE	X^2_2		N^b	%	SE	N^b	%	SE	N^b	%	SE	X^2_2
Mental disorders																					
Major depressive disorder or dysthymia	987	4.7	(0.2)	1,219	4.9	(0.2)	3,290	5.9	(0.1)	30.0*		61	6.3	(1.0)	186	14.0	(1.3)	945	27.4	(0.9)	196.5*
Bipolar	73	0.5	(0.1)	168	1.0	(0.1)	716	1.7	(0.1)	101.3*		12	18.1	(6.0)	38	17.4	(3.2)	204	29.9	(1.9)	13.9*
Generalized anxiety disorder	236	1.2	(0.1)	389	1.5	(0.1)	1,422	2.6	(0.1)	112.3*		7	2.2	(1.0)	63	15.8	(2.5)	431	29.2	(1.4)	102.2*
Panic disorder	168	0.7	(0.1)	187	0.7	(0.1)	792	1.4	(0.1)	64.0*		14	6.4	(2.0)	50	27.6	(3.5)	258	33.5	(2.0)	59.8*
Social phobia	200	1.3	(0.1)	431	2.0	(0.1)	1,805	3.9	(0.1)	219.5*		17	9.2	(3.2)	69	15.2	(2.1)	401	21.4	(1.0)	17.7*
Specific phobia	701	5.9	(0.3)	1,028	6.4	(0.3)	3,087	7.0	(0.3)	9.3*		35	3.4	(0.8)	127	9.9	(1.0)	476	13.2	(0.8)	69.7*
Post-traumatic stress	130	0.7	(0.1)	218	1.0	(0.1)	1,151	2.1	(0.1)	115.0*		4	3.0	(1.9)	30	11.9	(2.9)	352	28.0	(1.6)	50.2*
Attention-deficit/hyperactivity	1	0.1	(0.1)	87	0.6	(0.1)	266	1.0	(0.1)	39.3*		0	.	.	19	15.3	(4.1)	90	28.6	(3.5)	.
Intermittent explosive disorder	349	2.2	(0.1)	273	1.8	(0.2)	506	2.9	(0.2)	17.6*		21	5.0	(1.2)	26	7.5	(1.6)	91	16.4	(1.9)	23.6*
Oppositional-defiant disorder	16	0.4	(0.1)	42	0.4	(0.1)	89	0.3	(0.0)	0.6		2	28.9	(19.7)	7	13.0	(5.4)	32	32.9	(6.6)	4.7
Physical conditions																					
Arthritis	1,785	14.6	(0.5)	2,233	12.5	(0.3)	5,793	16.7	(0.3)	74.3*		349	45.0	(3.4)	349	42.9	(2.5)	1,416	50.0	(1.5)	6.6*
Asthma	263	2.1	(0.2)	561	3.3	(0.2)	3,212	9.2	(0.2)	624.6*		54	43.6	(6.6)	128	59.2	(6.6)	622	49.3	(3.1)	3.0
Cancer	74	0.5	(0.1)	134	0.8	(0.1)	1,228	3.7	(0.1)	338.0*		21	66.6	(13.2)	40	67.9	(7.3)	266	53.4	(3.9)	2.9
Chronic back/neck pain	2,526	21.8	(0.6)	3,308	19.4	(0.5)	6,754	18.4	(0.3)	25.4*		390	33.1	(2.4)	646	50.7	(2.1)	2,185	65.8	(1.3)	121.9*
Chronic pain	813	6.7	(0.3)	1,391	8.2	(0.3)	2,424	6.0	(0.2)	32.0*		135	46.4	(4.5)	326	61.7	(4.0)	682	71.8	(2.5)	22.6*
Diabetes	280	2.6	(0.2)	775	4.4	(0.2)	1,673	4.9	(0.2)	84.4*		160	77.5	(7.5)	260	77.8	(4.0)	591	93.3	(1.1)	16.5*
Headaches	1,806	15.2	(0.6)	3,298	19.4	(0.5)	4,515	11.1	(0.2)	232.3*		331	47.6	(3.3)	718	51.4	(2.0)	1,111	48.9	(1.5)	1.4
Heart disease	830	6.5	(0.3)	1,082	5.4	(0.2)	1,917	5.4	(0.2)	10.6*		123	46.5	(6.5)	264	70.7	(3.3)	514	74.7	(2.7)	12.1*
Hypertension	1,212	10.9	(0.5)	2,669	14.7	(0.4)	5,027	14.8	(0.3)	52.8*		301	67.9	(3.5)	872	73.0	(2.3)	1,791	86.4	(1.4)	34.9*
Ulcer	651	6.0	(0.4)	695	3.7	(0.2)	843	2.2	(0.1)	136.9*		162	63.0	(5.5)	156	60.9	(4.2)	198	65.9	(4.3)	0.7

^{a} Number of respondents with the disorder.
^{b} Number of participants receiving treatment.
* Significant at the 0.05 level, two-sided test.

difference found in treatment prevalence among low/lower-middle-income countries, upper-middle-income countries, and high-income countries was particularly pronounced for mental disorders.

Respondents reported receiving treatment for physical conditions more often than for mental disorders. In high-income countries, 65.3% ($n = 9,300$) of all the physical conditions were treated, versus 23.7% ($n = 2,841$) of all of the mental disorders. In low/lower-middle-income and upper-middle-income countries, only 5.7% ($n = 162$) and 13.6% ($n = 576$) of mental disorders were treated, versus 47.6% ($n = 2,007$) and 58.6% ($n = 3,683$) of the physical conditions. This pattern also holds true for severely disabling disorders (Appendix Table 13.3).

Individual-level disability

The mental disorders with the highest mean SDS global disability ratings in the three subsamples were bipolar disorder and MDD or dysthymia (Table 13.2). The lowest ratings were found for specific phobia. Six mental disorders were found to have significantly higher mean global disability ratings in high-income countries (MDD or dysthymia, bipolar disorder, GAD, panic disorder, PTSD, and IED). None had a significantly higher rating in low/lower-middle-income countries. A similar pattern of relative disability was found for the proportion of cases rated severely disabled in the total sample (Table 13.2) as well as among treated cases (Appendix Table 13.4).

The physical conditions with the highest mean SDS global disability ratings in all income subsamples were the pain disorders, although between-disorder variation in disability ratings was much greater in high-income than in low/lower-middle-income countries. Three physical conditions had significantly higher mean SDS global disability ratings in high-income countries (chronic back or neck pain, other chronic pain conditions, and frequent or severe headaches). Three others had significantly higher ratings in low/lower-middle-income or upper-middle-income countries (asthma, hypertension, ulcer). A similar pattern of relative disability was found for the proportion of cases rated severely disabled in the total sample (Table 13.2), as well as among treated cases (Appendix Table 13.4).

The SDS disability ratings for mental disorders were generally higher than for physical conditions. This was true, as verified by Mann–Whitney tests,

both for mean disability ratings and for proportions rated severely disabled, and for each income-level subsample (Appendix Table 13.5). Of the 100 logically possible pair-wise disorder-specific mental–physical comparisons, mean ratings were higher for mental disorders in 89 comparisons in low/lower-middle-income countries, 89 comparisons in upper-middle-income countries, and 88 comparisons in high-income countries (including 10 comparisons which were equal). Most exceptions were found for specific phobia: about 70% of the comparisons of specific phobia with physical conditions were higher for the physical condition. Most of the cases with higher mental ratings than physical ratings are statistically significant at the 0.05 level (Appendix Table 13.6). Comparable results were obtained for the proportion of severe disability ratings (Appendix Table 13.7) as well as for both mean and severe disability ratings when controlled for respondent age, sex, and education, and when the focus was exclusively on the subsamples of cases in treatment (Appendix Tables 13.8 and 13.9).

Consistently higher mental disability ratings than physical disability ratings were also found for each income-level subsample when individual SDS domains were considered instead of the global ratings of the total sample. The differences were much more pronounced for disability in social life and close relationships than in work or home management (Table 13.3). For example, the proportions of severe disability in work functioning associated with mental disorders in low/lower-middle-income, upper-middle-income, and high-income countries (15.0–23.9%) were similar to or only slightly higher than the proportions associated with physical conditions (16.3–21.6%). The proportions of severe disability in social life associated with mental disorders (13.9–28.6%), in comparison, were dramatically higher than those associated with physical conditions (7.4–12.6%). Similar patterns were found when we compared both means and proportions rated severe among cases in treatment (Appendix Table 13.10). In addition, an attenuated version of the same general pattern holds true when all physical conditions were compared to all (i.e., treated or not) mental disorders to address the possibility that a more superficial assessment of physical disorders than of mental disorders led to the inclusion of subthreshold cases of physical conditions that might be associated with a low degree of disability (Appendix Table 13.11).

Table 13.2 Disorder-specific global Sheehan Disability Scale ratings by country income level. The WMH surveys.

Disorders	Mean disability ratings											Proportion rated severely disabled									
	Country income level									Test for difference between income groups		Country income level									Test for difference between income groups
	Low/lower-middle			Upper-middle			High					Low/lower-middle			Upper-middle			High			
	N^a	Mean	(SE)	N^a	Mean	(SE)	N^a	Mean	(SE)	Numerator DF	F value	N^b	%	(SE)	N^b	%	(SE)	N^b	%	(SE)	χ^2
Mental disorders																					
Major depressive disorder or dysthymia	895	5.4	(0.1)	1,203	6.5	(0.1)	2,284	7.1	(0.1)	2	64.2*	354	39.2	(2.2)	651	54.2	(2.0)	1,488	64.5	(1.3)	88.04*
Bipolar	65	6.6	(0.5)	190	6.5	(0.3)	693	7.5	(0.1)	2	6.8*	35	54.2	(7.8)	118	58.3	(3.9)	506	71.1	(2.2)	10.89*
Generalized anxiety disorder	227	4.6	(0.3)	380	5.8	(0.2)	1,354	6.5	(0.1)	2	23.8*	66	28.9	(3.8)	163	46.9	(3.8)	760	54.9	(1.6)	35.47*
Panic disorder	157	4.5	(0.3)	173	5.5	(0.3)	750	5.8	(0.2)	2	8.0*	38	23.3	(3.4)	73	47.6	(4.7)	374	49.2	(2.3)	29.96*
Social phobia	200	4.9	(0.2)	449	5.5	(0.2)	1,830	5.1	(0.1)	2	3.4*	76	36.7	(4.5)	175	39.8	(3.5)	673	35.7	(1.3)	1.22
Specific phobia	701	3.0	(0.1)	1,103	3.5	(0.1)	3,127	3.3	(0.1)	2	3.7*	90	11.4	(1.4)	243	20.7	(1.6)	637	18.0	(0.9)	21.39*
Post-traumatic stress	72	5.9	(0.5)	116	4.9	(0.4)	726	6.7	(0.1)	2	9.4*	31	49.5	(9.5)	54	31.2	(5.1)	422	57.6	(2.4)	13.97*
Attention-deficit/hyperactivity disorder	0	–	–	85	5.6	(0.5)	254	5.6	(0.2)	1	0.0	0	–	–	35	39.5	(7.5)	101	41.0	(4.0)	.
Intermittent explosive disorder	341	3.7	(0.3)	278	4.2	(0.3)	501	4.6	(0.3)	2	3.8*	73	19.4	(2.8)	89	28.3	(3.6)	158	32.5	(2.5)	11.94*
Oppositional-defiant disorder	14	6.6	(0.8)	42	5.0	(0.5)	86	5.8	(0.2)	2	1.4	8	71.5	(10.5)	17	27.8	(8.2)	38	41.3	(7.2)	5.25
Physical conditions																					
Arthritis	737	3.2	(0.2)	949	3.8	(0.1)	2,723	3.8	(0.1)	2	3.0	123	19.3	(2.5)	229	24.6	(2.1)	720	26.5	(1.4)	6.13*
Asthma	114	3.1	(0.4)	210	3.8	(0.5)	1,336	2.2	(0.2)	2	6.9*	22	18.4	(5.5)	51	29.2	(5.5)	162	11.3	(1.6)	9.50*
Cancer	29	3.3	(0.7)	55	4.5	(1.3)	424	2.3	(0.2)	2	2.3	5	13.1	(5.7)	15	42.7	(14.3)	94	17.8	(2.4)	2.60
Chronic back/neck pain	1,066	3.5	(0.1)	1,352	4.3	(0.1)	3,377	5.2	(0.1)	2	52.8*	200	18.2	(1.9)	390	30.0	(1.9)	1,329	39.1	(1.3)	73.85*
Chronic pain	286	3.4	(0.3)	518	4.4	(0.3)	962	5.6	(0.2)	2	20.8*	76	23.6	(3.6)	178	32.8	(3.9)	435	45.1	(2.9)	20.51*
Diabetes	348	3.6	(0.7)	315	3.1	(0.4)	643	2.4	(0.3)	2	2.0	22	19.9	(8.3)	63	21.3	(4.5)	77	15.1	(3.3)	1.29
Headaches	729	4.6	(0.3)	1,549	4.4	(0.1)	2,278	5.7	(0.1)	2	29.7*	211	30.2	(3.2)	475	31.2	(1.8)	1,043	45.9	(1.6)	42.45*
Heart disease	242	3.6	(0.5)	374	3.7	(0.3)	685	3.8	(0.3)	2	0.1	43	24.1	(6.0)	101	26.0	(3.7)	158	28.9	(3.0)	0.68
Hypertension	458	3.6	(0.3)	1,129	3.0	(0.2)	2,079	1.6	(0.1)	2	32.9*	77	23.9	(3.2)	184	17.8	(2.0)	195	9.6	(1.3)	21.91*
Ulcer	256	2.4	(0.3)	262	3.7	(0.4)	280	3.1	(0.1)	2	3.9*	37	9.0	(2.2)	53	23.6	(4.3)	53	16.8	(3.3)	8.73*

[a] Number of respondents with valid Sheehan scores for the randomly selected physical disorder or the mental disorder. Note that the numbers for physical disorder are substantially lower than those in Table 13.1 because the prevalence estimates in Table 13.1 were based on all respondents who reported the disorder whereas the Sheehan scores were obtained only for the subsample of randomly selected physical disorders. The numbers for mental disorders in this table are slightly lower than those in Table 13.1 because participants with missing values on Sheehan scores were omitted from this table but not from Table 13.1. Skip errors in the Western European surveys led to the number of cases with missing Sheehan scores being higher than would normally be expected based on respondent refusals and interviewer recording errors.

[b] Number of participants rated as having a severely disabling disorder.

* Significant at the 0.05 level, two-sided test.

Table 13.3 Sheehan Disability Scale global and domain-specific ratings (proportion rated severely disabled) aggregated across physical (total and treated) and mental (total) disorders by country income level. The WMH surveys.

| Sheehan scale | Country income level | Proportion rated severely disabled | | | | | | | | | Test for difference between physical and mental disorders | |
| | | Mental disorders | | | Physical disorders | | | Treated physical disorders | | | Difference with mental disorders | |
		N^a	%	SE	N^a	%	SE	N^a	%	SE	Physical disorders χ^2_1	Treated physical disorders χ^2_1
Global	Low/lower-middle	771	26.9	(1.4)	816	21.6	(1.3)	435	24.7	(2.0)	49.6*	18.5*
	Upper-middle	1,618	38.7	(1.2)	1,739	27.0	(1.0)	1,114	32.2	(1.3)	71.7*	26.1*
	High	5,157	42.9	(0.7)	4,266	27.5	(0.6)	3,196	32.7	(0.9)	394.0*	166.9*
Home	Low/lower-middle	468	15.7	(1.1)	606	16.1	(1.2)	331	19.0	(1.8)	9.4*	0.6
	Upper-middle	959	22.7	(1.0)	1,213	19.2	(0.9)	771	22.6	(1.1)	19.6*	3.3
	High	2,668	22.2	(0.6)	3,252	21.4	(0.6)	2,454	25.4	(0.8)	14.4*	3.0
Work	Low/lower-middle	412	15.0	(1.0)	601	16.3	(1.2)	322	18.4	(1.6)	5.3*	0.0
	Upper-middle	892	22.3	(1.2)	1,252	21.0	(0.9)	814	25.3	(1.2)	5.9*	0.0
	High	2,811	23.9	(0.7)	3,097	21.6	(0.6)	2,372	26.2	(0.9)	31.5*	0.8
Social	Low/lower-middle	355	13.9	(1.0)	263	7.4	(0.8)	157	9.9	(1.5)	56.8*	20.5*
	Upper-middle	1,087	24.8	(1.0)	819	12.6	(0.7)	523	15.6	(0.9)	121.7*	59.6*
	High	3,434	28.6	(0.7)	1,708	10.9	(0.4)	1,288	13.1	(0.6)	589.8*	449.8*
Close relationships	Low/lower-middle	401	14.6	(1.0)	289	6.9	(0.7)	170	9.1	(1.3)	68.5*	30.3*
	Upper-middle	1,018	24.0	(1.0)	769	11.8	(0.7)	485	14.5	(0.9)	110.3*	61.1*
	High	2,979	24.8	(0.6)	1,309	8.6	(0.4)	969	10.3	(0.6)	575.6*	485.2*

^{a} Number of participants rated as having a severely disabling disorder.

* Significant at the 0.05 level, two-sided test.

Discussion

Four key findings emerge from our analyses. First, respondents generally attribute more disability to their mental than to their physical conditions. Second, the higher degree of disability associated with mental conditions than with physical conditions is similar in both low/lower-middle-income countries and high-income countries. Third, the higher aggregate disability of mental disorders than of physical conditions is much more pronounced for disability in social and personal relationships than in productive (work and housework) roles. Fourth, the proportion of cases in treatment at the time of the interview was much lower for mental than for physical conditions in all country income groups, both in the total sample and when we focused exclusively on cases rated severely disabling. These findings substantially expand upon the results of previous studies, none of which examined comparability among disabilities associated with such a varied a set of physical and mental disorders or disaggregated disability into the domains considered here to detect the greater relative impact of mental conditions compared to physical conditions in social–personal domains as opposed to productive role domains (Ware *et al.* 1986, Wells *et al.* 1989, Ormel *et al.* 1994, 1998, Hays *et al.* 1995, Spitzer *et al.* 1995, Verbrugge & Patrick 1995, Katschnig *et al.* 1997, Wells & Sherbourne 1999, Berto *et al.* 2000, Sprangers *et al.* 2000, Maetzel & Li 2002, Goetzel *et al.* 2003, Reed *et al.* 2004, Moussavi *et al.* 2007).

These results are limited by a number of sampling and measurement issues. With regard to sampling, the results may have been influenced by a truncation of the severity spectrum of physical conditions. For example, individuals facing the end stage of a chronic physical disease might be institutionalized or not willing or able to participate in an interview to a greater extent than people with severe mental disorders, leading to the underestimation of the relative disability of physical conditions compared to mental disorders. Whether such a difference in sample bias actually exists, however, is unknown.

There were a number of measurement problems in the analysis. One was that the physical conditions checklist did not include the infectious diseases that play such an important part in the morbidity of low/lower-middle-income countries. Our results consequently can be generalized only to chronic cardiovascular, digestive, metabolic, musculoskeletal, pain, and respiratory conditions. Despite this limitation, the conditions considered are important sources of morbidity in both low/lower-middle-income and upper-middle-income countries, and the results are therefore relevant to those countries despite the exclusion of infectious diseases.

Another measurement problem was that the physical conditions studied were assessed by simple self-reports rather than by abstracting medical records or administering medical examinations. Mental disorders were assessed more comprehensively with a fully structured lay-administered diagnostic interview. The more superficial assessment of physical conditions could have led to the inclusion of more subthreshold physical cases than mental disorder cases, introducing an artificial reduction in estimated disability. However, this was addressed in our analysis of treated physical conditions. It could also have led to an artificial overlap between the assessments of mental and physical conditions to the extent that core symptoms of some physical conditions (e.g., headache, unexplained chronic pain) are markers of underlying mental disorders, although this would have attenuated physical–mental differences by increasing the overlap between the two classes of disorders. In addition, the use of a self-report checklist almost certainly led to an underestimation of undiagnosed silent physical conditions. As the latter are likely to be less disabling than symptom-based conditions or diagnosed silent conditions, however, this bias presumably led to an artificial increase in the estimated disability of physical conditions.

Some of the WMH physical condition prevalence estimates are lower than those in gold-standard assessments. For example, the population prevalence of diabetes has been assessed in a number of community surveys using glucose tolerance tests from blood samples (e.g., King & Rewers 1993, Roglic *et al.* 2005). A meta-analysis of these studies suggests that the prevalence of diabetes is highest in North America (9.2%) and Europe (8.4%), lower in India and most of Latin America (5–8%), and lowest in most of Africa and China (2–5%) (International Diabetes Federation 2005). The WMH prevalence estimates, 2.6% in low/lower-middle-income countries, 4.4% in upper-middle-income countries, and 4.9% in high-income countries, are lower than these gold-standard estimates, presumably reflecting the fact that the gold-standard estimates include undiagnosed cases.

In other cases the WMH prevalence estimates are higher than those in gold-standard assessments. For example, cancer prevalence data have been assembled from various administrative databases and registries in a number of countries (Pisani *et al.* 2002). A meta-analysis of these data suggests that cancer is much more common in high-income than in low/lower-middle-income countries, with the highest prevalence in North America (1.5% of the population aged 15 and older diagnosed within the past five years), followed by Western Europe (1.2%), Australia and New Zealand (1.1%), Japan (1.0%), Eastern Europe (0.7%), Latin America, and the Caribbean (0.4%), with a much lower estimated prevalence in the rest of the world (0.2%). The much higher cancer prevalence estimates in the WMH data, 0.5% in low/lower-middle-income countries, 0.8% in upper-middle-income countries, and 3.7% in high-income countries, presumably reflect the fact that cancer survivors who were diagnosed and treated more than five years ago, although not counted in cancer prevalence estimates because they have the same survival rates as the general population, often consider themselves still to have cancer and report this in community surveys.

Based on comparisons such as these with gold-standard assessments, the WMH prevalence estimates of physical conditions should be interpreted with caution. However, the fact that the same general pattern of higher disability among sufferers of mental conditions than among individuals with physical conditions was also found in comparisons of treated physical conditions strongly suggests that the higher SDS disability associated with mental rather than physical conditions is not due to imprecision in the measurement of the latter.

Another measurement problem involves the fact that disability was assessed with brief self-report scales rather than clinical evaluations. This might have introduced upward bias in the reported disability caused by mental disorders compared to physical conditions to the extent that people with mental disorders gave overly pessimistic appraisals of their functioning. This would seem to be an unlikely interpretation, however, in that the associations of SDS ratings with reported numbers of days out of role – a more objective indicator of disability than the SDS ratings – were found to be equivalent for mental and physical conditions. Furthermore, within-person comparison, which controlled for individual differences in perceptions, found similar results (Appendix Table 13.12).

Another possibility is that the SDS questions may have been biased in the direction of assessing the disabilities associated with mental disorders as more severe than those associated with physical conditions. This would seem unlikely, however, as the SDS questions are quite broad and cover all the main areas of adult role functioning. Another possible limitation is that the SDS focused on the "worst month" in the past year, introducing recall error that is possibly more extreme for physical than for mental disorders. In addition, the persistence of between-disorder differences was not taken into consideration, which means that particular disorders might have been more dominant in the severity ratings than suggested here if they were more persistently severe than others. The aggregate disability estimates should be interpreted cautiously because of these limitations regarding the recall period.

A final measurement problem concerning the assessment of disability is related to our use of a condition-specific measurement approach. This is an attractive approach from a statistical perspective as compared to a non-condition-specific approach (i.e., one that simply assesses overall disability without asking the respondent to make inferences about the conditions that caused the disability), because it produces condition-specific estimates directly, avoiding the need to rely on multivariate equations that adjust for the effects of comorbidity in predicting overall disability. However, this advantage in analytic simplicity is achieved by requiring respondents with comorbid conditions to perform the difficult task of making judgments about the effects of individual conditions on their functioning.

Within the context of these limitations, the results reported here are consistent with previous comparative burden-of-illness studies in suggesting that musculoskeletal conditions, chronic pain, and major depressive episodes (unipolar and bipolar depression) are the disorders with the largest contribution to disability at the individual level both in high-income and in low/lower-middle-income countries. Previous studies have documented this pattern only in the USA (Druss *et al.* 2000, Manuel *et al.* 2002, Goetzel *et al.* 2003, Wang *et al.* 2003), although the importance of depression has also been documented throughout the world in the World Health Surveys (WHS) (Moussavi *et al.* 2007). This report replicates the WHS results regarding depression, and for the first time documents the cross-national significance of musculoskeletal conditions. As noted above, the WMH results also suggest that mental disorders are especially disabling to personal relationships and social life, which implies that they are disabling more because they create psychological barriers than because they create physical barriers to functioning. These barriers include limitations in cognitive and motivational capacities, affect regulation, embarrassment, and stigma (Buist-Bouwman *et al.* 2005), as well as a tendency of mental disorders to amplify physical symptoms (Barsky *et al.* 1988) and associated disability (Kessler *et al.* 2003).

Mediators and modifiers of the disorder–disability relationship

Considerable progress has been made in understanding the relationship between psychopathology and disability since the introduction of the International Classification of Impairments, Disabilities and Handicaps (ICIDH) in 1980 (World Health Organization 1980). The triad of impairment, disability, and handicap provided the framework for expanding disease concepts to include their impact on physical and psychosocial functioning. The ICIDH was replaced by the International Classification of Functioning, Disability, and Health (ICF) in 2001 (World Health Organization 2001). Both classifications provide a common language that was issued by the World Health Organization (WHO) to study the consequences of disease. Their underlying principles as a classification of health-related functioning and disability include: (a) their universality, i.e., they are applicable to all people regardless of country of origin; (b) their parity, i.e., no distinction should be drawn between mental and physical health conditions; (c) their neutrality, i.e., classifications can express both positive and negative aspects of functioning; and (d) the inclusion of contextual factors. Three levels of functioning are identified as: (1) body and structures, e.g., speech function, musculoskeletal function, structure and functioning of the nervous system; (2) activities, e.g., communication, mobility; and (3) participation, e.g., work, social life. Disability as assessed by the SDS – which asks the respondent to indicate on a scale of 1 to 10 the extent to which a particular disorder "interfered with" activities in one of four role domains – refers largely to limitations in participation as defined by the ICF. Within the ICF model, body function, activities, and participation are viewed as a single complex process in which pathology, personal characteristics, and context characteristics interact.

A better understanding of the interactions between psychopathology and participation could provide insight into how the burden of disease might be reduced (Buist-Bouwman *et al.* 2008). The ICF asserts that a disorder may lead to activity limitations which, in turn, lead to participation restrictions. The activity limitations through which mental and physical disorders cause limitations in participation are likely to differ. Physical conditions may produce participation restrictions because of limitations in physical capacities such as mobility, vision, aerobic capacity, lower and upper body strength, and manual dexterity, or because of incontinence, whereas mental disorders may produce participation restrictions via cognitive and motivational capacities, affect regulation, social perception, and a tendency to amplify physical symptoms such as fatigue and pain. For instance, Buist-Bouwman and colleagues (2008) examined the mediating effect of six domains of functioning on the association between severity of depression and the level of overall role functioning: (1) mobility, which included questions about difficulties related to standing for long periods, moving around inside the home, and walking long distances; (2) self-care, which included questions about difficulties with washing, getting dressed, and feeding; (3) cognition, which included questions about difficulties with concentration, memory, understanding, and ability to think clearly; (4) social interaction, which included questions associated with social interaction with people, maintaining a normal social life, and participating in social activities; (5) discrimination (1 item), which asked how much discrimination or unfair treatment the respondent had experienced due to health problems during the past 30 days; and (6) embarrassment (1 item), which asked how much embarrassment the respondent had experienced due to health problems during the past 30 days. Only concentration, attention problems, and embarrassment mediated a significant degree of association between depression and role functioning; the crude association dropped from 0.43 (SE = 0.04) to a residual association of 0.17 (SE = 0.10). Treatment may benefit from insight into which domains of functioning mediate the effects of a specific mental disorder on participation (work, social life).

The association between mental disorders and disability is strong but not perfect. Some mentally ill people seem to function rather well, although studies employing symptom-based severity measures of mental disorders show a strong linear association between the severity of the mental disorder and the degree of disability (Verboom *et al.* 2011). The question here is what environmental factors and personal characteristics dampen or enhance the impact of psychopathology on disability. Such knowledge may help enhance the effectiveness of treatments for mental illness itself, in addition to possible benefits for disability outcomes.

Treatment implications

Given the greater disability associated with mental disorders compared to physical conditions, it is disturbing to find that only a minority of patients with mental disorders, even severely debilitating conditions, receive treatment and that treatment is substantially more common among comparably severe physical conditions. In high-income countries, seriously disabling mental disorders were only about half as likely to be treated as seriously disabling physical conditions (34.7% vs. 77.4%), while they were only about 20% as likely to be treated as comparably severe physical conditions in low/lower-middle-income countries (11.4% vs. 54.4%). This low treatment rate is consistent with the low rate of recognition and treatment of mental disorders in primary care, especially if comorbid with physical conditions (Üstün & Sartorius 1995, Tiemens *et al.* 1999, Thompson *et al.* 2000). In combination with the burden of disability that mental disorders give rise to, the low treatment rates revealed in this study call for increased attention to mental disorders.

The implications of the WMH findings for treatment are not clear because, even though treatment effectiveness trials have shown that common mental disorders can often be successfully treated (Nathan & Gorman 1998, Hyman *et al.* 2006), uncertainties have emerged regarding long-term outcomes. In particular, it is important to track long-term functional outcomes, as residual disability and recurrence are major problems associated with chronic mental disorders (Ormel *et al.* 2004). Another limitation of treatment effectiveness trials is that they have typically focused on symptoms and have done little to assess the effects of treatment on reduced disability (Nathan & Gorman 1998, Hyman *et al.* 2006), although some notable exceptions suggest that the effective treatment of depression improves functional outcomes (Mintz *et al.* 1992, Mynors-Wallis *et al.* 1995, Coulehan *et al.* 1997, Katzelnick *et al.* 2000). Despite this uncertainty with regard to long-term outcomes, the results reported here argue strongly that,

on the basis of population disease burden associated with disorder-specific disability, more attention should be paid to the treatment of mental disorders in every country in the world, and that this need is particularly significant in low/lower-middle-income countries.

Future directions

What directions should be taken in future research on this subject? What research questions need to be addressed? What steps need to be taken to improve functional outcomes of psychological illness on a population basis? One promising direction is the conceptualization of disability in terms of social role performance. We have a basic lack of understanding about the development and course of the behavioral effects of mental disorders on social roles. Is there a hierarchical structure in the impairment of social roles? Work on severe mental illness suggests that social activities and family roles are the first to become impaired, followed by work roles, and finally the self-care role (Wiersma *et al.* 1988). Does recovery of social role performance – driven by remission of mental disorder – follow the reverse pattern? That is, when people recover, do self-care and work roles improve first, followed by family roles and social activities? We also know little about the lag times between onset and remission of mental disorders and associated social role disabilities.

The evidence that disability due to physical conditions is a risk factor for the onset of anxiety and depression raises intriguing questions on the bidirectional effects between mental disorders and disability. To what extent does disability, triggered by physical conditions, propel the onset and continuance of depression? In another study we examined the reciprocal effects between depressive symptoms and functional disability and their temporal character in a multi-wave community-based cohort of 753 older people with physical limitations (Ormel *et al.* 2002). We compared structural equation models that differed in terms of the direction and speed of effects between patient-reported disability in activities of daily living (ADLs) and depressive symptoms. The association between disability and depression could be separated into three components: (1) a strong contemporaneous effect of change in disability on depressive symptoms; (2) a weaker one-year lagged effect of change in depressive symptoms on disability (probably indirect via physical health); and (3) a weak correlation between the trait (or stable) components of depression and disability. These results were remarkably similar to the findings of Aneshensel and colleagues (1984) in a younger but unselected sample. Further research on the complex, possibly multi-directional interaction between physical disease, mental disorder, and social role functioning is needed.

Another aspect of the association between mental disorders and functional limitations that remains ambiguous is the amount of residual disability after the remission of the disorder. Some authors have reported that mean disability levels returned to normal levels among patients who had recovered from a major depressive episode (e.g., Von Korff *et al.* 1992, Ormel *et al.* 1993), while others found evidence of scarring, i.e., persistent disability after remission of the mental disorder (Wells *et al.* 1989, Coryell *et al.* 1993, Judd *et al.* 2000). More recently, a large multi-wave psychiatric epidemiologic survey in 4,796 Dutch adults from the general population who completed three measurement waves in a period of three years found evidence of trait and state effects, but not scarring effects. Major depressive episodes had temporary (*state*) but not enduring (*scar*) effects on self-reported role function (Ormel *et al.* 2004). According to the authors, the findings are best explained by the synchrony of change between depression and role function, superimposed on trait vulnerability which expresses itself in, among other ways, premorbid role dysfunction. The scarring reported in previous studies may well reflect trait vulnerability and residual symptom effects. Nonetheless, the issue of residual disability remains controversial.

Implications for public health and the organization of health care

Although the understanding of the causal relationships between mental disorders and disability is far from perfect, there is now substantial evidence to suggest that the effective treatment of mental disorders reduces social role disability, at least for depression. The public health challenge is now to organize healthcare systems so that they are capable of delivering effective treatment to everyone with depressive illnesses in the population who needs treatment. Effective treatments are not sufficient; we also need effective healthcare systems capable of disseminating those treatments to the population as a whole (Wagner *et al.* 1996). Beyond that, there remains

an urgent need for a greater understanding of the mechanisms and effective management of disability due to mental disorders.

Despite often higher disability, mental disorders are under-treated compared to physical conditions in all country income groups. Therefore, it does not make sense to introduce barriers to mental health treatment. To reduce healthcare costs, the Dutch government recently introduced co-payment for outpatient mental care but not for physical health care. This is in contrast to the parity legislation in the USA, by which insurers extend coverage to mental disorders as well as to physical conditions. Assuming similar treatment effectiveness, a not unreasonable assumption, the policy of barriers to mental health care is not only discriminatory but also illogical, given the often higher burden of disability associated with mental disorders.

Acknowledgments

Portions of this chapter are based on Ormel, J., Petukhova, M., Chatterji, S. *et al.* (2008). Disability and treatment of specific mental and physical disorders across the world. *British Journal of Psychiatry* **192**, 368–75. © 2008 The Royal College of Psychiatrists. Reproduced with permission.

References

Andrews, G., Henderson, S., & Hall, W. (2001). Prevalence, comorbidity, disability and service utilisation: overview of the Australian National Mental Health Survey. *British Journal of Psychiatry* **178**, 145–53.

Aneshensel, C. S., Frerichs, R. R., & Huba, G. J. (1984). Depression and physical illness: a multiwave, nonrecursive causal model. *Journal of Health and Social Behavior* **25**, 350–71.

Barsky, A. J., Goodson, J. D., Lane, R. S., & Cleary, P. D. (1988). The amplification of somatic symptoms. *Psychosomatic Medicine* **50**, 510–19.

Bertani, A., Perna, G., Migliarese, G., et al. (2004). Comparison of the treatment with paroxetine and reboxetine in panic disorder: a randomized, single-blind study. *Pharmacopsychiatry* **37**, 206–10.

Berto, P., D'Ilario, D., Ruffo, P., Di Virgilio, R., & Rizzo, F. (2000). Depression: cost-of-illness studies in the international literature, a review. *Journal of Mental Health Policy and Economics* **3**, 3–10.

Bijl, R. V., & Ravelli, A. (2000). Current and residual functional disability associated with psychopathology: findings from the Netherlands Mental Health Survey and Incidence Study (NEMESIS). *Psychological Medicine* **30**, 657–68.

Buist-Bouwman, M. A., de Graaf, R., Vollebergh, W. A., & Ormel, J. (2005). Comorbidity of physical and mental disorders and the effect on work-loss days. *Acta Psychiatrica Scandinavica* **111**, 436–43.

Buist-Bouwman, M. A., de Graaf, R., Vollebergh, W. A. M., *et al.* (2006). Functional disability of mental disorders and comparison with physical disorders: a study among the general population of six European countries. *Acta Psychiatrica Scandinavica* **113**, 492–500.

Buist-Bouwman M. A., Ormel J., de Graaf R., *et al.* (2008). Mediators of the association between depression and role functioning. *Acta Psychiatrica Scandinavica* **118**, 451–8.

Connor, K. M., & Davidson, J. R. (2001). SPRINT: a brief global assessment of post-traumatic stress disorder. *International Clinical Psychopharmacology* **16**, 279–84.

Coryell, W., Scheftner, W., Keller, M., *et al.* (1993). The enduring psychosocial consequences of mania and depression. *American Journal of Psychiatry* **150**, 720–27.

Coulehan, J. L., Schulberg, H. C., Block, M. R., Madonia, M. J., & Rodriquez, E. (1997). Treating depressed primary care patients improves their physical, mental, and social functioning. *Archives of Internal Medicine* **157**, 1113–20.

Davidson, J., Yaryura-Tobias, J., DuPont, R., *et al.* (2004). Fluvoxamine-controlled release formulation for the treatment of generalized social anxiety disorder. *Journal of Clinical Psychopharmacology* **24**, 118–25.

Druss, B. G., Rosenheck, R. A., & Sledge, W. H. (2000). Health and disability costs of depressive illness in a major U.S. corporation. *American Journal of Psychiatry* **157**, 1274–8.

Goetzel, R. Z., Hawkins, K., Ozminkowski, R. J., & Wang, S. (2003). The health and productivity cost burden of the "top 10" physical and mental health conditions affecting six large U.S. employers in 1999. *Journal of Occupational and Environmental Medicine* **45**, 5–14.

Hambrick, J. P., Turk, C. L., Heimberg, R. G., Schneier, R. F., & Liebowitz, M. R. (2004). Psychometric properties of disability measures among patients with social anxiety disorder. *Journal of Anxiety Disorders* **18**, 825–39.

Hays, R. D., Wells, K. B., Sherbourne, C. D., Rogers, W., & Spritzer, K. (1995). Functioning and well-being outcomes of patients with depression compared with chronic general medical illnesses. *Archives of General Psychiatry* **52**, 11–19.

Hudson, J. I., Perahia, D. G., Gilaberte, I., *et al.* (2007). Duloxetine in the treatment of major depressive disorder: an open-label study. *BMC Psychiatry* **7**, 43.

Hyman, S., Chisholm, D., Kessler, R. C., Patel, V., & Whiteford, H. (2006). Mental disorders. In D. T. Jamison, J. G. Breman, A. R. Measham, *et al.*, eds., *Disease Control Priorities in Developing Countries*. New York, NY: Oxford University Press, pp. 605–25.

International Diabetes Federation (2005). *2005 Diabetes Atlas*, 3rd edn. Brussels: International Diabetes Federation.

Judd, L. L., Akiskal, H. S., Zeller, P. J., *et al.* (2000). Psychosocial disability during the long-term course of unipolar major depressive disorder. *Archives of General Psychiatry* **57**, 375–80.

Katschnig, H., Freeman, H., & Sartorius, N. (1997). *Quality of Life in Mental Disorders*. Chichester: Wiley.

Katzelnick, D. J., Simon, G. E., & Pearson, S. D. (2000). Randomized trial of a depression management program in high utilizers of medical care. *Archives of Family Medicine* **9**, 345–51.

Kessler, R. C., & Frank, R. G. (1997). The impact of psychiatric disorders on work loss days. *Psychological Medicine* **27**, 861–73.

Kessler, R. C., Ormel, J., Demler, O., & Stang, P. E. (2003). Comorbid mental disorders account for the role impairment of commonly occurring chronic physical disorders: results from the National Comorbidity Survey. *Journal of Occupational and Environmental Medicine* **45**, 1257–66.

King, H., & Rewers, M. (1993). Global estimates for prevalence of diabetes mellitus and impaired glucose tolerance in adults. WHO Ad Hoc Diabetes Reporting Group. *Diabetes Care* **16**, 157–77.

Kish, L., & Frankel, M. R. (1974). Inferences from complex samples. *Journal of the Royal Statistical Society* **36**, 1–37.

Leon, A. C., Olfson, M., Portera, L., Farber, L., & Sheehan, D. V. (1997). Assessing psychiatric impairment in primary care with the Sheehan Disability Scale. *International Journal of Psychiatry in Medicine* **27**, 93–105.

Maetzel, A., & Li, L. (2002). The economic burden of low back pain: a review of studies published between 1996 and 2001. *Best Practice and Research Clinical Rheumatology* **16**, 23–30.

Manuel, D. G., Schultz, S. E., & Kopec, J. A. (2002). Measuring the health burden of chronic disease and injury using health adjusted life expectancy and the Health Utilities Index. *Journal of Epidemiology and Community Health* **56**, 843–50.

Mintz, J., Mintz, L. I., Arruda, M. J., & Hwang, S. S. (1992). Treatments of depression and the functional capacity to work. *Archives of General Psychiatry* **49**, 761–8.

Moussavi, S., Chatterji, S., Verdes, E., *et al.* (2007). Depression, chronic diseases, and decrements in health: results from the World Health Surveys. *Lancet* **370**, 851–8.

Murray, C. J. L., & López, A. D. (1996). *The Global Burden of Disease: a Comprehensive Assessment of Mortality and Disability from Diseases, Injuries and Risk Factors in 1990 and Projected to 2020*. Cambridge, MA: Harvard University Press.

Mynors-Wallis, L., Gath, D. H., Lloyd-Thomas, A. R., & Tomlinson, D. (1995). Randomised controlled trial comparing problem solving treatment with amitriptyline and placebo for major depression in primary care. *BMJ* **310**, 441–5.

Nathan, P. E., & Gorman, J. M. (1998). *A Guide to Treatment That Works*. Oxford: Oxford University Press.

Ormel, J., Von Korff, M., Van den Brink, W., *et al.* (1993). Depression, anxiety, and social disability show synchrony of change in primary care patients. *American Journal of Public Health* **83**, 385–90.

Ormel, J., Von Korff, M., Üstün, T. B., *et al.* (1994). Common mental disorders and disability across cultures. Results from the WHO Collaborative Study on Psychological Problems in General Health Care. *JAMA* **272**, 1741–8.

Ormel, J., Kempen, G. I., Deeg, D. J., *et al.* (1998). Functioning, well-being, and health perception in late middle-aged and older people: comparing the effects of depressive symptoms and chronic medical conditions. *Journal of the American Geriatrics Society* **46**, 39–48.

Ormel, J., Rijsdijk, F. V., Sullivan, M., Sonderen, E., & van Kempen, G. I. (2002). Temporal and reciprocal relationship between IADL/ADL disability and depressive symptoms in late life. *Journals of Gerontology B* **57**B, 338–47.

Ormel, J., Oldehinkel, A. J., Nolen, W. A., & Vollebergh, W. (2004). Psychosocial disability before, during, and after a major depressive episode: a 3-wave population-based study of state, scar, and trait effects. *Archives of General Psychiatry* **61**, 387–92.

Ormel, J., Petukhova, M., Chatterji, S. *et al.* (2008). Disability and treatment of specific mental and physical disorders across the world. *British Journal of Psychiatry* **192**, 368–75.

Pallanti, S., Bernardi, S., & Quercioli, L. (2006). The Shorter PROMIS Questionnaire and the Internet Addiction Scale in the assessment of multiple addictions in a high-school population: prevalence and related disability. *CNS Spectrum* **11**, 966–74.

Pisani, P., Bray, F., & Parkin, D. M. (2002). Estimates of the world-wide prevalence of cancer for 25 sites in the adult population. *International Journal of Cancer* **97**, 72–81.

Reed, S. D., Lee, T. A., & McCrory, D. C. (2004). The economic burden of allergic rhinitis: a critical evaluation of the literature. *Pharmacoeconomics* **22**, 345–61.

Reijneveld, S. A., & Stronks, K. (2001). The validity of self-reported use of health care across socioeconomic strata: a comparison of survey and registration data. *International Journal of Epidemiology* **30**, 1407–14.

Roglic, G., Unwin, N., Bennett, P. H., *et al.* (2005). The burden of mortality attributable to diabetes: realistic estimates for the year 2000. *Diabetes Care* **28**, 2130–5.

Spitzer, R. L., Kroenke, K., Linzer M., *et al.* (1995). Health-related quality of life in primary care patients with mental disorders. Results from the PRIME-MD 1000 Study. *JAMA* **274**, 1511–17.

Sprangers, M. A. G., de Regt, E. B., Andries, F., *et al.* (2000). Which chronic conditions are associated with better or poorer quality of life? *Journal of Clinical Epidemiology* **53**, 895–907.

Thompson, C., Kinmonth, A. L., Peveler, R., *et al.* (2000). Effects of a clinical-practice guideline and practice-based education on detection and outcome of depression in primary care: Hampshire Depression Project randomised controlled trial. *Lancet* **355**, 185–91.

Tiemens, B. G., Ormel, J., Jenner, J. A., *et al.* (1999). Training primary-care physicians to recognize, diagnose and manage depression: does it improve patient outcomes? *Psychological Medicine* **29**, 833–45.

Tylee, A., Lepine, J. P., Gastpar, M., & Mendlewicz, J. (1999). DEPRES II: a patient survey of the symptoms, disability and current management of depression in the community. *International Clinical Psychopharmacology* **3**, 139–51.

Üstün, T. B., & Sartorius, N. (1995). *Mental Illness in General Health Care: an International Study.* New York, NY: Wiley.

Verboom, C. E., Sentse, M., Sijtsema, J. J., *et al.* (2011). Explaining heterogeneity in disability with major depressive disorder: effects of personal and environmental characteristics. *Journal of Affective Disorders* **132**, 71–81.

Verbrugge, L. M., & Patrick, D. L. (1995). Seven chronic conditions: their impact on US adults' activity levels and use of medical services. *American Journal of Public Health* **85**, 173–82.

Von Korff, M., Ormel, J., Katon, W., & Lin, E. H. B. (1992). Disability and depression among high utilizers of health care: a longitudinal analysis. *Archives of General Psychiatry* **49**, 91–100.

Wagner, E. H, Austin, B. T., & Von Korff, M. (1996). Organizing care for patients with chronic illness. *Milbank Quarterly* **74**, 511–44.

Wang, P. S., Beck, A., Berglund, P., *et al.* (2003). Chronic medical conditions and work performance in the health and work performance questionnaire calibration surveys. *Journal of Occupational and Environmental Medicine* **45**, 1303–11.

Ware, J. E., Brook, R. H., Rogers, W. H., *et al.* (1986). Comparison of health outcomes at a health maintenance organisation with those of fee-for-service care. *Lancet* **1**, 1017–22.

Wells, K. B., & Sherbourne, C. D. (1999). Functioning and utility for current health of patients with depression or chronic medical conditions in managed, primary care practices. *Archives of General Psychiatry* **56**, 897–904.

Wells, K. B., Stewart, A., Hays, R. D., *et al.* (1989). The functioning and well-being of depressed patients. Results from the Medical Outcomes Study. *JAMA* **262**, 914–19.

Wiersma, D., De Jong, A., & Ormel, J. (1988). The Groningen Social Disabilities Schedule: development, relationship with I.C.I.D.H., and psychometric properties. *International Journal of Rehabilitation Research* **11**, 213–24.

World Health Organization (1980). *International Classification of Impairments, Disabilities and Handicaps.* Geneva: WHO.

World Health Organization (2001). *International Classification of Functioning, Disability and Health (ICF).* Geneva: WHO.

World Health Organization (2006). *World Health Statistics 2006.* Geneva: WHO.

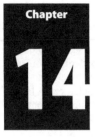

Chapter

14

Disability associated with common mental and physical disorders

Somnath Chatterji, Jordi Alonso, Maria V. Petukhova, Gemma Vilagut, Meyer Glantz, and Mohammad Salih Khalaf

Introduction

Chronic mental and physical disorders place a considerable burden on society. This is true even in low- and middle-income countries, where estimates from the World Health Organization (WHO) for the year 2004 reveal that almost half of the disease burden was caused by non-communicable diseases including mental disorders. In high-income countries, alcohol use disorders, major depression, ischemic heart disease, cerebrovascular disorders, chronic obstructive pulmonary disease (COPD), and diabetes together were responsible for 27.8 % of all burden (World Health Organization 2008). Disability, irrespective of the underlying health condition, is understood as a decrement in functioning in a given set of domains that arises out of an interaction between the health condition and the environment an individual lives in (World Health Organization 2001, Salomon *et al.* 2003). It provides a metric to compare the impact of different health conditions both at the individual and the population level (Moussavi *et al.* 2007). The WHO Disability Assessment Schedule (WHODAS) is based on the conceptual model of the International Classification of Functioning, Disability and Health (ICF) (World Health Organization 2000, 2001) and has been used in several previous studies to compare the impact of a range of health conditions (Chopra *et al.* 2004, 2008, Andrews *et al.* 2009, Garin *et al.* 2010, Üstün *et al.* 2010a, Velthorst *et al.* 2010, Honyashiki *et al.* 2011, Jittawisuthikul *et al.* 2011, Von Korff *et al.* 2011, Bonnín *et al.* 2012, Sosa *et al.* 2012). It measures difficulties in functioning reported by an individual, irrespective of the underlying health condition, over the preceding month in a variety of domains ranging from self-care to social participation and covers the breadth of mental and physical functioning. It also measures the impact of the health condition on the individual's family.

In this chapter we examine the variation in the average disability scores of all dimensions of a modified version of WHODAS in the month prior to the interview, associated with a wide range of mental and physical disorders.

Methods

Sample

We used all but one of the WMH surveys considered in this volume to examine the associations of mental and physical disorders with disability across different domains of functioning. The South African survey was excluded as disability was not measured in that survey. Disability was assessed in part 2 of the surveys, and thus the sample size used in this analysis across the remaining surveys is restricted to 58,656 respondents (see Appendix Table 2.1).

Measures

Disability was assessed with a modified version (Von Korff *et al.* 2008) of the WHO Disability Assessment Schedule 2.0 (WHODAS 2) (Üstün *et al.* 2010b). Questions were asked about difficulties in: (a) understanding and communication (*cognition*); (b) moving and getting around (*mobility*); (c) attending to personal hygiene, dressing and eating, and living alone (*self-care*); and (d) interacting with other people (*getting along*). In addition, a series of questions about activity limitations replaced the WHODAS life activities domain questions. In these questions, respondents were asked the number of days out of the past 30 that they were totally unable to carry out their normal activities or work, that they had to cut

The Burdens of Mental Disorders, ed. Jordi Alonso, Somnath Chatterji, and Yanling He. Published by Cambridge University Press. © World Health Organization 2013.

down in the activities, that they had to reduce their quality, or that they needed to exert an extreme effort to carry out their activities, due to physical or mental health problems (*role functioning*). Respondents were also asked about the extent of embarrassment (*stigma*) and discrimination or unfair treatment (*discrimination*) they experienced because of their health condition, and, finally, they were asked about the interference of their health condition on the day-to-day activities of family members (*family burden*). Scores on each dimension were obtained ranging from 0 to 100, where 0 indicated no disability and 100 indicated complete disability. Total scores on the eight WHODAS dimensions were considered the dependent variables.

It is important to note that WHODAS is different from the Sheehan Disability Scales (SDS) considered in Chapter 13. Whereas the SDS is disorder-specific (i.e., respondents are asked about disability that they think is due to a specific disorder) the WHODAS scales are not disorder-specific (i.e., respondents are asked about extent of disability irrespective of the underlying health condition/s). This is an important difference: since WHODAS is neutral to the underlying health condition, the scores can be used to address an important problem that has for the most part been neglected in the literature on health evaluation: the problem of disentangling the separate and joint impacts of comorbid mental and physical disorders. As noted in Chapters 11 and 12, comorbidity is very common and the disability due to individual disorders is affected by the co-occurrence of these different health conditions. We might expect, for example, that deafness would be much more disabling to a person who is blind than to those with normal vision, because of the special importance of hearing for people who cannot see. Comorbidity should therefore be accounted for when estimating individual- and population-level impacts of health conditions, in order to avoid overestimating the impact of any one condition. However, as noted in Chapters 11 and 12, very little previous research on the burden of illness took comorbidity into consideration. An important requirement for doing this is to begin with an outcome measure such as WHODAS that assesses disability regardless of specific disorders.

The mental and physical disorders considered here are identical to those in Chapters 11 and 12. The nine mental disorders are alcohol abuse with or without dependence, bipolar disorder (i.e., bipolar

I disorder, bipolar II disorder, and subthreshold bipolar disorder combined into a single variable), drug abuse with or without dependence, generalized anxiety disorder (GAD), major depressive disorder (MDD), panic disorder and/or agoraphobia, post-traumatic stress disorder (PTSD), social phobia, and specific phobia. The 10 physical conditions are arthritis, cancer, cardiovascular disorders (heart attack, heart disease, hypertension, and stroke), chronic pain (chronic back or neck pain and other chronic pain), diabetes, digestive disorders (stomach or intestine ulcer and irritable bowel disorder), frequent or severe headache or migraine, insomnia, neurological disorders (multiple sclerosis, Parkinson's disease, and epilepsy or seizures), and respiratory disorders (seasonal allergies such as hay fever, asthma, and COPD or emphysema). The focus was on mental and physical disorders that were present at some time in the 12 months prior to the interview.

Statistical analysis

The data analysis approach used in our analyses of the WMH surveys to take comorbidity into consideration has been illustrated in a number of previous chapters in this volume. Specifically, multiple regression analysis was used to estimate associations of each mental disorder and physical condition with each of the eight dimensions and the overall score of WHODAS. A wide range of model specifications was considered to choose the best-fitting model to predict the outcomes (see Chapter 2 for more information on model specifications). The best-fitting model specification to predict WHODAS scores was a generalized linear model (GLM) that assumed a logarithmic link function and a Poisson error distribution. Also, in order to account for comorbidity, five different models were compared that included different combinations of disorder indicators with increasing level of complexity. All models controlled for age, sex, employment status, and country. More details on the five models evaluated are described in Chapter 11. The model that provided the best fit for the eight dependent variables included the 19 mental and physical disorders, an additional term called the "importance score" of the disorder, and the interaction of this term with each disorder (Appendix Table 14.1). (See *Methods* in Chapter 11 for further information on the "importance score.")

As in earlier chapters of this volume, simulation was used to estimate the mean individual-level effect (i.e., increase in disability) on each of the domains of WHODAS and the combined disability score associated with each condition. See Chapter 2 for a detailed discussion of this simulation method. Also similar to previous chapters, both individual-level and societal-level associations are reported. Design-based standard errors of estimates were obtained using the Taylor Series Linearization (TSL) method (Wolter 1985) implemented in the SUDAAN software system (Research Triangle Institute 2005). Standard errors of individual- and societal-level effects were estimated using SAS macros for the Jackknife Repeated Replication (JRR) method for complex sample data (SAS Institute Inc. 2002). As in all other chapters in this volume, statistical significance was consistently evaluated at the 0.05 level with two-sided tests.

Results

Distribution of WHODAS scores

The mean scores of those respondents with any mental disorder, any physical disorder, either, or no disorder are shown separately for each dimension in Table 14.1. Overall, more than a half of all respondents (57%) with a mental disorder had some limitation in the WHODAS (score > 0), while around 46% of those with a physical condition reported some limitation. Respondents with any mental or physical disorders had significantly higher levels of disability on all dimensions than those with no health conditions. Moreover, those respondents with mental disorders had much higher scores on all dimensions than respondents with physical disorders.

Individual-level effects of disorders on WHODAS scores

Table 14.2 shows the relative effects of mental and physical disorders in the overall sample across dimensions at the individual level. Data combined from all the countries show that, in general, mental disorders are more disabling than physical disorders (3.8 vs. 3.4 for mental and physical disorders, respectively). Mental disorders produce significantly higher social and cognitive disability and lead to higher discrimination and family burden in the pooled sample, while physical conditions have a larger impact on mobility. Looking at specific disorders, bipolar disorder has the most disabling impact from all the conditions assessed in our study, comparable to neurological disorders

such as stroke and Parkinson's disease. In all the dimensions, except for mobility, bipolar disorder is the leading cause of disability (i.e., combined rate of 4.9). In addition, anxiety disorders such as PTSD and panic are also severely disabling mental disorders, followed by depression. Conditions like PTSD, insomnia, and pain had an important and significant impact on daily life activities. With regard to family burden, PTSD is associated as much disability as neurological disorders (5.7 and 5.9, respectively). Major depressive disorder causes moderate levels of disability across all dimensions (3.4), and its effect is comparable to the overall impact of physical health conditions.

Examination of results of individual-level effects by country income level, which are presented in the Appendix Table 14.2, shows that social dysfunction is significantly higher in the presence of a mental disorder in high-income countries than in the other two groups (high-income = 1.9; upper-middle-income = 1.5; low/lower-middle-income = 1.2). Cognitive dysfunction is significantly higher in the presence of a mental disorder in upper-middle-income and high-income countries than in low/lower-middle-income countries (upper-middle-income and high-income = 2.5; low/lower-middle-income = 1.3). In upper-middle-income countries, mental disorders cause significantly higher stigma (8.0 vs. 4.8) and discrimination (5.1 vs. 2.2–2.6) than in the other two country groups. More specifically, while drug abuse (6.0) and neurological disorders (7.1) are the most disabling conditions overall in low/lower-middle-income countries, panic (7.5) and bipolar disorder (6.6) are the most disabling in upper-middle-income countries, and bipolar disorder (4.4) and neurological disorders (4.3) are the most disabling in high-income countries. In low/lower-middle-income countries bipolar disorder (13.5), neurological disorders (11.1), and drug abuse (10.4) are the leading causes of problems with role functioning; neurological disorders are associated with significant stigma (13.7) and discrimination (8.9) comparable to drug abuse (9.5 and 8.9, respectively); these two conditions are also the ones that cause the largest burden. In low/lower-middle-income countries, drug abuse (6.0) is associated with overall disability almost twice as large as for physical disorders in general (3.1). In contrast, in upper-middle-income countries, physical health conditions cause little stigma and discrimination, while panic disorder is associated with high levels of disability with regard to role functioning (13.0), stigma (12.9), discrimination (5.1), and family burden (13.1). Panic disorder (7.5) is more than twice

Table 14.1 Distribution of WHODAS scores by type of disorders. The WMH surveys.

Dimensions	Any mental disorders				Any physical conditions				Any disorder (mental or physical)				No disorders	
	All		% with non-zero score		All		% with non-zero score		All		% with non-zero score		All	
	Mean	(SE)	%	(SE)	Mean	(SE)	%	(SE)	Mean	(SE)	%	SE	Mean	(SE)
Cognition	3.0	(0.1)	22.2	(0.5)	1.4	(0.0)	11.4	(0.2)	1.4	(0.0)	2.3	(0.2)	0.1	(0.0)
Mobility	6.1	(0.2)	22.9	(0.5)	5.5	(0.1)	19.0	(0.3)	5.2	(0.1)	3.4	(0.2)	0.7	(0.1)
Self-care	2.1	(0.1)	8.1	(0.3)	1.6	(0.1)	5.5	(0.2)	1.5	(0.1)	0.9	(0.1)	0.2	(0.0)
Getting along	2.2	(0.1)	13.2	(0.4)	1.0	(0.0)	6.4	(0.2)	1.0	(0.0)	1.1	(0.1)	0.1	(0.0)
Role functioning	18.8	(0.4)	48.9	(0.6)	13.5	(0.2)	38.8	(0.4)	13.1	(0.2)	22.3	(0.4)	3.4	(0.1)
Stigma	9.8	(0.3)	19.2	(0.5)	6.1	(0.1)	12.5	(0.2)	5.9	(0.1)	2.1	(0.1)	0.9	(0.1)
Discrimination	4.6	(0.2)	9.2	(0.3)	2.5	(0.1)	5.3	(0.2)	2.4	(0.1)	0.9	(0.1)	0.4	(0.0)
Family burden	9.3	(0.3)	19.6	(0.5)	5.7	(0.1)	12.5	(0.2)	5.5	(0.1)	2.1	(0.1)	0.9	(0.1)
Combined	7.3	(0.2)	57.0	(0.6)	4.9	(0.1)	46.2	(0.4)	4.8	(0.1)	24.6	(0.4)	0.9	(0.0)

Table 14.2 Individual-level effects of mental and physical disorder on WHODAS scores. The WMH surveys.

Disorders	Cognition		Mobility		Self-care		Getting along		Role functioning		Family burden		Stigma		Discrimination		Combined	
	Est[a]	(SE)	Est[a]	(SE)	Est[a]	(SE)	Est[a]	(SE)	Est[a]	(SE)	Est[a]	(SE)	Est[a]	(SE)	Est[a]	(SE)	Est[a]	(SE)
Alcohol abuse	0.5	(0.2)	−0.6	(0.3)	0.0	(0.0)	0.2	(0.3)	3.3	(0.9)	1.4	(0.6)	1.9	(0.6)	1.0	(0.5)	1.0	(0.3)
Bipolar	3.7	(0.6)	2.2	(0.6)	1.8	(0.7)	2.5	(0.5)	9.6	(1.3)	7.0	(1.1)	6.5	(0.9)	3.9	(0.9)	4.9	(0.6)
Drug abuse	1.2	(0.5)	0.6	(0.8)	−0.1	(0.5)	2.0	(0.8)	5.1	(1.8)	4.0	(1.4)	2.8	(1.2)	2.5	(1.1)	2.2	(0.8)
Generalized anxiety	1.6	(0.4)	1.5	(0.7)	0.5	(0.4)	1.7	(0.4)	5.5	(1.2)	4.0	(0.9)	3.5	(0.8)	1.0	(0.6)	2.5	(0.5)
Major depressive disorder	2.0	(0.2)	2.0	(0.3)	0.8	(0.2)	1.5	(0.2)	7.7	(0.6)	4.1	(0.4)	4.9	(0.4)	2.6	(0.3)	3.4	(0.2)
Panic and/or agoraphobia	2.7	(0.4)	2.2	(0.6)	0.9	(0.4)	1.9	(0.4)	7.7	(1.0)	4.5	(0.8)	6.3	(0.9)	1.9	(0.6)	3.7	(0.5)
Post-traumatic stress	3.1	(0.5)	4.3	(0.7)	1.8	(0.5)	1.7	(0.4)	8.9	(1.1)	5.7	(0.8)	5.1	(0.9)	2.8	(0.6)	4.2	(0.5)
Social phobia	2.1	(0.3)	1.0	(0.4)	0.0	(0.3)	1.8	(0.3)	4.7	(0.7)	4.4	(0.7)	4.1	(0.7)	2.6	(0.5)	2.7	(0.4)
Specific phobia	0.7	(0.2)	1.1	(0.4)	0.4	(0.2)	0.5	(0.2)	3.7	(0.7)	2.6	(0.5)	2.4	(0.5)	1.3	(0.4)	1.7	(0.3)
Arthritis	0.2	(0.2)	2.5	(0.4)	0.4	(0.2)	0.0	(0.1)	2.8	(0.5)	1.0	(0.4)	1.8	(0.4)	0.3	(0.3)	1.2	(0.2)
Cancer	0.4	(0.3)	1.4	(0.7)	0.7	(0.6)	0.4	(0.3)	4.8	(1.1)	1.6	(0.6)	1.0	(0.6)	0.0	(0.7)	1.4	(0.4)
Cardiovascular	0.2	(0.2)	2.1	(0.4)	0.5	(0.3)	0.1	(0.1)	3.9	(0.6)	2.1	(0.3)	1.9	(0.4)	1.0	(0.2)	1.6	(0.2)
Chronic pain	0.7	(0.1)	4.2	(0.3)	1.1	(0.2)	0.7	(0.1)	8.0	(0.5)	3.1	(0.3)	3.4	(0.3)	1.2	(0.2)	3.0	(0.2)
Diabetes	0.6	(0.2)	1.8	(0.6)	1.2	(0.4)	0.3	(0.2)	4.5	(0.9)	1.5	(0.5)	2.0	(0.6)	0.7	(0.3)	1.7	(0.3)
Digestive	0.2	(0.3)	1.8	(0.5)	0.3	(0.3)	0.7	(0.2)	4.6	(0.8)	2.3	(0.6)	2.7	(0.6)	0.7	(0.5)	1.8	(0.3)
Headache/migraine	1.3	(0.2)	0.7	(0.3)	0.8	(0.2)	0.4	(0.1)	3.7	(0.5)	2.8	(0.3)	2.2	(0.4)	1.4	(0.3)	1.7	(0.2)
Insomnia	1.2	(0.3)	2.9	(0.5)	1.1	(0.3)	0.9	(0.2)	6.6	(0.8)	4.0	(0.6)	4.4	(0.5)	2.7	(0.5)	3.1	(0.3)
Neurological	2.6	(0.6)	5.4	(1.4)	3.2	(0.9)	1.7	(0.5)	9.3	(1.6)	5.9	(1.4)	6.5	(1.4)	3.9	(1.2)	4.9	(0.9)
Respiratory	0.1	(0.1)	0.6	(0.2)	0.0	(0.7)	0.2	(0.1)	1.5	(0.4)	0.3	(0.3)	0.7	(0.3)	0.4	(0.2)	0.5	(0.1)
All mental	2.2	(0.1)	2.2	(0.2)	1.0	(0.1)	1.7	(0.1)	8.5	(0.3)	5.2	(0.2)	5.3	(0.2)	2.7	(0.2)	3.8	(0.1)
All physical	1.0	(0.1)	4.4	(0.2)	1.0	(0.1)	0.6	(0.1)	8.6	(0.3)	4.0	(0.1)	4.4	(0.1)	1.8	(0.1)	3.4	(0.1)
All disorders	1.5	(0.0)	4.4	(0.1)	1.3	(0.1)	1.0	(0.0)	10.3	(0.2)	5.0	(0.1)	5.4	(0.1)	2.3	(0.1)	4.1	(0.1)

[a] Individual-level estimate.

as disabling as physical disorders generally (3.4). Finally, in high-income countries, bipolar disorder (4.4) and PTSD (4.0) are the most disabling mental disorders, associated with levels of disability higher than physical disorders in general (3.5). Pain disorders (10.4) are responsible for the largest impact on role functioning in these countries, more than for neurological (7.9) and mental health disorders (9.0). Neurological disorders (4.9) are associated with higher stigma than depression (3.9) and discrimination (3.7 vs. 1.8, respectively), which is comparable to bipolar disorders (3.7).

Societal effects of disorders on WHODAS scores

Table 14.3 shows the population attributable risk proportions (PARPs) of the different dimensions of WHODAS for each condition pooled across all countries. Since PARPs combine information on the individual disability impact with the condition and the prevalence of the disorder, chronic pain conditions contribute the most to disability overall in the pooled sample, due, in part, to their high prevalence (PARP = 20.1%). They are followed by major depressive disorder (9.1%), cardiovascular disorders (8.0%), frequent or severe headaches or migraines (7.2%), and insomnia (5.8%). As opposed to levels of disability at the individual level, depression contributes to a large part of the burden in the social (18.4%), cognitive (17.9%), role functioning (7.4%), stigma (10.6%), and discrimination (13.4%) dimensions of WHODAS. Chronic pain conditions are responsible for 15–28% of the population-level burden across all the dimensions. The group of chronic disorders assessed in the WMH surveys together explain about 71.5% of all disability, 24.7% being associated with mental disorders and 53% with physical conditions. Note that together these two groups of disorders add up to less than the overall population-level burden due to comorbidity between these disorders and due to their sub-additive effect with regard to disability.

Generally speaking, and as a consequence of similar prevalence of the disorders in the different country types, PARPs for each condition tend to be similar across different country income levels. A detailed examination of these results (Appendix Table 14.3) reveals that between 67.1% (in low/lower-middle-income countries) and 74.3% (in upper-middle-income countries) of the overall population burden of health conditions is captured by those

measured in this analysis. Frequent or severe headaches or migraines (11.3%) and major depressive disorder (8.2%) are the most burdensome conditions overall in low/lower-middle-income countries, chronic pain conditions (17.2%) and major depressive disorder (15.5%) in upper-middle-income countries, and chronic pain conditions (23.3%), cardiovascular disorders (8.8%), and major depressive disorder (7.5%) in high-income countries. Across all country income levels, chronic pain conditions contribute to the largest amount of population-level disability on the self-care and mobility dimensions (24.2% and 28.0%, respectively). Of interest is also the finding that across all country groups, chronic pain is the largest factor contributing to stigma and embarrassment at the population level (18.8%). Social phobia is a significant determinant of the social dimension of disability in upper-middle-income (15.8%) and high-income countries (10.7%) while they contribute little in low/lower-middle-income countries (1.1%). It must be noted here that while neurological conditions are highly disabling at the individual level, because of their low prevalence they contribute to only about 2% of combined disability at the population level.

Discussion

The results reported here show that the commonly occurring mental and physical disorders considered here explain almost three-quarters of general population disability measured with a comprehensive instrument to assess disability, WHODAS. At the individual level, disability associated with mental disorders is higher than that of physical conditions. However, given that mental disorders are less prevalent than the physical conditions considered here, physical conditions explain a higher share of the population's disability than mental disorders. Among the mental disorders assessed in our study, bipolar disorder is the most disabling one at the individual level on all dimensions except mobility, followed by PTSD and panic disorder and/or agoraphobia. PTSD also causes the most individual-level disability in mobility and self-care. There is some international variation on the impact of mental disorders across different types of countries. For instance, substance disorders are most disabling in low/lower-middle-income countries, where they are associated with high stigma, discrimination, social dysfunction, and family burden. While bipolar disorder and panic disorder and/or

Table 14.3 Population attributable risk proportions (PARPs) of different WHODAS dimensions due to disorders. The WMH surveys.

Disorders	Cognition		Mobility		Self-care		Getting along		Role functioning		Family burden		Stigma		Discrimination		Combined	
	PARP (%)	SE	PARP (%)	SE	PARP (%)	SE	PARP (%)	SE	PARP (%)	SE	PARP (%)	SE	PARP (%)	SE	PARP (%)	SE	PARP (%)	SE
Alcohol abuse	1.1	(0.6)	-0.4	(-0.2)	0.0	(0.0)	0.8	(0.9)	0.8	(0.2)	0.9	(0.4)	1.1	(0.4)	1.3	(0.7)	0.7	(0.2)
Bipolar	4.9	(0.8)	0.9	(0.3)	2.4	(0.9)	4.8	(0.9)	1.4	(0.2)	2.4	(0.4)	2.1	(0.3)	3.0	(0.7)	1.9	(0.2)
Drug abuse	0.8	(0.3)	0.1	(0.2)	0.0	(0.3)	1.9	(0.7)	0.4	(0.1)	0.7	(0.3)	0.5	(0.2)	1.0	(0.4)	0.5	(0.2)
Generalized anxiety	3.4	(0.9)	1.0	(0.4)	1.1	(0.9)	4.9	(1.2)	1.2	(0.3)	2.2	(0.5)	1.8	(0.4)	1.3	(0.8)	1.6	(0.3)
Major depressive disorder	17.9	(1.8)	5.3	(0.9)	7.4	(1.8)	18.4	(2.1)	7.4	(0.5)	9.6	(0.9)	10.6	(0.9)	13.4	(1.5)	9.1	(0.6)
Panic disorder	7.3	(1.1)	1.8	(0.5)	2.5	(1.0)	7.2	(1.6)	2.2	(0.3)	3.1	(0.6)	4.1	(0.5)	2.9	(1.0)	3.0	(0.4)
Post-traumatic stress	7.2	(1.0)	2.9	(0.5)	4.2	(1.1)	5.7	(1.2)	2.2	(0.3)	3.4	(0.5)	2.8	(0.5)	3.7	(0.8)	2.9	(0.4)
Social phobia	7.6	(1.1)	1.1	(0.4)	-0.2	(1.0)	9.5	(1.6)	1.9	(0.3)	4.1	(0.6)	3.6	(0.6)	5.5	(1.0)	2.9	(0.4)
Specific phobia	5.5	(1.4)	2.5	(0.8)	3.1	(1.5)	5.1	(2.1)	3.1	(0.5)	5.1	(1.0)	4.4	(0.8)	5.8	(1.7)	3.8	(0.6)
Arthritis	3.6	(2.4)	11.4	(1.7)	6.1	(3.9)	1.0	(2.9)	4.7	(0.9)	3.9	(1.4)	6.7	(1.3)	2.7	(2.4)	5.6	(0.9)
Cancer	0.9	(0.7)	0.9	(0.5)	1.5	(1.2)	1.3	(0.8)	1.1	(0.3)	0.9	(0.4)	0.5	(0.3)	0.0	(0.9)	0.9	(0.2)
Cardiovascular	4.0	(2.9)	10.7	(1.9)	9.1	(4.2)	2.7	(2.9)	7.0	(1.0)	9.0	(1.5)	7.8	(1.6)	9.8	(2.3)	8.0	(1.1)
Chronic pain	16.8	(2.6)	28.0	(1.9)	24.2	(3.9)	22.0	(3.2)	19.3	(1.1)	18.1	(1.7)	18.8	(1.8)	15.1	(2.9)	20.1	(1.1)
Diabetes	2.2	(0.9)	2.2	(0.7)	4.8	(1.6)	2.0	(1.1)	1.9	(0.4)	1.6	(0.5)	2.0	(0.6)	1.7	(0.8)	2.0	(0.4)
Digestive	0.7	(0.9)	1.9	(0.5)	1.0	(1.1)	3.3	(1.2)	1.7	(0.3)	2.1	(0.5)	2.3	(0.5)	1.4	(0.9)	1.9	(0.3)
Headache/migraine	17.7	(2.2)	2.9	(1.2)	10.6	(2.8)	7.6	(2.7)	5.5	(0.7)	10.2	(1.2)	7.3	(1.3)	11.1	(2.4)	7.2	(0.8)
Insomnia	7.7	(1.8)	5.4	(0.8)	6.6	(1.7)	7.9	(1.9)	4.3	(0.5)	6.4	(0.9)	6.6	(0.8)	9.5	(1.6)	5.8	(0.6)
Neurological	3.2	(0.7)	2.0	(0.5)	4.0	(1.1)	2.9	(0.8)	1.2	(0.2)	1.9	(0.4)	1.9	(0.4)	2.7	(0.8)	1.8	(0.3)
Respiratory	2.5	(2.1)	2.8	(1.1)	0.1	(10.9)	3.8	(2.2)	2.6	(0.7)	1.3	(1.1)	2.8	(1.0)	3.6	(1.8)	2.3	(0.7)
All mental	47.3	(1.6)	14.1	(1.1)	21.7	(2.1)	50.6	(2.1)	19.8	(0.7)	28.9	(1.1)	28.1	(1.1)	33.8	(1.7)	24.7	(0.8)
All physical	52.7	(3.0)	66.9	(2.1)	54.4	(5.5)	47.1	(3.3)	47.2	(1.3)	53.5	(1.7)	55.2	(1.7)	53.3	(2.7)	53.0	(1.2)
All disorders	85.1	(1.1)	75.3	(1.8)	73.1	(3.8)	82.9	(1.7)	63.5	(1.0)	74.8	(1.3)	75.8	(1.2)	76.3	(1.8)	71.5	(0.9)

agoraphobia are the most disabling mental disorders in upper-middle-income countries, PTSD and bipolar disorder are the most disabling in high-income countries. Among physical conditions, neurological disorders are the most disabling conditions across all dimensions of disability consistently across the two higher country income levels. Taken together, these results suggest that there is an urgent need to reduce the impact of health conditions on people's lives.

As in previous chapters, a number of limitations must be taken into account when interpreting these results. First, physical conditions and mental disorders were differently assessed. The latter were measured with a standard diagnostic instrument, the WHO Composite International Diagnostic Interview (CIDI) version 3.0, with high levels of reliability and acceptable validity for research purposes. Conversely, chronic physical conditions were self-reported by respondents. Although we used standardized questions which have shown acceptable validity levels, misclassification cannot be ruled out, in particular, under-reporting of physical health conditions in countries with lower access to health care. Second, we did not assess some particularly disabling mental disorders such as non-affective psychotic disorders and dementia. Our study, therefore, likely underestimates disability caused by mental disorders. Third, while physical conditions and mental disorders were assessed in the 12 months previous to the interview, disability as assessed by WHODAS referred to the 30 days preceding the interview. The latter recall period is the standard for WHODAS. However, because of these different time frames it is not possible to definitively relate the disability reported by the respondents to their underlying mental or physical disorder for the preceding 12 months. Nevertheless, given that most conditions that were assessed are persistent disorders and the random occurrence of other acute conditions is likely to be spread over our large sample, it is very likely that what we assessed in WHODAS was indeed to a large extent explained by the health conditions we recorded here. It is nonetheless possible that these associations may be somewhat tenuous, especially for conditions that are episodic such as migraine. Finally, some caution is needed in the interpretation of the way we have estimated the marginal effects of conditions and disorders in disability. Our simulation assumed that it would be possible to "eliminate" the disability caused by removing the disorder, all other personal and health characteristics of the individual remaining

constant. This would only be plausible if all comorbid conditions were directly related to each other without the mediating effects of these other characteristics (Kraemer *et al.* 1997), and this hypothetical interpretation should be made cautiously.

Despite these limitations, it is clear from these results that, across all country income levels, mental disorders produce comparable levels of disability compared to physical conditions. At the individual level, bipolar disorders produce overall disability that is second only to neurological disorders. Conditions such as PTSD and panic disorder and/or agoraphobia, generally not considered to be associated with significant disability, also are amongst the most disabling conditions. There are variations by country groups among mental disorders: overall, drug use disorders rank below specific phobia as one of the least disabling mental conditions, but they are the most disabling condition in low/lower-middle-income countries. Among physical conditions also there are considerable variations between country income levels: while neurological disorders are the most disabling everywhere, cancer is the second most disabling condition in low/lower-middle-income countries, although it ranks near the bottom among upper-middle-income and high-income countries.

Within mental disorders the patterns across the difference dimensions of disability also show variations. While bipolar disorder shows the highest levels of disability across almost all the dimensions of WHODAS, PTSD is associated with the highest levels of disability in terms of self-care and mobility. Drug use disorders produce significant disability in social participation, next only to bipolar disorder. Alcohol use disorders rank near the bottom on almost all dimensions of disability.

Implications

These results show that, as regards disability associated with mental and physical disorders, there is no "one size that fits all." While mental disorders are all significantly disabling, the patterns of disability depend both on the country where the person resides and on the nature of the mental disorder. These variations, besides being inherently related to the condition, are also determined perhaps by the availability of health services for these conditions as well as by the societal acceptance of the conditions. Early diagnosis and intervention, associated with public awareness initiatives, perhaps alter the experience of disability.

Our results suggest that health systems must recognize the significant disability that mental disorders cause, comparable to physical health conditions. Interventions planned for these disorders at both the individual and the population level must take into account the patterns of disability and tailor the interventions accordingly. Matching interventions to the patterns of disability at individual and population levels is likely to be more cost-effective in reducing the impact of these conditions.

Acknowledgments

Portions of this chapter are based on Alonso, J., Vilagut, G., Chatterji, S., et al. (2011). Including information about co-morbidity in estimates of disease burden: results from the World Health Organization World Mental Health surveys. *Psychological Medicine* **41**, 873–86. © 2011. Cambridge University Press. Reproduced with permission.

References

Andrews, G., Kemp, A., Sunderland, M., Von Korff, M., & Üstün, T. B. (2009). Normative data for the 12 item WHO Disability Assessment Schedule 2.0. *PLoS One* **4**, e8343.

Bonnín, C. M., Sánchez-Moreno, J., Martínez-Arán, A., et al. (2012). Subthreshold symptoms in bipolar disorder: impact on neurocognition, quality of life and disability. *Journal of Affective Disorders* **136**, 650–9.

Chopra, P., Couper, J. W., & Herrman, H. (2004). The assessment of patients with long-term psychotic disorders: application of the WHO Disability Assessment Schedule II. *Australian and New Zealand Journal of Psychiatry* **38**, 753–9.

Chopra, P., Herrman, H., & Kennedy, G. (2008). Comparison of disability and quality of life measures in patients with long-term psychotic disorders and patients with multiple sclerosis: an application of the WHO Disability Assessment Schedule II and WHO Quality of Life-BREF. *International Journal of Rehabilitation Research* **31**, 141–9.

Garin, O., Ayuso-Mateos, J. L., Almansa, J., et al. (2010). Validation of the "World Health Organization Disability Assessment Schedule, WHODAS-2" in patients with chronic diseases. *Health and Quality of Life Outcomes* **19**, 51.

Honyashiki, M., Ferri, C. P., Acosta, D., et al. (2011). Chronic diseases among older people and co-resident psychological morbidity: a 10/66 Dementia Research Group population-based survey. *International Psychogeriatrics* 1–13.

Jittawisuthikul, O., Jirapramukpitak, T., & Sumpowthong, K. (2011). Disability and late-life depression: a prospective population-based study. *Journal of the Medical Association of Thailand* **94** (Suppl 7), S145–52.

Kraemer, H. C., Kazdin, A. E., Offord, D. R., et al. (1997). Coming to terms with the terms of risk. *Archives of General Psychiatry* **54**, 337–43.

Moussavi, S., Chatterji, S., Verdes, E., et al. (2007). Depression, chronic diseases, and decrements in health: results from the World Health Surveys. *Lancet* **370**, 851–8.

Research Triangle Institute (2005). *SUDAAN, Version 9.0.1.* [computer program]. Research Triangle Park, NC: Research Triangle Institute.

Salomon, J. A., Mathers, C. D., Chatterji, S., et al. (2003). Quantifying individual levels of health: definitions, concepts and measurement issues. In C. J. L. Murray & D. B. Evans, eds., *Health Systems Performance Assessment: Debates, Methods and Empricism*. Geneva: World Health Organization, pp. 301–18.

SAS Institute Inc. (2002). *SAS/STAT® Software, Version 9.1 for Windows*. Cary, NC: SAS Institute Inc.

Sosa, A. L., Albanese, E., Stephan, B. C., et al. (2012). Prevalence, distribution, and impact of mild cognitive impairment in Latin America, China, and India: a 10/66 population-based study. *PLoS Medicine* **9**, e1001170.

Üstün, T. B., Chatterji, S., Kostanjsek, N., et al. (2010a) WHO/NIH Joint Project. Developing the World Health Organization Disability Assessment Schedule 2.0. *Bulletin of the World Health Organization* **88**, 815–23.

Üstün, T. B., Kostanjsek, N., Chatterji, S., & Rehm, J. (2010b). *Measuring Health and Disability: Manual for WHO Disability Assessment Schedule (WHODAS 2.0)* Geneva: World Health Organization.

Velthorst, E., Nieman, D. H., Linszen, D., et al. (2010). Disability in people clinically at high risk of psychosis. *British Journal of Psychiatry* **197**, 278–84.

Von Korff, M., Crane, P. K., Alonso, J., et al. (2008). Modified WHODAS-II provides valid measure of global disability but filter items increased skewness. *Journal of Clinical Epidemiology* **61**, 1132–43.

Von Korff, M., Katon, W. J., Lin, E. H., et al. (2011). Functional outcomes of multi-condition collaborative care and successful ageing: results of randomised trial. *BMJ* **343**, d6612.

Wolter, K. M. (1985). *Introduction to Variance Estimation*. New York, NY: Springer-Verlag.

World Health Organization (2000). *WHO Disability Assessment Schedule II (WHODAS II)*. Geneva: WHO.

World Health Organization (2001). *International Classification of Functioning, Disability and Health (ICF)*. Geneva: WHO.

World Health Organization (2008). *The Global Burden of Disease 2004 Update*. Geneva: WHO.

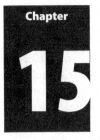

Chapter

15

Perceived health associated with common mental and physical disorders

Jordi Alonso, Gemma Vilagut, James Anthony, Evelyn J. Bromet, Oye Gureje, Carmen Lara, and Zhaorui Liu

Introduction

As discussed in previous chapters of this volume, it is becoming increasingly clear that no country can afford to provide universal healthcare coverage for all illnesses to all its citizens. Triage priority systems are needed to allocate available healthcare resources in order to best address the inevitable shortfall between resources and needs. Among the many types of information used to help develop these systems, comparative illness burden estimates have been especially valuable as a reference standard for government health policy planners (Murray & López 1996, Murray *et al.* 2001, López & Mathers 2007). A central component of these estimates is the condition-specific severity weight, a statistic obtained by means of the evaluations of expert raters on the relative burdens of different conditions using the person trade-off method (Murray & López, 1996, Murray *et al.* 2001, World Health Organization 2004). However, this approach is limited in that the vignettes represent single conditions rather than more realistic cases in which an individual simultaneously suffers from a number of different conditions (Fortin *et al.* 2007). This limitation is significant, because methodological research has shown that condition-specific severity weights vary as a function of the presence of comorbidity (Moussavi *et al.* 2007).

Previous attempts to consider comorbidity in estimating the condition-specific illness burden have been limited by the fact that simplistic models were used to estimate effects (Verbrugge *et al.* 1989, Maddigan *et al.* 2005). This chapter presents the results of an analysis aimed at generating condition-specific estimates of disease burden in a more realistic way. The method consists of the analysis of data on the joint associations of health conditions collected from the general population through a series of community epidemiologic surveys as well as overall respondent ratings of perceived health, although the same logic could be applied to the analysis of complex vignettes describing comorbid condition profiles. This approach has already been used in the analyses discussed in previous chapters of this volume, in particular Chapters 11, 12, and 14.

Methods

Sample

Our analysis is based on the data acquired from 23 WMH surveys. The two remaining WMH surveys in this volume, New Zealand and South Africa, were excluded because those surveys did not include the perceived health item. Country-specific response rates ranged from 45.9% (France) to 87.7% (Colombia), with a weighted (by sample size) average response rate across surveys of 69.6%. The total sample used in the analyses in this chapter is $n = 51,344$ (see Appendix Table 2.1).

As explained in Chapter 2, according to the World Bank (2008), seven of these 23 surveys were in countries classified as low/lower-middle-income (Colombia, India–Pondicherry, Iraq, Nigeria, People's Republic of China [PRC]–Beijing/Shanghai, PRC–Shenzhen, and Ukraine), five in upper-middle-income countries (Brazil–São Paulo, Bulgaria, Lebanon, Mexico, and Romania), and 11 in high-income countries (Belgium, France, Germany, Israel, Italy, Japan, the Netherlands, Northern Ireland, Portugal, Spain, and USA).

Measures

Overall perceived health was measured by means of a 0–100 visual analog scale (VAS) where 0 represented "the worst possible health a person can have" and 100 represented "perfect health" in the 30 days prior to the

---

interview. The VAS scores of overall mental and physical perceived health will be called simply "VAS scores" in the remainder of this chapter.

As detailed in Chapter 2, and as in other chapters of this book, 10 chronic physical conditions were considered: arthritis, cancer, cardiovascular disorders, chronic pain conditions, diabetes, digestive disorders, frequent or severe headaches or migraines, insomnia, neurological disorders, and respiratory disorders. The nine mental disorders considered in this chapter were alcohol abuse with or without dependence, bipolar disorder, drug abuse with or without dependence, generalized anxiety disorder (GAD), major depressive disorder (MDD), panic disorder and/or agoraphobia, post-traumatic stress disorder (PTSD), social phobia, and specific phobia. As with the chronic physical conditions, our focus was on mental disorders present at some time in the 12 months prior to the interview.

The control variables used in the analysis included age, sex, and country income groups.

Statistical analysis

As explained in greater detail in Chapter 2, in order to account for the skewed distribution of the VAS scores, 14 different specifications of two-part models (part 1 consists of a logistic regression equation predicting a VAS score of 100 versus a score of less than 100 in the total sample, and part 2 is a linear regression equation predicting scores in the 0–99 range) and generalized linear models (GLM) (including ordinary least squares [OLS] and different combinations of non-linear relationships and error structures) were fitted and compared using standard empirical model comparison procedures (Alonso *et al.* 2011). All models were estimated separately by country income groups. The OLS model was the best-fitting model of all the tests considered and was therefore the one selected (see Appendix Table 15.1).

A series of multiple regression models was used to estimate joint predictive associations of mental and physical disorders with VAS scores, controlling for age, sex, and country income groups. As the sample size was too small to allow each of the 524,268 (2^{19} – 20) logically possible multivariate condition profiles to be a separate predictor, the models necessarily made simplifying assumptions about the effects of comorbidity. To this end, four different models were proposed and compared. Model 1 was an additive model that included a separate predictor for each disorder without interactions. Model 2 included a series of

predictors for number of conditions (e.g., one predictor for having exactly one condition, another for exactly two, etc.) without information about type of disorder. Model 3 included 19 predictors for type, and predictors for number of conditions; the number-of-conditions dummies in this model represent aggregate patterns of comorbidity assumed regardless of types. Model 4 added interactions of types of conditions by number of conditions to model 3, allowing the effects of comorbidity to vary by type of condition as a linear function of the number of other conditions. All models were estimated separately in low/lower-middle-income, upper-middle-income, and high-income countries in an effort to obtain a rough indication of the variation in results by country level, but no attempt was made to estimate country-specific models. Model 4 was the best-fitting model in all country groups (see Appendix Table 15.2).

This is a model of intermediate complexity, in that it allows interactions to vary across conditions but not across particular pairs or across more than two disorders. Although this may not be the most optimal interaction model, the fact that it provides the best fit across the range of models considered suggests that it is a useful first approximation. One complication of the model, as in any interaction model, is that the coefficients have no intuitive interpretation. As explained in Chapter 2, we addressed this problem by using individual-level simulation to transform coefficients to a scale of average decrement in the VAS scores associated with each condition. We also calculated the population attributable risk proportion (PARP) to describe societal-level effects. PARPs can be interpreted as the proportion of instances of the outcome that would not have occurred in the absence of the predictor disorders. Further details of the methodology can be found in Chapter 2.

Because the WMH sample design featured weighting and clustering, all multiple regression analyses used the Taylor Series Linearization (TSL) method (Wolter 1985) implemented in the SUDAAN software system (Research Triangle Institute 2005). Standard errors of simulation estimates were obtained using the Jackknife Repeated Replication (JRR) method (Wolter 1985) implemented with a SAS macro (SAS Institute Inc. 2002). Statistical significance was consistently evaluated using two-sided 0.05-level tests.

Results

More than half of all respondents reported having one or more conditions in the 12 months prior to the

Table 15.1 12-month prevalence estimates of mental disorders and physical conditions by country income level. The WMH surveys.

Disorders	Country income level							
	All countries		Low/lower-middle		Upper-middle		High	
	%	(SE)	%	(SE)	%	(SE)	%	(SE)
Mental disorders	14.4	(0.2)	12.1	(0.3)	14.8	(0.4)	15.7	(0.3)
Alcohol abuse	1.7	(0.1)	1.8	(0.1)	1.9	(0.2)	1.6	(0.1)
Bipolar	0.7	(0.0)	0.4	(0.1)	0.8	(0.1)	0.9	(0.1)
Drug abuse	0.4	(0.0)	0.2	(0.0)	0.4	(0.1)	0.6	(0.1)
Generalized anxiety	1.3	(0.1)	1.1	(0.1)	1.0	(0.1)	1.6	(0.1)
Major depressive disorder	5.6	(0.1)	4.9	(0.2)	5.3	(0.2)	6.1	(0.2)
Panic and/or agoraphobia	1.6	(0.1)	1.1	(0.1)	1.5	(0.1)	1.9	(0.1)
Post-traumatic stress	1.3	(0.1)	0.7	(0.1)	1.1	(0.1)	1.9	(0.1)
Social phobia	2.1	(0.1)	1.1	(0.1)	2.0	(0.2)	2.7	(0.1)
Specific phobia	5.3	(0.1)	4.2	(0.2)	6.4	(0.3)	5.5	(0.2)
Physical conditions	51.4	(0.4)	45.6	(0.6)	49.3	(0.8)	56.0	(0.5)
Arthritis	14.5	(0.2)	13.1	(0.4)	13.5	(0.4)	15.8	(0.4)
Cancer	1.8	(0.1)	0.4	(0.1)	0.8	(0.1)	3.1	(0.2)
Cardiovascular	16.7	(0.2)	11.9	(0.4)	17.5	(0.5)	19.3	(0.3)
Chronic pain	21.5	(0.3)	21.9	(0.6)	20.5	(0.5)	21.6	(0.4)
Diabetes	4.0	(0.1)	2.5	(0.2)	3.9	(0.2)	5.1	(0.2)
Digestive	3.4	(0.1)	4.5	(0.2)	3.2	(0.2)	2.7	(0.1)
Headache/migraine	12.7	(0.2)	14.5	(0.4)	14.1	(0.5)	11.0	(0.3)
Insomnia	6.1	(0.1)	4.3	(0.2)	5.8	(0.3)	7.4	(0.2)
Neurological	1.0	(0.1)	0.8	(0.1)	1.1	(0.1)	1.1	(0.1)
Respiratory	15.2	(0.3)	11.9	(0.4)	10.7	(0.4)	19.2	(0.5)
Any condition	55.8	(0.4)	49.8	(0.6)	53.6	(0.7)	60.5	(0.5)
Exactly 1 condition	25.0	(0.3)	23.2	(0.4)	24.4	(0.6)	26.5	(0.4)
Exactly 2 conditions	14.9	(0.2)	13.1	(0.4)	14.6	(0.5)	16.3	(0.3)
3+ conditions	15.8	(0.2)	13.6	(0.4)	14.6	(0.4)	17.8	(0.4)

interview (Table 15.1). Twenty-five percent had exactly one condition, 14.9% exactly two, and 15.8% more than three. Most conditions became more prevalent as the income level of the country increased. Indeed, the percentage of respondents who reported experiencing any type of condition in high-income countries was more than 10 points higher than in low/lower-middle-income countries (60.5% vs. 49.8%). In all countries, chronic physical conditions (ranging from 1.0% in neurological to 21.5% in chronic pain) were much more prevalent than mental disorders (ranging from 0.4% in drug abuse to 5.6% in major depressive disorder). The same tendency was observed in each of the country income groups.

Overall perceived health VAS scores

The VAS scores were found to be quite homogeneously distributed across all country groups. As shown in Figure 15.1, fewer than 7% of respondents in any group of countries had scores below 50, while 15.8% in high-income and 29.0% in low/lower-middle-income

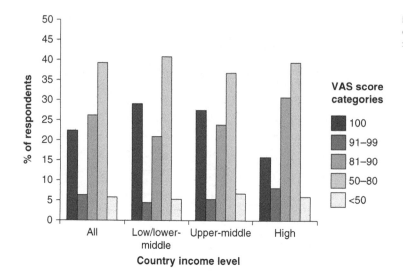

Figure 15.1 Distribution of VAS score categories by country income level. The WMH surveys.

VAS score categories

- 100
- 91–99
- 81–90
- 50–80
- <50

countries had scores of 100. In low/lower-middle-income countries, 4.3% of respondents had scores in the range 91–99, while scores in that range were found in 8.2% of respondents in high-income countries. The median score among respondents with scores of less than 100 was 80 (interquartile range [IQR] 70–90) in all three country income groups.

Individual-level effect of disorders on VAS scores

The coefficients in model 1 are significant as a set and show each condition to have a negative predictive association with VAS scores (Table 15.2). The coefficients in model 2 are also significant as a set and show that VAS scores decrease monotonically with the number of conditions. The model 3 results show that the individual conditions still have generally negative coefficients when controlling for number of conditions, and that the coefficients vary significantly across conditions. The coefficients associated with the number of conditions in model 3 are significantly positive. This indicates sub-additive interactions: that the joint adverse associations of comorbid condition clusters with VAS scores are less than the sum of the associations of the individual pure conditions in the clusters taken one at a time. Model 4 shows that these non-additive associations differ across conditions.

The transformation of the model 4 coefficients using simulation shows that the condition-specific, individual-level estimates are consistently negative

(Table 15.3). The magnitude of estimates is quite similar in all three types of countries, with absolute median (IQR) values of 5.4 (3.9–7.4) in low/lower-middle-income countries, 5.4 (4.4–6.1) in upper-middle-income countries, and 4.9 (3.2–6.5) in high-income countries. Disorders are ranked differently across the different income groups, with drug abuse with or without dependence being the most notable difference – ranked first in low/lower-middle-income countries and 19th in upper-middle-income countries, followed by cancer disorders – ranked fourth in low/lower-middle-income countries and 18th in high-income countries. The effect of bipolar disorder is consistently ranked high across all type of countries (second in low/lower-middle-income countries and third in upper-middle-income and high-income countries).

Coefficients based on the bivariate model (i.e., considering only one condition at a time in predicting VAS) are consistently higher than those in the multivariate model, with the condition-specific ratio of the latter to former in the range of 0.30–0.67 (social phobia – diabetes) (Table 15.4) and a median (IQR) ratio of 0.45 (0.37–0.58) (Appendix Table 15.3). Very similar results were found in low/lower-middle-income countries (0.51 [0.39–0.57]), upper-middle-income countries (0.49 [0.38–0.56]), and high-income countries (0.45 [0.35–0.56]) (Appendix Table 15.3). The influence of comorbidity can be seen in the fact that the correlation across conditions for the mean number of comorbid conditions and the ratio of the coefficient based on the multivariate model to the coefficient based on the bivariate model is –0.32.

Table 15.2 Coefficients of type of condition, number of conditions, and number by type of condition interactions for models 1 to 4. The WMH surveys.

	Model 1[a]		Model 2[b]		Model 3[c]		Model 4[d]	
	Coeff	(SE)	Coeff	(SE)	Coeff	(SE)	Coeff	(SE)
Alcohol abuse	−3.3*	(0.6)			−4.0*	(0.6)	−5.7*	(0.8)
Bipolar	−8.4*	(0.9)			−9.9*	(1.0)	−11.9*	(1.6)
Drug abuse	−3.8*	(1.2)			−5.0*	(1.2)	−4.3*	(1.8)
Generalized anxiety	−5.0*	(0.7)			−6.2*	(0.7)	−7.5*	(1.3)
Major depressive disorder	−8.1*	(0.3)			−9.0*	(0.4)	−9.9*	(0.6)
Panic and/or agoraphobia	−6.3*	(0.6)			−7.9*	(0.7)	−7.9*	(1.2)
Post-traumatic stress	−5.1*	(0.7)			−6.8*	(0.7)	−6.8*	(1.3)
Social phobia	−3.7*	(0.6)			−4.9*	(0.6)	−7.9*	(1.0)
Specific phobia	−2.7*	(0.4)			−3.6*	(0.4)	−4.3*	(0.5)
Arthritis	−4.9*	(0.2)			−5.7*	(0.3)	−5.8*	(0.4)
Cancer	−2.0*	(0.6)			−3.0*	(0.6)	−4.3*	(0.9)
Cardiovascular	−4.9*	(0.2)			−5.6*	(0.3)	−5.2*	(0.3)
Chronic pain	−6.5*	(0.2)			−7.1*	(0.3)	−6.7*	(0.3)
Diabetes	−5.2*	(0.4)			−6.1*	(0.4)	−5.1*	(0.6)
Digestive	−4.1*	(0.4)			−5.1*	(0.5)	−5.6*	(0.7)
Headache/migraine	−4.8*	(0.2)			−5.6*	(0.3)	−5.3*	(0.4)
Insomnia	−6.0*	(0.3)			−7.1*	(0.4)	−8.4*	(0.6)
Neurological	−9.4*	(0.8)			−10.6*	(0.8)	−12.0*	(1.2)
Respiratory	−1.7*	(0.2)			−2.4*	(0.3)	−2.7*	(0.3)
Exactly 1 condition			−5.6*	(0.2)				
Exactly 2 conditions			−10.4*	(0.2)	1.0*	(0.4)		
Exactly 3 conditions			−15.4*	(0.3)	1.9*	(0.6)		
4 or 5 conditions			−22.7*	(0.3)	2.6*	(0.8)		
6 or 7 conditions			−29.9*	(0.7)	7.8*	(0.3)		
8+ conditions			−37.3*	(1.4)	15.6*	(2.1)		
Number of conditions							0.8*	(0.3)
Number of conditions by Alcohol abuse							1.1*	(0.3)
Number of conditions by Bipolar							0.7	(0.5)
Number of conditions by Drug abuse							−0.5	(0.6)
Number of conditions by Generalized anxiety							0.5	(0.4)
Number of conditions by Major depressive disorder							0.5*	(0.2)
Number of conditions by Panic and/or agoraphobia							−0.1	(0.3)
Number of conditions by Post-traumatic stress							0.0	(0.3)
Number of conditions by Social phobia							1.1*	(0.3)
Number of conditions by Specific phobia							0.4	(0.2)
Number of conditions by Arthritis							0.2	(0.2)

Table 15.2 (cont.)

	Model 1[a]		Model 2[b]		Model 3[c]		Model 4[d]	
	Coeff	(SE)	Coeff	(SE)	Coeff	(SE)	Coeff	(SE)
Number of conditions by Cancer							0.7*	(0.3)
Number of conditions by Cardiovascular							−0.3	(0.2)
Number of conditions by Chronic pain							−0.3	(0.2)
Number of conditions by Diabetes							−0.4	(0.3)
Number of conditions by Digestive							0.4	(0.2)
Number of conditions by Headache/migraine							−0.2	(0.2)
Number of conditions by Insomnia							0.6*	(0.2)
Number of conditions by Neurological							0.8	(0.4)
Number of conditions by Respiratory							0.4*	(0.2)

[a] Model 1: Additive model that included a separate predictor for each disorder without interactions.
[b] Model 2: Included a series of predictors for number of conditions (e.g., one predictor for having exactly one condition, another for exactly two, etc.) without information about type of disorder.
[c] Model 3: Included 19 predictors for type of disorder and predictor dummies for number of conditions, starting with exactly 2 conditions.
[d] Model 4: Included 19 predictors for type and predictor dummies for number of conditions, starting with exactly 2 conditions and interactions of type of conditions by the number of conditions.
* Significant at the 0.05 level, two-sided test.

Societal-level impact of disorders on VAS scores

The PARPs for each condition and country level are shown in Table 15.5. The magnitude of the PARPs is low and similar in all three types of countries, and they increase with income level. The median PARPs (IQR) were 0.39 (0.25–1.85) for low/lower-middle-income countries, 0.67 (0.36–2.04) for upper-middle-income countries, and 0.79 (0.41–2.27) for high-income countries. Like individual-level estimates, the disorder types were ranked quite similarly, with chronic pain first and drug abuse last in all cases.

Discussion

As previous chapters of this volume have mentioned with regard to their specific focus of research, a number of limitations must be considered in interpreting the association between physical/mental disorders and overall perceived health using the visual analogue scale (VAS). First, only a restricted set of common conditions was included in the analysis and some were pooled to form larger disorder groups. A number of burdensome conditions, such as dementia and psychosis, were not included. Expansion and

disaggregation is clearly needed in future research. Second, diagnoses of chronic physical conditions were based on self-reports that could have been biased. Such bias might account for the generally higher prevalence estimates of these conditions in high-income countries than in low/lower-middle-income and upper-middle-income countries. Third, we focused not on the 12-month prevalence of conditions but 30-day health valuations, as these were the time frames included in the WMH surveys. This difference in recall periods would be expected to lead to an underestimation of the severity of the active phases of episodic conditions (e.g., migraine), although it should yield an accurate estimate of the average severity of conditions in a typical month (30-day period) of the year (12-month period). A related limitation is that even a 12-month time frame is relatively short compared to the time frames used in some other health valuation studies (e.g., 10-year period or lifetime).

Another limitation is that the highly skewed distribution of VAS scores and the non-additive effects of comorbid conditions might have led to instability in our results. Even though we explored the use of the GLM rather than the OLS and examined a number of different model specifications to capture the effects of comorbidity, it is possible that future research will

Table 15.3 Simulated individual-level condition-specific severity estimates based on the best-fitting regression model, by country income level. The WMH surveys.

Disorder	Country income level											
	All countries			Low/lower-middle			Upper-middle			High		
	Est[a]	(SE)	Rank	Est[a]	(SE)	Rank	Est[a]	(SE)	Rank	Est[a]	(SE)	Rank
Alcohol abuse	−3.1*	(0.8)	16	−3.7*	(1.4)	15	−5.4*	(2.5)	9	−1.7*	(0.8)	17
Bipolar	−8.6*	(1.3)	2	−11.3*	(3.8)	2	−8.3*	(2.3)	3	−7.5*	(1.5)	3
Drug abuse	−4.2*	(1.5)	13	−13.1*	(4.7)	1	−0.4	(4.0)	19	−3.2*	(1.6)	14
Generalized anxiety	−5.0*	(0.9)	9	−4.5*	(2.1)	13	−5.4*	(2.2)	10	−4.9*	(1.0)	11
Major depressive disorder	−7.8*	(0.4)	3	−7.6*	(0.9)	5	−8.5*	(1.0)	2	−7.8*	(0.5)	2
Panic and/or agoraphobia	−6.8*	(0.9)	4	−5.5*	(2.3)	9	−8.8*	(1.8)	1	−6.6*	(1.0)	5
Post-traumatic stress	−5.6*	(0.9)	7	−5.6*	(2.7)	8	−6.0*	(2.4)	6	−5.0*	(1.0)	9
Social phobia	−3.6*	(0.7)	15	−3.0	(1.7)	16	−4.8*	(1.5)	13	−3.0*	(0.9)	16
Specific phobia	−2.5*	(0.5)	17	−1.2	(1.1)	19	−2.7*	(0.9)	17	−3.1*	(0.6)	15
Arthritis	−4.8*	(0.4)	11	−5.2*	(0.8)	12	−4.4*	(0.8)	15	−4.6*	(0.5)	12
Cancer	−2.1*	(0.9)	18	−8.1*	(3.9)	4	−5.2	(2.8)	11	−1.5	(0.9)	18
Cardiovascular	−4.9*	(0.4)	10	−4.1*	(0.8)	14	−5.9*	(0.8)	7	−4.9*	(0.5)	10
Chronic pain	−6.4*	(0.3)	5	−5.6*	(0.7)	7	−6.2*	(0.7)	5	−6.6*	(0.4)	4
Diabetes	−5.3*	(0.6)	8	−5.4*	(1.4)	10	−5.4*	(1.5)	8	−5.1*	(0.8)	8
Digestive	−4.1*	(0.6)	14	−2.4*	(0.8)	17	−2.1	(−1.2)	18	−6.3*	(1.1)	6
Headache/migraine	−4.8*	(0.4)	12	−5.4*	(0.7)	11	−5.2*	(0.8)	12	−4.2*	(0.5)	13
Insomnia	−5.9*	(0.5)	6	−7.3*	(1.2)	6	−4.4*	(1.1)	14	−5.7*	(0.6)	7
Neurological	−9.4*	(1.1)	1	−8.8*	(2.2)	3	−7.0*	(2.5)	4	−10.5*	(1.4)	1
Respiratory	−1.6*	(0.3)	19	−2.2*	(0.7)	18	−3.1*	(1.0)	16	−0.8*	(0.4)	19
Mental disorders	−7.6*	(0.3)		−6.3*	(0.6)		−8.1*	(0.7)		−7.8*	(0.3)	
Physical disorders	−9.2*	(0.2)		−9.9*	(0.5)		−11.8*	(0.5)		−7.7*	(0.3)	
Any disorder	−10.9*	(0.2)		−11.0*	(0.5)		−13.9*	(0.5)		−9.4*	(0.3)	

[a] Individual-level estimate.
* Significant at the 0.05 level, two-sided test.

Table 15.4 Individual-level condition-specific estimates based on bivariate and the best-fitting multivariate model. The WMH surveys.

Disorder	Bivariate	Multivariate	Multivariate/bivariate	Number of comorbid disorders	
	Estimate	Estimate	Estimate	Mean	(SE)
Alcohol abuse	−7.3	−3.1	0.42	1.8	(0.07)
Bipolar	−16.5	−8.6	0.52	3.1	(0.11)
Drug abuse	−11.3	−4.2	0.37	2.6	(0.16)
Generalized anxiety	−13.6	−5.0	0.37	3.0	(0.08)
Major depressive disorder	−13.6	−7.8	0.57	2.4	(0.04)
Panic and/or agoraphobia	−16.2	−6.8	0.42	3.4	(0.08)
Post-traumatic stress	−15.1	−5.6	0.37	3.3	(0.10)
Social phobia	−12.1	−3.6	0.30	2.9	(0.07)
Specific phobia	−8.1	−2.5	0.31	2.1	(0.05)
Arthritis	−9.4	−4.8	0.51	1.9	(0.03)
Cancer	−3.6	−2.1	0.58	2.1	(0.07)
Cardiovascular	−8.2	−4.9	0.60	1.8	(0.03)
Chronic pain	−10.7	−6.4	0.60	1.8	(0.02)
Diabetes	−7.9	−5.3	0.67	2.0	(0.05)
Digestive	−9.5	−4.1	0.43	2.3	(0.06)
Headache/migraine	−10.2	−4.8	0.47	2.0	(0.03)
Insomnia	−13.1	−5.9	0.45	2.7	(0.05)
Neurological	−14.5	−9.4	0.65	2.5	(0.12)
Respiratory	−4.6	−1.6	0.35	1.6	(0.02)

discover better specifications, in terms of either functional form or joint associations of comorbid conditions with health valuations. In particular, the use of data-mining techniques such as regression tree analysis (Breiman *et al.* 1984, Friedman 1991, Breiman 2001, 2009) might provide useful insights into better specifications for the effects of interaction. A related limitation is that we considered the VAS as an interval scale. This assumption has been called into question in previous studies (Krabbe *et al.* 2006, Parkin & Devlin 2006), and non-linear monotonic transformations have been proposed to approximate interval-scale properties (Krabbe 2008, Craig *et al.* 2009). It would be very useful in future methodological research to explore the extent to which these different methods influence results. In addition, our VAS question used the anchors "best" and "worst" imaginable health. While this does not affect the main aim of our study (i.e., to estimate the relative burden of the conditions), it might certainly limit comparability with other measures which use "death" as their lowest anchor (Patrick & Erickson 1993).

Another limitation is that our estimates are based only on the overall adult population in aggregate groups of countries by income level. The ratings of the different conditions might be quite different in different population segments (e.g., the elderly, women, the poor) or in each individual country. Future research should look into these differing specifications, and the use of anchoring vignettes has been shown to help address this problem (Salomon *et al.* 2004). In addition, there are a number of statistical methods that improve the accuracy of comparisons across subsamples and populations and that could profitably be used in future applications (Tandon *et al.* 2002).

A further limitation is that our results are based on VAS scores assigned by respondents to their own states of health rather than to health states based on hypothetical vignettes (de Wit *et al.* 2000). While there is general agreement that perceptions of people in the general population should be taken into consideration in making health valuations (Gudex *et al.* 1996), concerns have been raised about bias in the perceptual

Table 15.5 Population attributable risk proportions (PARPs) of each condition based on the best-fitting regression model separately in WMH surveys by country income level. The WMH surveys.

Disorder	Country income level											
	All countries			Low/lower-middle			Upper-middle			High		
	PARP (%)	(SE)	Rank	PARP (%)	(SE)	Rank	PARP (%)	(SE)	Rank	PARP (%)	(SE)	Rank
Alcohol abuse	0.3*	(0.1)	17	0.4*	(0.1)	11	0.6*	(0.3)	11	0.1*	(0.1)	18
Bipolar	0.3*	(0.1)	16	0.2*	(0.1)	15	0.4*	(0.1)	14	0.3*	(0.1)	16
Drug abuse	0.1*	(0.0)	19	0.2*	(0.1)	19	0.0	(0.1)	19	0.1	(0.1)	19
Generalized anxiety	0.3*	(0.1)	15	0.3*	(0.1)	14	0.3*	(0.1)	17	0.4*	(0.1)	15
Major depressive disorder	2.3*	(0.1)	5	2.0*	(0.2)	5	2.4*	(0.3)	5	2.5*	(0.2)	4
Panic and/or agoraphobia	0.6*	(0.1)	11	0.3*	(0.1)	12	0.7*	(0.2)	10	0.6*	(0.1)	11
Post-traumatic stress	0.4*	(0.1)	13	0.2*	(0.1)	16	0.3*	(0.1)	16	0.5*	(0.1)	13
Social phobia	0.4*	(0.1)	14	0.2	(0.1)	18	0.5*	(0.2)	12	0.4*	(0.1)	14
Specific phobia	0.7*	(0.1)	10	0.3	(0.3)	13	0.9*	(0.3)	9	0.9*	(0.2)	9
Arthritis	3.7*	(0.3)	3	3.7*	(0.6)	3	3.1*	(0.6)	4	3.8*	(0.4)	3
Cancer	0.2*	(0.1)	18	0.2	(0.1)	17	0.2	(0.1)	18	0.2	(0.1)	17
Cardiovascular	4.3*	(0.3)	2	2.6*	(0.5)	4	5.5*	(0.7)	2	4.9*	(0.5)	2
Chronic pain	7.2*	(0.4)	1	6.7*	(0.8)	1	6.7*	(0.8)	1	7.4*	(0.5)	1
Diabetes	1.1*	(0.1)	8	0.7*	(0.2)	8	1.1*	(0.3)	8	1.4*	(0.2)	7
Digestive	0.7*	(0.1)	9	0.6*	(0.2)	9	0.4	(0.2)	15	0.9*	(0.2)	8
Headache/migraine	3.2*	(0.2)	4	4.3*	(0.6)	2	3.9*	(0.6)	3	2.4*	(0.3)	5
Insomnia	1.9*	(0.2)	6	1.7*	(0.3)	6	1.3*	(0.4)	7	2.2*	(0.3)	6
Neurological	0.5*	(0.1)	12	0.4*	(0.1)	10	0.4*	(0.2)	13	0.6*	(0.1)	12
Respiratory	1.3*	(0.3)	7	1.4*	(0.4)	7	1.7*	(0.6)	6	0.8*	(0.4)	10
Mental disorders	5.7*	(0.2)		4.1*	(0.4)		6.3*	(0.6)		6.4*	(0.3)	
Physical disorders	24.9*	(0.6)		24.4*	(1.2)		30.5*	(1.3)		22.2*	(0.9)	
Any disorder	31.9*	(0.7)		29.8*	(1.3)		39.4*	(1.4)		29.3*	(1.0)	

* Significant at the 0.05 level, two-sided test.

ratings of community respondents based on their own illness experiences (Stiggelbout & de Vogel-Voogt 2008) and their familiarity with the experiences of people close to them (Krabbe *et al.* 2006), resulting in a general preference for health valuations made by experts (Marquie *et al.* 2003). Furthermore, bias in self-reports in the WMH data might have been greater for mental than for physical conditions, because so many questions were asked in the survey about mental disorders and the VAS was administered only at the end of the survey. It would be useful to investigate this potential bias in future applications by randomizing the order of presentation of the VAS questions in the survey. Methods have been developed to integrate VAS responses with responses based on other valuation methods (e.g., time trade-off, willingness to pay) that might also effectively be used in future studies to evaluate these biases (Salomon & Murray 2004).

Finally, a less obvious limitation is that the simulation method evaluated *marginal* effects of individual conditions. This method can be faulted because it implicitly assumes that the presence versus absence of a single condition can be changed while all other conditions remain the same. This assumption would be plausible if all comorbid conditions were either causes or risk markers (Kraemer *et al.* 1997) of focal conditions. However, in cases where the comorbid condition is a consequence of the focal condition, or where two or more conditions are reciprocally related, the simulation method used here will underestimate the effect of the focal condition (assuming that comorbidity is positive) by controlling for one or more of the intervening pathways through which that condition influences VAS scores.

This underestimation could be remedied by deleting controls for all conditions that are thought to mediate the total effect of the focal condition. However, when these comorbid conditions are reciprocally related to the focal condition, exclusion of the comorbid conditions from the prediction equation will lead to an overestimation of the effect of the focal condition. The only plausible way to address that issue is to develop a *partial control* methodology, which would control for the subset of comorbid conditions that have causal effects on the focal conditions but not for the subset that occur as a consequence of the focal condition. An innovative methodology known as g-estimation has been developed to do this (Young *et al.* 2010), but this method requires access to large-scale longitudinal epidemiological data that monitor onset and course of comorbid conditions over time. As a result of this data requirement, use of g-estimation has been minimal (Taubman *et al.* 2009), and it has never to our knowledge been used to study health valuation. This method is nonetheless very promising and deserves to be explored in future studies aimed at sorting out the effects of comorbidity on health valuation.

Association of common physical and mental disorders with overall perceived health

Within the context of these limitations, our results clearly show that sensible estimates of condition-specific associations can be obtained with the overall perceived health VAS score without neglecting comorbidity. As noted above, a similar approach could be used to study informant ratings by using a series of hypothetical vignettes of people with comorbid conditions rather than pure conditions. We found that considering comorbidity has a substantial influence on ratings. In particular, condition-specific ratings are lower when comorbidity is taken into consideration, because of a general pattern of sub-additive interactions among comorbid conditions in predicting VAS scores. This sub-additive pattern is consistent with the findings of the one previous study that conducted a similar type of analysis (Verbrugge *et al.* 1989). Furthermore, we found substantial between-condition variation in the extent to which comorbidity influence estimates were adjusted for.

Although the substantive findings regarding the effects of individual conditions on VAS should be interpreted with caution, given the limitations enumerated above, it is noteworthy that neurological conditions, insomnia, and major depression were estimated to be the most severe conditions at the individual level. The neurological conditions we considered included epilepsy and seizure disorders, Parkinson's disease, and multiple sclerosis, all of which have been correlated with disability in previous studies (Singer *et al.* 1999, Jacoby & Baker 2008). The high ranking of insomnia is surprising, because previous studies, although documenting a high societal-level burden for insomnia, have generally found that its high prevalence is related to moderate rather than high individual-level burden (Roth *et al.* 2006). The high individual-level severity of insomnia in our study probably stems from the fact that a great sleep disruption was required (at least two hours of either delay in sleep onset or disruption in sleep maintenance per night most nights of the week for at least one month in the past year) in comparison to previous studies on insomnia (Ohayon 2002). Finally, the high individual-level impact estimate found here for depression is consistent with much previous research (Donohue & Pincus 2007, Wang *et al.* 2008, Gabilondo *et al.* 2010).

The rank ordering of the individual-level VAS impact estimates was found to be quite similar by country income groups, although there were several exceptions that should be investigated in future studies. Digestive disorders were rated as considerably more severe in high-income than in low/lower-middle-income and upper-middle-income countries, possibly reflecting a different combination of cases that might explain differences in estimated severity. The individual-level estimated severity of drug abuse, in comparison, was substantially higher in low/lower-middle-income countries than in the other two country income groups. Differential willingness to admit drug problems might have been involved in this result, as the reported prevalence of drug abuse was much lower in low/lower-middle-income than in high-income countries, possibly indicating that the cases we learned of in low/lower-middle-income countries were more severe than those in high-income countries (Schmidt & Room 1999).

When the individual-level disorder severity estimates presented here are compared with estimates from the WMH analysis of disorder-specific role impairment shown in Chapter 13, it is clear that the conditions rated most severe in that chapter were generally also rated among the most severe in this research. However, there are a number of differences in relative ratings that could be attributed either to differences in the outcome (i.e., a global VAS score versus a measure of condition-specific role impairment) or to the fact that the previous analysis did not adjust for comorbidity.

The results presented regarding societal-level associations are less novel because, consistent with previous studies, the prevalence estimates of the disorders was merely multiplied by the individual-level estimates of disorder severity to arrive at societal-level estimates of impact. As in previous studies that compared individual-level and societal-level estimates (Whiteford 2000, Andlin-Sobocki *et al.* 2005, Saarni *et al.* 2007), the rank ordering of conditions differs considerably between the two: societal-level estimates are considerably influenced by variations in prevalence, and the disorders estimated to be most burdensome at the societal level are dominated by high-prevalence conditions.

Implications

While our results make a clear argument for the importance of considering comorbidity when estimating disease burden, the best way to do this is not as obvious. The approach taken here has the advantage of considering comorbidities as they are actually distributed among the population rather than requiring the generation of hypothetical scenarios that might or might not adequately characterize the real distribution of complex comorbidities. However, other methods can also allow the effects of individual conditions to be estimated using expert ratings of hypothetical patient scenarios that include information about complex profiles of comorbidity (Jasso 2006, Saarni *et al.* 2007). Indeed, the actual distributions of comorbidity as revealed through community studies like the WMH surveys could be used to generate these vignettes to ensure that they represent the distribution and range of patterns in the population. Because many health policy researchers favor condition severity ratings given by experts over the ratings given by respondents in community surveys for a variety of other reasons (Insinga & Fryback 2003, Marquie *et al.* 2003, Ormel *et al.* 2008, Schnadig *et al.* 2008), the best approach might be to build information about comorbidity into conventional expert-rating scenarios. However, valuations of the sort presented here, based on community samples, would also seem to have value in representing the perceptions of actual people with real conditions in the population. It remains a challenge for the field to develop a way of integrating these different types of data.

Acknowledgments

Portions of this chapter are based on Alonso, J., Vilagut, G., Chatterji, S., *et al.* (2011). Including information about co-morbidity in estimates of disease burden: results from the World Health Organization World Mental Health Surveys. *Psychological Medicine* **41**, 873–86. © 2011. Cambridge University Press. Reproduced with permission.

References

Alonso, J., Vilagut, G., Chatterji, S., *et al.* (2011). Including information about co-morbidity in estimates of disease burden: results from the World Health Organization World Mental Health Surveys. *Psychological Medicine* **41**, 873–86.

Andlin-Sobocki, P., Jonsson, B., Wittchen, H. U., & Olesen, J. (2005). Cost of disorders of the brain in Europe. *European Journal of Neurology* **12** (Suppl 1), 1–27.

Breiman, L. (2001). Random forests. *Machine Learning* **45**, 32.

Breiman, L. (2009). Statistical modeling: the two cultures. *Statistical Science* **16**, 199–215.

Breiman, L., Friedman, J. H., Olshen, R. A., & Stone, C. J. (1984). *Classification and Regression Trees*. New York, NY: Chapman & Hall.

Craig, B. M., Busschbach, J. J., & Salomon, J. A. (2009). Modeling ranking, time trade-off, and visual analog scale values for EQ-5D health states: a review and comparison of methods. *Medical Care* **47**, 634–641.

De Wit, G. A., Busschbach, J. J., & De Charro, F. T. (2000). Sensitivity and perspective in the valuation of health status: whose values count? *Health Economics* **9**, 109–26.

Donohue, J. M., & Pincus, H. A. (2007). Reducing the societal burden of depression: a review of economic costs, quality of care and effects of treatment. *Pharmacoeconomics* **25**, 7–24.

Fortin, M., Soubhi, H., Hudon, C., Bayliss, E. A., & van den Akker, M. (2007). Multimorbidity's many challenges. *BMJ* **334**, 1016–17.

Friedman, J. H. (1991). Multivariate adaptive regression splines (with discussion). *Annals of Statistics* **19**, 1.

Gabilondo, A., Rojas-Farreras, S., Vilagut, G, et al. (2010). Epidemiology of major depressive episode in a southern European country: results from the ESEMeD-Spain project. *Journal of Affective Disorders* **120**, 76–85.

Gudex, C., Dolan, P., Kind, P., & Williams, A. (1996). Health state valuations from the general public using the visual analogue scale. *Quality of Life Research* **5**, 521–31.

Insinga, R. P., & Fryback, D. G. (2003). Understanding differences between self-ratings and population ratings for health in the EuroQOL. *Quality of Life Research* **12**, 611–19.

Jacoby, A., & Baker, G. A. (2008). Quality-of-life trajectories in epilepsy: a review of the literature. *Epilepsy Behavior* **12**, 557–71.

Jasso, G. (2006). Factorial survey methods for studying beliefs and judgments. *Sociological Methods and Research* **34**, 334–423.

Krabbe, P. F. (2008). Thurstone scaling as a measurement method to quantify subjective health outcomes. *Medical Care* **46**, 357–65.

Krabbe, P. F., Stalmeier, P. F., Lamers, L. M., & Busschbach, J. J. (2006). Testing the interval-level measurement property of multi-item visual analogue scales. *Quality of Life Research* **15**, 1651–61.

Kraemer, H. C., Kazdin, A. E., Offord, D. R., et al. (1997). Coming to terms with the terms of risk. *Archives of General Psychiatry* **54**, 337–43.

López, A. D., & Mathers, C. D. (2007). Inequalities in health status: findings from the 2001 Global Burden of Disease study. In S. Matlin, ed., *The Global Forum Update on Research for Health, Volume 4*. London: Pro-Brook Publishing, pp. 163–75.

Maddigan, S. L., Feeny, D. H., & Johnson, J. A. (2005). Health-related quality of life deficits associated with diabetes and comorbidities in a Canadian National Population Health Survey. *Quality of Life Research* **14**, 1311–20.

Marquie, L., Raufaste, E., Lauque, D., et al. (2003). Pain rating by patients and physicians: evidence of systematic pain miscalibration. *Pain* **102**, 289–96.

Moussavi, S., Chatterji, S., Verdes, E., et al. (2007). Depression, chronic diseases, and decrements in health: results from the World Health Surveys. *Lancet* **370**, 851–8.

Murray, C. J., & López, A. D. (1996). Evidence-based health policy: lessons from the Global Burden of Disease study. *Science* **274**, 740–3.

Murray, C. J. L., López, A. D., Mathers, C. D., & Stein, C. (2001). *The Global Burden of Disease 2000 Project: Aims, Methods and Data Sources*. Geneva: World Health Organization.

Ohayon, M. M. (2002). Epidemiology of insomnia: what we know and what we still need to learn. *Sleep Medicine Review* **6**, 97–111.

Ormel, J., Petukhova, M., Chatterji, S., et al. (2008). Disability and treatment of specific mental and physical disorders across the world. *British Journal of Psychiatry* **192**, 368–75.

Parkin, D., & Devlin, N. (2006). Is there a case for using visual analogue scale valuations in cost-utility analysis? *Health Economics* **15**, 653–64.

Patrick, D. L., & Erickson, P. 1993, *Health Status and Health Policy. Allocating Resources to Health Care*. New York, NY: Oxford University Press.

Research Triangle Institute (2005). *SUDAAN, Version 9.0.1*. [computer program]. Research Triangle Park, NC: Research Triangle Institute.

Roth, T., Jaeger, S., Jin, R., et al. (2006). Sleep problems, comorbid mental disorders, and role functioning in the national comorbidity survey replication. *Biological Psychiatry* **60**, 1364–71.

Saarni, S. I., Suvisaari, J., Sintonen, H., et al. (2007). Impact of psychiatric disorders on health-related quality of life: general population survey. *British Journal of Psychiatry* **190**, 326–32.

Salomon, J. A., & Murray, C. J. (2004). A multi-method approach to measuring health-state valuations. *Health Economics* **13**, 281–90.

Salomon, J. A., Tandon, A., & Murray, C. J. (2004). Comparability of self rated health: cross sectional multi-country survey using anchoring vignettes. *BMJ* **328**, 258.

SAS Institute Inc. (2002). *SAS/STAT® Software, Version 9.1 for Windows*. Cary, NC: SAS Institute Inc.

Schmidt, L., & Room, R. (1999). Cross-cultural applicability in international classifications and research on alcohol dependence. *Journal of Studies on Alcohol* **60**, 448–62.

Schnadig, I. D., Fromme, E. K., Loprinzi, C. L., et al. (2008). Patient-physician disagreement regarding performance status is associated with worse survivorship in patients with advanced cancer. *Cancer* **113**, 2205–14.

Singer, M. A., Hopman, W. M., & MacKenzie, T. A. (1999). Physical functioning and mental health in patients with chronic medical conditions. *Quality of Life Research* **8**, 687–91.

Stiggelbout, A. M., & de Vogel-Voogt, E. (2008). Health state utilities: a framework for studying the gap between the imagined and the real. *Value Health* **11**, 76–87.

Tandon, A., Murray, C. J. L., Salomon, J. A., & King, G. (2002). Statistical models for enhancing cross-population comparability. Paper No. 42. In *Global Programme on Evidence for Health Policy Discussion*. Geneva: World Health Organization.

Taubman, S. L., Robins, J. M., Mittleman, M. A., & Hernan, M. A. (2009). Intervening on risk factors for coronary heart disease: an application of the parametric g-formula. *International Journal of Epidemiology* **38**, 1599–611.

Verbrugge, L. M., Lepkowski, J. M., & Imanaka, Y. (1989). Comorbidity and its impact on disability. *Milbank Quarterly* **67**, 450–84.

Wang, P. S., Simon, G. E., & Kessler, R. C. (2008). Making the business case for enhanced depression care: the National Institute of Mental Health-Harvard Work Outcomes Research and Cost-effectiveness Study. *Journal of Occupational and Environmental Medicine* **50**, 468–75.

Whiteford, H. (2000). Unmet need: a challenge for governments. In G. Andrews & S. Henderson, eds., *Unmet Need in Psychiatry: Problems, Resources, Responses*. Cambridge: Cambridge University Press, pp. 8–10.

Wolter, K. M. (1985). *Introduction to Variance Estimation*. New York, NY: Springer-Verlag.

World Bank (2008). Data and statistics. http://go.worldbank.org/D7SN0B8YU0. Accessed May 12, 2009.

World Health Organization (2004). *The Global Burden of Disease: 2004 Update*. Geneva: WHO.

Young, J. G., Hernan, M. A., Picciotto, S., & Robins, J. M. (2010). Relation between three classes of structural models for the effect of a time-varying exposure on survival. *Lifetime Data Analysis* **16**, 71–84.

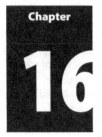

Chapter 16

Decomposing the total associations of common mental and physical disorders with perceived health

Jordi Alonso, Gemma Vilagut, Núria Duran Adroher, Somnath Chatterji, Yanling He, Nezar Ismet Taib, Daphna Levinson, and Siobhan O'Neill

Introduction

As was pointed out in Chapter 15, overall perceived health is widely recognized as an important indicator of health (Perruccio *et al.* 2007, Rohrer *et al.* 2007): it is often used to monitor health trends in the general population (Heistaro *et al.* 1996) as well as to assess patient-centered outcomes in clinical studies (Alonso 2000). Although the need to go beyond an exclusive focus on perceptions has been discussed (Sen 2002, Salomon *et al.* 2004), perceived health is nonetheless an important measure, because it has been shown to predict mortality independently of the presence and severity of disease and risk factors (Idler & Benyamini 1997), as well as to predict health services utilization, healthcare costs (DeSalvo *et al.* 2005), and future disability (Lee & Shinkai, 2003, Ashburner *et al.* 2011).

Mental and physical disorders are among the most important predictors of perceived health (Leinonen *et al.* 2001, Schultz & Kopec 2003, Alonso *et al.* 2004, Saarni *et al.* 2006, Damian *et al.* 2008). Some disorders, such as those causing pain, are known to be associated with great decrements in perceived health (van Dijk *et al.* 2008). In Chapter 15 we documented that substantial decrements in perceived health are associated with neurological conditions, major depressive disorder, and arthritis in the WMH survey data once the presence of other conditions is taken into account. A higher individual-level association of mental than physical disorders with the WHO Disability Assessment Schedule 2.0 (WHODAS 2) measures of disability was also documented in Chapter 14.

Most conceptual frameworks and models of health propose that disability mediates the effects of chronic disorders on perceived health (Guyatt *et al.* 1993,

Wilson & Cleary 1995, Valderas & Alonso 2008). A great deal of other evidence beyond the WMH survey findings is consistent with this possibility. It has been shown in a number of studies that disability is significantly associated with perceived health both cross-sectionally (Damian *et al.* 2008, Lee *et al.* 2008) and longitudinally (Leinonen *et al.* 2001, Lee, *et al.* 2008, Mavaddat *et al.* 2011). There is also evidence that chronic disorders are significantly associated with disability (Ormel *et al.* 2008, Blain *et al.* 2010, Boot *et al.* 2011). A few studies have assessed the mediating role of disability in the association of chronic disorders and mental health (Ormel *et al.* 1997, Buist-Bouwman *et al.* 2008). However, we are not aware of any systematic attempt to identify the extent to which different dimensions of disability mediate the overall associations of these disorders with perceived health in epidemiological samples. Such an analysis could have value in enhancing our understanding of the pathways that link chronic disorders to perceived health. This increased understanding, in turn, could help in customizing disorder-specific interventions aimed at ameliorating the disabilities that lead to significant decrements in perceived health. We explore this issue in the current chapter. Specifically, we examine the extent to which the associations documented in Chapter 15 between mental and physical disorders and the VAS measure of perceived health are mediated by the WHODAS measures described in Chapter 14. We focus not only on the overall importance of disability in mediating the total effects of each disorder, but also on variation in the relative importance of individual disability dimensions across disorders.

Methods

Sample

The same 23 surveys considered in Chapter 15 ($n = 51,344$) are the focus of analysis in the current chapter. These include seven surveys in countries classified by the World Bank (2008), at the time of data collection, as low-income or lower-middle-income (Colombia, India–Pondicherry, Iraq, Nigeria, People's Republic of China [PRC]–Beijing/Shanghai, PRC–Shenzhen, and Ukraine), five in upper-middle-income countries (Brazil–São Paulo, Bulgaria, Lebanon, Mexico, and Romania) and 11 in high-income countries (Belgium, France, Germany, Israel, Italy, Japan, the Netherlands, Northern Ireland, Portugal, Spain, and USA).

Measures

As in Chapter 15, perceived health was assessed using a visual analog scale (VAS) (Alonso *et al.* 2011). Respondents were asked to use a 0–100 scale, where 0 represents the worst possible health a person can have and 100 represents perfect health, to "describe your own overall physical and mental health during the past 30 days," taking into consideration all the mental and physical disorders reviewed in the survey.

Similar to the method described in Chapter 14, disability was assessed with a modified version of WHODAS 2 (Von Korff *et al.* 2008, Üstün *et al.* 2010). Questions were asked about difficulties in: (a) understanding and communication (*cognition*); (b) moving and getting around (*mobility*); (c) attending to personal hygiene, dressing and eating, and living alone (*self-care*); and (d) interacting with other people (*getting along*). In addition, a series of questions about activity limitations days replaced the WHODAS life activities domain questions. In these questions, respondents were asked the number of days out of the past 30 that they were totally unable to carry out their normal activities or work, that they had to cut down in the activities, that they had to reduce their quality, or that they needed to exert an extreme effort to carry out their activities, due to physical or mental health problems (*role functioning*). Respondents were also asked about the extent of embarrassment (*stigma*) and discrimination or unfair treatment (*discrimination*) they experienced because of their health condition and, finally, about the interference of their health condition on the day-to-day activities

of family members (*family burden*). Scores on each dimension were obtained, ranging from 0 to 100, where 0 indicated no disability and 100 indicated complete disability.

The same 12-month mental and physical disorders considered in Chapters 14 and 15 are used here as well. Thus the nine mental disorders considered here are: alcohol abuse with or without dependence, bipolar disorder (i.e., bipolar I disorder, bipolar II disorder, and subthreshold bipolar disorder combined into a single variable), drug abuse with or without dependence, generalized anxiety disorder (GAD), major depressive disorder (MDD), panic disorder and/or agoraphobia, post-traumatic stress disorder (PTSD), social phobia, and specific phobia. And the 10 physical disorders are: arthritis, cancer, cardiovascular disorders (heart attack, heart disease, hypertension, and stroke), chronic pain (chronic back or neck pain and other chronic pain), diabetes, digestive disorders (stomach or intestinal ulcer and irritable bowel disorder), frequent or severe headache or migraine, insomnia, neurological disorders (multiple sclerosis, Parkinson's disease, and epilepsy or seizures), and respiratory disorders (seasonal allergies such as hay fever, asthma, and chronic obstructive pulmonary disease [COPD] or emphysema). See Chapter 10 for a discussion of measurement issues. As in the earlier chapters, we focus on disorders present in the 12 months before interview.

We estimated condition prevalence and descriptive statistics for the distributions of the continuous variables using SUDAAN V10.0 (RTI International, USA). We then used MPlus 6.0 (Muthén and Muthén, Los Angeles, CA) to carry out multivariate analyses in parallel in the total sample and within three subsamples consisting of respondents in low/lower-middle-income, upper-middle-income, and high-income countries. Path analysis was used to estimate, through simultaneous regression models, the total, direct, and indirect effects through the WHODAS scores of each disorder in predicting VAS scores. The indirect effects were decomposed into separate components for each of the eight WHODAS dimensions. By the term "indirect effect" we mean the component of the overall association between a given disorder and VAS that is assumed to be mediated by a given WHODAS dimension, based on the fact that the gross association of the condition with the VAS score is reduced by the amount equal to the indirect effect when a statistical control is introduced for the WHODAS dimension.

All these models controlled for respondent age, gender, employment status, and country. For the purposes of comparing direct and indirect effects across conditions, components were standardized within a disorder to sum to 100%. The direct effect of each disorder on perceived health VAS was defined as the coefficient in the model that controlled for all WHODAS dimensions. To account for the complex sample design, standard errors and statistical tests were calculated using a sandwich estimator implemented in MPlus, which is equivalent to the Taylor Series Linearization (TSL) method.

Results

As noted in previous chapters, physical conditions were more prevalent than mental disorders, with prevalence ranging from 30.1% in PRC–Shenzhen to 71.3% in Ukraine and 70.1% in the USA. The prevalence of mental disorders ranged from 6% in PRC–Beijing/Shanghai to 27.3% in São Paulo and 24.5% in the USA. The prevalence of conditions was similar across all type of countries, but with a trend towards higher prevalence in higher-income countries. Chronic pain was the most common condition in low/lower-middle-income (21.9%), upper-middle-income (20.5%), and high-income countries (21.6%). In the third of these, cardiovascular disorders (19.3%) were also very common. Other common physical conditions in all countries were respiratory disorders, cardiovascular disorders, arthritis, and frequent or severe headaches or migraines. The prevalence of any physical condition ranged from 45.6% in low/lower-middle-income countries to 56% in high-income countries. Any mental disorder ranged from 12.1% in the former to 15.7% in the latter (see Chapter 15, Table 15.1).

Distribution of WHODAS scores

Table 16.1 shows the proportion of respondents with difficulties on each of the WHODAS dimensions for the overall sample and for each country income level. Over a third of respondents (35.7%) had some difficulty (score > 0), the frequency being considerably higher among respondents from high-income countries (46.5%) than for those in other countries (22.2% and 28.0% for upper-middle-income and low/lower-middle-income countries, respectively). The role functioning dimension was the most frequently affected (31.7%) in all country categories

(from 42.0% to 18.3%). Mobility and stigma showed the second most frequent difficulties (11.4% and 8.3%, respectively, in the overall sample), while self-care was the least frequently affected (3.4%).

Table 16.1 also shows the mean scores in each WHODAS dimension and the global score. For the latter, mean scores were higher for high-income countries (3.6) than for upper-middle-income and low/lower-middle-income countries (2.3). But mean global WHODAS scores across those with any difficulty tended to be higher for upper-middle-income (10.1) and low/lower-middle-income (8.2) than for high-income countries (7.8).

Distribution of perceived health VAS score

As shown in more detail in Chapter 15, the mean VAS score was 81.0 in the overall sample. Respondents with mental disorders showed lower mean perceived health (72.2) than those with physical conditions (75.0) (Table 16.2). These trends were consistent across all country income groups.

Direct and indirect (disability-mediated) effects of disorders on perceived health

Table 16.3 presents the association of mental and physical disorders with VAS score for the overall sample. Total effects are highest for neurological conditions, with an average decrement of 9.8 points on the VAS, major depressive disorder (8.2), and bipolar disorder (8.1). There is considerable variation across disorders in the extent to which total effects are mediated by WHODAS scores. The fourth column shows the proportion of overall indirect effects to total effects. Indirect effects tend to represent a lower proportion (among significant percentages in column four, ranging from 19.4% to 84.0%, with a median of 36.8%, interquartile range [IQR] = 31.2–51.5) of the total effect of the disorders on the VAS. Of note, some effects are non-significant. These proportions can be visualized in Figure 16.1, where the total effect of each disorder on the VAS is broken down into direct (shown in white) and indirect (in black) effects. In general, mental disorders tend to show higher proportions of indirect effects mediated by disability dimensions, with the highest values for PTSD (84.0%), GAD (63.7%), panic disorder and/or agoraphobia (53.1%), and bipolar disorder (47.0%). The physical conditions with the highest proportions of indirect

Table 16.1 Distribution of WHODAS dimension scores by income level. The WMH surveys.

Country income level	% with non-zero score	(SE)	Mean across all	(SE)	Across non-zero				
					Mean	(SE)	p25	median	p75
Overall sample									
Cognition	6.9	(0.14)	0.8	(0.03)	12.0	(0.3)	1.7	5.0	15.6
Mobility	11.4	(0.19)	3.2	(0.07)	28.2	(0.5)	5.0	16.7	50.0
Self-care	3.4	(0.10)	1.0	(0.05)	28.3	(1.1)	5.0	16.1	50.0
Getting along	3.9	(0.11)	0.6	(0.03)	15.8	(0.5)	2.3	7.5	22.2
Role functioning	31.7	(0.30)	9.0	(0.14)	28.5	(0.4)	3.2	10.8	46.7
Family burden	8.1	(0.15)	3.7	(0.08)	45.2	(0.5)	25.0	50.0	50.0
Stigma	8.3	(0.16)	4.0	(0.08)	48.7	(0.4)	25.0	50.0	75.0
Discrimination	3.5	(0.10)	1.7	(0.05)	47.1	(0.7)	25.0	50.0	50.0
Global WHODAS	35.7	(0.30)	2.9	(0.05)	8.2	(0.1)	0.6	2.5	10.0
Low/lower-middle									
Cognition	6.1	(0.27)	0.6	(0.05)	10.4	(0.7)	1.5	4.4	12.5
Mobility	8.7	(0.29)	2.0	(0.09)	22.4	(0.9)	3.9	11.1	33.3
Self-care	3.2	(0.20)	0.7	(0.09)	22.9	(2.2)	3.3	10.0	32.5
Getting along	3.5	(0.20)	0.5	(0.05)	13.1	(1.2)	2.0	5.3	16.7
Role functioning	24.6	(0.46)	7.8	(0.23)	31.6	(0.7)	6.7	16.7	49.2
Family burden	7.4	(0.28)	3.3	(0.15)	45.2	(0.9)	25.0	50.0	50.0
Stigma	8.9	(0.35)	4.3	(0.18)	48.7	(0.8)	25.0	50.0	75.0
Discrimination	4.3	(0.23)	1.9	(0.11)	45.8	(1.3)	25.0	50.0	50.0
Global WHODAS	28.0	(0.48)	2.3	(0.08)	8.2	(0.2)	1.3	3.5	10.3
Upper-middle									
Cognition	5.8	(0.30)	0.8	(0.06)	13.3	(0.8)	1.9	5.0	18.3
Mobility	7.8	(0.30)	2.2	(0.11)	28.8	(1.0)	5.6	16.7	50.0
Self-care	2.1	(0.17)	0.7	(0.06)	31.2	(2.4)	6.7	16.7	50.0
Getting along	2.2	(0.18)	0.5	(0.06)	22.8	(1.8)	4.0	15.0	36.7
Role functioning	18.3	(0.56)	7.1	(0.27)	38.8	(1.2)	8.3	25.0	60.0
Family burden	7.7	(0.27)	3.5	(0.14)	45.3	(0.9)	25.0	50.0	50.0
Stigma	9.1	(0.32)	4.8	(0.18)	52.3	(0.8)	25.0	50.0	75.0
Discrimination	4.3	(0.20)	2.0	(0.11)	47.3	(1.2)	25.0	50.0	75.0
Global WHODAS	22.2	(0.58)	2.3	(0.09)	10.1	(0.4)	1.3	5.0	13.3
High									
Cognition	7.9	(0.20)	1.0	(0.04)	12.5	(0.4)	1.7	5.0	16.7
Mobility	14.6	(0.30)	4.4	(0.13)	30.3	(0.6)	5.0	19.4	53.3
Self-care	4.1	(0.15)	1.3	(0.08)	30.3	(1.5)	5.0	16.7	50.0
Getting along	4.8	(0.17)	0.8	(0.04)	15.6	(0.6)	2.3	7.5	21.7
Role functioning	42.0	(0.43)	10.7	(0.21)	25.5	(0.5)	3.2	6.7	37.5
Family burden	8.7	(0.22)	3.9	(0.11)	45.2	(0.7)	25.0	50.0	50.0
Stigma	7.6	(0.19)	3.6	(0.10)	46.8	(0.7)	25.0	50.0	50.0
Discrimination	2.8	(0.11)	1.3	(0.06)	48.2	(1.1)	25.0	50.0	75.0
Global WHODAS	46.5	(0.43)	3.6	(0.08)	7.8	(0.2)	0.6	1.7	10.0

to total effects mediated by disability include cancer (78.9%), neurological disorders (57.6%), and insomnia (50.0%). Alcohol abuse with or without dependence and drug abuse with or without dependence are the only disorders considered here for which indirect effects through WHODAS scores are not statistically significant. The WHODAS dimensions most often associated with significant mediating effects across the 19 disorders are role functioning (89.5%), family burden (84.2%), stigma (79.0%), mobility (73.7%), cognition (68.4%), and self-care (42.1%).

Figure 16.2 shows the relative importance of each disability dimension in the indirect effects on VAS. Thus, the 100% is the overall indirect effect of each disorder, and the sections correspond to different disability dimensions. Only the disorders with significant overall indirect effects are considered. It can be observed that role functioning is the most important

Table 16.2 Perceived health visual analogue scale (VAS) scores by country income level. The WMH surveys.

| | Country income level | | | | | | | | | | | | | | | | | | | | | | |
| | All countries | | | | | Low/lower-middle | | | | | Upper-middle | | | | | High | | | | |
	Mean	(SE)	Q25	Median	Q75	Mean	(SE)	Q25	Median	Q75	Mean	(SE)	Q25	Median	Q75	Mean	(SE)	Q25	Median	Q75
Overall sample	81.0	(0.1)	70.0	90.0	95.0	81.6	(0.2)	70.0	90.0	99.8	81.0	(0.3)	70.0	89.9	99.5	80.7	(0.2)	74.4	89.8	90.0
Any mental disorder	72.2	(0.3)	59.9	79.9	89.9	71.9	(0.7)	59.8	79.1	89.2	71.6	(0.7)	59.1	79.9	89.7	72.6	(0.4)	60.0	79.9	89.9
Any physical condition	75.0	(0.2)	60.0	80.0	90.0	74.3	(0.4)	59.9	79.9	90.0	73.2	(0.5)	60.0	80.0	89.9	76.0	(0.2)	69.1	80.0	89.7
Any mental or physical disorder	75.5	(0.2)	64.9	80.0	90.0	74.9	(0.4)	60.0	79.9	90.0	73.8	(0.5)	60.0	80.0	89.9	76.4	(0.2)	69.2	80.0	89.9

Table 16.3 Effects (direct and indirect via WHODAS dimension scores) of conditions on perceived health VAS: overall sample. The WMH surveys.

| Disorders | Total effects of conditions on VAS | | Direct effects of conditions | | Indirect effects via WHODAS scales | | Percentage of indirect effects over total effects | | Indirect effects via each WHODAS dimension [a] | | | | | | | | | | | |
| | | | | | | | | | Cognition | | Mobility | | Self-care | | Role functioning | | Family burden | | Stigma | |
	Coeff	(SE)	Coeff	(SE)	Coeff	(SE)	Coeff	(SE)	Coeff	(SE)	Coeff	(SE)	Coeff	(SE)	Coeff	(SE)	Coeff	(SE)	Coeff	(SE)
Alcohol abuse	−2.9*	(0.8)	−3.0*	(0.8)	0.1	(0.3)	−3.2	(8.8)	0.00	(0.02)	0.32*	(0.06)	0.03	(0.02)	−0.1	(0.11)	−0.04	(0.06)	−0.10	(0.08)
Bipolar	−8.1*	(1.3)	−4.3*	(1.0)	−3.8*	(0.7)	47.0*	(7.4)	−0.48*	(0.13)	−0.26	(0.16)	−0.10	(0.08)	−1.2*	(0.24)	−0.86*	(0.19)	−0.77*	(0.20)
Drug abuse	−3.7*	(1.5)	−3.0*	(1.4)	−0.7	(0.6)	18.0	(14.7)	−0.09	(0.06)	0.13	(0.10)	0.03	(0.02)	−0.3	(0.22)	−0.28	(0.20)	−0.09	(0.17)
Generalized anxiety	−5.3*	(0.9)	−1.9*	(0.8)	−3.3*	(0.6)	63.7*	(9.8)	−0.28*	(0.08)	−0.49*	(0.15)	−0.06	(0.04)	−1.1*	(0.20)	−0.73*	(0.16)	−0.66*	(0.14)
Major depressive disorder	−8.2*	(0.4)	−5.2*	(0.4)	−3.0*	(0.2)	36.8*	(2.6)	−0.27*	(0.06)	−0.31*	(0.07)	−0.05*	(0.02)	−1.1*	(0.10)	−0.54*	(0.08)	−0.68*	(0.09)
Panic and/or agoraphobia	−6.3*	(0.9)	−3.0*	(0.7)	−3.3*	(0.5)	53.1*	(7.1)	−0.33*	(0.09)	−0.39*	(0.11)	−0.05	(0.03)	−1.1*	(0.17)	−0.61*	(0.13)	−0.80*	(0.14)
Post-traumatic stress	−5.2*	(0.9)	−0.8	(0.8)	−4.3*	(0.6)	84.0*	(13.5)	−0.43*	(0.11)	−0.79*	(0.16)	−0.10	(0.05)	−1.5*	(0.22)	−0.78*	(0.16)	−0.69*	(0.15)
Social phobia	−3.1*	(0.7)	−2.0*	(0.6)	−1.1*	(0.3)	34.6*	(9.8)	−0.18*	(0.06)	−0.01	(0.07)	0.03	(0.02)	−0.3*	(0.10)	−0.27*	(0.09)	−0.26*	(0.09)
Specific phobia	−2.3*	(0.5)	−1.7*	(0.4)	−0.6*	(0.2)	26.0	(8.9)	−0.03	(0.02)	0.00	(0.06)	0.01	(0.01)	−0.2*	(0.09)	−0.19*	(0.06)	−0.15*	(0.06)
Arthritis	−5.5*	(0.4)	−3.5*	(0.3)	−2.0*	(0.2)	36.8*	(2.8)	−0.04*	(0.01)	−0.65*	(0.07)	−0.05*	(0.02)	−0.6*	(0.07)	−0.24*	(0.04)	−0.36*	(0.05)
Cancer	−2.7*	(0.9)	−0.6	(0.8)	−2.1*	(0.4)	78.9*	(22.6)	−0.08	(0.05)	−0.64*	(0.14)	−0.05	(0.03)	−0.9*	(0.15)	−0.34*	(0.09)	−0.12	(0.08)
Cardiovascular	−5.8*	(0.4)	−3.6*	(0.3)	−2.2*	(0.2)	38.2*	(2.8)	−0.06*	(0.02)	−0.65*	(0.07)	−0.07*	(0.03)	−0.7*	(0.07)	−0.33*	(0.05)	−0.39*	(0.05)

Table 16.3 (cont.)

| Disorders | Total effects of conditions on VAS | | Direct effects of conditions | | Indirect effects via WHODAS scales | | Percentage of indirect effects over total effects | | Indirect effects via each WHODAS dimension [a] | | | | | | | | | | | |
| | | | | | | | | | Cognition | | Mobility | | Self-care | | Role functioning | | Family burden | | Stigma | |
	Coeff	(SE)	Coeff	(SE)	Coeff	(SE)	Coeff	(SE)	Coeff	(SE)	Coeff	(SE)	Coeff	(SE)	Coeff	(SE)	Coeff	(SE)	Coeff	(SE)
Chronic pain	-6.6*	(0.3)	-4.2*	(0.3)	-2.4*	(0.1)	36.8*	(1.9)	-0.07*	(0.02)	-0.62*	(0.06)	-0.04*	(0.02)	-1.0*	(0.07)	-0.32*	(0.04)	-0.40*	(0.05)
Diabetes	-5.9*	(0.7)	-3.8*	(0.6)	-2.1*	(0.3)	35.0*	(4.5)	-0.11*	(0.03)	-0.59*	(0.10)	-0.07*	(0.03)	-0.8*	(0.12)	-0.25*	(0.06)	-0.21*	(0.06)
Digestive	-4.1*	(0.6)	-2.8*	(0.5)	-1.3*	(0.3)	31.0*	(5.8)	-0.01	(0.02)	-0.22*	(0.08)	-0.02	(0.01)	-0.5*	(0.11)	-0.24*	(0.07)	-0.29*	(0.07)
Headache / migraine	-4.8*	(0.3)	-3.3*	(0.3)	-1.5*	(0.1)	31.4*	(2.9)	-0.12*	(0.03)	-0.08	(0.04)	-0.03*	(0.01)	-0.5*	(0.06)	-0.33*	(0.05)	-0.39*	(0.05)
Insomnia	-6.2*	(0.5)	-3.1*	(0.5)	-3.1*	(0.3)	50.0*	(4.3)	-0.21*	(0.06)	-0.64*	(0.08)	-0.07*	(0.03)	-1.0*	(0.11)	-0.56*	(0.08)	-0.52*	(0.08)
Neurological	-9.8*	(1.1)	-4.2*	(0.9)	-5.7*	(0.8)	57.6*	(6.8)	-0.37*	(0.10)	-1.45*	(0.29)	-0.24*	(0.11)	-1.6*	(0.26)	-0.84*	(0.18)	-1.06*	(0.21)
Respiratory	-1.5*	(0.3)	-1.2*	(0.2)	-0.3*	(0.1)	19.4*	(6.7)	-0.02	(0.01)	-0.10*	(0.04)	0.00	(0.01)	-0.2*	(0.05)	-0.02	(0.03)	0.01	(0.03)

Direct effects of scales

Cognition: −0.12 (0.03)* Mobility: −0.16 (0.03)* Self-care: −0.05 (0.02)* Getting along: −0.01 (0.03)
Role functioning: −0.12 (0.01)* Family burden: −0.11 (0.01)* Stigma: −0.11 (0.01)* Discrimination: −0.02 (0.02)

[a] Only dimensions with statistically significant direct effect are included. Getting along and Discrimination not statistically significant.
* Significant at the 0.05 level, two-sided test.

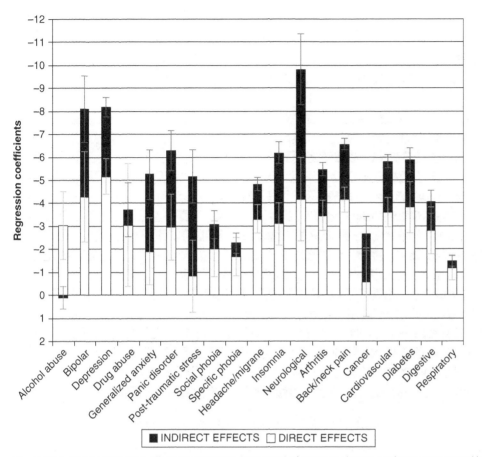

Figure 16.1 Direct and indirect effects (via WHODAS dimensions) of common chronic conditions on perceived health VAS; overall sample. Error bars show 95% confidence intervals (i.e., ± 1.96 SE). The WMH surveys.

mediator for all of the disorders with the exception of arthritis. The contribution of role functioning to the overall indirect effects ranges from 29% to 57%, and tends to be a bit more important among physical conditions (median 36.5%, IQR 32.4–39.3) than among mental disorders (median 32.9%, IQR 32.0–35.2).

The differential physical–mental disability mediation pattern is evident for mobility, with a median of 27.2% of indirect effects for physical conditions versus 10.3% for mental disorders. Conversely, stigma and family burden tend to be more important mediators of perceived health for mental disorders: the medians for stigma are 22.7% for mental disorders and 17.2% for physical disorders, and for family burden they are 21.7% and 15.0%, respectively. Cognition and self-care have a low contribution to the indirect effects (median across all disorders 6.6% and 1.85%, respectively).

Appendix Tables 16.1 to 16.3 are equivalent to Table 16.3 but show the sample for each of the three country income groups in turn. While all the total effects are statistically significant in the whole sample, not all of them are significant at the country income level. PTSD has the highest proportion of indirect over total effects across mental disorders in the three groups. Neurological disorders have the highest proportion for low/lower-middle-income and upper-middle-income countries across physical conditions, while the corresponding condition in high-income countries is cancer.

The overall contributions of indirect to total effects among the 19 conditions are shown in column four of each appendix table. These contributions range (among significant proportions) as follows: low/lower-middle-income 20.5–122.6%, median 38.7% (IQR 25.8–45.9); upper-middle-income 16.7–61.1%, median 33.2% (IQR 26.5–48.6); high-income 33.5–90.6%, median

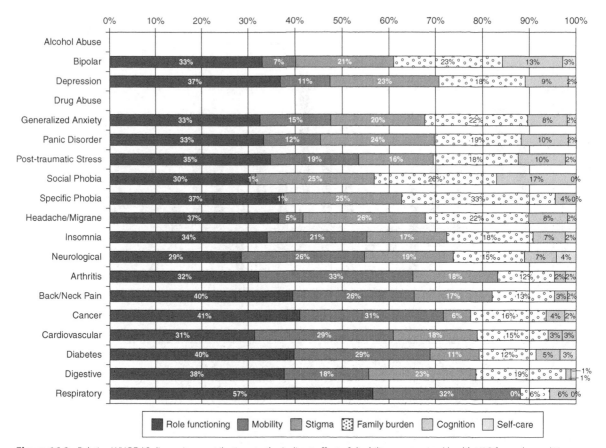

Figure 16.2. Relative WHODAS dimension contributions to the indirect effect of disability on perceived health VAS for each condition; overall sample. The WMH surveys. (Alcohol abuse and drug abuse are not represented because their respective overall indirect effect is not significant.)

42.6% (IQR 35.2–54.5). Hence, high-income countries show the highest contribution of indirect to total effects.

Country income-level information corresponding to Figure 16.2 (the proportion of indirect specific over the overall indirect effect) indicates that in all country income groups mobility has a higher contribution in physical conditions, and the indirect effects of family burden and stigma are higher among mental disorders. While role functioning is also the most important dimension for high-income and low/lower-middle-income countries (median percentages and IQRs 36.2% [32.9–40.8] and 35.9% [30.0–39.0], respectively), for upper-middle-income countries it is stigma (median percentage 38.8%, IQR = 31.4–45.1).

Discussion

We found that over a third (median of 36.8%, with an IQR of 31.2–51.5) of the total decrement in

perceived health associated with common mental and physical disorders is mediated by the disabilities assessed in WHODAS. We also found that role functioning is the predominant dimension which indirectly accounts for the association of all the disorders with perceived health. While mobility is the second most important mediator in the case of physical conditions, for mental disorders stigma and family burden are more important mediators. Taken together, these results suggest that there is a differential pattern of disability mediation of perceived health for mental and physical disorders. Of note, these results are very similar across the three levels of country income.

To our knowledge, the mediating role of disability on perceived health has never been reported for samples of the general population representing so many countries worldwide for the large range of disorders and disability dimensions assessed in this chapter. Many studies have previously shown an association between particular dimensions of disability and perceived health, in samples of patients with particular diseases. For instance, social functioning is an important determinant of perceived health among heart failure patients (Carlson *et al.* 2012), while physical ability has an important role on perceived health among spinal cord injury patients (Machacova *et al.* 2011). And for individuals with major depressive episode, cognition and embarrassment seem to be more relevant disability dimensions (Buist-Bouwman *et al.* 2008). The results presented in this chapter represent a first systematic attempt to disentangle the association between a range of chronic disorders and perceived health, considering a comprehensive range of disability indicators. And they indicate that, on average, the disability-mediated effect on perceived health is substantial and similar for the nine mental and the 10 physical disorders analyzed. Nevertheless, the type of disability dimension which mediates such effects tends to be different for mental and physical disorders. Moreover, there is variation across individual disorders in the extent to which their impact on perceived health is mediated by disability dimensions. More research is needed to further understand the underlying process of perceived health and disability evaluations and how they may differ by different levels of health.

Mobility disability is a frequent mediator of the effect of physical conditions on perceived health (median value of 10.2% of the total effect), while this dimension is much less important for mental disorders (3.2%). Many of the physical conditions considered in our study imply either pain (arthritis, back/neck pain) or impairment on the extremities and their functional performance (neurological, cardiovascular, and respiratory disorders), or general weakness (cancer and others). All of these have an impact on mobility function and modify the perception of health of the individual (Alonso *et al.* 2004, 2011, Garin *et al.* 2010). On the other hand, this disability dimension is not a very relevant mediator of the impact of mental disorders on perceived health, while family burden and stigma are. The empirical direct and indirect associations described here provide a textured picture of the ways health conditions impact on health perceptions and the role of functioning and disability. The importance of these findings may go beyond description, and may help in guiding therapeutic efforts towards particular disabilities. For instance, in a descriptive study of breast cancer survivors it was

estimated that potential interventions including physical mobility could prevent decreases in self-rated health among these patients (Schootman *et al.* 2012). Also, specific clinical problem-solving tools for physical and rehabilitation medicine could be used in conjunction with assessments of perceived health (Steiner *et al.* 2002). Consistent with previous work (Buist-Bouwman *et al.* 2008), the data presented in this chapter suggest that assessing stigma and family burden and trying to combat them can limit the decrements in perceived health of individuals with mental disorders.

As has been pointed out in the preceding chapters, the interpretation of these results must take into account several general and particular limitations. First, mental and physical disorders were differently assessed. The former were measured with a standard diagnostic instrument, the WHO Composite International Diagnostic Interview (CIDI), with high levels of reliability and acceptable validity for research purposes. In contrast, physical conditions were self-reported by respondents. Although we used standardized questions which have shown acceptable validity levels (Kriegsman *et al.* 1996, Baumeister *et al.* 2010), misclassification cannot be ruled out, in particular, under-reporting of physical conditions in countries with lower access to health care. Second, we did not assess some particularly disabling brain disorders such as non-affective psychoses and dementia (Murray & López 1996). Our study, therefore, likely underestimates disability caused by mental disorders. Third, as discussed in previous chapters, while mental and physical disorders were assessed in the 12 months prior to the interview, both overall perceived health (VAS) and the WHODAS questions referred to the 30 days preceding the interview. Because of these different time frames it is not possible to definitively relate either the health status or the disability reported by the respondents to their underlying mental or physical disorders for the preceding 12 months. Nevertheless, because both VAS and WHODAS use the same recall period, any such bias should not influence our analyses of the intermediating role of disability in the impact of conditions on perceived health. Similarly, we were not able to assess the duration of the disability. It has been suggested that age at disability onset may impact self-reported general health and should be considered when analyzing health-related quality of life (HRQOL) differences among people with disabilities (Jamoom *et al.* 2008). Finally, an important consideration is the difficulty of differentiating the nature of disorders, symptoms, function, and perceptions, as well as the need to refine the mediating and/or moderating nature of the described associations (Wang *et al.* 2006).

In conclusion, our results, which are basically descriptive, call attention to the need to consider both disability and perceived health in evaluating the impact of common mental and physical disorders. They suggest that there is a need to learn more about the strength and nature of indirect associations between chronic disorders and perceived health. In particular, it will be important to evaluate whether interventions addressed to improve specific disabilities may improve the perceived health of individuals with common chronic disorders beyond the benefits that would be obtained from the usual treatment for the disorder.

Acknowledgments

This chapter builds on and expands the analyses performed in Alonso J., Vilagut G., Duran N., *et al.* Decomposing the total effects of common mental and physical conditions on perceived health: results from the WHO World Mental Health surveys (*PLoS One*, in press).

References

Alonso, J. (2000). [The measurement of health-related quality of life in clinical research and practice]. *Gaceta Sanitaria* **14**, 163–7.

Alonso, J., Ferrer, M., Gandek, B., *et al.* (2004). Health-related quality of life associated with chronic conditions in eight countries. Results from the International Quality of Life Assessment (IQOLA) project. *Quality of Life Research* **13**, 283–98.

Alonso, J., Vilagut, G., Chatterji, S., *et al.* (2011). Including information about co-morbidity in estimates of disease burden: results from the World Health Organization World Mental Health Surveys. *Psychological Medicine* **41**, 873–86.

Ashburner, J. M., Cauley, J. A., Cawthon, P., *et al.* (2011). Self-ratings of health and change in walking speed over 2 years: results from the caregiver-study of osteoporotic fractures. *American Journal of Epidemiology* **173**, 882–9.

Baumeister, H., Kriston, L., Bengel, J., & Härter M. (2010). High agreement of self-report and physician-diagnosed somatic conditions yields limited bias in examining mental-physical comorbidity. *Journal of Clinical Epidemiology* **63**, 558–65.

Blain, H., Carriere, I., Sourial, N., *et al.* (2010). Balance and walking speed predict subsequent 8-year mortality independently of current and intermediate events in well-functioning women aged 75 years and older. *The Journal of Nutrition Health and Aging* **14**, 595–600.

Boot, C. R., Koppes, L. L., van den Bossche, S. N., Anema, J. R., & van der Beek, A. J. (2011). Relation between perceived health and sick leave in employees with a chronic illness. *Jounral of Occupational Rehabilitation* **21**, 211–19.

Buist-Bouwman, M. A., Ormel, J., de Graaf, R., *et al.* (2008). Mediators of the association between depression and role functioning. *Acta Psychiatrica Scandinavica* **118**, 451–8.

Carlson, B., Pozehl, B., Hertzog, M., Zimmerman, L., & Riegel, B. (2012). Predictors of overall perceived health in patients with heart failure. *Journal of Cardiovascular Nursing.* [Epub ahead of print].

Damian, J., Pastor-Barriuso, R., & Valderrama-Gama, E. (2008). Factors associated with self-rated health in older people living in institutions. *BMC Geriatrics* **8**, 5–10.

DeSalvo, K. B., Fan, V. S., McDonell, M. B., & Fihn, S. D. (2005). Predicting mortality and healthcare utilization with a single question. *Health Services Research* **40**, 1234–46.

Garin, O., Ayuso-Mateos, J. L., Almansa, J., *et al.* (2010). Validation of the World Health Organization Disability Assessment Schedule (WHODAS-2) in patients with chronic diseases. *Health and Quality of Life Outcomes* **8**, 51.

Guyatt, G. H., Feeny, D. H., & Patrick, D. L. (1993). Measuring health-related quality of life. *Annals of Internal Medicine* **118**, 622–9.

Heistaro, S., Vartiainen, E., & Puska, P. (1996). Trends in self-rated health in Finland 1972–1992. *Preventive Medicine* **25**, 625–32.

Idler, E. L., & Benyamini, Y. (1997). Self-rated health and mortality: a review of twenty-seven community studies. *Journal of Health and Social Behavior* **38**, 21–37.

Jamoom, E. W., Horner-Johnson, W., Suzuki, R., *et al.* (2008). Age at disability onset and self-reported health status. *BMC Public Health* **8**, 10–16.

Kriegsman, D. M., Penninx, B. W., van Eijk, J. T., Boeke, A. J. P., & Deeg, D. J. H. (1996). Self-reports and general practitioner information on the presence of chronic diseases in community dwelling elderly. A study on the accuracy of patients' self-reports and on determinants of inaccuracy. *Journal of Clinical Epidemiology* **49**, 1407–17.

Lee, H. Y., Jang, S. N., Lee, S., Cho, S. I., & Park, E. O. (2008). The relationship between social participation and self-rated health by sex and age: a cross-sectional survey. *International Journal of Nursing Studies* **45**, 1042–54.

Lee, Y., & Shinkai, S. (2003). A comparison of correlates of self-rated health and functional disability of older persons in the Far East: Japan and Korea. *Archives of Gerontology and Geriatrics* **37**, 63–76.

Leinonen, R., Heikkinen, E., & Jylha, M. (2001). Predictors of decline in self-assessments of health among older people: a 5-year longitudinal study. *Social Science and Medicine* **52**, 1329–41.

Machacova, K., Lysack, C., & Neufeld, S. (2011). Self-rated health among persons with spinal cord injury: what is the role of physical ability? *Journal of Spinal Cord Medicine* **34**, 265–72.

Mavaddat, N., Kinmonth, A. L., Sanderson, S., *et al.* (2011). What determines self-rated health (SRH)? A cross-sectional study of SF-36 health domains in the EPIC-Norfolk cohort. *Journal of Epidemiology and Community Health* **65**, 800–6.

Murray, C. J., & López, A. D. (1996). Evidence-based health policy. Lessons from the Global Burden of Disease study. *Science* **274**, 740–3.

Ormel, J., Kempen, G. I., Penninx, B. W., *et al.* (1997). Chronic medical conditions and mental health in older people: disability and psychosocial resources mediate specific mental health effects. *Psychological Medicine* **27**, 1065–77.

Ormel, J., Petukhova, M., Chatterji, S., *et al.* (2008). Disability and treatment of specific mental and physical disorders across the world. *British Journal of Psychiatry* **192**, 368–75.

Perruccio, A. V., Power, J. D., & Badley, E. M. (2007). The relative impact of 13 chronic conditions across three different outcomes. *Journal of Epidemiology and Community Health* **61**, 1056–61.

Rohrer, J. E., Young, R., Sicola, V., & Houston, M. (2007). Overall self-rated health: a new quality indicator for primary care. *Journal of Evaluation in Clinical Practice* **13**, 150–3.

Saarni, S. I., Harkanen, T., Sintonen, H., *et al.* (2006). The impact of 29 chronic conditions on health-related quality of life: a general population survey in Finland using 15D, and EQ-5D. *Quality of Life Research* **15**, 1403–14.

Salomon, J. A., Tandon, A., & Murray, C. J. (2004). Comparability of self rated health: cross sectional multi-country survey using anchoring vignettes. *BMJ* **328**, 258–63.

Schootman, M., Deshpande, A. D., Pruitt, S., Aft, R., & Jeffe, D. B. (2012). Estimated effects of potential interventions to prevent decreases in self-rated health among breast cancer survivors. *Annals of Epidemiology* **22**, 79–86.

Schultz, S. E., & Kopec, J. A. (2003). Impact of chronic conditions. *Health Reports* **14**, 41–53.

Sen, A. (2002). Health: perception versus observation. *BMJ* **324**, 860–1.

Steiner, W. A., Ryser, L., Huber, E., *et al.* (2002). Use of the ICF model as a clinical problem-solving tool in physical therapy and rehabilitation medicine. *Physical Therapy* **82**, 1098–107.

Üstün, T. B., Kostanjsek, N., Chatterji, S., & Rehm, J. (2010). *Measuring Health and Disability: Manual for WHO Disability Assessment Schedule (WHODAS 2.0)*. Geneva: World Health Organization.

Valderas, J. M., & Alonso, J. (2008). Patient reported outcome measures: a model-based classification system for research and clinical practice. *Quality of Life Research* **17**, 1125–35.

van Dijk, A., McGrath, P. A., Pickett, W., *et al.* (2008). Pain and self-reported health in Canadian children. *Pain Research & Management* **13**, 407–11.

Von Korff, M., Crane, P. K., Alonso, J., *et al.* (2008). Modified WHODAS-II provides valid measure of global disability but filter items increased skewness. *Journal of Clinical Epidemiology* **61**, 1132–43.

Wang, P. P., Badley, E. M., & Gignac, M. (2006). Exploring the role of contextual factors in disability models. *Disability and Rehabilitation* **28**, 135–40.

Wilson, I. B., & Cleary, P. D. (1995). Linking clinical variables with health-related quality of life. A conceptual model of patient outcomes. *JAMA* **273**, 59–65.

World Bank (2008). Data and statistics. http://go.worldbank.org/D7SN0B8YU0. Accessed May 12, 2009.

Chapter

17

The burdens of mental disorders in the Global Burden of Disease Study 2010 and the World Mental Health surveys: similarities, differences, and implications for mental health research

Harvey A. Whiteford and Alize J. Ferrari

Introduction

In its *World Development Report* of 1993 the World Bank introduced the concept of quantifying the global burden of different diseases using disability-adjusted life years (DALYs) (World Bank 1993). A DALY reflects the sum of years of life lived with a disability (YLD) and years of life lost to premature mortality (YLL). One DALY is equivalent to the loss of one healthy year of life (Murray & López 1996). The Global Burden of Disease (GBD) 1996 study and its update in 2000 greatly enhanced our understanding of the contribution made to disease burden by highly prevalent disorders, with relatively low mortality. Chief amongst this group are mental disorders (Murray & López 1996, World Health Organization 2008). In GBD 1996, depressive disorders were estimated to be the fourth leading cause of burden, explaining 3.7% of DALYs (Murray & López 1996). In GBD 2000 they were estimated to be the third leading cause of burden and the primary cause of disability (Üstün *et al.* 2004).

In 2007, work began on the GBD 2010 study, the findings of which will be launched in December 2012 (Lozano *et al.* 2012, Murray *et al.* 2012a, Vos *et al.* 2012). GBD 2010 is an all-inclusive revision of burden estimates for 291 diseases and 67 risk factors, across 21 world regions (see www.globalburden.org). The burden estimation process for each disease involves: conducting a systematic review of the literature to capture representative epidemiological data; using a Bayesian meta-regression approach to integrate these data; quantifying the associated disability and mortality; and calculating gender- and age-specific YLDs, YLLs, and DALYs for 21 world regions, for the years 1990, 2005, and 2010 (Vos *et al.* 2012, Flaxman *et al.* in press).

GBD 2010 is being carried out through four universities and the World Health Organization (WHO), supported by the Bill and Melinda Gates Foundation and over 50 international expert groups (Murray *et al.* 2007). One of these groups is the Mental Disorders and Illicit Drug Use Research Group (see www.global-burden.com.au), responsible for providing the epidemiological inputs (steps 1 and 2 of the GBD 2010 methodology) for 11 mental disorders and four illicit drug use disorders (Degenhardt *et al.* 2009).

The aim of this chapter is to compare how the burden of mental disorders is quantified in GBD 2010 and the World Mental Health (WMH) surveys, and to explain how each approach has contributed to mental health research. We will summarize the epidemiological data compiled for mental disorders in GBD 2010 and the contribution made by the WMH surveys. We will also compare the burden quantification process for mental disorders as used by GBD 2010 and by the WMH surveys.

Epidemiological inputs of burden estimates

For each of the 11 mental disorders included in GBD 2010 we required representative data on the incidence, prevalence, remission or duration, severity, age of onset, and excess mortality. These serve as inputs in the computation of YLDs which can be understood as a "meta-synthesis" of the available worldwide data, accommodating for changes in disability in the presentation of a disease (Vos *et al.* 2012).

Electronic databases (PsycInfo, Medline, and Embase) and the gray (published and unpublished) literature were searched. In order to ensure the comparability of epidemiological data across studies, we only included studies using a cross-sectional or longitudinal design, published from 1980 onwards. The epidemiological data collected also needed to be representative at a community, regional, or national level, and based on an internationally accepted classification system. For mental disorders, this meant either the *Diagnostic and Statistical Manual of Mental Disorders* (DSM-IV) (American Psychiatric Association 2000) or the *International Classification of Diseases* (ICD-10) (World Health Organization 1993).

This search strategy culminated in the inclusion of 1,249 studies for prevalence, 80 studies for incidence, 80 studies for remission, and 159 studies for excess mortality. Studies for all four parameters reported sex-specific and/or non-specific epidemiological estimates which were representative of specific age ranges (e.g., 10–20 years) and/or the entire lifespan (e.g., 0–99 years). The global coverage of the prevalence data ranged from 54 countries (for depressive and anxiety disorders) to 16 countries (for autism spectrum disorders). The WMH surveys made significant contributions to the GBD effort, as they provided representative prevalence estimates for eight out of the 11 mental disorders included in GBD 2010, from 28 countries (Kessler & Üstün 2008). For the most part, the WMH survey methodology for data collection and analysis (as described in Chapter 2) was similar to that required for GBD purposes.

The WMH surveys also allowed a mental disorder diagnosis using ICD-10 or DSM-IV criteria (World Health Organization 1993, American Psychiatric Association 2000, Kessler & Üstün 2008), which was a requirement for GBD 2010. Table 17.1 summarizes the disorders and disorder subtypes assessed in GBD 2010 and the WMH surveys. The aim of GBD 2010 was to estimate, to the greatest degree possible, the total population burden of all mental disorders. Consequently, disorders were only excluded where it was impossible to make defensible global epidemiological estimates. Unlike the WMH surveys, we collected data on low-prevalence disorders such as schizophrenia, which is typically not included in nationally representative

population samples (Ellenberg 1994) and was not assessed in the WMH surveys.

The type of disorders in GBD 2010 and the WMH surveys also varied. This is most noticeable in the case of illicit drug use disorders, for which the WMH surveys have a category for drug abuse and dependence whereas the GBD 2010 collected data on four drug use types separately (cannabis, opioid, cocaine, and amphetamine dependence); and also childhood disorders, where the WMH surveys collected information on oppositional-defiant disorder and intermittent explosive disorder and the GBD 2010 included the autistic spectrum and other pervasive developmental disorders. It is worth noting here that childhood disorders were not included in GBD 1996 and 2000, despite children making up a significant proportion of the population in developing regions. In Africa, for example, the proportion of the population under 15 years is 42%, compared to a world average of 27% (World Health Organization 2010). Consequently, excluding childhood disorders from GBD 1996's burden estimates grossly underestimated the burden attributable to mental disorders in this region.

Clearly GBD 2010 has also not been able to capture information on all mental disorders, because the information to make defensible global estimates is not always available. For example, personality disorders are not represented in GBD 2010 because of insufficient data to derive a representative epidemiological profile. With evolving work from research groups such as the WMH surveys, we are continually seeing new and high-quality epidemiological data published for mental disorders, and this can only benefit future work on the burden of diseases. In some WMH sampling sites, for instance, disorders not in GBD 2010 such as pathological gambling, intermittent explosive disorder, and neurasthenia were also captured (World Mental Health Survey Consortium 2005). This has started the process of providing information on a wider range of mental disorders, and it is important that this work should continue.

In contrast to many other epidemiological studies, the data from the WMH surveys can be pooled for comparability. Interpretation and synthesis of epidemiological data (as required for GBD) is usually complicated by variations in the methodology used by different studies to capture and analyze the data. Epidemiological studies are usually intended to inform local policy and practices rather than to generate data that can be systematically compared with those from

Table 17.1 The mental disorders assessed in GBD 2010 and the WMH surveys.

Mental disorder	GBD 2010	WMH surveys[a]
Schizophrenia	Yes	No
Depressive disorders	Major depressive disorder, dysthymia	Major depressive disorder, dysthymia, recurrent brief depression, irritable major/minor depression
Bipolar disorders	Bipolar I, bipolar II, bipolar NOS[b], cyclothymia	Bipolar I, bipolar II
Anxiety disorders	Obsessive–compulsive disorder (OCD), post-traumatic stress disorder (PTSD), panic disorder, agoraphobia, simple phobia, social phobia, generalized anxiety disorder (GAD), separation anxiety disorder, anxiety NOS[b]	Obsessive–compulsive disorder, post-traumatic stress disorder, panic disorder and/or agoraphobia, generalized anxiety disorder, specific phobia, social phobia, separation anxiety disorder
Eating disorders	Anorexia nervosa, bulimia nervosa	Anorexia nervosa, bulimia nervosa
Pervasive developmental disorders	Autistic disorder, Asperger's disorder, pervasive developmental disorders NOS[b]	No
Childhood behavioral disorders	Attention-deficit/hyperactivity disorder, conduct disorder	Attention-deficit/hyperactivity disorder, conduct disorder, oppositional-defiant disorder, intermittent explosive disorder
Illicit drug use disorders	Cannabis dependence, cocaine dependence, amphetamine dependence, opioid dependence	Drug abuse and dependence
Alcohol use disorders[c]	Alcohol dependence	Alcohol abuse and dependence
Nicotine dependence[c]	Yes	Yes
Premenstrual syndrome (PMS)[c]	Yes	Yes

[a] The WMH survey data summarized here were exported from http://www.hcp.med.harvard.edu/wmh/national_sample.php.
[b] Not otherwise specified.
[c] PMS, alcohol use and nicotine use disorders are being investigated for GBD 2010 by other research groups.

another country (Weich & Araya 2004). Consequently, the differences in the epidemiology of mental disorders reported across studies might be real or might be a result of bias introduced by variations in data collection and analysis. The GBD 2010 has had to put in place supplementary measures (e.g., meta-regression procedures), first to explore the sources of variability in these data and second to minimize those that are artifacts of study methodology and design (Baxter *et al.* 2012, Ferrari *et al.* 2013, Vos *et al.* 2012, Flaxman *et al.* in press). Although the inter-country variability within the WMH dataset is far from trivial – e.g., the 12-month prevalence of major depressive disorder ranges from 1.1% of adults in Nigeria to 10.4% of adults in Brazil–São Paulo (Kessler & Üstün 2008, Bromet *et al.* 2011), consistent with what had been previously reported (Weissman *et al.* 1996), and the reasons for this are not fully understood (Kessler & Üstün 2008) – its

dataset is more globally comparable than that from other epidemiological studies, as it has been assembled using a standardized protocol for sampling, interviewing, coding, and analysis. The emphasis on interviewer training and monitoring, adjusted to the cultural demands of different sampling sites, also enforced a higher standard of quality on the data, which is important for GBD purposes.

The WMH surveys placed strong emphasis on the geographic representativeness of the samples surveyed in each country. This was particularly relevant to GBD 2010 as it allowed for a more accurate depiction of each disorder's epidemiology. Although the national representativeness of WMH samples varied slightly in some of the sites sampled (e.g., Brazil, India, Japan, Nigeria, and the People's Republic of China used regionally rather than nationally representative samples), this was much easier to work with for GBD 2010 than clinical samples (based on those persons in contact with clinicians), which for some low-prevalence disorders such as schizophrenia are the only type of samples available in many countries (Saha *et al.* 2005).

The WMH surveys use lay interviewers to administer the WHO Composite International Diagnostic Interview (CIDI) across all sampling sites, which facilitates systematic comparison of estimates between settings. For GBD 2010, we included studies using any survey instrument that allowed a diagnosis using ICD or DSM nomenclature. GBD 2010 also included studies using both lay and clinically trained interviewers, the latter of which has been found to be more sensitive to detecting non-Western representations of mental disorders (Helzer *et al.* 1985, Carta & Angst 2005, Jorm 2006). Heterogeneity introduced in the dataset as a result of including studies with different methodological designs was investigated and where possible minimized. Publications illustrating how this was done for major depressive disorder and anxiety disorders are available (Baxter *et al.* 2012, Ferrari *et al.* 2013).

The CIDI assessed the lifetime prevalence of mental disorders. Current (or past-month) and past-year prevalence were retrospectively estimated using questions such as "when was the last time you had any symptoms of the disorder?" (Kessler & Üstün 2008). This has significant implications for GBD, which focuses on measuring current health loss. As acknowledged in previous chapters, retrospective prevalence data, particularly lifetime estimates, are susceptible to recall bias (Simon & Von Korff 1995, Kruijshaar *et al.* 2005, Moffitt *et al.* 2010, Susser & Shrout 2010). For this reason, lifetime estimates were not included in GBD 2010. Current prevalence estimates were the gold standard but, to maximize inclusion, past-year estimates were also accepted. These were then "cross-walked" toward current prevalence estimates using meta-regression techniques (Vos *et al.* 2012, Flaxman *et al.* in press) to minimize methodological heterogeneity in the dataset.

The WMH surveys were designed to assess adults aged from 16–21 years onwards. In some sampling sites (e.g., Beijing, Shanghai, Colombia, and Mexico), a maximum age of 65–70 years was also imposed. This means that the prevalence of childhood disorders occurring before 16 years was only captured retrospectively, through estimates of lifetime prevalence. As noted in the discussion of childhood mental disorders above, every effort needs to be made to better estimate the burden of childhood disorders, and the inclusion of child and adolescent surveys in GBD 2010 was

important in this regard. Furthermore, variations in the distribution of mental disorders in the older age group (particularly relevant to chronic disorders such as dysthymia and bipolar disorder) would not be fully captured in samples where a maximum age of 65 or 70 was imposed. GBD 2010 sought to include studies with older age groups, to help capture the burden of mental disorders across the entire lifespan and not underestimate the contribution to burden from mental disorders in the elderly.

Operationalization of burden

What constitutes burden and how it should be measured will depend on its function (Murray *et al.* 2000). This is an important consideration when comparing WMH surveys and GBD 2010 burden estimates. As previously explained, the GBD approach defines burden in terms of the disability (YLD) and mortality (YLL) attributable to a disease (Murray & López 1996, Murray *et al.* 2012b). Assessing the mortality attributed to mental disorders was not a focus of burden estimation in the WMH surveys. Consistent with what has been previously reported (Harris & Barraclough 1998), our literature review found evidence of excess mortality (from all causes) in all but five of the mental disorders included in GBD 2010 (attention-deficit/hyperactivity disorder, conduct disorder, dysthymia, bulimia nervosa, cannabis dependence). This reinforces the point that mortality is an important contributor to mental heath burden when burden is defined as years of life lost to premature mortality and disability. Driving this finding was the high proportion of suicides occurring as a result of mental disorders. This has been highlighted in a previous volume in the WMH Cambridge University Press series, which focused on understanding the association between suicidal behavior (e.g., suicide ideation, plans, attempts) and mental disorders (Nock *et al.* 2012). That said, given that the aim here is to compare the quantification of burden by GBD 2010 and the WMH surveys, the remainder of this chapter will focus on the non-fatal burden (i.e., disability) attributable to mental disorders.

Mental disorders have a major impact on the life of a person with the disorder, on family and carers, and on the community. For GBD purposes much of the wider impact of the disorder is not in scope. Disability, in the YLD component of the DALY, is restricted to measures of health loss such as body functions, senses, cognition, and ambulation. Welfare loss, such as quality of life or participation restrictions, while obviously important, is not what the DALY is intended to capture (Bland *et al.* 1988, Murray 1994, Hendrick *et al.* 2000, Salomon *et al.* 2003).

In GBD 2010, disability attributable to given mental disorder was measured across one or more health states (or disorder sequelae). To capture variations in how decrements in health are understood in a range of settings around the world, community-based household surveys were conducted in Tanzania, Bangladesh, Indonesia, and Peru, alongside a telephone survey in North America and a global internet survey. Participants were asked to make pair-wise comparisons regarding which of two health states has the worst impact on health: for instance, comparing who is the healthiest between an individual who is completely blind and another who suffers from severe back pain. Different combinations of health states were used for every participant. For each health state, responses were converted from pair-wise comparisons into discrete values (i.e., a disability weight) ranging from 0 (perfect health) to 1 (death) (Salomon 2010, Salomon *et al.* 2012). The disability attributable to bipolar disorder for instance, was measured across depressive, manic, and residual states separately. Then the overall proportion of bipolar disorder cases in each health state was used to pool the three disability weights into an average disability weight for the disorder which also adjusted for severity. This strategy for bipolar disorder and schizophrenia has been outlined elsewhere (Ferrari *et al.* 2012).

This approach to disability assessment has been criticized (Mont 2007) precisely because it does not capture the welfare impacts of mental disorders, including the environmentally dependent (and potentially correctable) impairment in functioning as described in the WHO's International Classification of Functioning (ICF) (Üstün *et al.* 2003). However, this limited conceptualization is necessary for the main purpose of the DALY, which is to compare the relative magnitude of disease burden across diseases, countries, and time (Murray 1994, Murray & López 1996, Murray *et al.* 2000). It is not technically possible to reliably collect and compare the welfare impacts of all 291 diseases and 67 risk factors across 21 world regions. Even trying to compare these diseases and risk factors using a limited health-based definition of disability is controversial, although feasible (Murray *et al.* 2012b, Salomon *et al.* 2012). This was illustrated in the work undertaken to develop the GBD 2010

disability weights. Results from the individual household surveys showed a high degree of consistency with overall pooled results in all cases apart from Bangladesh (Salomon *et al.* 2012).

In the previous chapters of this volume, data from the WMH surveys have been used to describe the much broader welfare impacts of mental disorders, incorporating societal/developmental outcomes in the domains of education, marital status, physical abuse, income, days out of role, comorbidity with physical disorders, and functional disability as defined by the Sheehan Disability Scale (SDS) (Sheehan *et al.* 1996, Kessler & Üstün 2008) and the WHO Disability Assessment Schedule 2.0 (WHODAS 2) (Von Korff *et al.* 2008, Üstün *et al.* 2010). Given the consistency in the definitions of mental disorders for GBD 2010 and the WMH surveys, a comparison of the YLD rankings of mental disorders in GBD 2010 and the corresponding "societal-level impact of disorders" rankings from the WMH surveys (as defined in Chapter 15) would help us better understand the extent to which the GBD 2010 disability underestimates the overall impact of mental disorders. This would also make a significant contribution to recent debates in the literature as to whether mental disorder symptoms (within the skin) and functional impairment (outside the skin) should be treated as mutually exclusive entities (Lehman 2009, Narrow *et al.* 2009, Njenga 2009, Phillips 2009, Sartorius 2009, Üstün & Kennedy 2009, Vazquez-Barquero 2009, Wakefield 2009, Weissman 2009, Whiteford 2009). This has salient implications for the formulation of disability in diagnoses where clinical significance requires the presence of both symptoms and functional impairment (American Psychiatric Association 2000).

Comparative risk analysis

GBD 2010 quantifies the burden attributable to mental disorders in two ways. First, the burden of mental disorders as an underlying cause is calculated. Second, the burden attributable to mental disorders as a risk factor for other health outcomes is calculated. The latter makes use of methodology from the comparative risk assessment (CRA) component of GBD 2010 and is focused on attributable burden (Lim *et al.* 2012). Counterfactual analysis is used to quantify the effect of risk factors on DALYs. This involves comparing the reduction in disability or mortality (termed *population attributable fractions*, PAFs) occurring as a result of an ideal reduction in the risk factor exposure, i.e., a

Table 17.2 The outcomes of mental disorders assessed in GBD 2010 and the WMH surveys.

GBD 2010
Mental and drug use disorders as independent risk factors for suicide
Major depressive disorder as a risk factor for ischemic heart disease
Cannabis use as a risk factor for schizophrenia
Injecting drug use as a risk factor for hepatitis B (HBV), hepatitis C (HCV), and human immunodeficiency virus (HIV)

WMH surveys
Mental disorders in parents as a risk factor for offspring psychopathology
Mental disorders as a risk factor for poor educational attainment
Mental disorders as a risk factor for marital problems/failure
Premarital mental disorder diagnosis as a risk factor for physical violence in the marriage
Serious mental illness as a risk factor for reductions in earnings
Early-life mental disorder diagnosis as a risk factor for reductions in adult household income
Early onset of mental disorders as a risk factor for chronic physical conditions (heart disease, adult-onset asthma, diabetes, arthritis, chronic back or spinal pain, chronic or severe headache) in adulthood
Mental disorders as a risk factor for days out of role

reduction in the prevalence of mental disorders (Ezzati *et al.* 2002, Lim *et al.* 2012).

The WMH surveys adopted a similar methodology in using counterfactual analysis to investigate mental disorders as a risk factor for specific outcomes. The WMH surveys' *population attributable risk proportion* (PARP), defined as "the proportion of respondents with a dichotomous outcome of interest who would not have had this outcome in the absence of a particular set of predictors" (Chapter 2), is comparable to the CRA approach used in GBD 2010. A point of difference lies in the selection of outcomes for which mental disorders were assessed. In keeping with GBD's focus on health-based losses, mental disorders were assessed as risk factors for outcomes such as suicide and ischemic heart disease. The WMH surveys were able to assess a wider range of welfare-based outcomes of mental disorders. When combined with the GBD 2010 CRA findings, these provide a comprehensive view of the consequences attributable to mental disorders. Table 17.2 summarizes the outcomes assessed across GBD 2010 and the WMH surveys. Note that mental disorders as a risk factor for physical disorders other than ischemic heart disease (e.g., cardiovascular disease, type 2 diabetes, and injuries) were initially investigated for inclusion in GBD 2010. They were later excluded as there was insufficient evidence, at the time, to confidently quantify this relationship (Baxter *et al.* 2011). Given the work presented in Chapter 7, it is our recommendation that the burden attributable to mental disorders as a risk factor for other chronic physical conditions be included in future GBD studies.

Previous chapters have clearly outlined the methodology and challenges in the measurement of disability

in the WMH surveys, so we will not repeat the details here. Of particular relevance to the GBD approach, however, is the period for which disability was assessed. Although CIDI captured mental disorders across participants' lifetimes, SDS and WHODAS assessed for the disability attributable to mental disorders in only the 30 days leading up to the interview (Kessler & Üstün 2008). Although this gets around the problem of recall bias, it likely underestimates the disability attributable to episodic disorders such as major depressive disorder and bipolar disorder, which involve patients transitioning through different health states with differing degrees of impairment, typically lasting for more than 30 days (American Psychiatric Association 2000).

Quantifying the proportional burden attributable to individual mental disorders also requires the disability attributable to comorbid disorders to be portioned out. Otherwise, disability quantification for an individual diagnosed with comorbid disorders may lead to disability weights in excess of 1, which would be interpreted as worse than death (Murray & López 1994). Both GBD 2010 and the WMH surveys used a comorbidity correction in their burden calculations. This involved multiplying prevalence estimates of each disorder by their corresponding comorbidity-adjusted disability weight (or estimates of disability and health as quantified by a range of measures in the WMH surveys) in order to capture the unique effect of different disorders on total disability (which includes the disability attributable to primary plus comorbid diagnoses). The WMH methodology for this has been outlined in Chapters 2 and 15.

In GBD 2010, disability weights were adjusted for comorbidity in three stages. First, micro-simulation techniques were used to estimate the number of individuals experiencing different combinations of the 291 diseases in GBD 2010. Second, a multiplicative model was used to estimate disability weights for each disease (or disease sequelae) combination. Third, the disability attributable to comorbid diseases was portioned out from the disability attributable to each disease (or disease sequelae) in GBD 2010. A more comprehensive explanation of this methodology can be accessed elsewhere (Vos *et al.* 2012).

Conclusion

The WMH surveys and GBD 2010 have different datasets, each with their strengths and limitations, and each can make valuable and unique contributions to the study of mental health. The WMH dataset is more comprehensive at the population level: i.e., it holds detailed information on the age pattern of different mental disorders in the population, the demographic profile and developmental status of those diagnosed, their access to treatment, and their comorbid diagnoses. This, coupled with higher methodological homogeneity between sampling sites, enables WMH investigators to make more meaningful interpretation of the cross-national differences in how mental disorders present, and who presents with them. The GBD 2010 epidemiological dataset, on the other hand, is more comprehensive at the disorder level. Unlike the WMH surveys, the GBD 2010 dataset also holds data on epidemiological estimates other than prevalence, such as incidence, remission, duration, and excess mortality. This allows for a clearer picture of the cross-national distribution of mental disorders, particularly in distinguishing between disorders with episodic and chronic courses. Although the GBD approach compromised the homogeneity between studies, it was able to capture epidemiological data for a wider range of countries.

Comparison of GBD 2010 YLDs and the WMH surveys' societal-level impact of disorders provides a comprehensive summary of the health and welfare loss attributable to mental disorders.

Acknowledgments

We acknowledge the work of members of the GBD core group and mental disorders and illicit drugs use research group for their work on this topic.

References

American Psychiatric Association (2000). *Diagnostic and Statistical Manual of Mental Disorders, Fourth Edition (DSM-IV)*. Washington, DC: American Psychiatric Association.

Baxter, A. J., Charlson, F. J., Somerville, A. J., & Whiteford, H. A. (2011). Mental disorders as risk factors: assessing the evidence for the Global Burden of Disease Study. *BMC Medicine* **9**, 134.

Baxter, A. J., Scott, K. M., Vos, T., & Whiteford, H. A. (2012). Global prevalence of anxiety disorders: a systematic review and meta-regression. *Psychological Medicine* 1–14. [Epub ahead of print].

Bland, R. C., Newman, S. C., & Orn, H. (1988). Prevalence of psychiatric disorders in the elderly in Edmonton. *Acta Psychiatrica Scandinavica Supplementum* **338**, 57–63.

Bromet, E., Andrade, L. H., Hwang, I., et al. (2011). Cross-national epidemiology of DSM-IV major depressive episode. *BMC Medicine* **9**, 90–105.

Carta, M. G., & Angst, J. (2005). Epidemiological and clinical aspects of bipolar disorders: controversies or a common need to redefine the aims and methodological aspects of surveys. *Clinical Practice and Epidemiology in Mental Health* **1**, 4.

Degenhardt, L., Whiteford, H., Hall, W., & Vos, T. (2009). Estimating the burden of disease attributable to illicit drug use and mental disorders: what is "Global Burden of Disease 2005" and why does it matter? *Addiction* **104**, 1466–71.

Ellenberg, J. H. (1994). Selection bias in observational and experimental studies. *Statistics in Medicine* **13**, 557–67.

Ezzati, M., López, A. D., Rodgers, A., et al. (2002). Selected major risk factors and global and regional burden of disease. *Lancet* **360**, 1347–60.

Ferrari, A. J., Saha, S., McGrath, J. J., et al. (2012). Health states for schizophrenia and bipolar disorder within the Global Burden of Disease 2010 Study. *Population Health Metrics* **10**, 16.

Ferrari, A. J., Somerville, A. J., Baxter, A. J., et al. (2013). Global variation in the prevalence and incidence of major depressive disorder: a systematic review of the epidemiological literature. *Psychological Medicine* **43**, 471–81.

Flaxman, A. D., Vos, T., & Murray, C. J. L., eds. (in press). *An Integrative Metaregression Framework for Descriptive Epidemiology*. Washington, DC: University of Washington Press.

Harris, E. C., & Barraclough, B. (1998). Excess mortality of mental disorder. *British Journal of Psychiatry* **173**, 11–53.

Helzer, J. E., Robins, L. N., McEvoy, L. T., et al. (1985). A comparison of clinical and diagnostic interview schedule diagnoses. Physician reexamination of lay-interviewed cases in the general population. *Archives of General Psychiatry* **42**, 657–66.

Hendrick, V., Altshuler, L. L., Gitlin, M. J., Delrahim, S., & Hammen, C. (2000). Gender and bipolar illness. *Journal of Clinical Psychiatry* **61**, 393–6.

Jorm, A. F. (2006). National surveys of mental disorders: are they researching scientific facts or constructing useful myths? *Australian and New Zealand Journal of Psychiatry* **40**, 830–4.

Kessler, R. C., & Üstün, T. B. (2008). *The WHO World Mental Health Surveys: Global Perspectives on the Epidemiology of Mental Disorders*. New York, NY: Cambridge University Press.

Kruijshaar, M. E., Barendregt, J., Vos, T., et al. (2005). Lifetime prevalence estimates of major depression: an indirect estimation method and a quantification of recall bias. *European Journal of Epidemiology* **20**, 103–11.

Lehman, A. F. (2009). Disentangle diagnosis and disability. *World Psychiatry* **8**, 89–90.

Lim, S. S., Vos, T., Flaxman. A. D., et al. (2012). A comparative risk assessment of burden of disease and injury attributable to 67 risk factors and risk factor clusters in 21 regions 1990–2010: a systematic analysis for the Global Burden of Disease Study 2010. *Lancet* **380**, 2224–60.

Lozano, R., Naghavi, M., Foreman, K., et al. (2012). Global and regional mortality from 235 causes of death for 20 age groups in 1990 and 2010: a systematic analysis for the Global Burden of Disease Study 2010. *Lancet* **380**, 2095–128.

Moffitt, T. E., Caspi, A., Taylor, A., et al. (2010). How common are common mental disorders? Evidence that lifetime prevalence rates are doubled by prospective versus retrospective ascertainment. *Psychological Medicine* **40**, 899–909.

Mont, D. (2007). Measuring health and disability. *Lancet* **369**, 1658–63.

Murray, C. J. (1994). Quantifying the burden of disease: the technical basis for disability-adjusted life years. *Bulletin of the World Health Organization* **72**, 429–45.

Murray, C. J. L., & López, A. D. (1994). Quantifying disability: data, methods and results. *Bulletin of the World Health Organization* **72**, 481–94.

Murray, C. J. L., & López, A. D., eds. (1996). *The Global Burden of Disease: a Comprehensive Assessment of Mortality and Disability from Diseases, Injuries and Risk Factors in 1990 and Projected to 2020*. Cambridge, MA: Harvard University Press.

Murray, C. J. L., Salomon, J. A., & Mathers, C. (2000). A critical examination of summary measures of population health. *Bulletin of the World Health Organization* **78**, 981–94.

Murray, C. J. L., López, A. D., Black, R., et al. (2007). Global burden of disease 2005: call for collaborators. *Lancet* **370**, 109–10.

Murray, C. J. L., Vos, T., Lozano, R., et al. (2012a). Disability-adjusted life years (DALYs) for 291 diseases and injuries in 21 regions, 1990–2010: a systematic analysis for the Global Burden of Disease Study 2010. *Lancet* **380**, 2197–223.

Murray, C. J. L., Ezzati, M., Flaxman, A., et al. (2012b). GBD 2010: design, definitions, and metrics. *Lancet* **380**, 2063–6.

Narrow, W. E., Kuhl, E. A., & Regier, D. A. (2009). DSM-V perspectives on disentangling disability from clinical significance. *World Psychiatry* **8**, 88–9.

Njenga, F. (2009). Factors that influence functional impairment and outcome of mental illness. *World Psychiatry* **8**, 95–6.

Nock, M. K., Borges, G., & Ono, Y. (2012). *Suicide: Global Perspective from the WHO World Mental Health Surveys*. New York, NY: Cambridge University Press.

Phillips, M. R. (2009). Is distress a symptom of mental disorders, a marker of impairment, both or neither? *World Psychiatry* **8**, 91–2.

Saha, S., Chant, D., Welham, J., & McGrath, J. (2005). A systematic review of the prevalence of schizophrenia. *PLoS Medicine* **2**, e141.

Salomon, J. A. (2010). New disability weights for the global burden of disease. *Bulletin of the World Health Organization* **88**, 879.

Salomon, J. A., Murray, C. J. L., Üstün, T. B., & Chatterji, S. (2003). Health state valuations in summary measures of population health. In C. J. L. Murray & D. B. Evans, eds., *Health Systems Performance Assessment: Debates, Methods and Empiricism*. Geneva: World Health Organization, pp. 409–36.

Salomon, J. A., Vos, T., Hogan, D. R., et al. (2012). Common values in assessing health outcomes from disease and injury: disability weights measurement study for the Global Burden of Disease Study 2010. *Lancet* **380**, 2129–43.

Sartorius, N. (2009). Disability and mental illness are different entities and should be assessed separately. *World Psychiatry* **8**, 86.

Sheehan, D. V., Harnett-Sheehan, K., & Raj, B. A. (1996). The measurement of disability. *International Clinical Psychopharmacology* **11** (Suppl 3), 89–95.

Simon, G. E., & Von Korff, M. (1995). Recall of psychiatric history in cross-sectional surveys: implications for epidemiologic research. *Epidemiologic Reviews* **17**, 221–7.

Susser, E., & Shrout, P. E. (2010). Two plus two equals three? Do we need to rethink lifetime prevalence? *Psychological Medicine* **40**, 895–7.

Üstün, B., & Kennedy, C. (2009). What is "functional impairment"? Disentangling disability from clinical significance. *World Psychiatry* **8**, 82–5.

Üstün, T. B., Ayuso-Mateos, J. L., Chatterji, S., Mathers, C., & Murray, C. J. (2004). Global burden of depressive disorders in the year 2000. *British Journal of Psychiatry* **184**, 386–92.

Üstün, T. B., Chatterji, S., Bickenbach, J., Kostanjsek, N., & Schneider, M. (2003). The International Classification of Functioning, Disability and Health: a new tool for understanding disability and health. *Disability and Rehabilitation* **25**, 565–71.

Üstün, T. B., Kostanjsek, N., Chatterji, S., & Rehm, J. (2010). *Measuring Health and Disability: Manual for WHO Disability Assessment Schedule (WHODAS 2.0)* Geneva: World Health Organization.

Vazquez-Barquero, L. J. (2009). The incorporation of the disability construct as an independent axis in the DSM-V and ICD-11 diagnostic systems. *World Psychiatry* **8**, 92–4.

Von Korff, M., Crane, P. K., Alonso, J., *et al.* (2008). Modified WHODAS-II provides valid measure of global disability but filter items increased skewness. *Journal of Clinical Epidemiology* **61**, 1132–43.

Vos, T., Flaxman, A. D., Naghavi, M., *et al.* (2012). Years lived with disability (YLDs) for 1160 sequelae of 289 diseases and injuries 1990–2010: a systematic analysis for the Global Burden of Disease Study 2010. *Lancet* **380**, 2163–96.

Wakefield, J. C. (2009). Disability and diagnosis: should role impairment be eliminated from DSM/ICD diagnostic criteria? *World Psychiatry* **8**, 87–8.

Weich, S., & Araya, R. (2004). International and regional variation in the prevalence of common mental disorders: do we need more surveys? *British Journal of Psychiatry* **184**, 289–90.

Weissman, M. M. (2009). Functional impairment can have different meanings. *World Psychiatry* **8**, 94.

Weissman, M. M., Bland, R. C., Canino, G. J., *et al.* (1996). Cross-national epidemiology of major depression and bipolar disorder. *JAMA* **276**, 293–9.

Whiteford, H. (2009). Clarifying the relationship between symptoms and disability: a challenge with practical implications. *World Psychiatry* **8**, 90–1.

World Bank (1993). *World Development Report 1993: Investing in Health*. Oxford: Oxford University Press.

World Health Organization (1993). *The ICD-10 Classification of Mental and Behavioural Disorders: Diagnostic Criteria for Research*. Geneva: WHO.

World Health Organization (2008). *The Global Burden of Disease: 2004 Update*. Geneva: WHO.

World Health Organization (2010). Demographic and socioeconomic statistics, population. http://apps.who.int/gho/data. Accessed November, 2010.

World Mental Health Survey Consortium (2005). WMH cross national sample: country compare document. http://www.hcp.med.harvard.edu/wmh/national_sample.php. Accessed December, 2012.

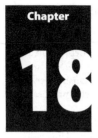

Chapter 18

The burdens of mental disorders: implications for policy

José Miguel Caldas de Almeida,
Sergio Aguilar-Gaxiola, and Gustavo Loera

Introduction

Mental disorders are commonly occurring, seriously impairing, and widely under-treated in both developed and developing countries. In short, they are a major cause of suffering, disability, and healthcare costs and they account for a great portion of the global burden of disease. For example, the landmark Global Burden of Disease (GBD) study demonstrated that, among the top 10 main causes of disability, five are mental disorders: major depression, schizophrenia, bipolar, alcohol abuse, and obsessive–compulsive disorders (Murray & López 1996). Most notably, all of these five mental disorders manifest by age 24 (Kessler *et al.* 2005). According to a 2009 report from the Committee on the Prevention of Mental Disorders and Substance Abuse, mental, emotional, and substance abuse disorders are common and costly. It is estimated that around one in five young people (14–20%) have a mental disorder, representing an estimated annual cost of $247 billion in the USA. These include costs to the individual and family, as well as to multiple sectors such as education, justice, health care, and social welfare (National Research Council & Institute of Medicine 2009).

The costs of mental illness

Despite the individual, family, community, and societal costs of mental illness, mental health continues to be a low priority on the public health agenda and for investment worldwide. Data collected by the World Health Organization (WHO) revealed that at the beginning of the new millennium 40.5% of the countries in the world had no mental health policy (World Health Organization 2001a) and that in many countries where there was a policy, the level of implementation was usually very low (Caldas de Almeida & Horvitz-Lennon 2010). Furthermore, the budget allocated to mental health has traditionally been, and still is in many countries, only a very small part of the overall health expenditure budget: the global median percentage of government health expenditure dedicated to mental health is 5.1% in high-income countries and 0.5% in low-income countries (World Health Organization 2011). The fact is that public as well as private institutions seem to lack the will to invest in improving the mental health of the population. For example, a recent report documenting a comprehensive assessment of development assistance for health (DAH) in order to promote economic, social, and political development in low-income and middle-income countries, from both public and private institutions, included no specific information on mental health financing, despite the fact that DAH grew from $5.6 billion in 1990 to $21.8 billion in 2007 (Ravishankar *et al.* 2009). Commitments to global health were made to HIV/AIDS, infectious disease control, reproductive health care, and tuberculosis control among several others, but mental health financing was not included (Institute for Health Metrics and Evaluation 2010).

This situation has been changing over the last 20 years, due in great part to the contributions from epidemiological studies showing that mental disorders (1) are highly prevalent, (2) are associated with higher levels of disability than chronic physical health conditions, and (3) affect a significant percentage of people who do not receive the treatment they need.

The Global Burden of Disease study, developed by the World Health Organization, the World Bank, and Harvard University's School of Public Health, showed that neuropsychiatric disorders are responsible for a

The Burdens of Mental Disorders, ed. Jordi Alonso, Somnath Chatterji, and Yanling He. Published by Cambridge University Press. © World Health Organization 2013.

significant proportion of the global burden of disease (Murray & López 1996, World Health Organization 2008), and this had a huge impact on policy. For the first time, it was possible to argue that there is an enormous disparity between the real burden of mental disorders and the public resources allocated for mental health care, based on data from a study conducted by some of the most credible institutions worldwide.

In keeping with the same argument on the need to invest significant resources to remedy the burden of mental disorders, the landmark book *World Mental Health Problems and Priorities in Low-Income Countries* (Desjarlais *et al.* 1995), which described the burden of mental health problems in low-income countries and highlighted the need to join efforts to decrease this burden, also played a key role in the provision of a framework for international policy makers to develop a specific agenda for action and further research on mental and social health.

These undertakings made major contributions and put the conditions in place to advance the WHO initiatives which, in 2001, gave new momentum to advocacy efforts to include mental health in the public health agenda: the 2001 World Health Day, the World Health Assembly mental health meetings and the *World Health Report* (World Health Organization 2001b). The subtitle of the World Health Report – *Mental Health: New Understanding, New Hope* – highlighted the urgency of developing new knowledge on the nature, causes, and epidemiology of mental disorders, as well as on the effectiveness of interventions and services, in order to decrease the treatment gap.

It was in this context, and acknowledging that the GBD study estimates and projections were based largely on literature reviews in conjunction with limited and isolated studies rather than on cross-national epidemiological survey data, that the World Mental Health (WMH) Survey Initiative was launched in the year 2000. Its main objective was to carry out rigorously implemented general population surveys in order to: (1) estimate the prevalence of mental disorders, (2) evaluate risk and protective factors for purposes of targeting interventions, (3) study patterns of and barriers to service use, and (4) validate estimates of disease burden worldwide (Kessler *et al.* 2006).

Purpose of this chapter

Using population-based, cross-national epidemiological data from both developed and developing countries, this volume adds to the body of scientific knowledge on the burden of mental illness. This chapter summarizes key findings from this volume that are relevant for policy, identifies and provides an overview of several components of policy development, and presents implications for public policy needed to promote the improved health and well-being of individuals with mental illness. This chapter also considers policy implications relevant to both developed and developing countries as they grapple with the challenges of the burden of mental disorders in their populations.

Key findings relevant for policy

The WMH survey results confirmed that, although some variations were found across countries, mental disorders are highly prevalent in both low- and high-income countries (Demyttenaere *et al.* 2004). Recent data from the WMH surveys on mental disorders show that low-income countries have an average 12-month prevalence of mental disorders of 14.8%, while high-income countries have an average 12-month prevalence of 16.7% (Wang *et al.* 2011).

As a result of the methodology used in the World Mental Health Survey Initiative (Kessler *et al.* 2012; see Chapter 2), the surveys' findings also made an important contribution toward better understanding of the impact of mental disorders, showing that the costs of these disorders for individuals, families, and society are extremely high, and in some areas significantly higher than the costs of physical conditions (see Chapter 14).

Disability impacts

Earlier research showed that mental disorders are associated with a significant portion of disability caused by disease (Bijl & Ravelli 2000, Andrews *et al.* 2001). The study of disability using the WHO Disability Assessment Schedule (WHODAS), included in the WMH surveys, helped to further understand the magnitude of this association, showing that mental disorders, although less prevalent than physical disorders, explain a higher share of the disability of a population than physical disorders.

Among the mental disorders included in the WMH surveys, bipolar disorder is one of the most disabling illnesses, which is not surprising given that psychotic disorders were not assessed. Then again, other conditions, such as post-traumatic stress disorder (PTSD) and panic disorder, which are usually not associated with significant disability, were also found to be amongst the most disabling conditions (see Chapter 14). The results of this study point to the inappropriateness of a "one size fits all" approach to disabilities associated with mental disorders. That is, the patterns of disability depend both on the context in which these individuals live as well as on the nature of the mental disorder from which they suffer.

The assessment of disability using the Sheehan Disability Scale (SDS) (Sheehan 1983) makes it possible to assess disability caused by a particular disorder and its interference with people's daily functioning. In particular, four role domains are examined with this scale: (1) home management, (2) ability to work, (3) social life, and (4) ability to maintain relationships with family and friends. Results obtained with SDS also showed that disability ratings for mental disorders are generally higher than for physical disorders, and this was found both in high- and low-income countries (see Chapter 13). In addition, the report by Ormel and colleagues (Chapter 13) showed that the effect of mental disorders is especially pronounced in terms of disability in social and personal relationships, which means that mental disorders have an impact that greatly exceeds the decrease in productivity, interfering with functions that are relevant for the establishment of meaningful relationships with family and friends, and for the development of social capital.

Days out of role due to mental disorders are a major source of lost human capital, as noted by Alonso *et al.* (2011), who provide clear evidence that mental disorders are among the health conditions most strongly associated with productivity loss (see Chapter 11). As mentioned earlier, bipolar disorder, PTSD, and panic disorder are related to the overall highest degree of disability, followed by generalized anxiety disorder (GAD) and social phobia. However, major depression has a unique importance from a societal perspective in terms of the impact on loss of productivity: it is one of the most important contributors to days out of role, combined with pain conditions, cardiovascular disorders, and migraine (Alonso *et al.* 2011).

The effects on productivity are not limited to full disability, and the WMH survey findings brought to light the impact of common mental disorders and physical disorders on the number of days in which individuals are partially unable to perform as usual (see Chapter 12). The study of the impact on partial disability showed that "mental disorders are associated with partial disability, over and above full disability" (Bruffaerts *et al.* 2012). This study also suggests that mental disorders are systematically associated, across countries, with about a one-third increase in partial-disability days per year compared to physical disorders. As with full disability, the impact at the population level of major depression on partial disability is especially important, given its high prevalence.

Individual and societal disadvantages

The studies included in this volume show that mental disorders can also affect many other aspects of the lives of individuals and families. For example, mental disorders are associated with a reduction in earnings. Using the human capital approach (Becker 1994, Kessler *et al.* 2008) to study the adverse individual- and societal-level effects of mental disorders in countries with different levels of income, an analysis focusing on the impact of serious mental disorders showed that, at the individual level, they are associated with a reduction in earnings equal to 29% of the median within-country earnings in high-income countries and 31% in low/lower-middle-income countries (Levinson *et al.* 2010; see Chapter 8). At the societal level, this reduction in earnings is equivalent to 1.0% of all earnings in high-income countries, 0.2% in upper-middle-income countries, and 0.4% in low/lower-middle-income countries (see Chapter 8).

Additionally, early-onset mental disorders can contribute to a higher prevalence of adult-onset physical disorders (see Chapter 7). Taking advantage of the data collected by the WMH surveys on the onset timing of mental disorders and physical disorders, it was possible to investigate the influence of early-onset mental disorders and childhood familial adversities on adult-onset physical disorders. Scott and Von Korff's study (Chapter 7) showed that early-onset mental disorders were independently associated with five of the six adult-onset chronic physical disorders studied (i.e., heart disease, asthma, arthritis, chronic back pain, severe headache), diabetes being the exception.

Common early-onset mental disorders are also strongly associated with low current household income after adjusting for education, in both high-income and upper-middle-income countries (Kawakami *et al.* 2012), and can affect the level of educational attainment (see

Chapter 4). These last findings showed that the impact on the level of educational attainment tends to be greater in high-income countries than in middle- and low-income countries, varies across countries, and is stronger for earlier educational milestones (i.e., primary and secondary school completion) than for later milestones (i.e., college entry and college graduation). Lee and colleagues (Chapter 4) emphasize that more needs to be done in secondary schools to reach out to youth and create an opportunity for teachers to work with parents and use a multi-domain developmental approach toward early detection to change the course of a mental disorder in children.

The study by McLaughlin and colleagues that examined the association of parent disorders with offspring disorders provides the first population-based estimates of the proportion of offspring mental disorders associated with parent mental disorders, suggesting that "parent disorders are associated with a meaningful proportion of disorder onset with little variation across country income groups in the overall pattern of associations" (McLaughlin *et al.* 2012). The implications from this study emphasize the importance of effective interventions for treating and improving the functioning of parents living with a mental disorder in order to prevent the development of mental disorders in their offspring (see Chapter 3).

Taken together, these new data suggest that the magnitude of the burden of mental disorders is even higher than that estimated before the WMH Survey Initiative. At the same time, the analysis of the data on the use of services has led to the realization that, despite all the efforts developed in the advancement of mental health policies (World Health Organization 2005), the treatment gap for mental disorders continues to be extremely high all over the world (Wang *et al.* 2011). The treatment gap represents the absolute difference between the true prevalence of a disorder and the treated proportion of individuals affected by the disorder. The treatment gap may also be articulated as the percentage of individuals who need care but do not receive treatment (Kohn *et al.* 2004). The treatment gap is further discussed later in this chapter.

Implications for mental health policy development

At the country level, a national mental health policy is essential for the reduction of the burden of mental disorders and the promotion of mental health in society. It expresses the values and the principles that each society considers fundamental in the sphere of mental health care, and defines the primary goals which that society strives to attain in terms of the mental health of its population in the future. Moreover, a national mental health policy: (1) states the level of priority that a government assigns to mental health in relation to other health and social policies, (2) helps to develop mental health services in a coordinated and systematic manner, and (3) identifies key stakeholders and allows different stakeholders to reach agreement (World Health Organization 2003).

Considering that a mental health policy is the best instrument to define priorities (Callahan 1995) and select the strategies indicated to systematically develop mental health services and other measures needed to address mental health problems, WHO has dedicated significant efforts to support countries in their development of national mental health policies over the last 15 years.

The WHO Mental Health Policy and Service Guidance Package (World Health Organization 2005) established the steps that governments should take in the process of mental health policy development: (1) gathering information about the mental health needs of populations, (2) gathering evidence for effective strategies, (3) consultation and negotiation, (4) exchange with other countries, (5) setting the vision, values, principles, and objectives, (6) determining areas for action, and (7) identifying the roles and responsibilities of different sectors (World Health Organization 2005).

The results of the studies in this volume have contributed to the increasing recognition of the need to complement mental health policy formulation with a mental health action plan and related performance measures, which detail the strategies, actions, and metrics that are required to realize the vision and put the objectives of the policy into practice (World Health Organization 2005). In line with this perspective, at its 65th session, held in May 2012, the World Health Assembly adopted a resolution on mental health – *the global burden of mental disorders and the need for a comprehensive, coordinated response from health and social sectors at the country level* – calling on WHO to "develop a comprehensive global mental health action plan with measurable outcomes, based on an assessment of vulnerabilities and risks, in consultation with and for consideration by Member States, covering services, policies, legislation, plans, strategies and programmes to provide treatment, facilitate recovery and prevent mental disorders, promote mental health and empower persons with mental disorders to live a full and productive life in the community" (World Health Organization 2012; p.3).

The results of the studies included in this volume have relevant implications for the way in which the different steps of mental health policy development are approached, particularly the collection of information on the needs of populations, the definition of objectives, and the selection of areas for action.

Information about the mental health needs of populations

Data-driven information about populations' needs for services is a fundamental cornerstone of mental health policy formulation. Without this information, it is not possible to identify the problems that will have to be addressed or establish priorities for action.

One of the best ways to assess needs for care is to collect information about the prevalence and incidence of mental disorders, their severity, their impact in terms of disability, and the social and economic costs. Based on a methodology that allows the collection of data about most of these factors in national representative samples of the adult population, the results from the WMH surveys offer participating countries the possibility of formulating or revising their national mental health policies based on more data-driven information. The new knowledge that the surveys have brought to light is crucial in facilitating agreements among stakeholders, generating the commitment of policy makers in the development of national mental health policies, and creating the knowledge base that must be at the core of policy formulation.

The number of countries that have joined the World Mental Health Survey Initiative illustrates the increasing recognition of the importance of sound epidemiologic data to support policy development. Furthermore, the fact that 76% of all countries which had a dedicated mental health policy in 2011 have updated or approved new mental health policies since 2005 (World Health Organization 2011) suggests that the availability of new epidemiologic data may have encouraged new efforts to develop mental health policies based on credible, data-driven information on the needs of populations.

Further efforts will now have to be made in order to acquire more accurate data on the needs for care in countries and regions that have been less thoroughly studied. Additional efforts are also needed to overcome the methodological and operational limitations that have contributed to the dearth of information regarding the specific needs of some population groups, such as people with long-term severe mental disorders.

Objectives in policy development

The three main objectives of any health policy – (1) improving the health of the population, (2) responding to people's health needs and expectations, and (3) providing financial protection against the cost of ill health (World Health Organization 2000) – can also be applied to mental healthcare policy development and advancement (World Health Organization 2005).

Having confirmed that mental disorders are not only highly prevalent, but also significant drivers of disability and largely untreated, the WMH survey results make a strong case for the inclusion of improving people's mental health as the top priority to be addressed by mental health policies.

At the same time, the results from the WMH surveys strongly suggest that mental health policies should also emphasize a set of specific objectives to address the problems that proved to have a unique importance in mental health, namely the treatment gap, comorbidity with physical disorders, and impact on disability. To do so, mental health policies should include, among their main specific objectives, issues such as decreasing the stigma associated with mental disorders, the allocation of more resources for mental health services and making better use of existing resources, the integration of mental health as part of primary care, the development of community-based care, rehabilitation through cooperation between the healthcare sector and other sectors, and the development of prevention and health promotion programs, among others.

Implications for action

Health policies, in general, address the various building blocks of mental health systems (World Health Organization 2007). Therefore, financing, leadership and governance, organization and delivery of services, information systems, human resources, and essential drug procurement must be the core components of mental health policy. Other important components include advocacy, legislation and human rights, promotion, prevention, treatment and rehabilitation, quality improvement, inter-sectoral collaboration, research and evaluation (World Health Organization 2005).

The results of the studies included in this volume reinforce the need for mental health policies that ensure the provision of financial resources commensurate with the real magnitude and impact of mental health problems. They also have important implications for other areas of action, especially leadership and governance, organization of services, workforce education and training, inter-sectoral collaboration, and prevention and health promotion. A brief description of each of these key areas for action follows.

Financing, leadership, and governance

The confirmation of the high burden of mental disorders yielded by the results of the studies discussed in this volume, together with the demonstration of the huge treatment gap in low-, middle-, and high-income countries (Wang *et al.* 2011), proves that mental health policies are urgently needed both at the national and the international level.

The WMH studies also have important implications for financing. The burden of mental disorders accounts for 7.9%, 9.5%, 14.6%, and 21.4% of the global burden of disease in low-income, lower-middle-income, upper-middle-income, and high-income countries, respectively (World Health Organization 2008), while in the same groups of countries, the median percentage of the health budget allocated to mental health is just 0.5%, 1.9%, 2.4%, and 5.1% (World Health Organization 2011). As a consequence of this huge disparity between the burden of mental disorders and the funding allocated to mental health treatment, a significant increase in financial resources for mental health is needed, particularly in low-income countries.

The allocation of more funds, however, is not enough to reduce the treatment gap of mental disorders. The analysis of barriers impeding the improvement of mental health services shows that inadequate governance and the lack of public mental health preparation of mental health leaders are also common obstacles to progress in this area (Saraceno *et al.* 2007). Furthermore, to respond to some of the issues revealed by studies resulting from the WMH surveys, such as high comorbidity between mental and physical disorders (Von Korff *et al.* 2009) and a high level of disability associated with mental disorders (Chapters 13 and 14), mental health services will have to undergo profound changes, requiring strong leadership and adequate governance.

Organization of services

Mental health services are the means by which effective interventions for mental health are organized, financed, and delivered, and the way they are organized has a strong influence on their effectiveness. It follows that the evidence that may be used to support the planning of mental services is of utmost importance. There are three significant challenges highlighted by the WMH results, each with key implications for the organization of services: (1) limited access to mental health care, (2) high comorbidity, and (3) a high level of disability associated with mental disorders.

Limited access to mental health care, found in both developed and developing countries, presents a significant challenge. According to the WMH surveys, the proportion of respondents who needed and made use of any mental health services in the 12 months before the interview was only 3.4% in low/lower-middle-income countries, and even in high-income countries the number rose only to 12% (Wang *et al.* 2011). This high prevalence of a lack of treatment, although more pronounced for the less severe mental disorders, is also unacceptably high among the serious mental disorders. For example, only 21.7%, 30.4%, and 44.4% of the people with severe mental disorders were treated in the 12 months before being interviewed in low/lower-middle-income countries, upper-middle-income countries, and high-income countries, respectively (Wang *et al.* 2011). It should be noted, however, that because of the high prevalence of mild and subthreshold cases, overall, the number of those who received treatment largely exceeds the number of untreated serious cases in every country. The treatment gap of mental disorders is a very serious problem that has no parallel with the treatment of physical disorders, as shown by the study conducted by Ormel and colleagues (Chapter 13). Although 47.6%, 58.6%, and 65.3% of physical conditions were treated in low/lower-middle-income, upper-middle-income, and high-income countries, only 5.7%, 13.6%, and 23.7% of the respondents with a mental disorder had access to treatment in the same groups of countries.

To address these problems, mental health policies have to include a range of strategies, including the allocation of more resources for the development of mental health services, the promotion of a more rational use of available resources, and the development of models of organization for services facilitating the provision of effective and efficient mental health care near the places where people usually live. This means that specific measures should be adopted to integrate mental health care into primary care services and to develop comprehensive community-based mental health services, in accordance with the specific characteristics and resources of each country.

Primary care services are less stigmatizing to people with mental disorders, and are generally more easily accessible and acceptable than specialized mental health services (World Health Organization & Wonca 2008). Moreover, for most common and acute mental disorders, they may have clinical outcomes that are as good as, or even better than, those of more specialized mental health services (World Health Organization & Wonca 2008).

The fact that a high percentage of people with serious mental disorders do not have access to treatment, while a significant number of people with mild and subthreshold disorders do receive mental health care (Wang et al. 2011), suggests that the problem is not only a lack of resources but also the inappropriate use of services and a misallocation of resources. More studies are needed in order to better understand the reasons why people with no diagnosis seek mental health care, and to better evaluate the benefits they may have received. It is very likely that, although not fulfilling all the diagnostic criteria for a mental disorder, many individuals do have significant symptoms of emotional suffering which would justify the use of some kind of intervention.

In any case, it is reasonable to think that strategies contributing to a more rational use of resources and a better organization of services, such as a clear definition of responsibilities at each level of care and an effective referral system, may lead to better treatment outcomes for less severe cases at the primary care level, while specialized services would be aimed at providing more differentiated care in the most serious cases.

In low- and middle-income countries, other strategies should also be adopted to tackle the problems of accessibility. Task shifting (i.e., the redistribution of clinical roles within health systems and healthcare teams) is one of the innovative strategies that has proven to be effective and efficient for increasing accessibility to effective mental health treatment (World Health Organization & Wonca 2008). The task-shifting approach has been used, for example, in the treatment of depression, through the development of programs including the provision of different types of intervention by community health workers (Rahman et al. 2008), non-medical health workers in primary care (Araya et al. 2003), and trained lay health workers (Rojas et al. 2007), with clinical benefits at least as significant as those seen with collaborative care programs for depression in higher-income countries.

Increasing availability and decreasing costs of new communication technologies such as telehealth/telemedicine can also open up new opportunities for increasing access to care for populations living in remote areas. Mental health policies in low/lower-middle-income and upper-middle-income countries should include specific strategies that promote the delivery of mental health interventions through cell phones, email, and other emerging technologies such as social media.

The **high comorbidity** found between mental and physical disorders (Von Korff et al. 2009) is the second key issue highlighted by the results of the WMH surveys with important implications for the organization of services. The high frequency of comorbidity suggests that mental health policies should include strategies that facilitate the development of integrated approaches to care. By diagnosing and treating both physical and mental illnesses, integrated care considers comorbidity and its effects on the individual as a whole, and meets the mental health needs of people with physical disorders, as well as the physical health needs of people with mental disorders.

Furthermore, most mental and physical disorders are chronic in course and require similar approaches to health management. There is evidence that collaborative models of care involving combinations of pharmacological and psychosocial interventions delivered in a stepped-care manner can be effective in the treatment of people with mental and physical comorbidities (Katon & Unützer 2006, Patel 2009). This evidence-based model of integrated care includes six key ingredients: (1) care management (i.e., patient education and empowerment, ongoing monitoring, and care-provider coordination); (2) evidence-based treatments (i.e., effective medication management and/or psychotherapy); (3) expert consultation for patients who are not improving; (4) systematic diagnosis and outcome tracking; (5) stepped care; and (6) technology support (i.e., creating and maintaining registries). Katon and Unützer (2006) have shown that the collaborative care model is most effective in treating depression, anxiety, and other common mental disorders in primary care settings. Research also indicates that the collaborative care model is effective in improving medical care for patients with severe mental illness (Katon & Unützer 2006). The collaborative care model has been shown to reduce suicidal ideation in depressed older patients, as well as to improve the rates of diminishing pain severity and depression in patients with arthritis (Lin *et al.* 2003).

Currently, the integration of mental health care into all levels of the general health system is consensually recognized as necessary to improve the quality of care and prevent the stigma associated with mental disorders and mental health care (World Health Organization 2001a). The results of the WMH surveys support the principle of the integration of mental health care into the general health system, suggesting that the adoption of coordinated models of care addressing the needs of people with comorbidities should be encouraged.

The rigorous identification of non-affective psychoses was not possible with the case ascertainment instruments used in the WMH surveys, a limitation that prevents us from drawing conclusions about the services specifically dedicated to patients with those mental disorders. Nevertheless, the high prevalence of non-treatment found in the group of the most severe mental disorders suggests that, along with the integration of mental health care into primary care services, it will also be necessary to develop community-based specialized services, prepared to respond to the specific needs of people with severe mental illness in locations that are not significantly remote from their homes.

Data collected for the *Mental Health Atlas* (World Health Organization 2011) show that most of the available financial resources allocated to mental health care (73% in low-income countries, 74% in middle-income countries, 54% in high-income countries) continue to be absorbed by mental hospitals, leaving very limited resources for community-based services. Therefore, community services are not regularly accessible for a significant part of the population in most countries. For instance, follow-up community care is provided by the majority of facilities in only 7%, 29%, 39%, and 45% in low-income, lower-middle-income, upper-middle-income, and high-income countries,

respectively (World Health Organization 2011). These figures emphasize the amount of work still needed in most countries to ensure the provision of community-based services to the population and to increase access to care and reduce the treatment gap.

The **high level of disability** associated with mental disorders, highlighted by the WMH surveys, shows that psychosocial rehabilitation needs to become a key component of mental health care. The huge negative impact of mental disorders on day-to-day functioning, together with the consequences this disability has for individuals, families, and society, shows that mental health services have to be designed to offer rehabilitation interventions and programs tailored to the specific challenges that people with mental disorders face. These programs may focus more on the recovery of personal or social skills, vocational rehabilitation, employment support, or housing, and in most cases they require a close collaboration between mental health services and services from other sectors (e.g., social services, criminal justice). Therefore, mental health policies should include specific strategies to integrate rehabilitation programs among the different components of mental health care.

Overall, the results from the WMH surveys support the principles of the organization of services recommended by WHO, underscoring the importance of integrating mental health care into primary care services, developing community-based care, combining prevention, treatment, and rehabilitation, and supporting early identification, intervention, and health promotion (World Health Organization 2003).

The application of these principles must be adapted to the existing level of resources. In accordance with the "balanced care model" of services proposed by Thornicroft and Tansella (2002), mental health policies should emphasize the priority of integrating mental health care into primary care services and community-based care with hospital back-up. In countries with a low level of resources, the large majority of mental disorder cases should be recognized and treated within the primary care setting, with specialist back-up to provide training, consultation for complex cases, and inpatient assessment and treatment of cases that cannot be managed in primary care. Meanwhile, countries with more resources may additionally include community mental health teams, acute inpatient care, community residential care, psychosocial rehabilitation programs, and differentiated specialized mental health services.

Human resource development

The findings in this volume provide valuable insight regarding the insufficient human resources for mental health in low- and middle-income countries, where between 76% and 85% of people with severe and persistent mental disorders receive no treatment (World Health Organization 2012). On a systems level, innovative, evidence-based educational pathways will need to be developed to meet the staffing needs for the WMH countries considered in this volume. For many people in these low-, middle-, and high-income countries, primary care professionals continue to be the main point of entry, and represent the place where their mental health journey begins and often ends. Providers of primary health care need to be trained in the current community-defined promising practices tailored to the general population (Aguilar-Gaxiola 2009). Moreover, emphasis should be placed on educational policies that focus on aligning integrated health and mental health content with secondary and higher education curricula to ensure that a well-trained workforce will be ready and competent to serve individuals in different capacities (Aguilar-Gaxiola *et al.* 2011). Given that most mental disorders have their roots in childhood and adolescence, and that the first symptoms typically occur 2–4 years before the onset of a full-blown mental disorder, thereby creating a window of opportunity when preventive programs might make a difference (National Research Council & Institute of Medicine 2009), early identification and intervention (for both physical and mental health) should be available for these high-risk children in normative environments such as school-based health programs as well as in primary care settings (Aguilar-Gaxiola 2009).

A recent recommendation for capacity building by the Latino Mental Health Concilio (Aguilar-Gaxiola *et al.* 2012) provides insight into workforce education and training resources for the development of grassroots community capacity-building strategies that focus on: (1) strengthening outreach and engagement, (2) building mental health leadership at the community level, (3) defining mental health outcomes at the community level and in terms that matter to the population being served, and (4) building local capacity aimed at reducing disparities and improving mental health outcomes.

Inter-sectoral collaboration

The associations found between mental disorders and physical disorders, especially non-communicable diseases, underscore the need for moving mental health policy forward, but they also suggest that mental health policies cannot be conceived and implemented without the participation of other sectors, particularly the social, work and employment sectors. As the results of the WMH surveys clearly show, not only is the comorbidity of mental and physical disorders very high, but these two types of disorder also share many determinants, characteristics, and consequences in terms of disability (see Chapter 14; Ormel *et al.* 2008). This is especially true for common mental disorders such as depression on the side of mental disorders, and for disorders such as chronic pain, arthritis, diabetes, and insomnia on the side of physical disorders (see Chapter 14).

One solution to improving the provision of quality care for mental disorders is to increase exposure to services by entering the physical environment of the people who are the most affected by mental disorders and organizing mental health care services in and around those environments. Being aware of the societal factors related to mental disorders, especially income, educational attainment, and employment stability, may help reduce the causes of global burden of disease. For example, school environments can provide a convenient venue for prevention and early identification, as well as for treatment programs, and this may help teachers to work more effectively with parents on the early detection of mental health symptoms in children and prevent the potential development of full-blown mental health disorders. Early identification of potential mental disorders is an important strategy, because it is during these sensitive periods of development (Barrett *et al.* 2006) that problems begin to manifest, and changing the course of a mental disorder with adequate treatment early on not only reduces health costs but also prevents unnecessary personal and family suffering. Furthermore, there is increasing evidence of the effectiveness and cost-effectiveness of interventions to prevent mental disorders, particularly in children and adolescents (World Health Organization 2012). For example, evidence has shown that the incidence of adolescent depression can be reduced and that full-blown schizophrenic episodes can be prevented (National Research Council & Institute of Medicine 2009). Hawkins and colleagues

(2008) demonstrated the long-term effects of an intervention in elementary schools in promoting positive functioning in school, work, and community. Specifically, teacher training in classroom instruction and management, child social and emotional skill development, and parent workshops produced a significant multi-varied effect across 16 primary outcome indices (e.g., preventing mental health problems, risky sexual behavior, substance misuse, and crime). Specific effects included significantly better educational and economic attainment, mental health, and sexual health 15 years after the intervention (Hawkins *et al.* 2008).

Establishing these types of links and commonalities between mental and physical disorders has helped to stimulate the development of joint approaches at the international level. The 2011 United Nations Summit on Non-Communicable Diseases represented a great opportunity to include mental health as a component of the non-communicable disease (NCDs) agenda. Due to the efforts led by the World Federation for Mental Health (WFMH), several organizations came together to promote the inclusion of mental health in the NCD agenda at that high-level meeting and in the global health and development agenda in the future. Unfortunately, in the end, mental health was briefly mentioned but was not formally included on the NCD agenda. Nonetheless, the available evidence is compelling and the outcome of other international initiatives with the same objective may be much more successful in the future. At the country level, the recognition of the links between mental and physical disorders has already had important implications in the fields of organization, coordination, and integration of services, leading to an increasing interest in the application of the chronic disease management and collaborative care models for mental disorders.

The integration of mental health into policies related to other sectors – e.g., social, education, and employment policies – is strongly reinforced by the results of the WMH surveys. In fact, given the impact of mental disorders on total and partial disability, a close articulation between mental health policy, social policies, and employment policy is of crucial importance to address the problems related to the recovery of people with mental disorders and to develop programs for the prevention of mental disorders in the workplace. The same principle applies to the integration of mental health awareness into education policies, in order to promote the mental health of children and adolescents through the collaboration of health services and schools, and to its integration with social policies related to the rights of ethnic minorities and other vulnerable groups.

One important conclusion that can be drawn from the links found between mental disorders and disability, income, education attainment, and employment is that it is not possible to address the prevention and treatment of mental disorders without an effective inter-sectoral collaboration, just as it is not possible to implement health-related development policies without the inclusion of mental health.

Societal investments in disease prevention and health promotion

The findings described in this volume emphasize the important role prevention plays in the social and economic impact of mental and later physical disorders in the general population. Clearly, multifaceted health promotion strategies that focus on disease prevention are essential to addressing the treatment gap for mental disorders in low- and middle-income countries.

Aguilar-Gaxiola (2009) noted the importance of understanding the determinants of health outcomes in populations across lifespans. Specifically, he emphasized optimizing health outcomes by balancing investments in different sectors of society (e.g., health care, education, economic development). The research presented in this volume suggests that a failure to invest in the treatment of children during the primary and secondary school years increases the likelihood of early school dropout and termination. Lack of schooling has been shown to be closely associated with an inadequate adulthood combined with limited financial opportunities, poor employment stability, low self-efficacy, diminished marital opportunities, and other later-life opportunities (Fronstin *et al.* 2005, Huurre *et al.* 2006, Freudenberg & Ruglis 2007).

Future research is needed to determine whether, and to what extent, the current poor world economy will have a long-term effect on treatment, and whether the treatment gap will continue to widen as treatment for mental disorders becomes scarce. Kawakami and colleagues (see Chapter 9) suggest carrying out longitudinal studies examining different developmental stages and different cultures to confirm findings from this volume and find developmental pathways linking early-onset mental disorders to household incomes.

Research

The results of the studies summarized in this volume underscore the importance of inter-sectoral collaborative work that focuses on the prevention and treatment of mental disorders. Many findings are noteworthy. First and foremost, consistent with previous volumes that examined data from the WMH surveys, there is an urgent need to respond to and reduce the negative impact that mental and physical health conditions have on the lives of people from different cultural and social settings. Secondly, prevention and early intervention strategies to address mental disorders and/or the course of a severe mental disorder lie at the individual and also the population level, in that such strategies must be tailored to the environment in which people live and interact. Third, in combination with the burden of disability that mental disorders create, low treatment rates suggest that more attention should be directed toward prioritizing health needs, prevention, and early intervention, and placing emphasis on social determinants of health. Finally, several of the chapters from this volume focus on the significant associations between marital and parental factors and mental disorders.

As noted by Breslau and colleagues in Chapter 5, mental disorders have a significant impact on the amount of time people devote to marital relationships. In other words, people with mental disorders have more difficulties managing interpersonal relationships over time, therefore increasing the likelihood of divorcing or separating after marriage. As a possible explanation for this negative association, previous researchers (e.g., Raj 2010) have stated that marriages between adolescents may sometimes be the result of an escape from a stressful home environment. This finding supports the notion of exploring early preventive solutions to address not only the life course of a mental disorder, but the negative impact that divorce has on the early life conditions of children and the subsequent risk for violence in marital relationships. Along similar lines, in Chapter 3 McLaughlin and colleagues explored parent psychopathology and offspring mental disorders. Their findings that a pervasive pattern of sub-additive interactions among comorbid parent disorders predicts offspring disorders contributes to the literature of the WMH surveys in that parents who live with a mental disorder are more likely to engage in negative parenting behaviors and create a stressful environment that leads to the continuation of the children's beliefs and motivations to marry in order to escape their stressful home environments.

Because the WMH survey data, examined in this comprehensive set of studies, were cross-sectional and did not explore causal mediators, the findings cannot be generalized to other populations. There are other limitations that should be noted. The first of these is that the WMH survey data has a limited capacity to advance our understanding of presumed causal mediators (see Kessler and colleagues in Chapter 2). Second, the WMH surveys did not assess which mental disorders (e.g., psychosis, substance abuse) are significantly associated with income and earnings. This is important, because such an assessment might shed light on the economic effects of early-onset mental disorders in low-income countries, where previous analyses have failed. The final limitation is the cross-sectional nature of the data presented in this volume. Future research with WMH survey data should investigate inter-sectoral collaborations with an emphasis on prevention and health promotion, rather than solely treatment, as potential solutions to the plight of mental illness. Moreover, future research should examine the social determinants of health and human capital as factors associated with reducing stigma and quality of care across multiple years.

Conclusions

The results of the WMH surveys included in this volume have important implications for policy. First, they strongly reinforce evidence supporting the urgent need to invest in the development and improvement of mental health systems, and they prove that this must be done across the board – in low-, middle-, and high-income countries. Second, they help us to understand why it is so important to integrate mental health policy into general health policy, as well as into social policies. Finally, they provide a new understanding of associated factors, course, comorbidity, impact, and treatment of mental disorders that is relevant for action in several areas of mental health policy (e.g., organization, financing and provision of services, prevention, psychosocial rehabilitation, child mental health services and interventions, inter-sectoral collaboration, workforce development and training).

The results of the surveys should strongly encourage governments to revise, update, and develop mental health policies and plans based on the existing knowledge of the burden of mental disorders, and taking into consideration the available evidence on the cost-effectiveness of services and interventions. They also call the attention of policy makers to the need to improve the provision of integrated mental health care, through strategies contributing to the development and provision of community-based services, the integration of mental health treatment and care into primary care services and general hospitals, the strengthening of psychosocial rehabilitation programs, the promotion of collaborative care models with task-shifting components, and the use of e-mental health programs. The surveys' findings also reinforce the need to further coordinate efforts at the global level to reduce the global burden of mental disorders and promote the mental health of the general population.

Finally, the surveys clearly show that further decisive efforts should be undertaken to increase the evidence base for mental health policies and plans. More epidemiological studies are needed to better understand the burden and associated factors of mental disorders, as well as the use of services by those who suffer from them, while cost-effectiveness studies will have to be developed to support evidence-based decisions related to the organization of mental health services. It has been nearly two decades since the Global Burden of Disease study demonstrated the tremendous burden of mental disorders in the functioning of individuals, a historical finding that has been replicated over and over again, and brought to light the significant treatment gap and lack of investment to remedy this huge public health challenge. The findings in this volume are a clear call to action for both public and private healthcare systems to muster political will to invest in an area of public health that has been too long neglected, in order to reduce the burden and improve people's health and quality of life in both developed and developing countries.

References

Aguilar-Gaxiola, S. (2009). Policy implications. In M. R. Von Korff, K. M. Scott, & O. Gureje, eds., *Global Perspectives on Mental–Physical Comorbidity in the WHO World Mental Health Surveys*. New York, NY: Cambridge University Press, pp. 302–12.

Aguilar-Gaxiola, S., Sribney, W. S., Raingruber, B., *et al.* (2011). Disparities in mental health status and care in the U.S. In N. Cohen & S. Galea, eds., *Population Mental Health: Evidence, Policy, and Public Health Practice*. London: Taylor and Francis, pp. 69–91.

Aguilar-Gaxiola, S., Loera, G., Méndez, L., Latino Mental Health Concilio, & Nakamoto, J. (2012). *Community-Defined Solutions for Latino Mental Health Care Disparities Project, Latino Strategic Planning Workgroup Population Report*. Sacramento, CA: UC Davis. http://www.ucdmc.ucdavis.edu/newsroom/pdf/latino_disparities.pdf. Accessed December 2012.

Alonso, J., Petukhova, M., Vilagut, G., *et al.* (2011). Days out of role due to common physical and mental conditions: results from the WHO World Mental Health surveys. *Molecular Psychiatry* **16**, 1234–46.

Andrews, G., Henderson, S., & Hall, W. (2001). Prevalence, comorbidity, disability and service uitlisation: overview of the Australian National Mental Health Survey. *British Journal of Psychiatry* **178**, 145–53.

Araya, R., Rojas, G., Fritsch, R., *et al.* (2003). Treating depression in primary care in low-income women in Santiago, Chile. *Lancet* **361**, 995–1000.

Barrett, P. M., Farrell, L. J., Ollendick, T. H., & Dadds, M. (2006). Long-term outcomes of an Australian universal prevention trial of anxiety and depression symptoms in children and youth: an evaluation of the Friends Program. *Journal of Clinical Child and Adolescent Psychology* **35**, 403–11.

Becker, G. (1994). *Human Capital: a Theoretical and Empirical Analysis with Special Reference to Education*. Chicago, IL: University of Chicago Press.

Bijl, R. V., & Ravelli, A. (2000). Current and residual functional disability associated with psychopathology: findings from the Netherlands Mental Health Survey and Incidence Study (NEMESIS). *Psychological Medicine* **30**, 657–68.

Bruffaerts, R., Vilagut, G., Demyttenaere, K., *et al.* (2012). The role of mental and physical health in partial disability around the world. *British Journal of Psychiatry* **200**, 454–61.

Caldas de Almeida, J. M., & Horvitz-Lennon, M. (2010). Mental health care reforms in Latin America: an overview of mental health care reforms in Latin America and the Caribbean. *Psychiatric Services* **61**, 218–21.

Callahan, D. (1995). Setting mental health priorities. In P. J. Boyle & D. Callahan, eds., *What Price Mental Health? The Ethics and Politics of Setting Priorities*. Washington, DC: Georgetown University Press, pp. 175–192.

Demyttenaere, K., Bruffaerts, R., Posada-Villa, J., *et al.* (2004). Prevalence, severity and unmet need for treatment of mental disorders in the World Health Organization World Mental Health (WMH) Surveys. *JAMA* **291**, 2581–90.

Desjarlais, R., Eisenberg, L., Good, B., & Kleinman, A. (1995). *World Mental Health Problems and Priorities in Low-Income Countries*. Oxford: Oxford University Press.

Freudenberg, N., & Ruglis, J. (2007). Reframing school dropout as a public health issue. *Preventing Chronic Disease* **4**, A107.

Fronstin, P., Greenberg, D. H., & Robins, P. K. (2005). The labor market consequences of childhood maladjustment. *Social Science Quarterly* **86**, 1170–95.

Hawkins, J. D., Kosterman, R., Catalano, R. F., Hill, K. G., & Abbott, R. D. (2008). Effects of social development intervention in childhood 15 years later. *Archives of Pediatric and Adolescent Medicine* **162**, 1133–41.

Huurre. T., Junkkari, H., & Aro, H. (2006). Long-term psychosocial effects of parental divorce: a follow-up study from adolescence to adulthood. *European Archives of Psychiatry and Clinical Neuroscience* **256**, 256–63.

Institute for Health Metrics and Evaluation (2010). *Financing Global Health 2010: Development Assistance and Country Spending in Economic Uncertainty*. Seattle, WA: IHME.

Katon, W., & Unützer, J. (2006). Collaborative care models for depression: time to move from evidence to practice. *Archives of Internal Medicine* **166**, 2304–6.

Kawakami, N., Abdulghani, E. A., Alonso, J., *et al.* (2012). Early-life mental disorders and adult household income in the World Mental Health surveys. *Biological Psychiatry* **72**, 228–37.

Kessler, R. C., Berglund, P., Demler, O., *et al.* (2005). Lifetime prevalence and age-of-onset distributions of DSM-IV disorders in the National Comorbidity Survey Replication. *Archives of General Psychiatry* **62**, 593–602.

Kessler, R. C., Haro, J. M., Heeringa, S. G., Pennell, B.-E., & Üstün, B. T. (2006). The World Health Organization World Mental Health Survey Initiative. *Epidemiologia e Psichiatria Sociale* **15**, 161–6.

Kessler, R. C., Heeringa, S., Lakoma, M. D., *et al.* (2008). The individual-level and societal-level effects of mental disorders on earnings in the United States: results from the National Comorbidity Survey Replication. *American Journal of Psychiatry* **165**, 703–11

Kessler, R. C., Harkness, J., Heeringa, S. G., *et al.* (2012). Methods of the World Mental Health surveys. In M. K. Nock, G. Borges, & Y. Ono, eds., *Suicide: Global Perspectives from the WHO World Mental Health Surveys*. New York, NY: Cambridge University Press, pp. 35–62.

Kohn R., Saxena, S., Levav, I., & Saraceno, B. (2004). The treatment gap in mental health care. *Bulletin of the World Health Organization* **82**, 858–66.

Levinson, D., Lakoma, M. D., Petukhova, M., *et al.* (2010). Associations of serious mental illness with earnings: results from the WHO World Mental Health surveys. *British Journal of Psychiatry* **197**, 114–21.

Lin, E. H., Katon, W., Von Korff, M., *et al.* (2003). Effect of improving depression care on pain and functional outcomes among older adults with arthritis: a randomized controlled trial. *JAMA* **290**, 2428–9.

McLaughlin, K. A., Gadermann, A. M., Hwang, I., *et al.* (2012). Parent psychopathology and offspring mental disorders in the WHO World Mental Health Surveys. *British Journal of Psychiatry* **200**, 290–9.

Murray, C. J. L., & López, A. D. (1996). *The Global Burden of Disease: a Comprehensive Assessment of Mortality and Disability from Diseases, Injuries and Risk Factors in 1990 and Projected to 2020*. Cambridge, MA: Harvard University Press.

National Research Council & Institute of Medicine. (2009). *Preventing Mental, Emotional, and Behavioral Disorders Among Young People: Progress and Possibilities*. Washington, DC: National Academies Press.

Ormel, J., Petukhova, M., Chatterji, S., *et al.* (2008). Disability and treatment of specific mental and physical disorders across the world: results from the WHO World Mental Health Surveys. *British Journal of Psychiatry* **192**, 368–75.

Patel, V. (2009). Integrating mental health care with chronic diseases in low-resource settings. *International Journal of Public Health* **54**, 1–3.

Rahman, A., Malik, A., Sikander, S., Roberts, C., & Creed, F. (2008). Cognitive behaviour therapy based intervention by community health workers for mothers with depression and their infants in rural Pakistan: a cluster-randomised controlled trial. *Lancet* **372**, 902–9.

Raj, A. (2010). When the mother is a child: the impact of child marriage on the health and human rights of girls. *Archives of Disease in Childhood* **95**, 931–5.

Ravishankar, N., Gubbins, P., Cooley, R. J., *et al.* (2009). Financing of global health: tracking development assistance for health from 1990 to 2007. *Lancet* **373**, 2113–24.

Rojas, G., Fritsch, R., Solis, J., *et al.* (2007). Treatment of postnatal depression in low-income mothers in primary-care clinics in Santiago, Chile: a randomised controlled trial. *Lancet* **370**, 1629–37.

Saraceno, B., van Ommeren, M., Batniji, R., *et al.* (2007). Barriers to improvement of mental health services in low-income and middle-income countries. *Lancet* **370**, 1164–74.

Sheehan, D. V. (1983). *The Anxiety Disease*. New York, NY: Charles Scribner's Sons.

Thornicroft, G., & Tansella, M. (2002). Balancing community-based and hospital-based mental health care. *World Psychiatry* **1**, 84–90.

Von Korff, M. R., Scott, K. M., & Gureje, O., eds. (2009). *Global Perspectives on Mental–Physical Comorbidity in the WHO World Mental Health Surveys*. New York, NY: Cambridge University Press.

Wang, P. S., Aguilar-Gaxiola, S., Al-Hamzawi, A. O., *et al.* (2011). Treated and untreated prevalence of mental disorders: results from the World Health Organization World Mental Health (WMH) surveys. In G. Thornicroft, G. Szmukler, K. Mueser, & R. Drake, eds., *Oxford Textbook of Community Mental Health*. London: Oxford University Press, pp. 50–66.

World Health Organization (2000) *World Health Report 2000 – Health Systems: Improving Performance*. Geneva: WHO.

World Health Organization (2001a). *Mental Health Resources in the World*. Geneva: WHO.

World Health Organization (2001b). *The World Health Report 2001 – Mental Health: New Understanding, New Hope.* Geneva: WHO.

World Health Organization (2003). *Organization of Services for Mental Health.* Geneva: WHO.

World Health Organization (2005). *Mental Health Policy, Plans and Programmes (updated version 2).* Mental Health Policy and Service Guidance Package. Geneva: WHO.

World Health Organization (2007). *Everybody's Business: Strengthening Health Systems to Improve Health Outcomes. WHO's Framework for Action.* Geneva: WHO.

World Health Organization (2008). *The Global Burden of Disease: 2004 Update.* Geneva: WHO.

World Health Organization (2011). *Mental Health Atlas 2011.* Geneva: WHO.

World Health Organization (2012). The global burden of mental disorders and the need for a comprehensive, coordinated response from health and social sectors at the country level. WHA65.4. Geneva: WHO.

World Health Organization & World Organization of Family Doctors (Wonca) (2008). *Integrating Mental Health into Primary Care: a Global Perspective.* Geneva: WHO & Wonca.

Chapter 19

Conclusions and future directions

Somnath Chatterji, Yanling He, and Jordi Alonso

The last three decades have seen increasing, and deserved, attention in the scientific literature focused on the impact that mental disorders have on the lives of the millions who are affected by these conditions directly or indirectly. The Global Burden of Disease (GBD) study and its periodic updates (World Health Organization 2008) have consistently shown that these groups of health conditions, traditionally relegated to "Cinderella" status, need to be recognized for the burden they produce and need the health systems to gear up and respond accordingly (World Health Organization 2012). Over these last three decades the quality of evidence underpinning these observations has increasingly improved, in large measure due to the data provided by the World Mental Health (WMH) surveys.

What have we learned?

The various chapters in this volume have examined the issues related to the impact of mental disorders from a wide variety of perspectives, both individual and societal. They have addressed the direct impacts that these disorders have on the lives of people who have them at some point in their lives in terms of the disability and stigma they experience, as well as the impacts these disorders produce on their family and the wider society at large by affecting their marriages, their earnings, and their performance in the workplace.

In summary, the key messages from this large cross-national dataset, reaffirming earlier findings and providing new evidence, are: (1) mental disorders across the world are associated with large burdens at individual and societal levels; (2) the burden of mental disorders is comparable to and often larger than that of chronic physical conditions such as arthritis, cancers, cardiovascular

disorders, diabetes, neurological disorders, chronic pain, and respiratory disorders; (3) not only are mental disorders associated with disability in a range of functioning domains that is comparable to physical health conditions, but they also lead to a large number of days of work lost due to being absent or not performing at peak levels; (4) mental disorders occurring earlier on in life lead to significantly lower earnings later during the most productive years, substantially reducing the human capital of countries; (5) mental disorders beginning early in life substantially increase the risk of physical health conditions later on (a fact that has not heretofore been adequately appreciated); (6) mental disorders, when combined with physical health conditions, produce significantly increased disability, as shown earlier in other large-scale studies (Moussavi *et al.* 2007); and (7) a range of adversities in childhood, such as having broken homes and being a victim of abuse, significantly raise the risks of a mental disorder in adulthood.

What are the strengths and limitations of this study?

The major strengths of the World Mental Health Survey Initiative are: (1) the implementation of a large-scale general population survey to capture the magnitude and impact of mental disorders in a range of high-, medium-, and low-income countries from across the world; (2) the use of a uniform methodology, not just a common instrument, but all stages of planning, training, implementation, generation of data, monitoring of quality, and analysis; (3) a methodology that allows comparisons across countries in terms of the impacts of mental and physical disorders within the same study;

(4) an epidemiological design that goes beyond prevalence to tease apart the determinants and impacts over the course of the individual's life; and (5) a study that provides systematic evidence on patterns of treatment seeking, identifies gaps, and indicates possible reasons for the discrepancies between need and receipt of care.

However, the study is not without limitations. Despite the use of standard approaches to measurements and efforts to reduce recall bias, there remains a possibility that retrospective recall of onset of mental health symptoms and conditions, adversities experienced in earlier periods in life, including traumatic events, and the severity associated with the episodes may not result in completely accurate reports. We relied on self-reports for all our chronic conditions, either as experienced by the respondent in conditions such as pain, or as told to the respondent by a healthcare provider in the case of, for example, non-communicable diseases such as heart disease or diabetes. The availability of health services has been known to influence the self-report of these conditions across and within countries where health systems may be at different levels of development (Sen 2002). Although the WHO Composite International Diagnostic Interview (CIDI) is a structured interview that was administered by trained lay interviewers in our study, and we validated the instrument against clinician assessments, it is possible that the difference we obtained in the prevalence of these conditions could to some extent be a function of how these questions are understood in different populations with different levels of exposure to surveys in general. In addition, the exercises we carried out to estimate the value that people place on a range of health conditions, and the health states associated with them, were limited by the trade-off made in the collection of this data using different methods (such as, the visual analog scale) and the time devoted to other pieces of information deemed more central to this exercise. This also highlights the fact that an exercise such as this is resource-intensive and needs to be monitored carefully when implemented. This is perhaps the reason why the WMH surveys are yet to be carried out in certain sections of the world such as sub-Saharan Africa (other than Nigeria and South Africa, which were included) and other parts of South and Southeast Asia.

What should be the response?

The preceding two chapters (Chapters 17 and 18) have pointed to some possible responses to the magnitude of the burden of mental disorders. It is abundantly clear that health systems need to gear up and scale up their response to a range of, at least, priority health conditions. These conditions have been identified by the World Health Organization, and a set of evidence-based guidelines have been recommended to bridge this gap by integrating the care of mental health disorders in primary care (World Health Organization 2010). This will require the training of healthcare professionals at all levels and a holistic people-centered approach that does not manage diseases in silos. This scale-up will need to be carefully monitored and evaluated to ensure adequate returns on investment and adequate quality, and to make mid-stream corrections as needed.

Early detection and intervention is where we are likely to have the most pay-offs. As previous results from this study show, there is a substantial gap between the first occurrence of symptoms of a mental disorder and the first contact with and treatment by health services. One major bottleneck that can be readily addressed by the health system is the early recognition of these disorders and initiation of appropriate treatment to reduce subsequent disability.

The need to intervene during the most vulnerable periods of childhood and adolescence requires engaging school health systems and educating parents to identify early signs and to manage risks in childhood that increase the likelihood of mental disorders later in life. Life skills training during early years and mental health promotion strategies can likely prevent some of these disorders in adulthood (World Health Organization 2004, Herrman et al. 2005).

It is also imperative that health systems across the world set up a regular surveillance system that is integrated within national health information systems such that the situation can be monitored over time to detect trends and drivers. These surveillance systems will need to identify a range of priority conditions for prevalence and incidence, the coverage of interventions, the quality and effectiveness of interventions, and will need to be capable of providing data that are disaggregated by age, sex, and a range of stratifiers that have been shown in this and other studies to be related to differences in the prevalence, impact, and access to treatment of mental disorders, such as education, income, geographical location, and belonging to a minority population. Such a system will have to link administrative data and that gathered from healthcare facilities with other systematic data collection efforts through periodic surveys such as the World Mental Health surveys. Finally, health information systems will need to track health expenditures for mental health and the human resources that are available to address this burden.

Where do we go from here?

In recognition of the burden of mental disorders, the global mental health community has identified a series of barriers that, if addressed through appropriate research, could be removed. The interventions resulting from this research would also be expected to be feasibly scaled up to the point where they would have a large impact. One of the key goals of this exercise was to raise the awareness of the global burden of mental disorders, and among the top 25 challenges was the need to generate cross-national evidence to understand the variance in the incidence, treatment, and outcomes of mental disorders and to develop appropriate measurement approaches to quantify the impact of these conditions (Collins *et al.* 2011).

Thus a key requirement in future exercises will be to continue to refine our measurement methods and to improve their precision and validity in making comparisons across diverse populations. The World Mental Health Survey Initiative continues to carry out research on these aspects.

Future studies also need to include children and adolescents, as well as older adults. There remain major gaps in understanding the patterns of mental disorders in children and their impacts on the lives of children and their families internationally, especially in low- and middle-income countries. These studies will be critical in targeting interventions in schools to promote mental health and prevent disorders later in life. Similarly, as the global population ages at an unprecedented rate, there is a need to understand the patterns of mental disorders in this segment of the population. The maintenance of the mental health and well-being of older adults will be imperative, if we are to capitalize on the longevity dividend. Evidence from these studies will point to the management of mental disorders coupled with chronic physical conditions, which is the rule rather than the exception in this age group.

A key strategy to address recall bias is to carry out longitudinal cohort studies that will not only track respondents over time in terms of the prevalence and incidence of mental disorders and identify risk and protective factors, but that will also monitor the evolution of disability over time to enable early identification of those at risk for disability. Ideally, if these studies could be linked to administrative data related to a range of indicators from income, employment, insurance, and healthcare utilization, they would provide a wealth of information that is currently just not available in most settings.

A major gap in the World Mental Health surveys is the lack of inclusion of major non-affective psychotic illnesses such as schizophrenia. These are some of the most disabling conditions, and they have been identified as priority public mental disorders, and yet little is known about their magnitude and their impacts in the general population, especially in low- and middle-income countries. Such studies will identify those most at risk and possibly point to non-pharmacological interventions that may prevent or delay the onset of these severely disabling conditions.

Finally, there is a need to adapt and transfer some of the methodologies developed in these general population surveys in the World Mental Health Survey Initiative to clinical settings. While general population surveys capture the entire spectrum of disorders and are reflective of the public health impact, they need to be brought to the clinic to integrate care in these settings. Strategies to rapidly screen attendees at healthcare services and provide diagnoses using standardized measurement approaches have great appeal in translating early recognition into appropriate intervention and preventing disability. The creation of such a clinical epidemiology is the need of the hour, to complement larger population-based periodic surveys and thereby truly understand and address the burden of mental disorders.

References

Collins, P. Y., Patel, V., Joestl, S. S., *et al.* (2011). Grand challenges in global mental health. *Nature* **475**, 27–30.

Herrman, H., Saxena, S., & Moodie, R. (2005). *Promoting Mental Health: Concepts, Emerging Evidence, Practice: Report of the World Health Organization, Department of Mental Health and Substance Abuse in Collaboration with the Victoria Health Promotion Foundation and the University of Melbourne.* Geneva: World Health Organization.

Moussavi, S., Chatterji, S., Verdes, E., *et al.* (2007). Depression, chronic diseases, and decrements in health: results from the World Health Surveys. *Lancet* **370**, 851–8.

Sen, A. (2002). Health: perception versus observation. *BMJ* **324**, 860–1.

World Health Organization (2004). *Prevention of Mental Disorders: Effective Interventions and Policy Options: Summary Report*. Geneva: WHO.

World Health Organization (2008). *The Global Burden of Disease: 2004 Update*. Geneva: WHO.

World Health Organization (2010). *mhGAP Intervention Guide for Mental, Neurological and Substance Use Disorders in Non-Specialized Health Settings*. Geneva: WHO.

World Health Organization (2012). *Development of a Global Mental Health Action Plan 2013–2020*. Geneva: WHO.

Appendices

Appendix Table 2.1 Sample characteristics for each of the chapters of this volume. The WMH surveys.

Chapter number and title	N	Number of surveys	Sample restrictions	Surveys excluded (reason)	Females		Not married		High school or more		Not working		Age	
					%[a]	SE	%[a]	SE	%[a]	SE	%[a]	SE	Mean	SE
3. Parent psychopathology and offspring MDs[b]	51,509	23	none	Israel, New Zealand (no parent psychopathology)	52.0	(0.3)	37.2	(0.3)	55.0	(0.4)	43.8	(0.3)	41.7	(0.1)
4. Associations between MDs and early termination of education	62,242	24	none	France (no education)	52.0	(0.3)	36.8	(0.3)	57.4	(0.3)	42.1	(0.3)	42.1	(0.1)
5. MDs, marriage, and divorce														
Marriage analysis subsample	46,126	20	none	Iraq, S. Africa, Israel, Portugal, N. Ireland (no age at first marriage)	52.1	(0.3)	36.1	(0.4)	57.9	(0.4)	38.8	(0.4)	42.6	(0.1)
Divorce analysis subsample	30,020	13	none	Iraq, S. Africa, Israel, Portugal, N. Ireland, New Zealand, ESEMeD countries[c] (no age at first marriage or age at first divorce)	52.2	(0.4)	37.6	(0.4)	57.0	(0.5)	39.1	(0.4)	41.0	(0.2)
6. Premarital MDs and risk for marital violence														
Married respondents subsample	8,766	11	Married	Colombia, PRC–Beijing/Shanghai, Ukraine, Iraq, Mexico, Romania, S. Africa, Germany, Israel, Japan, Netherlands, New Zealand, N. Ireland, Portugal (no couples sample)	50.4	(0.7)	0.0	–	52.5	(0.8)	35.6	(0.7)	45.8	(0.2)
Couples subsample	3,642		1,841 couples (couples samples)		47.3	(0.8)	0.0	–	54.6	(1.1)	34.1	(1.1)	45.9	(0.4)
7. Early-onset MDs and their links to chronic physical conditions in adulthood	25,715	13	21+ year olds; 278 respondents in N. Ireland not included (chronic conditions not assessed)	India–Pondicherry, Nigeria, PRC–Beijing/Shanghai, PRC–Shenzhen, Ukraine, Iraq, Brazil, Bulgaria, Lebanon, S. Africa, Israel, New Zealand	52.5	(0.4)	32.3	(0.5)	61.8	(0.6)	40.8	(0.5)	46.2	(0.2)
8. Association between serious mental illness and personal earnings	52,275	23	Age 18–64	Ukraine, Romania (no personal earnings)	51.2	(0.3)	36.9	(0.3)	59.9	(0.3)	34.4	(0.3)	37.4	(0.1)

Appendix Table 2.1 (cont.)

Chapter number and title	N	Number of surveys	Sample restrictions	Surveys excluded (reason)	Females		Not married		High school or more		Not working		Age	
					%	SE	%[a]	SE	%[a]	SE	%[a]	SE	Mean	SE
9. Early-onset MDs and adult household income Disability analysis subsample	44,527	23	Age 18–64, non-retired, not students	France (no education), S. Africa (no personal and/or spouse earnings)	51.2	(0.3)	31.6	(0.3)	60.6	(0.4)	25.2	(0.3)	38.0	(0.1)
Household income subsample	37,741	21	Age 18–64, non-retired, not students	France (no education), Ukraine, New Zealand, S. Africa (no personal and/or spouse earnings)	51.2	(0.4)	32.1	(0.4)	59.2	(0.4)	27.0	(0.3)	37.6	(0.1)
10. Family burden associated with mental and physical disorders	43,732	19	In most countries, random sample of respondents selected to assess family burden	PRC–Beijing/Shanghai, India–Pondicherry, New Zealand, Israel and S. Africa (no family burden information)	51.7	(0.3)	37.4	(0.3)	55.6	(0.3)	37.6	(0.3)	40.1	(0.1)
11. Days out of role associated with common mental and physical disorders	62,971	25	429 from Lebanon and 278 from N. Ireland excluded (chronic conditions not assessed)	None	51.9	(0.3)	36.5	(0.3)	57.4	(0.3)	42.0	(0.3)	42.2	(0.1)
12. Partial disability associated with common mental and physical disorders	61,259	25	429 from Lebanon and 278 from N. Ireland excluded (chronic conditions not assessed)	None	51.9	(0.3)	36.5	(0.3)	57.8	(0.3)	41.3	(0.3)	41.9	(0.1)
13. Disorder-specific disability and treatment of common mental and physical disorders	56,164	23	429 from Lebanon and 278 from N. Ireland excluded (chronic conditions not assessed); individuals with full disability excluded	Iraq, PRC–Shenzhen (no random chronic condition)	52.2	(0.3)	36.3	(0.3)	59.5	(0.3)	42.2	(0.3)	43.2	(0.1)
14. Disability associated with common mental and physical disorders	58,656	24	429 from Lebanon and 278 from N. Ireland excluded (chronic conditions not assessed)	S. Africa (no WHODAS)	51.8	(0.3)	35.6	(0.3)	58.9	(0.3)	40.3	(0.3)	42.6	(0.1)
15. Perceived health associated with common mental and physical disorders	51,344	23	429 from Lebanon and 278 from N. Ireland excluded (chronic conditions not assessed)	New Zealand, S. Africa (no perceived health variable)	51.8	(0.3)	35.7	(0.3)	58.6	(0.4)	41.6	(0.3)	42.3	(0.1)
16. Decomposing the total associations of common mental and physical disorders with perceived health	51,344	23	429 from Lebanon and 278 from N. Ireland excluded (chronic conditions not assessed)	New Zealand, S. Africa (no perceived health variable)	51.8	(0.3)	35.7	(0.3)	58.6	(0.4)	41.6	(0.3)	42.3	(0.1)

[a] Weighted %.
[b] MDs, mental disorders.
[c] ESEMeD countries: Belgium, France, Germany, Italy, the Netherlands, Spain.

Appendix Table 2.2 Design effects of 12-month prevalence estimates of major mental disorder categories by country income level. The WMH surveys.[a]

Country income level	Mood	Anxiety	Disruptive behavior	Substance	Any disorder
I. All countries	1.3	1.2	1.1	1.2	1.4
II. Cross-national combination of countries					
Low/lower-middle	1.0	1.0	0.7	1.2	1.0
Upper-middle	1.2	0.9	1.0	1.3	1.2
High	1.3	1.4	1.6	1.3	1.6
III. Low/lower-middle					
Colombia	1.1	1.1	0.8	0.9	1.2
India–Pondicherry	1.2	0.8	1.2	1.4	1.0
Iraq	0.9	1.0	0.6	1.0	0.9
Nigeria	1.1	0.9	0.9	1.0	1.0
PRC–Beijing/Shanghai	1.0	0.9	0.5	1.1	1.2
PRC–Shenzhen	0.7	1.5	0.7	–	1.0
PRC (all sites combined)	0.8	1.3	0.6	1.1	1.1
Ukraine	1.6	1.0	0.9	1.1	1.2
IV. Upper-middle					
Brazil–São Paulo	1.3	0.5	1.2	1.2	0.8
Bulgaria	1.0	1.0	1.1	1.2	0.9
Lebanon	1.2	1.0	1.4	1.0	0.9
Mexico	1.2	1.3	0.9	1.1	1.5
Romania	0.8	1.0	1.3	0.4	1.1
South Africa	1.4	1.3	0.6	1.5	1.9
V. High					
Belgium	1.2	2.0	1.6	1.0	1.6
France	1.2	0.9	0.5	0.9	1.0
Germany	0.8	1.6	1.0	1.0	1.8
Israel	1.1	0.9	–	0.6	1.1
Italy	0.8	1.0	0.8	1.0	1.1
Japan (11 cities)	1.0	1.0	0.7	1.0	0.9
Netherlands	1.1	0.8	1.0	0.9	0.6
New Zealand	1.4	1.0	–	1.2	1.2
Northern Ireland	1.2	1.0	1.0	0.8	1.4
Portugal	1.2	1.2	0.7	0.7	0.8
Spain	1.0	1.2	1.0	1.0	1.0
USA	1.3	1.6	1.4	1.8	1.8
VI. Mean D^2 across countries	1.2	1.2	1.0	1.1	1.3

[a] As described in more detail in the text, the design effect (D^2) is the square of the ratio of the standard error of the prevalence estimate using design-based methods divided by the standard error of the prevalence estimate assuming a simple random sample. D^2 represents the extent to which the design-based sample would have to increase in size to obtain the same standard error as that obtained in a simple random sample of the observed size. For example, the D^2 of 1.2 in Colombia means that the part 2 sample of 2,381 respondents would have to be 2,857 (i.e., $1.2 \times 2,381$) to achieve a design-based standard error equal in size to the standard error in a simple random sample of 2,381 respondents. – This group of disorders was not evaluated.

Appendix Table 3.1 Bivariate associations of parent psychopathology with subsequent onset of offspring lifetime mental disorders by country income level. The WMH surveys.[a]

Country income level	Types of parent disorder	Offspring disorders									
		Mood disorder		Anxiety disorder		Disruptive behavior disorder		Substance disorder		Any disorder	
		OR	(95% CI)	OR	(95% CI)	OR	(95% CI)	OR	(95% CI)	OR	(95% CI)
Low/lower-middle	I. Major depressive episode										
	Exactly 1 parent	3.3*	(2.5–4.5)	3.6*	(2.6–5.0)	4.5*	(3.0–6.7)	2.0*	(1.2–3.4)	3.3*	(2.5–4.3)
	Both parents	5.2*	(2.9–9.5)	6.6*	(3.2–13.4)	8.0*	(3.7–17.4)	0.1*	(0.1–0.1)	6.2*	(3.7–10.4)
	χ^2_2	85.7*		93.5*		71.7*		347.6*		139.7*	
	II. Generalized anxiety										
	Exactly 1 parent	3.1*	(2.2–4.4)	3.3*	(2.3–4.8)	3.8*	(2.3–6.3)	1.6	(0.8–3.1)	3.0*	(2.2–4.1)
	Both parents	5.7*	(3.0–11.0)	5.9*	(3.0–11.5)	6.5*	(1.7–24.4)	3.4*	(1.2–9.4)	5.3*	(2.5–11.0)
	χ^2_2	73.9*		61.2*		34.4*		8.1*		69.5*	
	III. Panic disorder										
	Exactly 1 parent	2.9*	(2.4–3.4)	2.8*	(2.3–3.4)	3.2*	(2.4–4.2)	2.1*	(1.7–2.6)	2.7*	(2.3–3.1)
	Both parents	3.4*	(2.2–5.2)	4.8*	(3.5–6.6)	4.7*	(2.5–8.7)	3.6*	(2.0–6.5)	4.0*	(2.9–5.5)
	χ^2_2	177.1*		182.7*		93.9*		58.9*		243.4*	
	IV. Substance abuse										
	Exactly 1 parent – mother	2.8*	(1.5–5.3)	2.5*	(1.5–4.2)	4.5*	(2.3–8.8)	6.2*	(4.0–9.5)	3.4*	(2.4–4.8)
	Exactly 1 parent – father	1.6*	(1.3–2.1)	1.7*	(1.4–2.2)	2.2*	(1.6–3.0)	2.1*	(1.5–3.1)	1.8*	(1.5–2.2)
	Both parents	2.6	(0.4–14.8)	3.3*	(1.5–7.0)	1.0	(0.1–8.6)	1.0	(0.2–5.4)	2.2*	(1.2–4.0)
	χ^2_3	26.7*		38.5*		46.1*		80.8*		84.1*	
	V. Antisocial personality disorder										
	Exactly 1 parent	2.0*	(1.4–2.9)	2.6*	(2.1–3.4)	3.3*	(2.2–4.9)	2.5*	(1.6–3.9)	2.4*	(1.9–3.2)
	Both parents	3.9*	(1.5–9.6)	7.8*	(4.9–12.5)	4.6*	(1.4–14.9)	3.2	(0.7–14.5)	5.1*	(2.7–9.9)
	χ^2_2	22.7*		131.1*		44.2*		18.4*		69.7*	
	VI. Suicide attempt										
	Exactly 1 parent	1.5*	(1.0–2.2)	1.4*	(1.0–2.0)	1.7*	(1.1–2.7)	1.6*	(1.1–2.5)	1.5*	(1.1–2.0)
	Both parents	2.0	(0.5–7.6)	0.2	(0.0–1.5)	3.6	(0.8–16.2)	0.0*	(0.0–0.0)	1.0	(0.3–4.0)
	χ^2_2	5.2		6.5*		8.8*		567.4*		8.8*	

VII. Suicide (death from suicide)[b]

Upper-middle					
Any	1.0 (0.4–2.1)	1.6 (0.8–3.1)	3.5* (1.3–9.2)	1.9 (0.8–4.3)	1.6 (0.9–2.8)
χ^2_1	0.0	1.6	6.6*	2.1	2.6
I. Major depressive episode					
Exactly 1 parent	2.3* (1.8–2.9)	2.9* (2.4–3.5)	3.7* (2.6–5.2)	2.3* (1.6–3.4)	2.7* (2.2–3.3)
Both parents	4.6* (2.5–8.5)	3.0* (1.7–5.1)	7.2* (3.8–13.8)	1.6 (0.7–4.1)	3.3* (2.1–5.4)
χ^2_2	63.4*	113.0*	89.8*	19.0*	117.0*
II. Generalized anxiety					
Exactly 1 parent	2.5* (2.0–3.1)	3.0* (2.4–3.6)	3.1* (2.1–4.7)	2.3* (1.7–3.0)	2.8* (2.3–3.3)
Both parents	3.3* (2.0–5.5)	3.5* (2.2–5.5)	7.1* (4.4–11.6)	3.0* (1.4–6.7)	3.8* (2.4–5.9)
χ^2_2	83.1*	160.6*	79.1*	39.5*	147.0*
III. Panic disorder					
Exactly 1 parent	2.1* (1.8–2.6)	2.5* (2.1–2.9)	3.1* (2.2–4.2)	2.0* (1.6–2.6)	2.4* (2.0–2.8)
Both parents	2.7* (2.0–3.6)	3.1* (2.3–4.2)	5.3* (3.4–8.5)	3.2* (2.0–5.0)	3.2* (2.5–4.0)
χ^2_2	101.8*	146.1*	84.8*	44.9*	179.6*
IV. Substance abuse					
Exactly 1 parent – mother	2.1* (1.3–3.3)	2.5* (1.6–3.9)	2.6* (1.3–5.1)	2.1* (1.1–4.1)	2.4* (1.6–3.5)
Exactly 1 parent – father	1.5* (1.2–1.8)	1.5* (1.3–1.8)	2.3* (1.6–3.3)	2.3* (1.7–2.9)	1.8* (1.5–2.1)
Both parents	1.5 (0.7–2.9)	2.1* (1.1–3.9)	3.8* (1.7–8.5)	3.6* (1.9–6.6)	2.3* (1.3–3.9)
χ^2_3	27.3*	46.6*	32.7*	54.1*	76.5*
V. Antisocial personality disorder					
Exactly 1 parent	1.8* (1.4–2.2)	1.9* (1.5–2.4)	2.8* (1.9–4.1)	2.3* (1.8–2.9)	2.1* (1.7–2.5)
Both parents	0.9 (0.3–3.4)	1.0 (0.3–3.9)	2.2 (0.5–10.2)	1.4 (0.5–4.4)	1.2 (0.4–3.7)
χ^2_2	25.6*	30.5*	29.2*	50.1*	60.7*
VI. Suicide attempt					
Exactly 1 parent	1.8* (1.3–2.3)	1.8* (1.4–2.4)	2.2* (1.3–3.7)	1.3 (0.9–1.9)	1.7* (1.4–2.2)
Both parents	0.8 (0.2–3.6)	0.7 (0.2–3.2)	1.2 (0.1–9.6)	0.9 (0.3–2.6)	0.8 (0.3–2.7)
χ^2_2	17.0*	20.7*	9.2*	2.5	22.0*

Appendix Table 3.1 (cont.)

Country income level	Types of parent disorder	Offspring disorders									
		Mood disorder		Anxiety disorder		Disruptive behavior disorder		Substance disorder		Any disorder	
		OR	(95% CI)	OR	(95% CI)	OR	(95% CI)	OR	(95% CI)	OR	(95% CI)
	VII. Suicide (death from suicide)[b]										
	Any	2.1*	(1.3–3.4)	1.3	(0.5–3.3)	0.2	(0.0–1.2)	0.6	(0.1–2.8)	1.4	(0.8–2.4)
	χ^2_1	8.9*		0.4		3.2		0.4		1.2	
High	I. Major depressive episode										
	Exactly 1 parent	2.5*	(2.2–2.8)	2.6*	(2.3–3.0)	3.3*	(2.7–4.1)	2.6*	(2.1–3.2)	2.7*	(2.3–3.0)
	Both parents	3.6*	(2.3–5.7)	4.0*	(2.6–6.0)	4.7*	(2.8–7.9)	2.8*	(1.4–5.7)	3.8*	(2.5–5.6)
	χ^2_2	185.8*		211.0*		138.3*		92.0*		248.1*	
	II. Generalized anxiety										
	Exactly 1 parent	2.7*	(2.4–3.0)	3.0*	(2.6–3.4)	3.8*	(3.1–4.6)	2.5*	(2.1–3.1)	2.9*	(2.6–3.3)
	Both parents	4.3*	(3.3–5.8)	5.2*	(4.0–6.8)	6.3*	(4.3–9.1)	5.4*	(3.2–8.9)	5.1*	(4.0–6.6)
	χ^2_2	362.7*		489.0*		220.0*		132.9*		570.6*	
	III. Panic disorder										
	Exactly 1 parent	2.2*	(1.9–2.4)	2.5*	(2.3–2.7)	2.6*	(2.1–3.1)	2.4*	(2.0–2.8)	2.4*	(2.2–2.6)
	Both parents	3.7*	(2.3–5.8)	4.9*	(3.2–7.5)	4.2*	(2.8–6.5)	3.2*	(1.9–5.2)	4.1*	(2.9–6.0)
	χ^2_2	229.8*		452.7*		126.0*		115.6*		416.6*	
	IV. Substance abuse										
	Exactly 1 parent – mother	2.1*	(1.6–2.8)	2.0*	(1.6–2.5)	3.2*	(2.3–4.4)	3.3*	(2.5–4.2)	2.5*	(2.0–3.1)
	Exactly 1 parent – father	2.0*	(1.8–2.3)	2.1*	(1.9–2.3)	2.5*	(1.9–3.3)	2.6*	(2.2–3.1)	2.2*	(2.0–2.5)
	Both parents	2.8*	(2.0–4.0)	3.5*	(2.5–4.8)	3.8*	(2.6–5.7)	5.0*	(3.3–7.6)	3.6*	(2.7–5.0)
	χ^2_3	238.4*		308.0*		106.8*		329.4*		361.2*	
	V. Antisocial personality disorder										
	Exactly 1 parent	2.3*	(2.0–2.8)	2.6*	(2.3–2.9)	3.7*	(2.9–4.7)	2.8*	(2.4–3.4)	2.8*	(2.4–3.1)
	Both parents	3.1*	(2.3–4.1)	4.0*	(3.2–5.1)	4.7*	(2.8–7.7)	5.8*	(2.9–11.4)	4.3*	(3.1–5.8)
	χ^2_2	128.8*		326.8*		128.1*		144.4*		286.8*	

VI. Suicide attempt

Exactly 1 parent	1.8*	(1.6–2.1)	1.8*	(1.5–2.1)	2.5*	(1.9–3.2)	2.1*	(1.6–2.7)	1.9*	(1.7–2.2)
Both parents	3.9*	(1.8–8.8)	4.8*	(2.2–10.7)	5.5*	(2.6–11.9)	1.3	(0.4–4.5)	4.1*	(2.1–8.1)
χ^2_2	80.8*		63.1*		62.2*		38.8*		86.0*	

VII. Suicide (death from suicide)[b]

Any	1.7*	(1.1–2.8)	1.3	(0.7–2.3)	0.2*	(0.0–0.5)	2.0	(0.8–5.0)	1.5	(0.9–2.5)
χ^2_1	5.2*		0.6		8.7*		2.4		2.8	

[a] Assessed in the part 2 sample. Models control for country, person-year, age, and sex.
[b] Parent death from suicide is a time-varying predictor; all other parent disorders are considered time-invariant.
* Significant at the 0.05 level, two-sided test.

Appendix Table 3.2 Multivariate associations of parent psychopathology with subsequent onset of offspring lifetime mental disorders based on an additive model by country income level. The WMH surveys.[a]

Country income level	Types of parent disorder	Offspring disorders									
		Mood disorder		Anxiety disorder		Disruptive behavior disorder		Substance disorder		Any disorder	
		OR	(95% CI)	OR	(95% CI)	OR	(95% CI)	OR	(95% CI)	OR	(95% CI)
Low/lower-middle											
	I. Major depressive episode										
	Exactly 1 parent	1.8*	(1.3–2.7)	1.9*	(1.4–2.6)	2.3*	(1.4–3.6)	1.7	(0.9–3.2)	1.9*	(1.5–2.4)
	Both parents	2.1	(0.9–4.5)	3.1*	(1.4–7.0)	4.0*	(1.6–10.0)	0.1*	(0.0–0.1)	3.1*	(1.6–6.0)
	χ^2_2	11.0*		23.4*		16.3*		237.5*		32.9*	
	II. Generalized anxiety										
	Exactly 1 parent	1.2	(0.8–1.9)	1.2	(0.8–1.8)	1.2	(0.6–2.3)	0.7	(0.2–1.8)	1.1	(0.8–1.6)
	Both parents	1.4	(0.6–3.6)	1.1	(0.5–2.3)	1.0	(0.2–4.9)	1.1	(0.3–4.2)	1.1	(0.5–2.5)
	χ^2_2	1.1		0.8		0.2		0.9		0.4	
	III. Panic disorder										
	Exactly 1 parent	2.4*	(2.0–2.9)	2.3*	(1.8–2.8)	2.4*	(1.8–3.3)	1.8*	(1.4–2.4)	2.2*	(1.9–2.6)
	Both parents	2.4*	(1.5–3.8)	3.3*	(2.2–4.8)	3.0*	(1.5–5.8)	3.2*	(1.7–6.1)	2.8*	(2.0–4.1)
	χ^2_2	86.9*		64.0*		36.9*		30.0*		104.1*	
	IV. Substance abuse										
	Exactly 1 parent – mother	1.9*	(1.0–3.6)	1.7	(0.9–3.2)	3.0*	(1.5–6.0)	5.4*	(3.4–8.5)	2.5*	(1.6–3.7)
	Exactly 1 parent – father	1.2	(1.0–1.6)	1.2	(1.0–1.5)	1.5*	(1.1–2.0)	1.7*	(1.2–2.5)	1.3*	(1.1–1.6)
	Both parents	0.8	(0.1–6.0)	0.6*	(0.4–0.9)	0.2	(0.0–2.9)	0.2	(0.0–3.4)	0.5	(0.2–1.2)
	χ^2_3	7.0		17.0*		17.3*		58.8*		32.1*	
	V. Antisocial personality disorder										
	Exactly 1 parent	1.1	(0.7–1.6)	1.5*	(1.1–2.0)	1.6	(0.9–2.6)	1.4	(0.8–2.4)	1.3	(1.0–1.8)
	Both parents	1.9	(0.7–5.6)	5.1*	(2.9–9.0)	3.3*	(1.5–7.4)	3.4	(0.8–14.9)	3.3*	(1.7–6.2)
	χ^2_2	1.5		33.7*		10.4*		4.5		15.6*	
	VI. Suicide attempt										
	Exactly 1 parent	1.1	(0.7–1.6)	0.9	(0.6–1.2)	0.9	(0.5–1.5)	1.1	(0.6–1.8)	0.9	(0.7–13)
	Both parents	1.1	(0.3–3.5)	0.1*	(0.0–0.7)	1.4	(0.3–5.4)	0.0*	(0.0–0.0)	0.5	(0.1–1.8)
	χ^2_2	0.2		6.3*		0.4		628.8*		1.2	
	VII. Suicide (death from suicide)[b]										
	Any	0.9	(0.4–1.9)	1.5	(0.8–3.1)	3.2*	(1.1–9.0)	1.5	(0.6–3.8)	1.5	(0.9–2.6)
	χ^2_1	0.1		1.5		4.9*		0.8		2.0	
	Global χ^2_{14}	279.0*		498.5*		254.1*		1161.0*		485.2*	

Upper-middle					
I. Major depressive episode					
Exactly 1 parent	1.2 (0.9-1.6)	1.4* (1.1-1.8)	1.5* (1.0-2.3)	1.1 (0.7-1.9)	1.3* (1.0-1.7)
Both parents	2.0* (1.0-3.7)	1.1 (0.5-2.1)	1.6 (0.8-3.6)	0.5 (0.2-1.8)	1.2 (0.7-2.1)
χ^2_2	4.9	8.7*	4.8	1.9	5.3
II. Generalized anxiety					
Exactly 1 parent	1.6* (1.2-2.1)	1.6* (1.3-2.1)	1.4 (0.9-2.1)	1.3 (0.9-1.9)	1.6* (1.3-2.0)
Both parents	1.5 (0.8-2.8)	1.4 (0.8-2.5)	1.7 (0.9-3.3)	1.3 (0.5-3.3)	1.5 (0.8-2.6)
χ^2_2	13.5*	18.5*	3.4	1.9	15.8*
III. Panic disorder					
Exactly 1 parent	1.7* (1.4-2.0)	1.9* (1.5-2.2)	2.1* (1.5-2.9)	1.7* (1.3-2.2)	1.8* (1.5-2.1)
Both parents	1.8* (1.3-2.5)	2.1* (1.5-2.9)	2.9* (1.6-5.2)	2.4* (1.4-4.1)	2.1* (1.6-2.7)
χ^2_2	32.8*	54.0*	24.6*	17.5*	67.3*
IV. Substance abuse					
Exactly 1 parent – mother	1.2 (0.8-1.8)	1.3 (0.8-2.0)	1.1 (0.5-2.4)	1.1 (0.5-2.6)	1.2 (0.8-1.9)
Exactly 1 parent – father	1.2 (0.9-1.4)	1.1 (0.9-1.4)	1.6* (1.1-2.5)	1.8* (1.4-2.4)	1.3* (1.1-1.6)
Both parents	1.1 (0.6-2.1)	1.5 (0.9-2.8)	2.3* (1.0-5.0)	3.2* (1.7-6.0)	1.7* (1.0-2.8)
χ^2_3	2.5	4.1	8.6*	25.3*	15.2*
V. Antisocial personality disorder					
Exactly 1 parent	1.3* (1.0-1.7)	1.4* (1.1-1.8)	1.6* (1.1-2.4)	1.6* (1.2-2.1)	1.5* (1.2-1.7)
Both parents	0.7 (0.3-1.9)	0.9 (0.4-2.0)	1.3 (0.5-3.8)	1.0 (0.3-3.0)	0.9 (0.5-1.9)
χ^2_2	6.2*	8.4*	5.6	12.7*	16.8*
VI. Suicide attempt					
Exactly 1 parent	1.2 (0.9-1.5)	1.1 (0.9-1.4)	1.1 (0.7-1.8)	0.9 (0.6-1.3)	1.1 (0.9-1.3)
Both parents	0.6 (0.2-1.8)	0.5 (0.2-1.5)	0.4 (0.1-2.2)	0.4 (0.1-1.4)	0.5 (0.2-1.1)
χ^2_2	1.8	2.5	1.4	2.6	3.4
VII. Suicide (death from suicide)[b]					
Any	2.0* (1.2-3.5)	1.4 (0.6-3.0)	0.2 (0.0-1.2)	0.7 (0.1-3.1)	1.4 (0.8-2.3)
χ^2_1	6.2*	0.6	3.0	0.3	1.3
Global χ^2_{14}	201.0*	300.2*	223.9*	152.2*	328.2*
High					
I. Major depressive episode					
Exactly 1 parent	1.2* (1.0-1.4)	1.1 (1.0-1.3)	1.2 (0.9-1.6)	1.2 (0.8-1.6)	1.1 (1.0-1.3)
Both parents	1.1 (0.7-1.9)	1.0 (0.6-1.7)	1.0 (0.6-1.5)	0.7 (0.3-2.1)	1.0 (0.6-1.6)
χ^2_2	4.8		1.9	1.6	3.1
II. Generalized anxiety					
Exactly 1 parent	1.7* (1.5-2.0)	1.8* (1.6-2.1)	2.0* (1.6-2.5)	1.4* (1.1-1.8)	1.7* (1.5-2.0)
Both parents	1.7* (1.0-2.9)	1.9* (1.1-3.1)	1.8* (1.0-3.2)	1.6 (0.7-3.9)	1.7* (1.1-2.8)
χ^2_2	42.9*	72.8*	31.0*	5.7	68.8*

Appendix Table 3.2 (cont.)

Country income level / Types of parent disorder	Offspring disorders									
	Mood disorder		Anxiety disorder		Disruptive behavior disorder		Substance disorder		Any disorder	
	OR	(95% CI)	OR	(95% CI)	OR	(95% CI)	OR	(95% CI)	OR	(95% CI)
III. Panic disorder										
Exactly 1 parent	1.6*	(1.5–1.9)	1.9*	(1.7–2.1)	1.7*	(1.4–2.0)	1.8*	(1.5–2.2)	1.8*	(1.6–2.0)
Both parents	1.9*	(1.2–3.0)	2.6*	(1.7–3.8)	1.6*	(1.1–2.4)	2.0*	(1.2–3.5)	2.2*	(1.6–3.1)
χ^2_2	63.3*		159.7*		41.1*		36.9*		143.9*	
IV. Substance abuse										
Exactly 1 parent – mother	1.2	(0.8–1.6)	1.1	(0.9–1.4)	1.5*	(1.1–2.2)	2.1*	(1.5–2.9)	1.4*	(1.1–1.8)
Exactly 1 parent – father	1.5*	(1.3–1.7)	1.4*	(1.3–1.6)	1.5*	(1.1–2.1)	2.0*	(1.6–2.4)	1.5*	(1.4–1.7)
Both parents	1.7*	(1.1–2.4)	1.9*	(1.4–2.6)	1.8*	(1.1–2.7)	3.5*	(2.4–5.2)	2.1*	(1.6–2.9)
χ^2_3	44.9*		42.9*		12.0*		109.6*		65.7*	
V. Antisocial personality disorder										
Exactly 1 parent	1.4*	(1.1–1.7)	1.5*	(1.3–1.8)	2.1*	(1.6–2.8)	1.5*	(1.2–1.8)	1.6*	(1.4–1.8)
Both parents	1.2	(0.7–2.0)	1.4	(0.9–2.3)	1.8	(0.9–3.4)	2.1	(0.9–5.0)	1.6	(0.9–2.7)
χ^2_2	9.7*		35.5*		26.0*		18.2*		44.1*	
VI. Suicide attempt										
Exactly 1 parent	1.1	(0.9–1.3)	1.0	(0.8–1.2)	1.2	(0.9–1.5)	1.1	(0.8–1.5)	1.1	(0.9–1.3)
Both parents	1.4	(0.6–3.2)	1.4	(0.6–3.0)	1.3	(0.5–3.4)	0.4	(0.1–1.2)	1.1	(0.5–2.5)
χ^2_2	1.3		0.6		1.5		3.2		0.6	
VII. Suicide (death from suicide)[b]										
Any	1.4	(0.9–2.1)	1.0	(0.6–1.7)	0.1*	(0.0–0.3)	1.7	(0.7–4.1)	1.2	(0.8–1.8)
χ^2_1	1.9		0.0		21.6*		1.7		0.9	
Global χ^2_{14}	655.2*		1084.4*		714.0*		638.1*		1188.2*	

[a] Assessed in the part 2 sample. Models include dummy variables for all parent mental disorders and control for country, person-year, age, and sex.

[b] Parent death from suicide is a time-varying predictor; all other parent disorders are not time-varying.

* Significant at the 0.05 level, two-sided test.

Appendix Table 3.3 Multivariate associations between number of parent mental disorders and subsequent onset of offspring lifetime mental disorders. The WMH surveys.[a]

Country income level	Number of parent disorders	Offspring disorders									
		Mood disorder		Anxiety disorder		Disruptive behavior disorder		Substance disorder		Any disorder	
		OR	(95% CI)	OR	(95% CI)	OR	(95% CI)	OR	(95% CI)	OR	(95% CI)
Low/lower-middle	I. Number of maternal disorders[b]										
	1	2.2*	(1.8–2.7)	2.2*	(1.9–2.7)	2.2*	(1.6–3.0)	2.3*	(1.8–2.9)	2.2*	(1.9–2.6)
	2	2.9*	(2.0–4.4)	2.5*	(1.6–3.8)	3.4*	(1.9–6.1)	2.0*	(1.2–3.4)	2.5*	(1.8–3.7)
	3+	3.7*	(2.5–5.5)	3.8*	(2.6–5.6)	5.7*	(3.5–9.1)			3.8*	(2.8–5.2)
	χ^2_3	111.2*		102.6*		67.7*		50.0*		162.0*	
	II. Number of paternal disorders[b]										
	1	1.4*	(1.1–1.7)	1.4*	(1.2–1.7)	1.8*	(1.3–2.5)	1.7*	(1.3–2.2)	1.5*	(1.3–1.7)
	2	1.9*	(1.2–3.0)	2.6*	(1.6–4.5)	2.1*	(1.2–3.7)	1.4	(0.9–2.4)	2.2*	(1.5–3.4)
	3	1.6	(0.8–3.3)	2.1*	(1.4–3.3)					1.4	(0.7–2.7)
	4+	3.0*	(1.9–4.6)	3.2*	(2.1–4.9)					2.5*	(1.6–3.8)
	χ^2_4	15.9*		28.5*		20.3*		12.7*		49.7*	
	Global χ^2_7	225.5*		268.7*		185.4*		91.4*		372.5*	
Upper-middle	I. Number of maternal disorders[b]										
	1	1.9*	(1.6–2.3)	2.1*	(1.8–2.5)	2.1*	(1.4–2.9)	1.6*	(1.2–2.1)	2.0*	(1.7–2.3)
	2	1.8*	(1.3–2.6)	1.7*	(1.1–2.6)	1.8*	(1.1–2.9)	1.6	(1.0–2.8)	1.7*	(1.2–2.4)
	3	2.7*	(1.8–4.2)	3.3*	(2.3–4.9)	4.4*	(2.8–6.9)	1.7	(1.0–2.9)	2.9*	(2.0–4.1)
	4+	3.0*	(1.9–4.6)	3.2*	(2.1–4.9)					3.3*	(2.3–4.8)
	χ^2_4	73.9*		116.2*		47.3*		16.3*		111.4*	
	II. Number of paternal disorders[b]										
	1	1.3*	(1.1–1.5)	1.4*	(1.2–1.6)	1.7*	(1.2–2.3)	1.7*	(1.3–2.2)	1.4*	(1.3–1.6)
	2	1.4*	(1.1–1.9)	1.8*	(1.3–2.3)	2.5*	(1.7–3.7)	2.3*	(1.6–3.4)	1.9*	(1.5–2.3)
	3	1.7*	(1.1–2.5)	1.5*	(1.0–2.3)	2.6*	(1.6–4.4)	2.6*	(1.4–5.0)	2.2*	(1.5–3.3)
	4+									1.1	(0.6–2.2)
	χ^2_4	15.2*		26.5*		28.2*		32.6*		55.0*	
	Global χ^2_8	157.5*		222.9*		171.1*		95.8*		265.9*	
High	I. Number of maternal disorders[b]										
	1	1.7*	(1.5–1.9)	1.9*	(1.7–2.1)	1.9*	(1.5–2.3)	1.9*	(1.5–2.2)	1.8*	(1.7–2.0)
	2	2.1*	(1.8–2.5)	2.2*	(1.9–2.6)	2.5*	(1.9–3.4)	2.3*	(1.7–3.1)	2.3*	(1.9–2.7)
	3	3.0*	(2.4–3.7)	3.1*	(2.5–3.9)	4.1*	(3.0–5.6)	2.5*	(1.5–4.2)	3.2*	(2.6–3.9)
	4	2.0*	(1.5–2.7)	2.2*	(1.5–3.2)	3.7*	(2.4–5.8)	4.5*	(3.1–6.4)	2.5*	(1.7–3.6)
	5			3.2*	(2.1–4.8)					3.6*	(2.2–5.8)
	6+									3.2	(0.9–10.6)
	χ^2_5	214.3*		356.5*		161.3*		148.7*		377.9*	

Appendix Table 3.3 (cont.)

Country income level	Number of parent disorders	Offspring disorders									
		Mood disorder		Anxiety disorder		Disruptive behavior disorder		Substance disorder		Any disorder	
		OR	(95% CI)	OR	(95% CI)	OR	(95% CI)	OR	(95% CI)	OR	(95% CI)
	II. Number of paternal disorders[b]										
	1	1.8*	(1.6–2.0)	1.8*	(1.6–2.0)	1.8*	(1.5–2.1)	1.9*	(1.6–2.2)	1.8*	(1.7–2.0)
	2	1.8*	(1.5–2.2)	2.0*	(1.7–2.3)	2.5*	(1.7–3.8)	2.2*	(1.8–2.7)	2.0*	(1.7–2.4)
	3	2.6*	(1.8–3.6)	2.5*	(1.9–3.4)	2.6*	(1.8–3.8)	1.9*	(1.1–3.4)	2.4*	(1.8–3.2)
	4	2.8*	(2.0–4.1)	3.6*	(2.9–4.4)	3.1*	(2.0–4.8)	3.2*	(1.8–5.7)	3.7*	(2.7–5.1)
	5			1.8	(0.9–3.4)					1.8	(0.9–3.7)
	6+									2.0*	(1.1–3.7)
	X^2_5	161.4*		384.5*		72.9*		109.5*		328.0*	
	Global X^2_{10}	710.3*		1412.0*		393.0*		372.8*		1048.6*	

[a] Assessed in the part 2 sample. Models include dummy variables for number of parent mental disorders and control for country, person-year, age, and sex.

[b] For number of parental disorders, the last odds ratio represents the odds of that number or more. For example, for mood disorders, the last odds ratio for number of maternal disorders in high-income countries represents 4 or more maternal disorders.

* Significant at the 0.05 level, two-sided test.

Appendix Table 3.4 Multivariate associations of types and number of parent mental disorders and offspring mental disorders by country income level. The WMH surveys.[a]

Country income level		Mood disorder		Anxiety disorder		Disruptive behavior disorder		Substance disorder		Any disorder	
		OR	(95% CI)	OR	(95% CI)	OR	(95% CI)	OR	(95% CI)	OR	(95% CI)
Low/lower-middle	Types of parent disorder										
	I. Major depressive episode										
	Exactly 1 parent	2.3*	(1.5–3.5)	2.5*	(1.6–3.8)	2.2*	(1.3–3.8)	2.0*	(1.2–3.4)	2.3*	(1.7–3.2)
	Both parents	3.1*	(1.4–6.7)	4.3*	(2.0–9.3)	4.4*	(1.6–12.1)	0.1*	(0.0–0.1)	4.4*	(2.3–8.2)
	χ^2_2	16.0*		24.9*		12.3*		179.9*		37.2*	
	II. Generalized anxiety										
	Exactly 1 parent	1.7*	(1.0–2.7)	1.5	(1.0–2.5)	1.3	(0.6–2.8)	1.0	(0.3–3.4)	1.5	(1.0–2.4)
	Both parents	3.0	(1.0–9.1)	1.8	(0.7–4.4)	1.4	(0.2–8.6)	2.2	(0.4–12.2)	1.9	(0.7–5.2)
	χ^2_2	5.1		3.3		0.3		1.7		3.3	
	III. Panic disorder										
	Exactly 1 parent	2.5*	(2.1–3.0)	2.4*	(1.9–3.0)	2.4*	(1.7–3.4)	1.9*	(1.4–2.4)	2.3*	(2.0–2.7)
	Both parents	2.7*	(1.9–4.0)	3.8*	(2.6–5.4)	3.1*	(1.6–6.0)	3.9*	(2.2–6.9)	3.4*	(2.5–4.6)
	χ^2_2	114.9*		88.1*		33.9*		42.8*		144.3*	
	IV. Substance abuse										
	Exactly 1 parent – mother	2.4*	(1.3–4.7)	2.2*	(1.2–4.2)	2.9*	(1.4–6.0)	5.7*	(3.5–9.2)	2.9*	(1.9–4.5)
	Exactly 1 parent – father	1.3	(1.0–1.6)	1.2	(1.0–1.5)	1.6*	(1.2–2.2)	1.9*	(1.3–2.8)	1.4*	(1.1–1.7)
	Both parents	1.2	(0.2–8.9)	1.2	(0.5–2.5)	0.2	(0.0–3.1)	0.4	(0.0–6.9)	1.0	(0.4–2.5)
	χ^2_3	10.6*		9.2*		19.7*		62.3*		41.3*	
	V. Antisocial personality disorder										
	Exactly 1 parent	1.3	(0.8–2.0)	1.6*	(1.1–2.3)	1.9*	(1.1–3.1)	2.2*	(1.3–3.8)	1.7*	(1.2–2.3)
	Both parents	3.2*	(1.3–8.2)	7.4*	(3.8–14.3)	3.7*	(1.4–10.0)	5.8*	(1.0–32.4)	5.3*	(2.6–10.9)
	χ^2_2	6.5*		35.9*		11.4*		11.9*		25.6*	
	VI. Suicide attempt										
	Exactly 1 parent	1.2	(0.8–1.8)	1.0	(0.7–1.5)	0.9	(0.5–1.7)	1.4	(0.8–2.2)	1.1	(0.8–1.5)
	Both parents	1.4	(0.4–4.5)	0.1*	(0.0–0.8)	1.5	(0.3–7.0)	0.0*	(0.0–0.0)	0.6	(0.2–2.3)
	χ^2_2	1.3		4.7		0.5		270.1*		1.0	
	VII. Suicide (death from suicide)[b]										
	Any	1.0	(0.5–2.2)	1.7	(0.9–3.2)	3.3*	(1.2–9.2)	1.7	(0.6–4.5)	1.7	(1.0–3.0)
	χ^2_1	0.0		2.3		5.3*		1.2		3.8	
	VIII. Global tests for types										
	Global χ^2_{14}	174.6*		179.5*		88.1*		802.1*		256.0*	
	χ^2_{12} for difference among types	20.7		35.4*		15.0		570.9*		38.1*	

Appendix Table 3.4 (cont.)

Country income level		Offspring disorders									
		Mood disorder		Anxiety disorder		Disruptive behavior disorder		Substance disorder		Any disorder	
		OR	(95% CI)	OR	(95% CI)	OR	(95% CI)	OR	(95% CI)	OR	(95% CI)
Number of parent disorders											
I. Number of maternal disorders[c]											
	2	0.7	(0.4–1.2)	0.6	(0.3–1.1)	1.2	(0.6–2.3)	0.7	(0.3–1.8)	0.7	(0.4–1.1)
	3+	0.4*	(0.2–0.9)	0.5	(0.2–1.0)	1.0	(0.4–2.5)			0.5*	(0.3–1.0)
	χ^2_2	5.4		4.1		0.3		0.6		4.3	
II. Number of paternal disorders[c]											
	2	0.9	(0.5–1.5)	1.2	(0.7–2.0)	0.7	(0.3–1.4)	0.4*	(0.2–0.8)	0.9	(0.6–1.5)
	3	0.4	(0.2–1.0)	0.5*	(0.2–0.9)					0.3*	(0.1–0.7)
	4+									0.4*	(0.2–0.8)
	χ^2_3	3.6		6.2*		1.1		5.7*		10.5*	
III. Global test for number											
	Global χ^2_5	6.8		6.5		1.8		6.4*		10.7	
Upper-middle	**Types of parent disorder**										
I. Major depressive episode											
	Exactly 1 parent	1.5*	(1.1–2.1)	2.1*	(1.6–2.7)	1.7	(1.0–3.0)	1.3	(0.8–2.3)	1.8*	(1.4–2.4)
	Both parents	3.1*	(1.6–6.3)	2.1*	(1.1–4.1)	2.1	(0.7–5.9)	0.7	(0.2–2.8)	2.2*	(1.3–4.0)
	χ^2_2	13.2*		30.2*		3.6		2.2		18.6*	
II. Generalized anxiety											
	Exactly 1 parent	1.9*	(1.5–2.5)	2.3*	(1.8–2.8)	1.6*	(1.0–2.4)	1.5	(1.0–2.2)	2.1*	(1.7–2.5)
	Both parents	2.5*	(1.2–5.0)	3.1*	(1.7–5.6)	2.8*	(1.4–5.2)	1.6	(0.6–4.1)	2.9*	(1.7–4.9)
	χ^2_2	27.3*		55.2*		10.1*		3.8		57.4*	
III. Panic disorder											
	Exactly 1 parent	1.8*	(1.5–2.1)	2.1*	(1.7–2.5)	2.2*	(1.5–3.2)	1.7*	(1.3–2.3)	2.0*	(1.7–2.3)
	Both parents	2.2*	(1.6–3.1)	2.7*	(1.9–3.9)	3.3*	(1.7–6.5)	2.5*	(1.4–4.6)	2.7*	(2.0–3.6)
	χ^2_2	41.7*		70.7*		21.1*		16.9*		82.9*	
IV. Substance abuse											
	Exactly 1 parent – mother	1.4	(0.8–2.6)	1.8*	(1.1–3.2)	1.1	(0.5–2.5)	1.2	(0.5–3.2)	1.5	(0.9–2.7)
	Exactly 1 parent – father	1.2	(1.0–1.5)	1.2	(0.9–1.4)	1.7*	(1.1–2.7)	1.9*	(1.3–2.6)	1.4*	(1.2–1.7)
	Both parents	1.3	(0.7–2.6)	2.1*	(1.1–3.8)	2.6*	(1.2–5.4)	3.4*	(1.7–6.8)	2.2*	(1.3–3.9)
	χ^2_3	6.3		11.4*		9.6*		20.6*		23.4*	

V. Antisocial personality disorder					
Exactly 1 parent	1.5* (1.1–2.0)	1.6* (1.2–2.0)	1.7* (1.2–2.5)	1.7* (1.2–2.2)	1.7* (1.4–2.0)
Both parents	0.9 (0.3–2.4)	1.2 (0.5–2.8)	1.4 (0.4–4.2)	1.2 (0.4–3.7)	1.2 (0.5–2.5)
χ^2_2	8.5*	11.9*	7.7*	12.3*	30.7*
VI. Suicide attempt					
Exactly 1 parent	1.4* (1.0–1.8)	1.5* (1.1–2.0)	1.2 (0.8–2.0)	1.0 (0.6–1.5)	1.3* (1.1–1.7)
Both parents	1.0 (0.3–2.7)	1.0 (0.3–2.9)	0.6 (0.1–3.1)	0.4 (0.1–1.7)	1.1 (0.5–2.6)
χ^2_2	4.4	7.6*	1.2	1.5	5.9
VII. Suicide (death from suicide)[b]					
Any	2.3* (1.4–3.9)	1.7 (0.7–3.9)	0.3 (0.1–1.4)	0.7 (0.2–3.3)	1.6 (1.0–2.8)
χ^2_1	10.3*	1.4	2.4	0.2	3.2
VIII. Global tests for types					
Global χ^2_{14}	103.9*	169.9*	48.1*	61.2*	192.0*
χ^2_{12} for difference among types	24.7*	64.4*	17.3	21.7*	37.0*
Number of parent disorders					
I. Number of maternal disorders[c]					
2	0.7 (0.5–1.0)	0.5* (0.3–0.7)	0.7 (0.4–1.1)	0.9 (0.5–1.5)	0.6* (0.4–0.8)
3	0.6* (0.3–0.9)	0.4* (0.3–0.7)	0.8 (0.3–1.8)	0.7 (0.3–1.6)	0.5* (0.3–0.7)
4+	0.4* (0.2–0.9)	0.2* (0.1–0.5)			0.3* (0.2–0.6)
χ^2_3	6.4	30.5*	2.4	1.0	19.2*
II. Number of paternal disorders[c]					
2	0.8 (0.6–1.1)	0.9 (0.7–1.2)	0.9 (0.5–1.5)	0.9 (0.6–1.5)	0.8 (0.6–1.0)
3	0.5* (0.3–0.8)	0.4* (0.2–0.6)	0.5 (0.2–1.2)	0.8 (0.4–1.7)	0.6* (0.4–0.9)
4+					0.2* (0.1–0.5)
χ^2_3	6.9*	14.4*	2.9	0.5	17.4*
III. Global test for number					
Global χ^2_6	10.3	38.6*	5.0	1.3	27.9*
Types of parent disorder					
I. Major depressive episode					
Exactly 1 parent	1.6* (1.3–1.9)	1.7* (1.4–2.0)	1.5* (1.1–2.0)	1.3 (0.9–1.8)	1.6* (1.4–1.9)
Both parents	1.9* (1.2–3.1)	2.4* (1.6–3.6)	1.4 (0.7–2.8)	0.9 (0.3–3.0)	2.0* (1.3–3.1)
χ^2_2	23.3*	36.3*	6.8*	2.7	32.4*
II. Generalized anxiety					
Exactly 1 parent	2.1* (1.8–2.5)	2.5* (2.1–2.9)	2.3* (1.7–3.2)	1.5* (1.1–2.0)	2.2* (1.9–2.6)
Both parents	2.9* (1.7–4.9)	3.9* (2.4–6.3)	2.7* (1.3–5.4)	2.3 (0.8–6.9)	3.2* (2.0–5.2)
χ^2_2	68.7*	132.6*	29.4*	7.5*	101.5*

High

Appendix Table 3.4 (cont.)

Country income level

	Offspring disorders									
	Mood disorder		Anxiety disorder		Disruptive behavior disorder		Substance disorder		Any disorder	
	OR	(95% CI)	OR	(95% CI)	OR	(95% CI)	OR	(95% CI)	OR	(95% CI)
III. Panic disorder										
Exactly 1 parent	1.8*	(1.6–2.1)	2.1*	(1.9–2.4)	1.8*	(1.5–2.2)	1.9*	(1.5–2.3)	2.0*	(1.8–2.2)
Both parents	2.5*	(1.6–3.8)	4.2*	(2.9–6.2)	1.9*	(1.2–3.0)	2.2*	(1.2–4.1)	3.3*	(2.4–4.6)
χ^2_2	76.9*		216.3*		36.3*		36.2*		171.0*	
IV. Substance abuse										
Exactly 1 parent – mother	1.7*	(1.2–2.4)	1.7*	(1.3–2.2)	1.8*	(1.1–3.0)	2.1*	(1.5–2.9)	1.9*	(1.5–2.5)
Exactly 1 parent – father	1.6*	(1.4–1.8)	1.6*	(1.5–1.8)	1.6*	(1.2–2.1)	2.1*	(1.7–2.6)	1.7*	(1.5–1.9)
Both parents	2.2*	(1.5–3.2)	2.9*	(2.1–4.0)	2.0*	(1.1–3.5)	3.8*	(2.5–5.9)	3.0*	(2.2–4.1)
χ^2_3	77.5*		94.4*		14.8*		90.5*		127.0*	
V. Antisocial personality disorder										
Exactly 1 parent	1.7*	(1.4–2.1)	2.1*	(1.8–2.4)	2.3*	(1.7–3.1)	1.7*	(1.4–2.2)	2.1*	(1.8–2.4)
Both parents	2.1*	(1.3–3.4)	3.3*	(2.3–4.9)	2.6*	(1.4–5.0)	2.5*	(1.1–5.5)	3.1*	(2.1–4.6)
χ^2_2	30.9*		111.2*		31.6*		22.8*		115.3*	
VI. Suicide attempt										
Exactly 1 parent	1.4*	(1.2–1.6)	1.4*	(1.2–1.6)	1.4*	(1.0–2.0)	1.2	(0.9–1.6)	1.4*	(1.3–1.7)
Both parents	2.8*	(1.3–5.9)	3.2*	(1.9–5.6)	2.2	(0.8–5.8)	0.4	(0.1–1.5)	2.3*	(1.3–4.0)
χ^2_2	21.2*		31.7*		5.7		3.1		29.8*	
VII. Suicide (death from suicide)[b]										
Any	1.6*	(1.0–2.5)	1.4	(0.8–2.4)	0.1*	(0.0–0.3)	2.0	(0.8–4.9)	1.6	(1.0–2.5)
χ^2_1	3.9*		1.1		19.3*		2.5		3.7	
VIII. Global tests for types										
Global χ^2_{14}	235.4*		430.8*		119.9*		152.3*		521.1*	
χ^2_{12} for difference among types	25.5*		46.8*		52.2*		35.1*		38.0*	
Number of parent disorders[c]										
I. Number of maternal disorders[c]										
2	0.7*	(0.6–0.9)	0.6*	(0.5–0.8)	0.9	(0.6–1.2)	1.0	(0.7–1.5)	0.7*	(0.6–0.8)
3	0.6*	(0.4–0.9)	0.4*	(0.3–0.6)	0.8	(0.4–1.4)	0.7	(0.4–1.2)	0.5*	(0.4–0.7)
4	0.2*	(0.1–0.4)	0.2*	(0.1–0.3)	0.3*	(0.1–0.9)	0.7	(0.4–1.5)	0.2*	(0.2–0.4)
5			0.1*	(0.1–0.3)					0.2*	(0.1–0.4)
6+									0.1*	(0.0–0.4)
χ^2_5	35.8*		60.1*		5.8		2.7		47.4*	

II. Number of paternal disorders[c]

	OR	(95% CI)	OR	(95% CI)	OR	(95% CI)	OR	(95% CI)	OR	(95% CI)
2	0.7*	(0.5–0.9)	0.8	(0.5–1.2)	0.6*	(0.5–0.8)	0.8	(0.6–1.1)	0.6*	(0.5–0.8)
3	0.6*	(0.4–0.8)	0.6*	(0.3–1.0)	0.4*	(0.3–0.6)	0.5	(0.2–1.1)	0.4*	(0.3–0.6)
4	0.3*	(0.2–0.5)	0.4	(0.1–1.2)	0.3*	(0.2–0.5)	0.6	(0.2–1.8)	0.5*	(0.3–0.7)
5					0.1*	(0.0–0.2)			0.1*	(0.1–0.3)
6+									0.1*	(0.0–0.2)
χ^2_5	21.6*		4.1		49.8*		5.8		54.9*	

III. Global test for number

Global χ^2_{10}	44.5*		7.6		81.5*		7.4		72.6*	

[a] Assessed in the part 2 sample. Models include dummy variables for both type and number of parent mental disorders and control for country, person-year, age, and sex.

[b] Parent death from suicide is a time-varying predictor; all other parent disorders are not time-varying.

[c] For number of parental disorders, the last odds ratio represents the odds of that number or more. For example, for mood disorders, the last odds ratio for maternal disorders in high-income countries represents 4 or more maternal disorders. No variable for exactly one parent disorder is included in the model, as this value is redundant with the information on types of disorders.

* Significant at the 0.05 level, two-sided test.

Appendix 7

Respondents were classified as having experienced **physical abuse** when they indicated that, when they were growing up, their father or mother (includes biological, step, or adoptive parent) slapped, hit, pushed, grabbed, shoved, or threw something at them, or that they were beaten up as a child by the persons who raised them.

For **sexual abuse**, the following questions were asked: "The next two questions are about sexual assault. The first is about rape. We define this as someone either having sexual intercourse with you or penetrating your body with a finger or object when you did not want them to, either by threatening you or using force, or when you were so young that you didn't know what was happening. Did this ever happen to you?"; and "Other than rape, were you ever sexually assaulted or molested?" Sexual abuse was the only adversity where information was not collected that would distinguish whether the perpetrator was a family member or someone else. However, previous research using a similar measure but which did allow such a distinction showed that a good indirect way to distinguish family versus non-family sexual abuse is to ask about number of instances of victimization, with cases involving one or two instances typically perpetrated by a stranger and those involving three or more instances typically perpetrated by a family member. In the WMH surveys, therefore, respondents who reported that any of these experiences occurred to them three times or more were coded as having experienced sexual abuse (within the family context).

For the assessment of **neglect**, two neglect scales were created. These were based on responses to the neglect items: "How often were you made to do chores that were too difficult or dangerous for someone your age?"; "How often were you left alone or unsupervised when you were too young to be alone?"; "How often did you go without things you needed like clothes, shoes, or school supplies because your parents or caregivers spent the money on themselves?"; "How often did your parents or caregivers make you go hungry or not prepare regular meals?"; "How often did your parents or caregivers ignore or fail to get you medical treatment when you were sick or hurt?" The **serious** neglect scale was the sum of the number of neglect items where the respondent replied "often" or "sometimes," plus 1 if the respondent rated either of his/her parents as having spent little or no effort in watching over them to ensure they had a good upbringing. The **severe** neglect scale was the sum of the

number of neglect items where respondents replied "often," plus 1 if the respondent rated either of his/her parents as having spent no effort in watching over them to ensure they had a good upbringing. Both the serious and severe neglect scales ranged from 0 to 6. For the final definition of **neglect**, the respondent had to have a score of at least 1 on the severe neglect scale and at least 2 on the serious neglect scale.

(Note that the coding of the **neglect** domain was determined empirically on the basis of frequency distributions, to derive estimates in keeping with existing literature on the prevalence of these experiences in the general population.)

For **parental death**, **parental divorce**, or **other parental loss**, respondents were first asked whether they lived with both of their parents when they were being brought up. If respondents replied in the negative, they were asked: "Did your biological mother or father die, were they separated or divorced, or was there some other reason?" According to their answers to these questions, respondents were classified as having experienced parental death (when they indicated that one or both parents died), parental divorce (when they indicated that their parents divorced), or other parental loss (when they replied that they were adopted, went to boarding school, were in foster care, or left home before the age of 16).

For **parental mental disorder** the following questions were asked. **Parental depression** was assessed with: "During the years you were growing up, did (*woman/man who raised the respondent*) ever have periods lasting two weeks or more where (*she/he*) was sad or depressed most of the time?"; and "During the time when (*his/her*) depression was at its worst, did (*he/she*) also have other symptoms like low energy, changes in sleep or appetite, and problems with concentration?" **Parental generalized anxiety disorder** (GAD) was assessed with: "During the time you were growing up, did (*woman/man who raised the respondent*) ever have periods of a month or more when (*she/he*) was constantly nervous, edgy, or anxious?"; and "During the time (*her/his*) nervousness was at its worst, did (*she/he*) also have other symptoms like being restless, irritable, easily tired, and difficulty falling asleep?" **Parental panic disorder** was assessed with: "Did (*woman/man who raised the respondent*) ever complain about anxiety attacks where all of a sudden (*she/he*) felt frightened, anxious, or panicky?" Respondents who replied positively on the diagnostic items for any of these mental disorders were then asked: (a) whether these symptoms occurred all or most of the time, (b) whether these symptoms interfered a lot with the life or activities of the parent or the person who raised the respondent, and (c) whether their parents sought professional help for this problem. If respondents replied affirmatively on (c), and either on (a) or (b), they were coded as respondents with parental depression, parental GAD, or parental panic disorder.

Similarly, **parental substance use disorder** was assessed with the following items: (criterion a) "Did (*woman/man who raised the respondent*) ever have a problem with alcohol or drugs?"; and (criterion b) "Did (*he/she*) have this problem during all, most, some, or only a little of your childhood?" Respondents who replied positively on the first and "all" or "most" on the second item were then asked whether the problem interfered a lot with life or activities of the man or woman who raised the respondent (criterion c), or whether they had sought professional help for this problem (criterion d). Those respondents who replied affirmatively on criteria (a) and (b), and on either (c) or (d), were coded as having had parents with a substance use disorder.

Parental criminal behavior was assessed by the following questions: "Was (*woman/man who raised the respondent*) ever involved in criminal activities like burglary or selling stolen property?"; and "Was (*woman/man who raised the respondent*) ever arrested or sent to prison?" Respondents who replied positively on either question were classified as having experienced criminal behaviour in the family.

Respondents were coded as having experienced **family violence** when they indicated that they "were often hit, shoved, pushed, grabbed, or slapped while growing up" or "witnessed physical fights at home, like when your father beat up your mother."

Family economic adversity was coded positive if there was a positive response to either item (a) or item (b). Item (a) was: "During your childhood and adolescence, was there ever a period of six months or more when your family received money from a government assistance program like Welfare, Aid to Families with Dependent Children, General Assistance, or Temporary Assistance for Needy Families?" (This item was modified to be relevant to the welfare programs in each country where the survey was administered). Item (b) was: If there was no male head of the family and the female head did *not* work all or most of the time during the respondent's childhood; or, if there was no female head of the family and the male head did *not* work all or most of the respondent's childhood; or, if there was no female head and no male head of the family.

Appendix 8

Chapter 8 updates the analyses from an earlier report (Levinson *et al.* 2010), but uses the same GLM specification based on analysis of competing models in the new surveys, which showed that no other model considered here out-performed that initially preferred model. Based on this result, we did not rerun the simulations reported here with the larger set of surveys. At the time these simulations were carried out, the number of countries available for analysis was too small to allow results to be decomposed into the three income groups (high, upper-middle, low/lower-middle) considered in this volume. As a result, the tables and figures reported in this appendix present results only for two country income groups (high-income countries on the one hand, and low/lower-middle/upper-middle-income countries on the other) rather than the three used in the chapter.

Appendix Table 8.1 Goodness-of-fit tests for the competing models by country income level. The WMH surveys.

Country income level	Mean squared error (MSE)	Kurtosis[a]	Park test Estimate	(SE)
Low/lower-middle/upper-middle				
I. One-part models				
OLS: constant variance, linear link function	102.8	3.3	1.9	(0.02)
GLM: constant variance, ln link function	102.3	3.8	1.1	(0.02)
GLM: constant variance, sqrt link function	266.8	3.3	1.5	(0.02)
GLM: variance proportional to mean, ln link function	102.2	6.0	2.1	(0.02)
GLM: variance proportional to mean, sqrt link function	102.4	2.8	1.9	(1.9)
GLM: variance proportional to mean-sq, ln link function	102.5	3.6	2.1	(0.02)
GLM: variance proportional to mean-sq, sqrt link function	102.8	3.7	2.0	(0.02)
II. Two-part models				
OLS: constant variance, linear link function	165.6	6.4	2.0	(0.04)
GLM: constant variance, ln link function	166.0	7.1	0.9	(0.02)
GLM: constant variance, sqrt link function	201.6	6.2	0.8	(0.02)
GLM: variance proportional to mean, ln link function	165.4	4.3	2.5	(0.02)
GLM: variance proportional to mean, sqrt link function	165.4	5.9	2.4	(0.03)
GLM: variance proportional to mean-sq, ln link function	166.2	9.8	2.5	(0.02)
GLM: variance proportional to mean-sq, sqrt link function	165.6	11.3	2.5	(0.03)
High				
I. One-part models				
OLS: constant variance, linear link function	2.0	5.8	1.1	(0.06)
GLM: constant variance, ln link function	2.0	4.9	1.1	(0.04)
GLM: constant variance, sqrt link function	2.0	4.3	1.1	(0.04)
GLM: variance proportional to mean, ln link function	2.0	5.4	1.2	(0.04)
GLM: variance proportional to mean, sqrt link function	2.0	5.0	1.1	(0.04)
GLM: variance proportional to mean-sq, ln link function	2.0	4.8	1.2	(0.03)
GLM: variance proportional to mean-sq, sqrt link function	2.0	6.8	1.2	(0.03)
II. Two-part models				
OLS: constant variance, linear link function	2.4	7.4	1.5	(0.04)
GLM: constant variance, ln link function	2.4	23.4	1.6	(0.05)
GLM: constant variance, sqrt link function	2.4	6.9	1.6	(0.05)
GLM: variance proportional to mean, ln link function	2.4	9.9	1.6	(0.05)
GLM: variance proportional to mean, sqrt link function	2.4	8.0	1.6	(0.06)
GLM: variance proportional to mean-sq, ln link function	2.4	13.7	1.6	(0.05)
GLM: variance proportional to mean-sq, sqrt link function	2.4	7.2	1.6	(0.05)

[a] Log of the residuals.

Appendix Table 8.2 Coefficients for the best-fitting model of the association between SMI and normalized earnings by country income level. The WMH surveys.

Country income level	Females		Males	
	Coeff[a]	(95% CI)	Coeff[a]	(95% CI)
Model 1: any earnings in previous 12 months				
Low/lower-middle	0.8	(0.6 – 1.3)	0.3*	(0.2 – 0.7)
Upper-middle	0.8*	(0.6 – 1.0)	0.8	(0.5 – 1.4)
High	0.5*	(0.4 – 0.6)	0.4*	(0.3 – 0.5)
Model 2: amount of earnings in the total sample				
Low/lower-middle	−0.1	(−0.3 – 0.2)	−0.6*	(−0.8 – −0.3)
Upper-middle	−0.6*	(−1.1 – −0.1)	0.1	(−0.3 – 0.4)
High	−0.4*	(−0.5 – −0.3)	−0.4*	(−0.6 – −0.3)
Model 3: amount of earnings among those with any earnings				
Low/lower-middle	0.03	(−0.2 – 0.2)	−0.3*	(−0.6 – 0.0)
Upper-middle	−0.5	(−1.2 – 0.1)	0.03	(−0.3 – 0.4)
High	−0.2*	(−0.3 – −0.1)	−0.2*	(−0.4 – −0.1)

[a] The coefficients reported here come from multiple regression equations in which SMI was the predictor of primary interest and the outcomes were a dichotomous measure of having any earnings (yes/no) in the total sample (model 1), amount of earnings in the total sample (model 2), or amount of earnings among those with any earnings (model 3). Model 1 used a logistic link function. Models 2–3 were generalized linear models (GLMs) that used a logarithmic link function and assumed that outcome prediction error variance was proportional to predicted values. Controls were included in all models for respondent age, age-squared, education, marital status, household size, country, four dummy variables defining substance abuse dependence in the 12 months before interview (alcohol dependence, alcohol abuse without dependence, drug dependence, drug abuse without dependence), and four dummy variables defining lifetime prevalence of the same substance abuse dependence variables. The model 1 coefficients are odds ratios (ORs) produced by exponentiation of the regression coefficients based on model 1. The models 2–3 coefficients are GLM coefficients.
* Significant at the 0.05 level, two-sided test.

Appendix Table 9.1 Goodness-of-fit tests for the competing models. The WMH surveys.

Model	MSE	Kurtosis	Park test Estimate	(SE)
Normalized total household income				
OLS: constant variance, linear link function	0.406	15.6	1.09	(0.05)
GLM: constant variance, ln link function	0.406	17.5	0.98	(0.06)
GLM: constant variance, square root link function	0.406	14.2	1.03	(0.06)
GLM: variance proportional to mean, ln link function	0.407	20.0	1.01	(0.06)
GLM: variance proportional to mean, square root link function	0.406	16.2	1.07	(0.06)
GLM: variance proportional to mean squared, ln link function	0.406	13.6	2.33	(0.13)
GLM: variance proportional to mean squared, square root link function	0.406	13.6	2.38	(0.12)
Normalized other household income				
OLS: constant variance, linear link function	0.830	57.0	1.39	(0.06)
GLM: constant variance, ln link function	0.828	32.0	1.34	(0.06)
GLM: constant variance, square root link function	0.829	58.0	1.37	(0.06)
GLM: variance proportional to mean, ln link function	0.828	47.8	1.37	(0.06)
GLM: variance proportional to mean, square root link function	0.829	45.1	1.40	(0.06)
GLM: variance proportional to mean squared, ln link function	0.829	83.9	3.76	(0.17)
GLM: variance proportional to mean squared, square root link function	0.830	44.2	3.79	(0.17)
Normalized personal earnings				
OLS: constant variance, linear link function	0.674	13.3	0.99	(0.03)
GLM: constant variance, ln link function	0.679	19.2	1.02	(0.03)
GLM: constant variance, square root link function	0.671	13.9	1.14	(0.02)
GLM: variance proportional to mean, ln link function	0.685	12.9	0.92	(0.03)
GLM: variance proportional to mean, square root link function	0.677	11.4	1.05	(0.02)
GLM: variance proportional to mean squared, ln link function	0.677	18.9	2.48	(0.07)
GLM: variance proportional to mean squared, square root link function	0.676	14.3	2.54	(0.06)
Normalized spouse's earnings				
OLS: constant variance, linear link function	1.224	25.4	1.49	(0.04)
GLM: constant variance, ln link function	1.224	13.1	1.56	(0.02)
GLM: constant variance, square root link function	1.222	34.8	1.58	(0.02)
GLM: variance proportional to mean, ln link function	1.230	21.4	1.54	(0.02)
GLM: variance proportional to mean, square root link function	1.228	16.4	1.58	(0.02)
GLM: variance proportional to mean squared, ln link function	1.227	14.8	4.00	(0.06)
GLM: variance proportional to mean squared, square root link function	1.227	21.3	4.09	(0.06)

Appendix Table 9.2 Lifetime prevalence estimates of early-onset disorders among male respondents who were in the age range 18–64 at the time of interview by country income level. The WMH surveys.

Types of disorder	Country income level							
	All countries		Low/lower-middle		Upper-middle		High	
	%	(SE)	%	(SE)	%	(SE)	%	(SE)
Mood disorders								
Bipolar	0.8	(0.1)	0.4	(0.1)	0.7	(0.1)	1.4	(0.2)
Major depression or dysthymia	2.5	(0.1)	1.5	(0.2)	1.3	(0.2)	3.7	(0.2)
Anxiety disorders								
Agoraphobia	0.3	(0.0)	0.3	(0.1)	0.3	(0.1)	0.3	(0.1)
Generalized anxiety	0.6	(0.1)	0.3	(0.1)	0.4	(0.1)	0.9	(0.1)
Panic disorder	0.6	(0.1)	0.3	(0.1)	0.3	(0.1)	0.8	(0.1)
Post-traumatic stress	0.7	(0.1)	0.1	(0.0)	0.4	(0.1)	1.1	(0.1)
Separation anxiety[a]	2.7	(0.2)	2.0	(0.4)	2.4	(0.3)	3.3	(0.3)
Social phobia	3.0	(0.1)	1.0	(0.1)	1.8	(0.2)	5.5	(0.3)
Specific phobia	5.2	(0.2)	4.3	(0.3)	4.3	(0.4)	6.5	(0.4)
Disruptive behavior disorders								
Attention-deficit/hyperactivity[b]	2.6	(0.2)	0.7	(0.1)	2.1	(0.3)	5.0	(0.5)
Conduct disorder[c]	3.4	(0.2)	1.9	(0.4)	2.1	(0.3)	5.3	(0.4)
Intermittent explosive disorder	3.7	(0.2)	2.3	(0.2)	2.2	(0.3)	6.9	(0.5)
Oppositional-defiant disorder[d]	3.3	(0.2)	4.3	(0.7)	1.5	(0.3)	4.3	(0.4)
Substance disorders								
Alcohol abuse[e]	4.0	(0.2)	1.5	(0.2)	2.5	(0.3)	6.2	(0.3)
Alcohol abuse with dependence	0.8	(0.1)	0.3	(0.1)	0.6	(0.1)	1.1	(0.1)
Drug abuse[e]	2.0	(0.1)	0.4	(0.1)	0.8	(0.1)	4.4	(0.3)
Drug abuse with dependence	0.5	(0.1)	0.1	(0.0)	0.3	(0.1)	1.1	(0.2)
Total number of disorders								
Exactly 1 disorder	9.6	(0.3)	7.7	(0.4)	8.4	(0.6)	11.5	(0.5)
Exactly 2 disorders	3.3	(0.1)	1.8	(0.2)	3.0	(0.3)	4.5	(0.2)
Exactly 3 disorders	1.4	(0.1)	0.7	(0.1)	1.0	(0.2)	2.1	(0.2)
Exactly 4 disorders	0.6	(0.1)	0.2	(0.1)	0.5	(0.1)	0.9	(0.1)
5+ disorders	0.9	(0.1)	0.1	(0.0)	0.4	(0.2)	1.7	(0.1)
(n)		(16,564)		(5,654)		(3,310)		(7,600)

[a] Age is restricted to ≤ 44 for India, Lebanon, Belgium, Germany, Italy, Netherlands, and Spain; age is restricted to ≤ 39 for Nigeria and PRC–Beijing/Shanghai.
[b] Age is restricted to ≤ 44 for Colombia, India, Bulgaria, Lebanon, Mexico, Belgium, Germany, Italy, Netherlands, Portugal, Spain, and USA.
[c] Age is restricted to ≤ 44 for Colombia, India, Bulgaria, Lebanon, Mexico, Belgium, Germany, Italy, Netherlands, Portugal, Spain, and USA; age is restricted to ≤ 39 for Nigeria and PRC–Beijing/Shanghai.
[d] Age is restricted to ≤ 44 for Colombia, Mexico, Belgium, Germany, Italy, Netherlands, Portugal, Spain, and USA.
[e] With or without dependence.

Appendix Table 9.3 Lifetime prevalence estimates of early-onset DSM-IV/CIDI disorders among female respondents who were in the age range 18–64 at the time of interview by country income level. The WMH surveys.

Types of disorder	Country income level							
	All countries		Low/lower-middle		Upper-middle		High	
	%	(SE)	%	(SE)	%	(SE)	%	(SE)
Mood disorders								
Bipolar	0.7	(0.1)	0.3	(0.1)	0.5	(0.1)	1.2	(0.1)
Major depression or dysthymia	4.0	(0.1)	2.0	(0.2)	3.6	(0.3)	5.6	(0.2)
Anxiety disorders								
Agoraphobia	0.8	(0.1)	0.9	(0.2)	1.2	(0.2)	0.6	(0.1)
Generalized anxiety	1.1	(0.1)	0.5	(0.2)	0.8	(0.2)	1.6	(0.1)
Panic disorder	0.9	(0.1)	0.5	(0.1)	0.7	(0.1)	1.3	(0.1)
Post-traumatic stress	1.7	(0.1)	0.2	(0.1)	1.2	(0.2)	2.8	(0.2)
Separation anxiety[a]	4.3	(0.2)	2.7	(0.3)	3.4	(0.3)	5.8	(0.3)
Social phobia	3.9	(0.2)	1.3	(0.2)	3.3	(0.2)	6.6	(0.3)
Specific phobia	1.2	(0.3)	7.7	(0.5)	10.9	(0.6)	11.9	(0.4)
Disruptive behavior disorders								
Attention-deficit/hyperactivity[b]	1.6	(0.1)	0.4	(0.1)	1.1	(0.2)	3.3	(0.3)
Conduct disorder[c]	1.6	(0.1)	0.5	(0.1)	0.7	(0.1)	3.1	(0.3)
Intermittent explosive disorder	2.0	(0.1)	1.3	(0.1)	1.8	(0.2)	3.3	(0.2)
Oppositional-defiant disorder[d]	2.7	(0.2)	2.4	(0.4)	1.5	(0.3)	3.6	(0.4)
Substance disorders								
Alcohol abuse[e]	1.1	(0.1)	0.1	(0.0)	0.7	(0.1)	1.8	(0.1)
Alcohol abuse with dependence	0.2	(0.0)	0.0	(0.0)	0.1	(0.0)	0.4	(0.1)
Drug abuse[e]	0.8	(0.1)	0.1	(0.1)	0.3	(0.1)	1.8	(0.2)
Drug abuse with dependence	0.3	(0.0)	0.0	(0.0)	0.1	(0.1)	0.6	(0.1)
Total number of disorders								
Exactly 1 disorder	12.2	(0.3)	10.0	(0.5)	13.6	(0.6)	13.1	(0.4)
Exactly 2 disorders	3.6	(0.1)	1.9	(0.2)	4.1	(0.3)	4.5	(0.2)
Exactly 3 disorders	1.6	(0.1)	0.5	(0.1)	1.8	(0.2)	2.2	(0.1)
Exactly 4 disorders	0.7	(0.1)	0.2	(0.1)	0.4	(0.1)	1.1	(0.1)
5+ disorders	0.7	(0.1)	0.0	(0.0)	0.3	(0.1)	1.3	(0.1)
(n)		(21,177)		(6,508)		(4,745)		(9,924)

[a] Age is restricted to ≤ 44 for India, Lebanon, Belgium, Germany, Italy, Netherlands and Spain; age is restricted to ≤ 39 for Nigeria and PRC–Beijing/Shanghai.
[b] Age is restricted to ≤ 44 for Colombia, India, Bulgaria, Lebanon, Mexico, Belgium, Germany, Italy, Netherlands, Portugal, Spain, and USA.
[c] Age is restricted to ≤ 44 for Colombia, India, Bulgaria, Lebanon, Mexico, Belgium, Germany, Italy, Netherlands, Portugal, Spain, and USA; age is restricted to ≤ 39 for Nigeria and PRC–Beijing/Shanghai.
[d] Age is restricted to ≤ 44 for Colombia, Mexico, Belgium, Germany, Italy, Netherlands, Portugal, Spain, and USA.
[e] With or without dependence.

Appendix Table 9.4 Model fit statistics (Akaike's information criterion; AIC) of total family income and continuous income component measures on type and number of early-onset mental disorders among respondents who were in the age range 18–64 at the time of interview. The WMH surveys.

	DF	Total household income	Personal earnings	Spouse earnings	Other household income
Type of disorder + controls[a]	46	80,094.2	66,600.6	54,890.3	81,481.3
Number of disorders + controls	34	80,081.2	66,599.3	54,875.5	81,488.8
Type + number of disorders + controls	50	80,099.9	66,604.5	54,890.8	81,485.9
Type + number of disorders + type*number + controls	63	80,119.0	66,627.2	54,909.8	81,484.7
Type of disorder + score + type*score[b]	63	80,120.6	66,619.7	54,910.0	81,480.5

[a] Controls include country, sex, level of education, and time since completing education.
[b] This model is a refinement of the model listed above it (i.e., type + number of disorders + type*number + controls) that adjusts the terms for number of disorders to take into consideration the fact that some disorders are associated with greater decrements in income or earnings than other disorders. This is done by assigning respondents with a given number of disorders a score that equals the sum of the regression coefficients for the types of disorders they have. This means that rather than all people with a given number of disorders having a score of 1 on a dummy variable that represents that number of disorders (which is the way number of disorders is characterized in the earlier model), the people with a given number of disorders vary in their scores depending on the precise types of disorders they have. For example, one person with exactly three disorders might have a score of −0.50 on the variable for having three disorders, whereas another person with exactly three disorders might have a score of 1.80 on the same variable, because the three disorders of the second person have a larger sum of type regression coefficients than the disorders of the first person. It is noteworthy that iterative estimation is needed to identify this model, as the number-of-disorders scores have to be constructed from the type-of-disorder coefficients in an earlier iteration of the equation. This iterative approach is continued until the number-of-disorder scores converge.

Appendix Table 9.5 Model fit statistics (Akaike's information criterion; AIC) of dichotomous income component measures on type and number of early-onset mental disorders among respondents who were in the age range 18–64 at the time of interview. The WMH surveys.

	DF	Employed Y/N	Married Y/N	Spouse employed Y/N	Any current disability
Type of disorder + controls[a]	48	37768.4	42320.8	27564.4	23169.1
Number of disorders + controls	36	37778.8	42355.0	27560.8	23132.6
Type + number of disorders + controls	52	37774.8	42326.7	27571.6	23134.8
Type + number of disorders + type*number + controls	65	37774.4	42333.5	27586.2	23082.8
Type of disorder + score + type*score[b]	65	37770.8	42338.7	27584.7	23075.2

[a] Controls include country, sex, level of education, and time since completing education.
[b] See footnote b from Appendix Table 9.4 for a description of this model.

Appendix Table 9.6 Regression of components of total household income on number of early-onset mental disorders with associated controls among respondents who were in the age range 18–64 at the time of interview. All countries. The WMH surveys (continued).[a]

All countries	Disabled		Employed		Married		Spouse employed among the married		Personal earnings among the employed		Spouse earnings among those with an employed spouse		Other household income	
	Coeff	(SE)	Coeff	(SE)	Coeff	(SE)	Coeff	(SE)	Coeff	(SE)	Coeff	(SE)	Coeff	(SE)
Female (n = 21,177)														
Exactly 1 disorder	−0.02	(0.02)	−0.02	(0.02)	−0.02	(0.02)	−0.02	(0.02)	−0.00	(0.02)	−0.01	(0.02)	−0.04*	(0.02)
Exactly 2 disorders	0.01	(0.03)	−0.01	(0.03)	−0.00	(0.03)	−0.00	(0.03)	0.00	(0.03)	0.01	(0.03)	−0.01	(0.03)
Exactly 3 disorders	−0.04	(0.04)	−0.06	(0.04)	−0.04	(0.04)	−0.04	(0.04)	−0.04	(0.04)	−0.01	(0.04)	−0.07*	(0.03)
Exactly 4 disorders	−0.18*	(0.06)	−0.20*	(0.05)	−0.20*	(0.06)	−0.19*	(0.06)	−0.18*	(0.04)	−0.16*	(0.05)	−0.18*	(0.05)
5+ disorders	−0.24*	(0.06)	−0.26*	(0.07)	−0.26*	(0.06)	−0.25*	(0.06)	−0.22*	(0.06)	−0.20*	(0.05)	−0.24*	(0.06)
X^2_5	19.1*		24.7*		25.1*		23.7*		23.9*		22.2*		28.4*	
Male (n = 16,564)														
Exactly 1 disorder	−0.00	(0.02)	0.00	(0.02)	−0.02	(0.02)	−0.02	(0.02)	0.01	(0.02)	−0.02	(0.02)	−0.01	(0.02)
Exactly 2 disorders	−0.01	(0.03)	0.01	(0.03)	−0.02	(0.03)	−0.03	(0.03)	0.01	(0.02)	−0.04	(0.03)	−0.01	(0.03)
Exactly 3 disorders	−0.07	(0.04)	−0.05	(0.04)	−0.08	(0.04)	−0.08*	(0.04)	−0.00	(0.04)	−0.08	(0.04)	−0.10*	(0.04)
Exactly 4 disorders	−0.08	(0.06)	−0.04	(0.06)	−0.09	(0.06)	−0.09	(0.06)	−0.01	(0.05)	−0.07	(0.06)	−0.14*	(0.05)
5+ disorders	−0.06	(0.05)	−0.05	(0.05)	−0.09	(0.05)	−0.09	(0.05)	0.04	(0.04)	−0.07	(0.05)	−0.16*	(0.05)
X^2_5	5.2		3.0		8.2		8.9		1.1		6.9		29.8*	
Female and male combined (n = 37,741)														
Exactly 1 disorder	−0.01	(0.02)	−0.01	(0.02)	−0.02	(0.02)	−0.02	(0.02)	0.00	(0.01)	−0.02	(0.01)	−0.03*	(0.01)
Exactly 2 disorders	−0.00	(0.02)	−0.00	(0.02)	−0.01	(0.02)	−0.02	(0.02)	0.01	(0.02)	−0.02	(0.02)	−0.01	(0.02)
Exactly 3 disorders	−0.06	(0.03)	−0.06*	(0.03)	−0.06*	(0.03)	−0.07*	(0.03)	−0.02	(0.03)	−0.05	(0.03)	−0.09*	(0.02)
Exactly 4 disorders	−0.13*	(0.04)	−0.14*	(0.04)	−0.15*	(0.04)	−0.15*	(0.04)	−0.10*	(0.03)	−0.12*	(0.04)	−0.16*	(0.03)
5+ disorders	−0.12*	(0.04)	−0.13*	(0.04)	−0.15*	(0.04)	−0.15*	(0.04)	−0.06	(0.03)	−0.12*	(0.04)	−0.19*	(0.03)
X^2_5	21.0*		25.2*		29.5*		28.9*		13.2*		21.6*		55.5*	

[a] Controls used in the model include country, sex, educational level, and time since completing education.
* Significant at the 0.05 level, two-sided test.

Appendix Table 9.7 Regression of components of total household income on number of early-onset mental disorders with associated controls among respondents who were in the age range 18–64 at the time of interview. Low/lower-middle-income countries. The WMH surveys (continued).[a]

Low/lower-middle-income countries	Disabled		Employed		Married		Spouse employed among the married		Personal earnings among the employed		Spouse earnings among those with an employed spouse		Other household income	
	Coeff	(SE)	Coeff	(SE)	Coeff	(SE)	Coeff	(SE)	Coeff	(SE)	Coeff	(SE)	Coeff	(SE)
Female (n = 6,508)														
Exactly 1 disorder	0.01	(0.04)	0.01	(0.04)	0.00	(0.04)	0.00	(0.04)	0.05	(0.04)	-0.01	(0.04)	0.00	(0.03)
Exactly 2 disorders	0.07	(0.10)	0.05	(0.10)	0.05	(0.10)	0.05	(0.10)	0.03	(0.09)	0.05	(0.09)	0.08	(0.08)
Exactly 3 disorders	-0.23*	(0.12)	-0.21*	(0.12)	-0.26*	(0.13)	-0.29*	(0.13)	-0.19*	(0.09)	-0.26*	(0.10)	-0.19*	(0.08)
Exactly 4 disorders	-0.02	(0.16)	-0.08	(0.12)	-0.08	(0.14)	-0.07	(0.15)	-0.02	(0.09)	-0.06	(0.18)	-0.05	(0.10)
5+ disorders	-0.15	(0.42)	-0.17	(0.42)	-0.23	(0.40)	-0.25	(0.39)	.01	(0.41)	-0.38	(0.38)	-0.04	(0.26)
χ^2_5	4.9		5.3		5.2		5.8		6.2		7.0		8.7	
Male (n = 5,654)														
Exactly 1 disorder	0.02	(0.05)	0.04	(0.05)	0.02	(0.05)	0.00	(0.05)	0.02	(0.04)	-0.03	(0.05)	0.04	(0.04)
Exactly 2 disorders	0.18*	(0.08)	0.19*	(0.08)	0.18*	(0.08)	0.18*	(0.07)	0.05	(0.06)	0.12	(0.06)	.16*	(0.07)
Exactly 3 disorders	0.06	(0.15)	0.08	(0.14)	0.05	(0.16)	0.07	(0.15)	0.02	(0.11)	0.06	(0.16)	-0.07	(0.10)
Exactly 4 disorders	-0.14	(0.18)	-0.15	(0.19)	-0.13	(0.18)	-0.08	(0.18)	0.12	(0.21)	-0.07	(0.17)	-0.28*	(0.07)
5+ disorders	-0.38	(0.41)	-0.32	(0.38)	-0.38	(0.41)	-0.41	(0.37)	-0.17	(0.26)	-0.40	(0.35)	-0.22	(0.28)
χ^2_5	6.8		8.1		6.2		6.9		1.5		4.4		22.9*	
Female and male combined (n = 12,162)														
Exactly 1 disorder	0.01	(0.03)	0.03	(0.03)	0.01	(0.03)	-0.01	(0.03)	0.04	(0.03)	-0.02	(0.03)	0.02	(0.03)
Exactly 2 disorders	0.12	(0.07)	0.12	(0.07)	0.11	(0.07)	0.09	(0.06)	0.08	(0.05)	0.06	(0.06)	0.12*	(0.06)
Exactly 3 disorders	-0.07	(0.12)	-0.04	(0.11)	-0.08	(0.12)	-0.10	(0.12)	-0.03	(0.09)	-0.10	(0.12)	-0.12	(0.07)
Exactly 4 disorders	-0.09	(0.11)	-0.10	(0.11)	-0.11	(0.11)	-0.10	(0.11)	0.06	(0.11)	-0.10	(0.12)	-0.16*	(0.06)
5+ disorders	-0.31	(0.30)	-0.27	(0.29)	-0.32	(0.29)	-0.35	(0.26)	-0.10	(0.24)	-0.40	(0.25)	-0.16	(0.21)
χ^2_5	6.2		6.8		6.2		6.7		4.7		6.7		18.0*	

[a] Controls used in the model include country, sex, educational level, and time since completing education.

* Significant at the 0.05 level, two-sided test.

Appendix Table 9.8 Regression of components of total household income on number of early-onset mental disorders with associated controls among respondents who were in the age range 18–64 at the time of interview. Upper-middle-income countries. The WMH surveys (continued).[a]

Upper-middle-income countries	Disabled		Employed		Married		Spouse employed among the married		Personal earnings among the employed		Spouse earnings among those with an employed spouse		Other household income	
	Coeff	(SE)	Coeff	(SE)	Coeff	(SE)	Coeff	(SE)	Coeff	(SE)	Coeff	(SE)	Coeff	(SE)
Female (n = 4,745)														
Exactly 1 disorder	−0.03	(0.05)	−0.03	(0.05)	−0.03	(0.05)	−0.02	(0.05)	−0.04	(0.04)	−0.02	(0.04)	−0.03	(0.04)
Exactly 2 disorders	0.08	(0.06)	0.09	(0.06)	0.09	(0.06)	0.09	(0.06)	0.07	(0.06)	0.10	(0.06)	0.00	(0.04)
Exactly 3 disorders	−0.08	(0.09)	−0.06	(0.09)	−0.08	(0.09)	−0.06	(0.08)	−0.03	(0.09)	−0.05	(0.07)	−0.04	(0.08)
Exactly 4 disorders	−0.02	(0.16)	−0.02	(0.15)	−0.05	(0.16)	−0.08	(0.16)	−0.02	(0.10)	−0.07	(0.13)	−0.08	(0.08)
5+ disorders	−0.39*	(0.17)	−0.38*	(0.17)	−0.39*	(0.17)	−0.37*	(0.17)	−0.29*	(0.13)	−0.28	(0.15)	−0.27*	(0.13)
χ^2_5	10.6		11.1*		11.5*		10.5		10.4		9.9		6.7	
Male (n = 3,310)														
Exactly 1 disorder	0.02	(0.06)	0.02	(0.06)	0.00	(0.06)	0.02	(0.06)	0.04	(0.05)	0.04	(0.06)	0.02	(0.05)
Exactly 2 disorders	0.18*	(0.07)	0.18*	(0.07)	0.17*	(0.07)	0.14*	(0.07)	0.08	(0.07)	0.11	(0.07)	0.16*	(0.07)
Exactly 3 disorders	−0.02	(0.12)	−0.04	(0.11)	−0.07	(0.12)	−0.06	(0.12)	0.10	(0.12)	−0.06	(0.12)	−0.05	(0.07)
Exactly 4 disorders	0.19	(0.14)	0.20	(0.13)	0.17	(0.14)	0.12	(0.15)	0.11	(0.10)	0.11	(0.15)	0.09	(0.11)
5+ disorders	−0.16	(0.14)	−0.06	(0.10)	−0.18	(0.13)	−0.14	(0.12)	0.16	(0.14)	−0.10	(0.12)	−0.20*	(0.10)
χ^2_5	10.1		10.6		10.4		6.6		4.4		3.7		10.6	
Female and male combined (n = 8,055)														
Exactly 1 disorder	−0.02	(0.04)	−0.02	(0.04)	−0.02	(0.04)	−0.01	(0.04)	−0.01	(0.03)	−0.00	(0.04)	−0.02	(0.03)
Exactly 2 disorders	0.12*	(0.04)	0.12*	(0.05)	0.11*	(0.04)	0.12*	(0.04)	0.08	(0.05)	0.11*	(0.04)	0.06	(0.04)
Exactly 3 disorders	−0.06	(0.07)	−0.06	(0.07)	−0.08	(0.07)	−0.07	(0.07)	0.01	(0.07)	−0.06	(0.06)	−0.05	(0.05)
Exactly 4 disorders	0.12	(0.09)	0.12	(0.08)	0.10	(0.09)	0.06	(0.10)	0.06	(0.07)	0.05	(0.10)	0.03	(0.07)
5+ disorders	−0.25*	(0.11)	−0.21*	(0.10)	−0.25*	(0.11)	−0.23*	(0.10)	−0.04	(0.09)	−0.17	(0.10)	−0.23*	(0.08)
χ^2_5	19.8*		19.3*		20.5*		15.8*		4.7		10.5		14.1*	

[a] Controls used in the model include country, sex, educational level, and time since completing education.
* Significant at the 0.05 level, two-sided test.

Appendix Table 9.9 Regression of components of total household income on number of early-onset mental disorders with associated controls among respondents who were in the age range 18–64 at the time of interview. High-income countries. The WMH surveys (continued).[a]

High-income countries	Disabled		Employed		Married		Spouse Employed among the married		Personal Earnings among the employed		Spouse Earnings among those with an employed spouse		Other Household Income	
	Coeff	(SE)	Coeff	(SE)	Coeff	(SE)	Coeff	(SE)	Coeff	(SE)	Coeff	(SE)	Coeff	(SE)
Female (n = 9,924)														
Exactly 1 disorder	−0.02	(0.02)	−0.03	(0.02)	−0.02	(0.02)	−0.02	(0.02)	−0.02	(0.02)	−0.00	(0.02)	−0.05*	(0.02)
Exactly 2 disorders	−0.04	(0.04)	−0.06	(0.04)	−0.06	(0.03)	−0.05	(0.03)	−0.04	(0.04)	−0.04	(0.03)	−0.05	(0.04)
Exactly 3 disorders	0.02	(0.05)	−0.03	(0.05)	0.02	(0.04)	0.02	(0.04)	−0.01	(0.04)	0.06	(0.04)	−0.06	(0.04)
Exactly 4 disorders	−0.22*	(0.07)	−0.25*	(0.06)	−0.23*	(0.07)	−0.21*	(0.07)	−0.23*	(0.05)	−0.17*	(0.06)	−0.23*	(0.06)
5+ disorders	−0.22*	(0.07)	−0.25*	(0.07)	−0.24*	(0.06)	−0.22*	(0.06)	−0.22*	(0.07)	−0.17*	(0.05)	−0.26*	(0.07)
X^2_5	19.4*		25.9*		23.6*		21.1*		29.1*		22.7*		30.2*	
Male (n = 7,600)														
Exactly 1 disorder	−0.02	(0.03)	−0.02	(0.03)	−0.04	(0.03)	−0.05	(0.03)	−0.01	(0.02)	−0.04	(0.03)	−0.04*	(0.02)
Exactly 2 disorders	−0.13*	(0.03)	−0.10*	(0.03)	−0.13*	(0.03)	−0.14*	(0.03)	−0.05	(0.02)	−0.13*	(0.03)	−0.13*	(0.03)
Exactly 3 disorders	−0.11*	(0.04)	−0.08	(0.05)	−0.10*	(0.04)	−0.12*	(0.04)	−0.02	(0.04)	−0.11*	(0.04)	−0.12*	(0.04)
Exactly 4 disorders	−0.17*	(0.07)	−0.12	(0.07)	−0.17*	(0.07)	−0.16*	(0.07)	−0.08	(0.06)	−0.14*	(0.07)	−0.21*	(0.06)
5+ disorders	−0.04	(0.06)	−0.04	(0.06)	−0.08	(0.05)	−0.08	(0.05)	0.03	(0.04)	−0.06	(0.05)	−0.15*	(0.04)
X^2_5	27.4*		16.4*		30.2*		36.4*		7.4		30.7*		40.6*	
Female and male combined (n = 17,524)														
Exactly 1 disorder	−0.02	(0.02)	−0.03	(0.02)	−0.03	(0.02)	−0.04	(0.02)	−0.01	(0.02)	−0.02	(0.02)	−0.05*	(0.02)
Exactly 2 disorders	−0.08*	(0.03)	−0.08*	(0.02)	−0.09*	(0.02)	−0.10*	(0.02)	−0.04*	(0.02)	−0.08*	(0.02)	−0.09*	(0.03)
Exactly 3 disorders	−0.05	(0.03)	−0.06	(0.03)	−0.04	(0.03)	−0.05	(0.03)	−0.02	(0.03)	−0.03	(0.03)	−0.09*	(0.03)
Exactly 4 disorders	−0.19*	(0.04)	−0.20*	(0.04)	−0.20*	(0.05)	−0.19*	(0.05)	−0.17*	(0.04)	−0.16*	(0.04)	−0.22*	(0.04)
5+ disorders	−0.10*	(0.04)	−0.12*	(0.04)	−0.13*	(0.04)	−0.14*	(0.04)	−0.06	(0.03)	−0.10*	(0.04)	−0.20*	(0.04)
X^2_5	32.3*		36.7*		36.3*		36.2*		27.3*		30.0*		66.3*	

[a] Controls used in the model include country, sex, educational level, and time since completing education.
* Significant at the 0.05 level, two-sided test.

Appendix Table 11.1 Model comparison by country income level. The WMH surveys.

Country income level	Model	MSE whole sample	MAPE whole sample
Low/lower-middle	OLS	10.659	1.240
	GLM constant variance, link = log	10.272	1.122
	GLM constant variance, link = square root	10.550	1.263
	GLM variance proportional to mean, link = log	10.481	1.170
	GLM variance proportional to mean squared, link = log	10.539	1.178
	GLM variance proportional to mean, link = square root	10.518	1.183
	GLM variance proportional to mean squared, link = square root	54.016	1.493
Upper-middle	OLS	17.334	1.629
	GLM constant variance, link = log	17.015	1.589
	GLM constant variance, link = square root	17.172	1.541
	GLM variance proportional to mean, link = log	17.194	1.592
	GLM variance proportional to mean squared, link = log	17.267	1.597
	GLM variance proportional to mean, link = square root	17.250	1.601
	GLM variance proportional to mean squared, link = square root	17.883	1.594
High	OLS	23.058	2.117
	GLM constant variance, link = log	22.107	1.966
	GLM constant variance, link = square root	22.198	1.863
	GLM variance proportional to mean, link = log	22.699	1.939
	GLM variance proportional to mean squared, link = log	22.725	1.960
	GLM variance proportional to mean, link = square root	22.550	1.987
	GLM variance proportional to mean squared, link = square root	23.282	2.032

Appendix Table 11.2 Odds ratios between pairs of disorders. The WMH surveys.

Disorders	Alcohol abuse	Bipolar	Drug abuse	Generalized anxiety	Major depressive disorder	Panic disorder and/or agoraphobia	Post-traumatic stress	Social phobia	Specific phobia	Arthritis	Cancer	Cardiovascular	Chronic pain	Diabetes	Digestive	Headache/migraine	Insomnia	Neurological
Bipolar	7.09 (3.89, 12.90)**																	
Drug abuse	32.97 (18.50, 58.76)**	8.95 (5.34, 15.00)**																
Generalized anxiety	2.04 (1.09, 3.80)*	5.30 (3.16, 8.88)**	3.02 (1.58, 5.78)*															
Major depressive disorder	3.52 (2.55, 4.86)**	15.45 (10.69, 22.32)**	4.41 (2.75, 7.09)**	6.60 (4.69, 9.28)**														
Panic disorder and/or agoraphobia	3.44 (2.03, 5.83)**	12.15 (8.42, 17.51)**	2.45 (1.04, 5.76)*	5.64 (3.85, 8.26)**	8.57 (6.37, 11.52)**													
Post-traumatic stress	3.96 (2.67, 5.90)**	8.35 (5.26, 13.24)**	2.23 (1.17, 4.24)*	0.77 (0.35, 1.72)	8.17 (6.24, 10.69)**	9.42 (6.61, 13.43)**												
Social phobia	3.37 (2.26, 5.02)**	9.00 (6.50, 12.44)**	4.00 (2.33, 6.87)**	4.86 (3.33, 7.07)**	6.43 (5.25, 7.88)**	10.87 (8.24, 14.33)**	6.27 (5.03, 7.82)**											
Specific phobia	1.86 (1.26, 2.73)*	5.75 (4.14, 7.97)**	1.76 (0.92, 3.34)	3.84 (2.82, 5.23)**	4.58 (3.61, 5.82)**	10.63 (7.98, 14.15)**	6.16 (4.54, 8.35)**	7.38 (5.75, 9.46)**										
Arthritis	0.55 (0.35, 0.84)*	1.14 (0.88, 1.48)	0.48 (0.26, 0.89)*	1.65 (1.25, 2.17)**	1.18 (0.97, 1.44)	1.63 (1.23, 2.15)**	1.84 (1.39, 2.43)**	1.19 (0.97, 1.46)	1.56 (1.28, 1.91)**									
Cancer	0.49 (0.26, 0.93)*	0.75 (0.40, 1.43)	0.54 (0.18, 1.66)	1.48 (0.91, 2.41)	0.84 (0.53, 1.32)	0.86 (0.45, 1.65)	1.14 (0.66, 1.95)	0.91 (0.59, 1.38)	1.24 (0.91, 1.68)	3.48 (2.65, 4.56)**								

Appendix Table 11.2 (cont.)

Disorders	Alcohol abuse	Bipolar	Drug abuse	Generalized anxiety	Major depressive disorder	Panic disorder and/or agoraphobia	Post-traumatic stress	Social phobia and/or agoraphobia	Specific phobia	Arthritis	Cancer	Cardiovascular	Chronic pain	Diabetes	Digestive	Headache/migraine	Insomnia	Neurological
Cardiovascular	0.46 (0.30, 0.70)**	1.05 (0.76, 1.45)	0.67 (0.36, 1.27)	1.03 (0.77, 1.37)	1.03 (0.81, 1.30)	1.37 (1.02, 1.83)*	1.63 (1.24, 2.13)**	1.02 (0.83, 1.26)	1.18 (0.97, 1.42)	3.94 (3.40, 4.56)**	2.83 (2.20, 3.64)**							
Chronic pain	1.27 (0.94, 1.72)	2.67 (1.81, 3.95)**	1.13 (0.69, 1.84)	2.87 (2.08, 3.96)**	2.72 (2.22, 3.33)**	2.11 (1.67, 2.66)**	3.21 (2.51, 4.09)**	1.72 (1.39, 2.13)**	2.23 (1.92, 2.60)**	3.63 (3.02, 4.36)**	1.90 (1.45, 2.49)**	1.88 (1.59, 2.21)**						
Diabetes	0.13 (0.03, 0.52)*	1.11 (0.59, 2.10)	0.08 (0.01, 0.61)*	1.20 (0.64, 2.25)	1.00 (0.63, 1.60)	1.49 (0.91, 2.43)	1.33 (0.88, 2.01)	0.93 (0.61, 1.43)	1.22 (0.88, 1.70)	3.16 (2.29, 4.37)**	1.64 (1.04, 2.59)*	7.99 (5.79, 11.02)**	1.89 (1.40, 2.54)**					
Digestive	1.90 (0.91, 3.96)	4.28 (2.12, 8.61)**	3.95 (1.92, 8.15)**	2.64 (1.49, 4.67)**	3.26 (2.15, 4.95)**	2.82 (1.52, 5.25)*	2.94 (1.63, 5.32)**	2.44 (1.65, 3.59)**	2.42 (1.70, 3.45)**	2.59 (1.96, 3.41)**	1.56 (0.94, 2.59)	2.65 (1.68, 4.17)**	4.95 (3.35, 7.32)**	2.38 (1.35, 4.17)*				
Headache/migraine	1.52 (1.06, 2.16)*	3.87 (2.68, 5.59)**	1.71 (0.95, 3.08)	2.66 (1.94, 3.65)**	3.80 (2.92, 4.94)**	3.97 (3.10, 5.09)**	4.47 (3.56, 5.62)**	2.75 (2.24, 3.38)**	2.78 (2.37, 3.26)**	1.50 (1.30, 1.73)**	1.07 (0.77, 1.47)	0.99 (0.75, 1.30)	4.04 (3.34, 4.89)**	0.63 (0.44, 0.92)*	3.00 (2.15, 4.20)**			
Insomnia	2.19 (1.48, 3.24)**	3.92 (2.79, 5.52)**	2.03 (1.16, 3.55)*	4.16 (3.08, 5.61)**	3.93 (3.20, 4.82)**	4.68 (3.70, 5.92)**	5.37 (4.09, 7.05)**	3.82 (3.23, 4.52)**	3.10 (2.53, 3.81)**	2.04 (1.68, 2.48)**	1.64 (1.20, 2.22)*	1.50 (1.11, 2.03)*	2.91 (2.46, 3.46)**	1.96 (1.40, 2.76)**	3.11 (2.04, 4.72)**	3.97 (3.22, 4.90)**		
Neurological	1.74 (0.80, 3.78)	0.76 (0.24, 2.41)	0.97 (0.11, 8.25)	0.92 (0.30, 2.84)	1.93 (1.13, 3.30)*	1.86 (0.94, 3.70)	2.99 (1.81, 4.95)**	1.69 (0.98, 2.91)	2.01 (1.15, 3.50)*	1.50 (0.96, 2.33)	1.01 (0.43, 2.35)	1.23 (0.69, 2.21)	2.34 (1.46, 3.74)**	1.66 (0.50, 5.54)	2.91 (0.82, 10.31)	1.49 (0.83, 2.70)	1.31 (0.85, 2.04)	
Respiratory	1.14 (0.81, 1.61)	1.59 (1.13, 2.22)*	1.23 (0.83, 1.82)	2.05 (1.45, 2.92)**	1.55 (1.26, 1.92)**	1.72 (1.31, 2.25)**	1.84 (1.45, 2.34)**	1.45 (1.18, 1.79)**	1.57 (1.31, 1.90)**	1.47 (1.22, 1.76)**	0.92 (0.73, 1.16)	1.06 (0.89, 1.26)	2.04 (1.72, 2.41)**	0.93 (0.61, 1.42)	1.67 (1.15, 2.43)*	2.17 (1.80, 2.61)**	1.66 (1.38, 2.00)**	1.77 (1.10, 2.87)*

* Significant at the 0.05 level, two-sided test.

** Significant at the 0.0001 level, two-sided test.

Appendix Table 11.3 Coefficients from the best model (score plus interactions with disorders). The WMH surveys.

Variables	Coeff	(SE)	χ^2
Score	−0.45	0.15	8.56*
Alcohol abuse	0.24	0.11	4.43*
Bipolar	1.29	0.14	85.88**
Drug abuse	0.03	0.22	0.01
Generalized anxiety	0.66	0.11	38.27**
Major depressive disorder	1.05	0.07	224.39**
Panic disorder	0.77	0.10	61.00**
Post-traumatic stress	1.21	0.08	205.81**
Social phobia	0.45	0.10	19.71**
Specific phobia	0.18	0.09	4.17*
Arthritis	0.45	0.05	89.90**
Cancer	0.47	0.08	31.91**
Cardiovascular	0.43	0.05	69.98**
Chronic pain	0.89	0.07	175.29**
Diabetes	0.49	0.07	52.84**
Digestive	0.60	0.08	58.96**
Headache/migraine	0.67	0.06	119.23**
Insomnia	0.79	0.07	136.42**
Neurological	1.04	0.10	98.66**
Respiratory	0.25	0.05	24.46**
Score*Alcohol abuse	−0.17	0.11	2.27
Score*Bipolar	−0.45	0.11	16.10**
Score*Drug abuse	0.33	0.19	3.20
Score*Generalized anxiety	−0.28	0.09	9.22*
Score*Major depressive disorder	−0.67	0.06	107.56**
Score*Panic disorder	−0.17	0.09	4.02*
Score*Post-traumatic stress	−0.67	0.08	78.7**
Score*Social phobia	−0.09	0.09	1.00
Score*Specific phobia	0.15	0.08	3.34
Score*Arthritis	−0.43	0.05	75.35**
Score*Cancer	−0.33	0.09	14.15*
Score*Cardiovascular	−0.12	0.05	6.29*

Appendix Table 11.3 (cont.)

Variables	Coeff	(SE)	χ^2
Score*Chronic pain	0.32	0.08	18.03**
Score*Diabetes	−0.11	0.06	2.99
Score*Digestive	−0.26	0.07	13.29*
Score*Headache/migraine	−0.24	0.05	20.54**
Score*Insomnia	−0.43	0.06	52.20**
Score*Neurological	−0.34	0.09	14.46*
Score*Respiratory	−0.06	0.05	1.68
Scale	4.54	0.01	–

* Significant at the 0.05 level, two-sided test.
** Significant at the 0.001 level, two-sided test.

Appendix Table 12.1 Models comparison using Bayesian information criterion (BIC). The WMH surveys.

Partial-disability variables	Models[a]	BIC
Quantity cut-down days	Model 1. Disorders only	397,886.6
	Model 2. Number of disorders only	398,050.5
	Model 3. Disorders + number	397,875.4
	Model 4. Disorders + number*disorder	397,958.2
	Model 5. With scores	397,965.1
Quality cut-back days	Model 1. Disorders only	362,881.7
	Model 2. Number of disorders only	364,970.0
	Model 3. Disorders + number	362,833.4
	Model 4. Disorders + number*disorder	362,950.7
	Model 5. With scores	362,953.5
Extreme-effort days	Model 1. Disorders only	374,051.0
	Model 2. Number of disorders only	374,434.4
	Model 3. Disorders + number	373,958.8
	Model 4. Disorders + number*disorder	374,011.5
	Model 5. With scores	374,029.3
Days with partial disability	Model 1. Disorders only	378,678.9
	Model 2. Number of disorders only	379,088.0
	Model 3. Disorders + number	378,663.2
	Model 4. Disorders + number*disorder	378,688.5
	Model 5. With scores	378,698.9

[a] All models are GLM models with constant variance and link square root.

Appendix Table 12.2 Mean number of partial-disability days per month by country income level. The WMH surveys.

Country income level/Disorder	Quantity cut-down days		Quality cut-back days		Extreme-effort days		Any days with partial disability	
	Mean	(SE)	Mean	(SE)	Mean	(SE)	Mean	(SE)
Low/lower-middle								
Alcohol abuse	1.9	(0.3)	1.4	(0.2)	1.4	(0.2)	1.9	(0.3)
Bipolar	1.9	(0.4)	2.0	(0.3)	2.1	(0.6)	2.5	(0.4)
Drug abuse	3.3	(0.9)	3.8	(1.1)	2.2	(0.7)	4.1	(1.0)
Generalized anxiety	5.1	(1.0)	3.7	(0.9)	3.3	(0.6)	5.0	(0.9)
Major depressive disorder	3.2	(0.3)	2.8	(0.2)	3.1	(0.3)	3.7	(0.3)
Panic and/or agoraphobia	3.8	(0.8)	2.5	(0.4)	2.9	(0.5)	3.8	(0.6)
Post-traumatic stress	7.1	(1.0)	5.7	(0.8)	6.5	(0.8)	7.8	(0.9)
Social phobia	2.3	(0.7)	1.7	(0.3)	2.1	(0.3)	2.5	(0.5)
Specific phobia	1.4	(0.2)	1.3	(0.2)	1.4	(0.2)	1.7	(0.2)
Arthritis	2.5	(0.2)	2.1	(0.1)	2.2	(0.2)	2.7	(0.2)
Cancer	3.1	(0.8)	3.4	(1.0)	3.0	(0.8)	3.7	(0.9)
Cardiovascular	2.9	(0.2)	2.2	(0.2)	2.3	(0.2)	3.0	(0.2)
Chronic pain	2.5	(0.2)	1.9	(0.1)	2.1	(0.1)	2.7	(0.1)
Diabetes	2.8	(0.4)	2.2	(0.3)	2.4	(0.4)	2.9	(0.3)
Digestive	1.9	(0.3)	1.3	(0.2)	1.5	(0.2)	2.0	(0.2)
Headache/migraine	3.0	(0.2)	2.4	(0.2)	2.4	(0.2)	3.2	(0.2)
Insomnia	4.8	(0.5)	3.7	(0.3)	4.2	(0.5)	5.1	(0.4)
Neurological	3.5	(0.8)	2.6	(0.7)	3.2	(0.8)	3.9	(0.8)
Respiratory	2.0	(0.2)	1.5	(0.2)	1.6	(0.2)	2.1	(0.2)
Any mental	2.6	(0.2)	2.0	(0.1)	2.2	(0.2)	2.8	(0.2)
Any physical	1.9	(0.1)	1.5	(0.1)	1.5	(0.1)	2.0	(0.1)
Any disorder	1.9	(0.1)	1.4	(0.1)	1.5	(0.1)	2.0	(0.1)
Upper-middle								
Alcohol abuse	2.0	(0.3)	1.0	(0.2)	1.3	(0.2)	1.8	(0.3)
Bipolar	2.5	(0.6)	2.8	(0.7)	3.1	(0.5)	3.4	(0.7)
Drug abuse	1.7	(0.7)	1.4	(0.5)	1.1	(0.3)	1.8	(0.5)
Generalized anxiety	4.0	(0.6)	2.9	(0.5)	3.4	(0.5)	4.1	(0.6)
Major depressive disorder	3.7	(0.3)	2.9	(0.3)	3.2	(0.3)	4.0	(0.3)
Panic and/or agoraphobia	3.6	(0.5)	2.5	(0.4)	3.2	(0.4)	3.7	(0.4)
Post-traumatic stress	3.8	(0.7)	3.7	(0.7)	4.0	(0.8)	4.4	(0.8)
Social phobia	3.4	(0.6)	2.9	(0.5)	3.4	(0.6)	3.8	(0.6)
Specific phobia	2.6	(0.3)	2.2	(0.3)	2.6	(0.3)	2.9	(0.3)
Arthritis	2.5	(0.2)	1.6	(0.1)	1.7	(0.1)	2.3	(0.2)
Cancer	3.3	(0.9)	2.1	(0.7)	2.8	(0.9)	3.3	(0.9)
Cardiovascular	2.8	(0.2)	1.7	(0.1)	1.7	(0.1)	2.6	(0.2)
Chronic pain	2.5	(0.2)	1.7	(0.1)	1.9	(0.1)	2.5	(0.2)
Diabetes	2.8	(0.3)	1.7	(0.2)	2.2	(0.3)	2.7	(0.3)
Digestive	2.6	(0.4)	1.9	(0.3)	1.8	(0.3)	2.5	(0.3)
Headache/migraine	2.1	(0.2)	1.5	(0.1)	1.6	(0.1)	2.1	(0.1)
Insomnia	2.6	(0.3)	2.1	(0.2)	2.9	(0.3)	3.0	(0.3)
Neurological	4.0	(0.7)	2.7	(0.5)	2.7	(0.5)	3.9	(0.6)
Respiratory	1.8	(0.2)	1.2	(0.1)	1.4	(0.2)	1.8	(0.2)
Any mental	2.6	(0.2)	2.0	(0.1)	2.3	(0.2)	2.8	(0.2)
Any physical	2.0	(0.1)	1.2	(0.1)	1.3	(0.1)	1.9	(0.1)
Any disorder	1.9	(0.1)	1.2	(0.1)	1.3	(0.1)	1.8	(0.1)
High								
Alcohol abuse	2.6	(0.2)	2.4	(0.2)	2.5	(0.3)	3.0	(0.3)
Bipolar	4.6	(0.4)	4.1	(0.4)	4.3	(0.4)	5.3	(0.4)
Drug abuse	3.4	(0.4)	3.0	(0.4)	3.7	(0.5)	4.0	(0.5)
Generalized anxiety	4.7	(0.3)	3.8	(0.3)	4.6	(0.3)	5.2	(0.3)
Major depressive disorder	4.3	(0.2)	3.6	(0.2)	4.3	(0.2)	4.8	(0.2)
Panic and/or agoraphobia	4.7	(0.3)	4.2	(0.3)	4.7	(0.3)	5.4	(0.3)
Post-traumatic stress	5.3	(0.3)	4.4	(0.3)	5.0	(0.3)	5.8	(0.3)
Social phobia	3.8	(0.2)	3.1	(0.2)	3.8	(0.2)	4.3	(0.2)
Specific phobia	3.4	(0.2)	2.7	(0.2)	3.3	(0.2)	3.8	(0.2)
Arthritis	3.8	(0.2)	2.6	(0.1)	3.2	(0.1)	3.8	(0.1)
Cancer	3.7	(0.3)	2.6	(0.2)	3.2	(0.3)	3.8	(0.3)

Appendix Table 12.2 (cont.)

Country income level/Disorder	Quantity cut-down days		Quality cut-back days		Extreme-effort days		Any days with partial disability	
	Mean	(SE)	Mean	(SE)	Mean	(SE)	Mean	(SE)
Cardiovascular	3.2	(0.1)	2.3	(0.1)	2.8	(0.1)	3.3	(0.1)
Chronic pain	4.0	(0.1)	2.9	(0.1)	3.6	(0.1)	4.2	(0.1)
Diabetes	3.2	(0.3)	2.6	(0.2)	3.0	(0.3)	3.4	(0.2)
Digestive	5.0	(0.4)	4.1	(0.4)	5.1	(0.4)	5.5	(0.4)
Headache/migraine	3.6	(0.1)	2.8	(0.1)	3.4	(0.1)	3.9	(0.1)
Insomnia	4.3	(0.2)	3.8	(0.2)	4.4	(0.2)	4.9	(0.2)
Neurological	4.2	(0.5)	3.5	(0.4)	4.3	(0.6)	4.6	(0.5)
Respiratory	2.5	(0.1)	1.9	(0.1)	2.1	(0.1)	2.6	(0.1)
Any mental	3.5	(0.1)	2.8	(0.1)	3.4	(0.1)	3.9	(0.1)
Any physical	2.6	(0.1)	1.8	(0.1)	2.2	(0.1)	2.6	(0.1)
Any disorder	2.5	(0.1)	1.8	(0.1)	2.1	(0.1)	2.6	(0.1)

Appendix Table 13.1 Cronbach's alpha for the four Sheehan Disability Scale domains pooled across all mental disorders and all physical conditions by country income level. The WMH surveys.

Country income level	Mental disorder	Physical condition	Overall
I. Low/lower-middle	0.88	0.92	0.91
Colombia	0.87	0.89	0.88
India–Pondicherry	0.97	0.97	0.97
Nigeria	0.93	0.94	0.94
PRC–Beijing/Shanghai	0.86	0.91	0.90
Ukraine	0.86	0.90	0.88
II. Upper-middle	0.90	0.92	0.91
Brazil–São Paulo	0.91	0.91	0.91
Bulgaria	0.91	0.94	0.93
Lebanon	0.84	0.90	0.85
Mexico	0.88	0.91	0.90
Romania	0.91	0.92	0.92
South Africa	0.87	0.93	0.92
III. High	0.87	0.90	0.88
Belgium	0.81	0.85	0.82
France	0.81	0.89	0.85
Germany	0.82	0.88	0.85
Israel	0.86	0.91	0.91
Italy	0.81	0.92	0.89
Japan	0.83	0.89	0.88
Netherlands	0.88	0.86	0.85
New Zealand	0.88	0.90	0.89
Northern Ireland	0.88	0.90	0.90
Portugal	0.85	0.89	0.86
Spain	0.89	0.90	0.89
USA	0.87	0.89	0.88

Appendix Table 13.2 Multiple correlations of the four Sheehan disability domain scores predicting days out of role due to the focal disorder pooled for mental disorders and physical conditions by country income level. The WMH surveys.

Country income level	Mental disorders	Physical conditions
All countries	0.52	0.46
Low/lower-middle	0.38	0.34
Upper-middle	0.42	0.37
High	0.56	0.50

Appendix Table 13.3 Treatment prevalence among all cases and severe cases (i.e., rated severe on at least one SDS domain) pooled across all mental disorders and all physical conditions by country income level. The WMH surveys.

		Country income level								
		Low/lower-middle			Upper-middle			High		
		N	%	(SE)	N	%	(SE)	N	%	(SE)
Severe cases	Mental	76	11.4	(2.0)	311	19.1	(1.5)	1,765	34.7	(1.2)
	Physical	435	54.4	(3.2)	1,114	69.8	(1.6)	3,196	77.4	(0.9)
Total cases	Mental	162	5.7	(0.9)	576	13.6	(0.9)	2,841	23.7	(0.7)
	Physical	2,007	47.6	(1.4)	3,683	58.6	(1.1)	9,300	65.3	(0.8)

Appendix Table 13.4. Disorder-specific global Sheehan Disability Scale ratings for disorders in treatment by country income level. The WMH surveys.

	Mean disability ratings										Proportion rated severely disabled										
	Country income level									Test for significant difference between groups of countries	Country income level									Test for significant difference between groups of countries
	Low/lower-middle			Upper-middle			High				Low/lower-middle			Upper-middle			High			
Mental disorders	N^a	Mean	(SE)	N^a	Mean	(SE)	N^a	Mean	(SE)	χ_2^2	N^b	%	(SE)	N^b	%	(SE)	N^b	%	(SE)	χ_2^2
Major depressive disorder or dysthymia	54	7.3	(0.3)	177	7.4	(0.2)	644	7.8	(0.1)	5.4	30	70.7	(6.1)	117	66.8	(4.1)	484	75.8	(2.1)	4.0
Bipolar	12	7.3	(1.3)	37	7.4	(0.6)	202	8.3	(0.2)	2.5	8	69.5	(15.7)	28	76.5	(9.2)	167	82.6	(3.4)	1.1
Generalized anxiety disorder	6	7.2	(0.5)	55	7.0	(0.4)	409	7.4	(0.1)	0.8	5	85.4	(14.0)	32	61.4	(7.1)	285	70.1	(2.6)	2.3
Panic disorder	12	6.2	(1.1)	47	7.2	(0.5)	244	7.2	(0.2)	0.9	6	54.0	(16.7)	29	70.2	(6.1)	176	72.6	(3.3)	1.2
Social phobia	17	5.8	(1.1)	69	6.0	(0.4)	401	6.0	(0.2)	0.0	9	49.2	(18.2)	30	47.0	(7.0)	223	55.9	(2.6)	1.5
Specific phobia	35	3.5	(0.5)	127	3.7	(0.3)	476	4.3	(0.2)	4.6	7	16.6	(6.6)	35	24.6	(4.6)	151	31.7	(2.5)	4.7
Post-traumatic stress	3	7.5	(2.2)	15	6.4	(1.6)	261	7.5	(0.2)	0.5	1	70.3	(25.7)	12	60.0	(17.6)	181	70.0	(3.4)	0.3
Attention-deficit/ hyperactivity	–	–	–	17	7.0	(0.4)	86	6.2	(0.4)	1.8	0	–	–	10	65.3	(13.3)	45	49.9	(6.9)	–
Intermittent explosive disorder	21	5.8	(0.9)	25	4.7	(0.9)	89	5.5	(0.4)	0.9	8	38.8	(11.7)	12	37.4	(10.7)	36	40.5	(5.4)	0.1
Oppositional-defiant disorder	2	9.1	(0.2)	7	7.6	(0.7)	29	5.8	(0.8)	20.5*	2	100.0	(0.0)	6	69.0	(23.3)	17	42.2	(10.6)	.

Physical disorders																			
Arthritis	344	3.9	(0.3)	341	4.8	(0.2)	1,409	5.1	(0.1)	15.2*	67	20.0	(3.6)	130	35.6	(3.6)	546	40.1	(2.1)	16.2*
Asthma	53	3.9	(0.5)	126	4.8	(0.5)	615	3.3	(0.3)	6.1*	12	19.1	(8.1)	38	39.1	(7.2)	124	18.4	(3.1)	5.1
Cancer	21	4.4	(0.6)	37	5.5	(1.7)	262	3.1	(0.3)	5.4	4	15.7	(7.4)	13	55.0	(17.1)	75	25.1	(3.5)	2.7
Chronic back/ neck pain	386	4.1	(0.2)	634	5.0	(0.2)	2,178	5.9	(0.1)	72.8*	85	20.4	(3.0)	224	37.1	(3.0)	1,039	46.8	(1.7)	46.2*
Other chronic pain	135	3.8	(0.4)	321	4.9	(0.4)	677	6.2	(0.2)	38.1*	45	27.4	(5.5)	130	38.9	(4.1)	357	51.9	(3.6)	13.6*
Diabetes	159	4.2	(0.8)	250	3.3	(0.4)	585	2.4	(0.3)	5.4	18	24.9	(10.0)	58	25.3	(5.2)	74	15.8	(3.5)	2.5
Headaches	330	5.0	(0.4)	710	5.2	(0.2)	1,106	6.6	(0.1)	52.9*	103	33.0	(5.3)	258	37.4	(2.5)	619	56.9	(2.1)	41.2*
Heart disease	122	5.0	(0.5)	258	4.0	(0.4)	510	4.2	(0.3)	3.0	31	38.7	(8.3)	78	27.7	(4.5)	143	33.3	(3.4)	1.6
Hypertension	298	3.9	(0.4)	850	3.4	(0.2)	1,764	1.7	(0.1)	73.6*	45	26.4	(4.2)	148	20.0	(2.3)	174	9.8	(1.4)	20.7*
Ulcer	159	2.5	(0.5)	156	4.3	(0.5)	194	3.3	(0.4)	7.4*	25	8.0	(2.4)	37	27.1	(6.2)	45	19.2	(4.3)	8.0*

[a] Number of respondents with valid Sheehan scores for the randomly selected physical disorder or the mental disorder.
[b] Number of participants rated as having a severely disabling disorder.
* Significant at the 0.05 level, two-sided test.

Appendix Table 13.5 Mann–Whitney tests for the pooled significance of all 100 logically possible pair-wise differences between each mental disorder and each physical condition in mean Sheehan Disability Scale scores and in percentages of cases rated severely impaired, separately for all cases, for cases in treatment, and for all physical disorders in treatment compared to all mental disorders (whether or not in treatment) by country income level. The WMH surveys.

Country income level	Mean SDS						% severely impaired					
	All cases		Cases in treatment		Physical in treatment		All cases		Cases in treatment		Physical in treatment	
	Z	Two-sided Pr > |Z|	Z	Two-sided Pr > |Z|	Z	Two-sided Pr > |Z|	Z	Two-sided Pr > |Z|	Z	Two-sided Pr > |Z|	Z	Two-sided Pr > |Z|
Low/lower-middle	2.7	0.006	2.9	0.004	1.7	0.094	2.1	0.037	3.0	0.003	1.7	0.094
Upper-middle	2.8	0.005	2.7	0.007	2.2	0.031	2.0	0.045	2.8	0.006	1.3	0.186
High	2.8	0.005	2.8	0.006	1.9	0.054	2.6	0.009	2.7	0.007	1.8	0.076

All comparisons showed mental disorders to have higher aggregate means and percentages rated severe than physical disorders. The positive values of the z tests consequently refer to higher mental than physical.

Appendix **Table 13.6** Pair-wise differences in mean global Sheehan Disability Scale disability ratings for all mental–physical disorder pairs by country income level. The WMH surveys.[a]

Country income level	Physical conditions	Mental disorders																		
		Major depressive disorder or dysthymia		Bipolar disorder		Generalized anxiety disorder		Panic disorder		Social phobia		Specific phobia		Post-traumatic stress		Attention-deficit/hyperactivity		Intermittent explosive disorder		Oppositional-defiant disorder	
		Diff	Sig*	Diff	Sig*	Diff	Sig*	Diff	Sig*	Diff	Sig*	Diff	Sig*	Diff	Sig*	Diff	Sig*	Diff	Sig*	Diff	Sig*
Low/lower-middle	Arthritis	2.2	1	3.3	1	1.4	1	1.2	1	1.6	1	−0.2	0	2.7	1	.	0	0.5	0	3.4	1
	Asthma	2.3	1	3.5	1	1.5	1	1.4	1	1.8	1	−0.1	0	2.8	1	.	0	0.6	0	3.5	1
	Cancer	2.1	1	3.2	1	1.3	0	1.2	0	1.6	1	−0.3	0	2.6	1	.	0	0.4	0	3.3	1
	Chronic back/neck pain	2.0	1	3.1	1	1.2	1	1.0	1	1.4	1	−0.5	0	2.5	1	.	0	0.3	0	3.1	1
	Chronic pain	2.0	1	3.1	1	1.2	0	1.0	1	1.5	1	−0.4	0	2.5	1	.	0	0.3	0	3.2	1
	Diabetes	1.9	1	3.0	1	1.1	0	0.9	0	1.3	0	−0.6	0	2.4	1	.	0	0.2	0	3.0	1
	Headaches	0.9	1	2.0	1	0.1	0	−0.1	0	0.3	1	−1.6	0	1.4	1	.	0	−0.8	0	2.0	1
	Heart disease	1.8	1	2.9	1	1.0	0	0.9	0	1.3	1	−0.6	0	2.3	1	.	0	0.1	0	3.0	1
	Hypertension	1.8	1	3.0	1	1.0	0	0.9	1	1.3	1	−0.6	0	2.4	1	.	0	0.2	0	3.0	1
	Ulcer	3.1	1	4.2	1	2.3	1	2.1	1	2.5	1	0.7	0	3.6	1	.	0	1.4	1	4.2	1
Upper-middle	Arthritis	2.6	1	2.7	1	2.0	1	1.6	1	1.7	1	−0.4	0	1.0	1	1.8	1	0.4	0	1.2	1
	Asthma	2.7	1	2.7	1	2.1	1	1.7	1	1.8	1	−0.3	0	1.1	1	1.8	1	0.5	0	1.3	0
	Cancer	2.0	0	2.0	0	1.3	0	1.0	1	1.0	0	−1.0	0	0.4	0	1.1	1	−0.3	0	0.5	0
	Chronic back/neck pain	2.2	1	2.3	1	1.6	1	1.2	1	1.3	1	−0.8	0	0.6	0	1.4	1	0.0	0	0.8	0
	Chronic pain	2.1	1	2.1	1	1.4	1	1.1	1	1.1	1	−0.9	0	0.5	0	1.2	1	−0.2	0	0.6	0
	Diabetes	3.4	1	3.4	1	2.7	1	2.4	1	2.4	1	0.4	0	1.8	1	2.5	1	1.1	0	1.9	1
	Headaches	2.1	1	2.1	1	1.4	1	1.1	1	1.1	1	−0.9	0	0.5	0	1.2	1	−0.2	0	0.6	0
	Heart disease	2.7	1	2.8	1	2.1	1	1.7	1	1.8	1	−0.3	1	1.1	1	1.9	1	0.5	0	1.3	1
	Hypertension	3.4	1	3.5	1	2.8	1	2.4	1	2.5	1	0.4	1	1.8	1	2.6	1	1.2	1	2.0	1
	Ulcer	2.8	1	2.8	1	2.1	1	1.7	1	1.8	1	−0.3	0	1.1	1	1.9	1	0.5	0	1.3	1
High	Arthritis	3.3	1	3.7	1	2.7	1	2.0	1	1.2	1	−0.5	0	2.9	1	1.8	1	0.8	1	2.0	1
	Asthma	4.9	1	5.4	1	4.3	1	3.6	1	2.9	1	1.1	1	4.5	1	3.4	1	2.4	1	3.6	1
	Cancer	4.8	1	5.3	1	4.2	1	3.5	1	2.8	1	1.1	1	4.4	1	3.4	1	2.4	1	3.6	1
	Chronic back/neck pain	1.9	1	2.4	1	1.3	1	0.6	1	−0.1	0	−1.9	0	1.5	1	0.4	0	−0.6	0	0.6	0
	Chronic pain	1.6	1	2.0	1	1.0	1	0.2	0	−0.5	0	−2.2	0	1.2	1	0.1	0	−0.9	0	0.3	0
	Diabetes	4.8	1	5.2	1	4.2	1	3.4	1	2.7	1	1.0	1	4.4	1	3.3	1	2.3	1	3.5	1

Appendix Table 13.6 (cont.)

Country income level	Physical conditions	Major depressive disorder or dysthymia		Bipolar		Generalized anxiety disorder		Panic disorder		Social phobia		Specific phobia		Post-traumatic stress		Attention-deficit/hyperactivity		Intermittent explosive disorder		Oppositional-defiant disorder	
		Diff	Sig*	Diff	Sig*	Diff	Sig*	Diff	Sig*	Diff	Sig*	Diff	Sig*	Diff	Sig*	Diff	Sig*	Diff	Sig*	Diff	Sig*
	Headaches	1.4	1	1.8	1	0.8	1	0.1	0	-0.7	0	-2.4	0	1.0	1	-0.1	0	-1.1	0	0.1	0
	Heart disease	3.3	1	3.7	1	2.7	1	2.0	1	1.3	1	-0.5	0	2.9	1	1.8	1	0.8	1	2.0	1
	Hypertension	5.5	1	5.9	1	4.9	1	4.2	1	3.4	1	1.7	1	5.1	1	4.0	1	3.0	1	4.2	1
	Ulcer	4.0	1	4.4	1	3.4	1	2.7	1	1.9	1	0.2	0	3.6	1	2.5	1	1.5	1	2.7	1

[a] Each coefficient represents the difference in the mean global disability rating between the mental disorder in the column and the physical disorder in the row. A positive coefficient means that the mental disorder has a higher mean than the physical disorder.

* Significance at the 0.05 level of difference between the pairs of mental and physical disorders, two-sided test. 1 = yes; 0 = no.

Appendix Table 13.7 Pair-wise differences in proportion of cases rated severely disabled in the global Sheehan Disability Scale disability ratings for all mental–physical disorder pairs by country income level. The WMH surveys.[a]

Country income level	Physical conditions	Mental conditions																		
		Major depressive disorder or dysthymia		Bipolar		Generalized anxiety disorder		Panic disorder		Social phobia		Specific phobia		Post-traumatic stress		Attention-deficit/ hyperactivity		Intermittent explosive disorder		Oppositional-defiant disorder	
		Diff	Sig*	Diff	Sig*	Diff	Sig*	Diff	Sig*	Diff	Sig*	Diff	Sig*	Diff	Sig*	Diff	Sig*	Diff	Sig*	Diff	Sig*
Low/ lower-middle	Arthritis	20.0	1	35.0	1	9.6	1	4.0	0	17.4	1	−7.9	0	30.3	1	.	0	0.1	0	52.2	1
	Asthma	20.8	1	35.8	1	10.5	0	4.8	0	18.3	1	−7.0	0	31.1	1	.	0	1.0	0	53.1	1
	Cancer	26.1	1	41.1	1	15.7	1	10.1	0	23.5	1	−1.7	0	36.4	1	.	0	6.3	0	58.4	1
	Chronic back/ neck pain	21.0	1	36.0	1	10.6	1	5.0	0	18.4	1	−6.8	0	31.3	1	.	0	1.2	0	53.3	1
	Other chronic pain	15.7	1	30.7	1	5.3	0	−0.3	0	13.1	1	−12.2	0	26.0	1	.	0	−4.2	0	47.9	1
	Diabetes	19.4	1	34.4	1	9.0	0	3.4	0	16.8	0	−8.4	0	29.7	1	.	0	−0.4	0	51.6	1
	Headaches	9.1	1	24.1	1	−1.3	0	−6.9	0	6.5	0	−18.8	0	19.4	0	.	0	−10.8	0	41.3	1
	Heart disease	15.1	1	30.1	1	4.8	0	−0.9	0	12.6	0	−12.7	0	25.4	1	.	0	−4.7	0	47.4	1
	Hypertension	15.3	1	30.3	1	4.9	0	−0.7	0	12.7	1	−12.5	0	25.6	1	.	0	−4.5	0	47.6	1
	Ulcer	30.2	1	45.2	1	19.8	1	14.2	0	27.6	1	2.4	0	40.5	1	.	0	10.4	1	62.5	1
Upper-middle	Arthritis	29.6	1	33.7	1	22.3	1	23.0	1	15.2	0	−3.9	0	6.6	0	14.9	0	3.6	0	3.2	0
	Asthma	25.0	1	29.1	1	17.7	1	18.4	1	10.6	0	−8.5	0	2.0	0	10.3	0	−0.9	0	−1.4	0
	Cancer	11.4	0	15.5	0	4.2	0	4.8	0	−3.0	0	−22.1	0	−11.6	0	−3.3	0	−14.5	0	−14.9	0
	Chronic back/ neck pain	24.2	1	28.3	1	16.9	1	17.6	1	9.8	0	−9.3	0	1.2	0	9.5	0	−1.7	0	−2.2	0
	Other chronic pain	21.4	1	25.5	1	14.1	1	14.7	1	7.0	0	−12.2	0	−1.6	0	6.6	0	−4.6	0	−5.0	0
	Diabetes	32.9	1	37.0	1	25.6	1	26.3	1	18.5	1	−0.6	0	9.9	0	18.2	1	7.0	0	6.5	0
	Headaches	23.0	1	27.1	1	15.7	1	16.4	1	8.6	0	−10.5	0	0.0	0	8.3	0	−2.9	0	−3.4	0
	Heart disease	28.1	1	32.2	1	20.9	1	21.5	1	13.8	0	−5.4	0	5.1	0	13.4	0	2.2	0	1.8	0
	Hypertension	36.4	1	40.5	1	29.1	1	29.8	1	22.0	1	2.9	0	13.4	0	21.7	1	10.5	1	10.0	0
	Ulcer	30.6	1	34.7	1	23.3	1	24.0	1	16.2	0	−2.9	0	7.6	0	15.8	0	4.6	0	4.2	0

Appendix Table 13.7 (cont.)

Country income level	Physical conditions	Mental conditions																		
		Major depressive disorder or dysthymia		Bipolar		Generalized anxiety disorder		Panic disorder		Social phobia		Specific phobia		Post-traumatic stress		Attention-deficit/hyperactivity		Intermittent explosive disorder		Oppositional-defiant disorder	
		Diff	Sig*	Diff	Sig*	Diff	Sig*	Diff	Sig*	Diff	Sig*	Diff	Sig*	Diff	Sig*	Diff	Sig*	Diff	Sig*	Diff	Sig*
High	Arthritis	38.0	1	44.6	1	28.4	1	22.6	1	9.2	1	-8.5	0	31.1	1	14.4	1	6.0	1	14.8	1
	Asthma	53.2	1	59.8	1	43.6	1	37.9	1	24.5	1	6.8	1	46.3	1	29.7	1	21.2	1	30.0	1
	Cancer	46.7	1	53.3	1	37.1	1	31.3	1	17.9	1	0.2	0	39.8	1	23.2	1	14.7	1	23.5	1
	Chronic back/neck pain	25.4	1	32.0	1	15.7	1	10.0	1	-3.4	0	-21.1	0	18.4	1	1.8	0	-6.7	0	2.1	0
	Other chronic pain	19.4	1	26.0	1	9.8	1	4.1	0	-9.3	0	-27.0	0	12.5	1	-4.1	0	-12.6	0	-3.8	0
	Diabetes	49.5	1	56.1	1	39.8	1	34.1	1	20.7	1	3.0	0	42.5	1	25.9	1	17.4	1	26.2	1
	Headaches	18.6	1	25.2	1	9.0	1	3.3	0	-10.1	0	-27.9	0	11.7	1	-4.9	0	-13.4	0	-4.6	0
	Heart disease	35.6	1	42.2	1	25.9	1	20.2	1	6.8	1	-10.9	0	28.6	1	12.0	1	3.6	0	12.3	0
	Hypertension	55.0	1	61.6	1	45.3	1	39.6	1	26.2	1	8.5	1	48.0	1	31.4	1	22.9	1	31.7	1
	Ulcer	47.7	1	54.3	1	38.1	1	32.4	1	19.0	1	1.3	0	40.8	1	24.2	1	15.7	1	24.5	1

[a] Each coefficient represents the difference in the proportion of cases rated severely disabled on the global disability rating between the mental disorder in the column and the physical disorder in the row. A positive coefficient means that the mental disorder has a higher proportion rated severe than the physical disorder.

* Significance at the 0.05 level of difference between the pairs of mental and physical disorders, two-sided test. 1 = yes; 0 = no.

Appendix Table 13.8 Pair-wise differences in mean global Sheehan Disability Scale disability ratings for all mental–physical disorder pairs in treatment by country income level. The WMH surveys.

Country income level	Physical conditions	Mental disorders																		
		Major depressive disorder or dysthymia		Bipolar		Generalized anxiety disorder		Panic disorder		Social phobia		Specific phobia		Post-traumatic stress		Attention-deficit/ hyperactivity		Intermittent explosive disorder		Oppositional-defiant disorder	
		Diff	Sig*	Diff	Sig*	Diff	Sig*	Diff	Sig*	Diff	Sig*	Diff	Sig*	Diff	Sig*	Diff	Sig*	Diff	Sig*	Diff	Sig*
Low/lower-middle	Arthritis	3.4	1	3.4	1	3.3	1	2.2	0	1.8	0	−0.4	0	3.6	0	–	–	1.9	1	5.2	1
	Asthma	3.4	1	3.4	1	3.3	1	2.2	0	1.9	0	−0.4	0	3.6	0	–	–	1.9	0	5.2	1
	Cancer	2.9	1	2.9	1	2.8	1	1.8	0	1.4	0	−0.9	0	3.1	0	–	–	1.5	0	4.7	1
	Chronic back/ neck pain	3.2	1	3.2	1	3.2	1	2.1	0	1.7	0	−0.6	0	3.5	0	–	–	1.8	1	5.1	1
	Other chronic pain	3.5	1	3.5	1	3.4	1	2.4	1	2.0	0	−0.3	0	3.7	0	–	–	2.1	1	5.3	1
	Diabetes	3.1	1	3.1	1	3.1	1	2.0	0	1.6	0	−0.7	0	3.3	0	–	–	1.7	0	5.0	1
	Headaches	2.3	1	2.3	0	2.3	1	1.2	0	0.8	0	−1.5	0	2.5	0	–	–	0.9	0	4.2	1
	Heart disease	2.3	1	2.3	0	2.2	1	1.2	0	0.8	0	−1.5	0	2.5	0	–	–	0.9	0	4.1	1
	Hypertension	3.4	1	3.4	1	3.4	1	2.3	0	1.9	0	−0.4	0	3.6	0	–	–	2.0	1	5.3	1
	Ulcer	4.8	1	4.8	1	4.7	1	3.6	1	3.3	1	1.0	0	5.0	1	–	–	3.3	1	6.6	1
Upper-middle	Arthritis	2.6	1	2.6	1	2.2	1	2.4	1	1.2	0	−1.1	0	1.6	0	2.2	1	−0.2	0	2.8	1
	Asthma	2.6	1	2.6	1	2.3	1	2.4	1	1.2	0	−1.1	0	1.7	0	2.2	1	−0.1	0	2.9	1
	Cancer	1.9	0	1.9	0	1.6	0	1.7	0	0.5	0	−1.8	0	1.0	0	1.5	0	−0.8	0	2.2	0
	Chronic back/ neck pain	2.3	1	2.4	1	2.0	1	2.1	1	1.0	1	−1.3	0	1.4	0	2.0	1	−0.4	0	2.6	1
	Other chronic pain	2.5	1	2.5	1	2.2	1	2.3	1	1.1	1	−1.2	0	1.6	0	2.1	1	−0.2	0	2.8	1
	Diabetes	4.1	1	4.1	1	3.7	1	3.9	1	2.7	1	0.4	0	3.1	0	3.7	1	1.4	0	4.3	1
	Headaches	2.2	1	2.2	1	1.8	1	2.0	1	0.8	0	−1.5	0	1.2	0	1.8	0	−0.6	0	2.4	1
	Heart disease	3.4	1	3.4	1	3.0	1	3.2	1	2.0	1	−0.3	0	2.4	0	3.0	1	0.7	0	3.6	1
	Hypertension	3.9	1	4.0	1	3.6	1	3.7	1	2.6	1	0.3	0	3.0	0	3.6	1	1.2	0	4.2	1
	Ulcer	3.0	1	3.1	1	2.7	1	2.9	1	1.7	1	−0.6	0	2.1	0	2.7	1	0.3	0	3.3	1
High	Arthritis	2.7	1	3.2	1	2.3	1	2.1	1	0.9	0	−0.8	0	2.4	1	1.1	1	0.4	0	0.7	0
	Asthma	4.5	1	5.0	1	4.1	1	3.9	1	2.7	1	1.0	1	4.2	1	2.8	1	2.1	1	2.5	1
	Cancer	4.7	1	5.2	1	4.3	1	4.1	1	2.9	1	1.2	1	4.4	1	3.0	1	2.3	1	2.7	1
	Chronic back/ neck pain	1.9	1	2.5	1	1.6	1	1.4	1	0.1	0	−1.5	0	1.7	1	0.3	0	−0.4	0	−0.1	0

Appendix Table 13.8 (cont.)

Country income level	Physical conditions	Mental disorders																		
		Major depressive disorder or dysthymia		Bipolar		Generalized anxiety disorder		Panic disorder		Social phobia		Specific phobia		Post-traumatic stress		Attention-deficit/hyperactivity		Intermittent explosive disorder		Oppositional-defiant disorder	
		Diff	Sig*	Diff	Sig*	Diff	Sig*	Diff	Sig*	Diff	Sig*	Diff	Sig*	Diff	Sig*	Diff	Sig*	Diff	Sig*	Diff	Sig*
	Other chronic pain	1.6	1	2.2	1	1.3	1	1.1	1	-0.2	0	-1.9	0	1.4	1	0.0	0	-0.7	0	-0.4	0
	Diabetes	5.4	1	5.9	1	5.0	1	4.8	1	3.6	1	1.9	1	5.1	1	3.7	1	3.0	1	3.4	1
	Headaches	1.2	1	1.8	1	0.8	1	0.6	1	-0.6	0	-2.3	0	0.9	1	-0.4	0	-1.1	0	-0.8	0
	Heart disease	3.6	1	4.1	1	3.2	1	3.0	1	1.8	1	0.1	0	3.3	1	2.0	1	1.3	1	1.6	0
	Hypertension	6.1	1	6.6	1	5.7	1	5.5	1	4.3	1	2.6	1	5.8	1	4.5	1	3.8	1	4.1	1
	Ulcer	4.5	1	5.0	1	4.1	1	3.9	1	2.7	1	1.0	1	4.2	1	2.8	1	2.1	1	2.5	1

[a] Each coefficient represents the difference in the mean global disability rating between the mental disorder in the column and the physical disorder in the row. A positive coefficient means that the mental disorder has a higher mean than the physical disorder.

* Significance at the 0.05 level of difference between the pairs of mental and physical disorders, two-sided test. 1 = yes; 0 = no.

Appendix Table 13.9 Pair-wise differences in proportion of cases rated severely disabled in the global Sheehan Disability Scale disability ratings for all mental–physical disorder pairs in treatment by country income level. The WMH surveys.[a]

Country income level	Physical conditions	Major depressive disorder or dysthymia		Bipolar		Generalized anxiety disorder		Panic disorder		Social phobia		Specific phobia		Post-traumatic stress		Attention-deficit/hyperactivity		Intermittent explosive disorder		Oppositional-defiant disorder	
		Diff	Sig*	Diff	Sig*	Diff	Sig*	Diff	Sig*	Diff	Sig*	Diff	Sig*	Diff	Sig*	Diff	Sig*	Diff	Sig*	Diff	Sig*
Low/lower-middle	Arthritis	50.7	1	49.5	1	65.4	1	34.0	1	29.2	0	-3.4	0	50.3	0	.	0	18.8	0	80.0	1
	Asthma	51.6	1	50.4	1	66.3	1	34.9	0	30.1	0	-2.5	0	51.2	0	.	0	19.8	0	80.9	1
	Cancer	55.0	1	53.8	1	69.7	1	38.3	1	33.4	0	0.9	0	54.5	1	.	0	23.1	0	84.3	1
	Chronic back/neck pain	50.3	1	49.1	1	65.1	1	33.6	1	28.8	0	-3.7	0	49.9	0	.	0	18.5	0	79.6	1
	Other chronic pain	43.3	1	42.1	1	58.0	1	26.6	0	21.8	0	-10.8	0	42.8	0	.	0	11.4	0	72.6	1
	Diabetes	45.8	1	44.6	1	60.5	1	29.1	0	24.3	0	-8.3	0	45.3	0	.	0	13.9	0	75.1	1
	Headaches	37.7	1	36.5	1	52.5	1	21.0	0	16.2	0	-16.4	0	37.3	0	.	0	5.9	0	67.0	1
	Heart disease	32.0	1	30.8	0	46.7	1	15.3	0	10.5	0	-22.1	0	31.6	0	.	0	0.2	0	61.3	1
	Hypertension	44.3	1	43.1	1	59.0	1	27.6	0	22.8	0	-9.8	0	43.8	0	.	0	12.4	0	73.6	1
	Ulcer	62.7	1	61.5	1	77.4	1	45.9	1	41.1	1	8.6	1	62.2	1	.	0	30.8	1	92.0	1
Upper-middle	Arthritis	31.1	1	40.9	1	25.8	1	34.5	1	11.4	0	-11.0	0	24.4	0	29.7	1	1.8	0	33.3	0
	Asthma	27.7	1	37.4	1	22.3	1	31.0	1	7.9	0	-14.5	0	20.9	0	26.2	0	-1.7	0	29.9	0
	Cancer	11.8	0	21.5	0	6.4	0	15.1	0	-8.0	0	-30.4	0	5.0	0	10.3	0	-17.6	0	14.0	0
	Chronic back/neck pain	29.7	1	39.4	1	24.3	1	33.1	1	10.0	0	-12.5	0	22.9	0	28.2	1	0.3	0	31.9	0
	Other chronic pain	27.9	1	37.6	1	22.5	1	31.2	1	8.1	0	-14.3	0	21.1	0	26.4	0	-1.5	0	30.1	0
	Diabetes	41.4	1	51.2	1	36.1	1	44.8	1	21.7	1	-0.7	0	34.7	0	40.0	1	12.1	0	43.6	0
	Headaches	29.4	1	39.1	1	24.0	1	32.8	1	9.7	0	-12.8	0	22.6	0	27.9	1	0.0	0	31.6	0
	Heart disease	39.1	1	48.8	1	33.7	1	42.4	1	19.3	1	-3.1	0	32.3	0	37.6	1	9.7	0	41.3	0
	Hypertension	46.8	1	56.5	1	41.4	1	50.1	1	27.0	1	4.6	0	40.0	1	45.3	1	17.4	0	49.0	1
	Ulcer	39.7	1	49.4	1	34.4	1	43.1	1	20.0	1	-2.4	0	33.0	0	38.3	1	10.3	0	41.9	0
High	Arthritis	35.7	1	42.5	1	30.0	1	32.5	1	15.8	1	-8.4	0	29.9	1	9.8	0	0.5	0	2.1	0
	Asthma	57.4	1	64.1	1	51.7	1	54.2	1	37.5	1	13.2	1	51.5	1	31.5	1	22.1	1	23.8	1
	Cancer	50.7	1	57.5	1	45.0	1	47.5	1	30.8	1	6.6	0	44.9	1	24.8	1	15.4	1	17.1	0

Appendix Table 13.9 (cont.)

Country income level	Physical conditions	Mental disorders																		
		Major depressive disorder or dysthymia		Bipolar disorder		Generalized anxiety disorder		Panic disorder		Social phobia		Specific phobia		Post-traumatic stress		Attention-deficit/ hyperactivity		Intermittent explosive disorder		Oppositional-defiant disorder	
		Diff	Sig*	Diff	Sig*	Diff	Sig*	Diff	Sig*	Diff	Sig*	Diff	Sig*	Diff	Sig*	Diff	Sig*	Diff	Sig*	Diff	Sig*
	Chronic back/neck pain	29.0	1	35.7	1	23.3	1	25.8	1	9.1	1	−15.2	0	23.1	1	3.1	0	−6.3	0	−4.6	0
	Other chronic pain	23.9	1	30.7	1	18.2	1	20.7	1	4.1	0	−20.2	0	18.1	1	−2.0	0	−11.3	0	−9.7	0
	Diabetes	60.0	1	66.7	1	54.3	1	56.8	1	40.1	1	15.8	1	54.1	1	34.1	1	24.7	1	26.4	1
	Headaches	18.9	1	25.7	1	13.2	1	15.7	1	−1.0	0	−25.2	0	13.0	1	−7.0	0	−16.4	0	−14.7	0
	Heart disease	42.5	1	49.3	1	36.9	1	39.3	1	22.7	1	−1.6	0	36.7	1	16.7	1	7.3	0	8.9	0
	Hypertension	65.9	1	72.7	1	60.3	1	62.8	1	46.1	1	21.8	1	60.1	1	40.1	1	30.7	1	32.4	1
	Ulcer	56.6	1	63.4	1	51.0	1	53.4	1	36.8	1	12.5	1	50.8	1	30.8	1	21.4	1	23.0	1

[a] Each coefficient represents the difference in the proportion of cases rated severely disabled on the global disability rating between the mental disorder in the column and the physical disorder in the row. A positive coefficient means that the mental disorder has a higher proportion rated severe than the physical disorder.

* Significance at the 0.05 level of difference between the pairs of mental and physical disorders, two-sided test. 1 = yes; 0 = no.

Appendix Table 13.10 Sheehan Disability Scale global and domain-specific ratings for aggregated physical and mental disorders in treatment by country income level. The WMH surveys.

Sheehan Disability Scale	Country income level	Mean disability rating								Proportion rated severely disabled							
		Treated mental disorders			Treated physical conditions			Difference between treated mental and physical disorders		Treated mental disorders			Treated physical conditions			Difference between treated mental and physical disorders
		N	Mean	(SE)	N	Mean	(SE)	χ^2_1		N	%	(SE)	N	%	(SE)	χ^2_1
Global	Low/lower-middle	162	6.2	(0.4)	2,007	4.1	(0.1)	44.4*		76	53.8	(5.5)	435	24.7	(2.0)	18.2*
	Upper-middle	576	6.2	(0.2)	3,683	4.5	(0.1)	82.1*		311	54.1	(2.8)	1,114	32.2	(1.3)	42.4*
	High	2,841	6.8	(0.1)	9,300	4.3	(0.1)	798.1*		1,765	62.8	(1.2)	3,196	32.7	(0.9)	302.9*
Home	Low/lower-middle	159	4.9	(0.4)	1,986	3.6	(0.1)	13.5*		53	36.9	(6.4)	331	19.0	(1.8)	8.6*
	Upper-middle	565	4.9	(0.2)	3,565	3.8	(0.1)	39.3*		213	36.7	(2.5)	771	22.6	(1.1)	27.8*
	High	2,817	4.8	(0.1)	9,144	3.7	(0.1)	134.8*		1,011	36.7	(1.3)	2,454	25.4	(0.8)	67.7*
Work	Low/lower-middle	154	4.5	(0.4)	1,915	3.6	(0.1)	12.0*		42	27.2	(6.1)	322	18.4	(1.6)	3.5
	Upper-middle	541	5.3	(0.2)	3,504	3.9	(0.1)	53.5*		220	39.3	(2.9)	814	25.3	(1.2)	21.4*
	High	2,754	5.2	(0.1)	8,660	3.5	(0.1)	230.4*		1,145	41.7	(1.5)	2,372	26.2	(0.9)	97.7*
Social	Low/lower-middle	147	4.4	(0.4)	1,897	2.2	(0.1)	35.0*		37	30.1	(6.4)	157	9.9	(1.5)	10.1*
	Upper-middle	574	5.2	(0.2)	3,604	2.7	(0.1)	170.3*		242	40.7	(2.7)	523	15.6	(0.9)	63.1*
	High	2,815	5.5	(0.1)	9,107	2.1	(0.1)	1,205.4*		1,280	46.2	(1.3)	1,288	13.1	(0.6)	306.2*
Close relationships	Low/lower-middle	159	4.6	(0.4)	1,990	2.2	(0.1)	48.9*		46	32.3	(5.3)	170	9.1	(1.3)	13.3*
	Upper-middle	575	5.0	(0.2)	3,620	2.6	(0.1)	234.4*		223	37.1	(2.3)	485	14.5	(0.9)	55.3*
	High	2,837	5.1	(0.1)	9,107	1.7	(0.1)	1,325.1*		1,115	40.4	(1.3)	969	10.3	(0.6)	271.3*

* Significant at the 0.05 level, two-sided test.

Appendix Table 13.11 Sheehan Disability Scale global and domain-specific mean SDS ratings aggregated across physical (total and treated) and mental disorders (total and treated) by country income level. The WMH surveys.

Sheehan Disability Scale	Country income level	Mean disability rating						
		Mental disorders			Physical conditions			Difference between mental and physical disorders
		N	Mean	(SE)	N	Mean	(SE)	χ^2_1
Global	Low/lower-middle	2,672	4.3	(0.1)	4,265	3.6	(0.1)	119.3*
	Upper-middle	4,019	5.1	(0.1)	6,713	3.9	(0.1)	152.7*
	High	11,605	5.4	(0.0)	14,787	3.8	(0.1)	952.2*
Home	Low/lower-middle	2,624	3.3	(0.1)	4,226	3.1	(0.1)	30.8*
	Upper-middle	3,890	3.7	(0.1)	6,507	3.3	(0.1)	34.2*
	High	11,521	3.5	(0.1)	14,547	3.3	(0.0)	61.2*
Work	Low/lower-middle	2,520	3.2	(0.1)	4,052	3.1	(0.1)	31.7*
	Upper-middle	3,758	3.7	(0.1)	6,376	3.4	(0.1)	23.3*
	High	11,284	3.7	(0.1)	13,883	3.1	(0.1)	171.5*
Social	Low/lower-middle	2,413	3.0	(0.1)	3,933	1.7	(0.1)	231.0*
	Upper-middle	3,978	3.8	(0.1)	6,591	2.3	(0.1)	331.8*
	High	11,500	4.1	(0.1)	14,480	1.8	(0.0)	1,576.8*
Close relationships	Low/lower-middle	2,625	3.0	(0.1)	4,218	1.7	(0.1)	272.1*
	Upper-middle	3,991	3.8	(0.1)	6,607	2.2	(0.1)	310.6*
	High	11,566	3.8	(0.1)	14,500	1.4	(0.0)	1,978.0*

* Significant at the 0.05 level, two-sided test.

Appendix Table 13-12 Mental and physical within-person mean Sheehan Disability Scale scores by country income level. The WMH surveys.[a]

Country income level	Physical disorders	Mental disorders	Global Mental Mean (SE)	Global Physical Mean (SE) Sig*	Home Mental Mean (SE)	Home Physical Mean (SE) Sig*	Work Mental Mean (SE)	Work Physical Mean (SE) Sig*	Social Mental Mean (SE)	Social Physical Mean (SE) Sig*	Close relationships Mental Mean (SE)	Close relationships Physical Mean (SE) Sig*
All countries	Arthritis	MDD or dysthymia	6.6 (0.2)	5.0 (0.2) 1	5.2 (0.2)	4.4 (0.2) 1	5.2 (0.2)	4.2 (0.3) 1	5.2 (0.2)	2.5 (0.2) 1	4.8 (0.2)	2.3 (0.2) 1
		Bipolar	7.8 (0.3)	5.2 (0.6) 1	6.5 (0.4)	4.0 (0.6) 1	6.6 (0.5)	4.0 (0.7) 1	6.5 (0.4)	3.4 (0.6) 1	6.6 (0.4)	2.8 (0.5) 1
		GAD	6.3 (0.3)	5.5 (0.3) 1	4.4 (0.3)	4.7 (0.4) 0	4.9 (0.3)	4.7 (0.4) 0	5.1 (0.3)	3.0 (0.4) 1	4.7 (0.3)	2.4 (0.3) 1
		Panic	6.1 (0.5)	6.2 (0.5) 0	4.4 (0.5)	4.9 (0.6) 0	4.9 (0.5)	5.1 (0.6) 0	4.6 (0.5)	4.3 (0.6) 0	4.3 (0.5)	3.4 (0.6) 0
		Social phobia	5.4 (0.3)	4.4 (0.4) 1	2.3 (0.2)	3.5 (0.3) 0	3.4 (0.3)	3.6 (0.4) 0	4.9 (0.3)	2.0 (0.3) 1	4.2 (0.2)	1.8 (0.3) 1
		Specific phobia	3.5 (0.2)	4.4 (0.2) 0	2.4 (0.2)	3.9 (0.3) 0	2.3 (0.2)	3.5 (0.3) 0	2.1 (0.2)	1.8 (0.2) 0	2.0 (0.2)	1.5 (0.2) 0
		PTSD	6.5 (0.4)	5.8 (0.5) 0	4.1 (0.5)	4.7 (0.5) 0	4.6 (0.5)	4.4 (0.7) 0	5.5 (0.5)	3.5 (0.5) 1	5.1 (0.4)	3.2 (0.5) 1
		IED	4.4 (0.4)	4.8 (0.4) 0	3.6 (0.4)	4.4 (0.4) 0	3.4 (0.4)	4.4 (0.5) 0	2.6 (0.4)	2.3 (0.4) 0	3.4 (0.4)	2.3 (0.4) 1
	Asthma	MDD or dysthymia	6.2 (0.3)	2.9 (0.5) 1	4.5 (0.3)	2.3 (0.4) 1	4.5 (0.3)	1.9 (0.4) 1	4.7 (0.3)	1.3 (0.3) 1	4.0 (0.3)	0.8 (0.2) 1
		Bipolar	7.0 (0.5)	3.1 (0.9) 1	4.9 (0.6)	2.9 (1.0) 0	5.1 (0.5)	1.3 (0.7) 1	5.2 (0.6)	0.6 (0.2) 1	5.2 (0.6)	0.6 (0.3) 1
		GAD	6.2 (0.3)	3.0 (0.7) 1	4.4 (0.4)	2.7 (0.8) 0	3.8 (0.5)	1.2 (0.4) 1	4.7 (0.4)	0.7 (0.3) 1	4.5 (0.4)	0.5 (0.2) 1
		Panic	5.9 (0.7)	4.3 (1.0) 0	3.4 (0.6)	4.0 (1.1) 0	3.8 (0.8)	1.3 (0.4) 1	4.4 (0.6)	2.1 (1.2) 0	4.7 (0.7)	1.9 (1.2) 0
		Social phobia	5.1 (0.3)	2.8 (0.6) 1	2.0 (0.3)	2.5 (0.6) 0	3.1 (0.3)	1.3 (0.4) 1	4.4 (0.4)	0.9 (0.3) 1	3.7 (0.3)	0.7 (0.2) 1
		Specific phobia	3.1 (0.3)	2.5 (0.5) 0	2.1 (0.3)	2.1 (0.5) 0	1.5 (0.3)	1.3 (0.3) 1	2.0 (0.3)	1.1 (0.3) 1	1.6 (0.3)	0.8 (0.2) 1
		IED	5.3 (0.6)	2.9 (0.6) 1	2.1 (0.6)	2.5 (0.5) 0	2.9 (0.5)	2.3 (0.5) 0	2.9 (0.6)	2.0 (0.4) 0	3.7 (0.8)	1.5 (0.3) 1
	Cancer	MDD or dysthymia	7.5 (0.4)	3.5 (1.0) 1	5.4 (0.8)	3.1 (1.0) 0	6.1 (0.5)	3.0 (0.9) 1	5.6 (0.7)	2.1 (0.8) 1	5.1 (0.6)	1.9 (0.7) 1
		Specific phobia	3.5 (0.5)	2.9 (0.6) 0	2.3 (0.4)	2.4 (0.6) 0	2.2 (0.5)	2.4 (0.6) 0	2.6 (0.5)	1.4 (0.4) 0	2.3 (0.4)	0.9 (0.2) 1
	Chronic back/neck pain	MDD or dysthymia	6.7 (0.1)	5.9 (0.2) 1	5.2 (0.2)	5.3 (0.2) 0	5.0 (0.2)	5.2 (0.2) 0	5.2 (0.2)	3.3 (0.2) 1	4.8 (0.2)	2.7 (0.2) 1
		Bipolar	7.3 (0.3)	6.7 (0.4) 0	5.9 (0.4)	5.9 (0.4) 0	5.7 (0.4)	5.6 (0.4) 0	6.0 (0.4)	3.8 (0.4) 1	5.8 (0.3)	3.6 (0.5) 1
		GAD	6.0 (0.2)	6.4 (0.2) 0	4.3 (0.2)	5.7 (0.2) 0	4.7 (0.2)	5.7 (0.3) 0	4.8 (0.2)	3.8 (0.3) 1	4.3 (0.2)	3.1 (0.2) 1
		Panic	5.3 (0.3)	6.2 (0.3) 0	3.9 (0.3)	5.6 (0.3) 0	4.4 (0.4)	5.4 (0.4) 0	3.7 (0.3)	3.4 (0.4) 0	3.3 (0.4)	2.8 (0.4) 0
		Social phobia	4.9 (0.2)	5.8 (0.2) 0	2.3 (0.2)	5.0 (0.2) 0	3.3 (0.2)	5.0 (0.3) 1	4.2 (0.2)	3.1 (0.3) 0	3.7 (0.2)	2.4 (0.3) 1
		Specific phobia	3.2 (0.2)	5.4 (0.2) 0	2.2 (0.2)	4.7 (0.2) 0	2.1 (0.2)	4.6 (0.2) 0	2.0 (0.2)	2.7 (0.2) 0	1.7 (0.1)	2.1 (0.2) 0
		PTSD	6.2 (0.4)	6.7 (0.5) 0	4.1 (0.4)	5.7 (0.5) 0	4.7 (0.6)	6.0 (0.6) 0	5.0 (0.5)	4.5 (0.7) 0	4.3 (0.4)	3.2 (0.7) 0
		ADHD	3.9 (0.6)	6.3 (0.6) 0	3.6 (0.5)	5.5 (0.6) 0	2.9 (0.6)	4.8 (0.8) 0	3.3 (0.5)	3.3 (0.8) 0	2.9 (0.5)	2.3 (0.7) 0
		IED	4.3 (0.4)	5.0 (0.4) 0	2.9 (0.3)	3.9 (0.3) 0	2.9 (0.3)	4.5 (0.4) 0	2.6 (0.3)	2.9 (0.4) 0	3.1 (0.4)	2.3 (0.3) 0

Appendix Table 13.12 (cont.)

Country income level	Physical disorders	Mental disorders	Global Mental Mean (SE)	Global Physical Mean (SE)	Sig*	Home Mental Mean (SE)	Home Physical Mean (SE)	Sig*	Work Mental Mean (SE)	Work Physical Mean (SE)	Sig*	Social Mental Mean (SE)	Social Physical Mean (SE)	Sig*	Close relationships Mental Mean (SE)	Close relationships Physical Mean (SE)	Sig*
	Other chronic pain	MDD or dysthymia	6.9 (0.2)	6.2 (0.3)	0	5.4 (0.3)	5.5 (0.3)	0	5.3 (0.3)	5.5 (0.3)	0	5.6 (0.3)	3.9 (0.3)	1	5.5 (0.3)	3.6 (0.3)	1
		Bipolar	7.4 (0.5)	6.8 (0.9)	0	5.8 (0.5)	6.1 (0.8)	0	6.0 (0.5)	6.5 (0.9)	0	6.3 (0.6)	5.2 (0.8)	0	6.1 (0.6)	4.8 (0.8)	0
		GAD	6.8 (0.3)	6.1 (0.5)	0	5.3 (0.4)	5.3 (0.5)	0	5.7 (0.5)	5.3 (0.5)	0	5.1 (0.4)	3.7 (0.5)	1	4.9 (0.4)	3.4 (0.5)	1
		Panic	5.5 (0.6)	5.9 (0.5)	0	4.8 (0.8)	5.3 (0.5)	0	4.2 (0.6)	5.2 (0.6)	0	4.1 (0.7)	3.3 (0.6)	0	4.1 (0.7)	2.9 (0.6)	0
		Social phobia	5.8 (0.4)	7.0 (0.3)	0	3.4 (0.4)	6.0 (0.4)	0	4.1 (0.3)	6.1 (0.3)	0	4.9 (0.4)	4.5 (0.6)	0	4.3 (0.4)	3.9 (0.6)	0
		Specific phobia	3.8 (0.3)	5.8 (0.5)	0	2.6 (0.3)	5.0 (0.4)	0	2.7 (0.3)	5.0 (0.5)	0	2.4 (0.3)	3.1 (0.4)	0	1.9 (0.3)	2.8 (0.4)	0
		PTSD	5.9 (0.6)	6.7 (0.5)	0	4.6 (0.6)	6.4 (0.5)	0	4.3 (0.6)	6.0 (0.7)	0	5.0 (0.7)	3.6 (0.8)	0	3.7 (0.7)	2.8 (0.7)	0
		IED	5.4 (0.5)	5.4 (0.8)	0	3.3 (0.5)	4.5 (0.6)	0	2.5 (0.6)	5.5 (0.7)	0	2.7 (0.5)	2.2 (0.7)	0	4.1 (0.6)	2.3 (0.6)	1
	Diabetes	MDD or dysthymia	6.3 (0.5)	3.7 (0.6)	1	5.1 (0.4)	3.2 (0.5)	1	5.2 (0.5)	3.1 (0.5)	1	4.8 (0.5)	1.7 (0.4)	1	4.9 (0.5)	1.8 (0.4)	1
		Specific phobia	2.6 (0.4)	5.3 (0.9)	0	1.5 (0.2)	4.6 (1.0)	0	1.9 (0.3)	4.2 (1.2)	0	2.0 (0.4)	1.9 (0.9)	0	1.8 (0.4)	1.7 (0.8)	0
	Headaches	MDD or dysthymia	7.0 (0.1)	6.3 (0.2)	1	5.3 (0.2)	5.5 (0.2)	0	5.3 (0.1)	5.4 (0.2)	0	5.4 (0.2)	4.8 (0.2)	1	5.2 (0.1)	4.4 (0.2)	1
		Bipolar	7.4 (0.3)	6.1 (0.4)	1	5.9 (0.4)	4.7 (0.4)	1	5.8 (0.4)	5.7 (0.4)	0	5.9 (0.4)	3.6 (0.5)	1	5.2 (0.3)	3.5 (0.5)	1
		GAD	6.4 (0.2)	6.4 (0.2)	0	3.9 (0.2)	5.5 (0.3)	0	4.5 (0.3)	5.2 (0.3)	0	5.0 (0.3)	4.7 (0.3)	0	4.8 (0.3)	4.3 (0.3)	0
		Panic	5.4 (0.4)	6.1 (0.5)	0	3.6 (0.3)	5.1 (0.5)	0	3.8 (0.3)	5.3 (0.5)	0	4.4 (0.4)	4.8 (0.5)	0	4.2 (0.4)	4.1 (0.5)	0
		Social phobia	5.5 (0.2)	6.3 (0.2)	0	2.2 (0.2)	5.1 (0.2)	0	3.1 (0.2)	5.4 (0.3)	0	4.9 (0.2)	4.7 (0.3)	0	4.2 (0.2)	3.8 (0.3)	0
		Specific phobia	3.2 (0.2)	5.8 (0.2)	0	2.2 (0.1)	5.1 (0.2)	0	2.2 (0.2)	5.1 (0.2)	0	2.0 (0.1)	4.4 (0.2)	0	1.8 (0.1)	3.8 (0.2)	0
		PTSD	6.1 (0.4)	7.2 (0.2)	0	3.7 (0.4)	6.0 (0.4)	0	3.8 (0.4)	6.4 (0.3)	0	5.2 (0.4)	5.3 (0.4)	0	4.8 (0.5)	4.3 (0.4)	0
		ADHD	5.9 (0.6)	7.1 (0.4)	0	4.8 (0.5)	6.0 (0.4)	0	4.1 (0.6)	6.4 (0.5)	0	4.1 (0.6)	5.5 (0.7)	0	4.1 (0.5)	4.8 (0.7)	0
		IED	4.6 (0.3)	5.9 (0.4)	0	2.8 (0.3)	4.6 (0.4)	0	2.7 (0.3)	4.8 (0.4)	0	3.7 (0.3)	4.2 (0.4)	0	3.6 (0.3)	4.4 (0.3)	0
	Heart disease	MDD or dysthymia	6.7 (0.3)	5.1 (0.5)	1	5.1 (0.4)	4.5 (0.4)	0	5.5 (0.4)	4.8 (0.5)	0	5.1 (0.4)	2.2 (0.4)	1	5.0 (0.4)	2.5 (0.4)	1
		GAD	6.2 (0.4)	5.1 (0.7)	0	5.0 (0.5)	4.4 (0.6)	0	4.4 (0.5)	4.7 (0.8)	0	4.5 (0.5)	3.1 (0.6)	0	4.2 (0.5)	2.8 (0.5)	0
		Panic	5.9 (0.7)	5.0 (0.9)	0	4.8 (0.8)	4.1 (1.0)	0	4.5 (0.7)	4.3 (1.0)	0	.	.		4.6 (0.6)	3.0 (0.7)	0
		Social phobia	6.6 (0.5)	3.9 (1.1)	1	3.0 (0.7)	3.1 (1.1)	0	3.1 (0.7)	3.8 (1.2)	0	5.4 (0.5)	2.8 (0.5)	1	5.0 (0.6)	2.6 (0.8)	1
		Specific phobia	2.5 (0.4)	3.9 (0.6)	0	1.6 (0.3)	2.9 (0.6)	0	1.4 (0.3)	3.7 (0.6)	0	1.2 (0.3)	1.8 (0.3)	0	1.1 (0.3)	1.5 (0.3)	0

Hypertension										
MDD or dysthymia	6.5 (0.2)	4.3 (0.3) 1	5.0 (0.3)	3.8 (0.3) 1	4.9 (0.3)	3.6 (0.3) 1	5.1 (0.2)	2.6 (0.3) 1	4.9 (0.2)	2.6 (0.3) 1
Bipolar	7.5 (0.5)	4.2 (0.5) 1	6.6 (0.6)	3.7 (0.5) 1	6.1 (0.5)	3.6 (0.5) 1	6.8 (0.5)	2.5 (0.6) 1	5.9 (0.5)	2.3 (0.5) 1
GAD	5.5 (0.4)	4.0 (0.5) 1	4.4 (0.4)	3.7 (0.4) 0	4.8 (0.4)	3.3 (0.6) 1	4.1 (0.4)	2.4 (0.5) 1	4.0 (0.4)	2.4 (0.4) 1
Panic	6.4 (0.5)	4.6 (0.5) 1	4.8 (0.6)	4.1 (0.5) 0	4.4 (0.6)	3.5 (0.6) 0	4.8 (0.5)	2.1 (0.5) 0	4.0 (0.5)	2.3 (0.4) 1
Social phobia	5.7 (0.4)	3.0 (0.4) 1	2.2 (0.3)	2.5 (0.4) 0	3.5 (0.4)	2.6 (0.4) 0	4.7 (0.3)	1.6 (0.4) 0	4.4 (0.3)	1.5 (0.4) 1
Specific phobia	3.3 (0.2)	2.9 (0.3) 0	2.3 (0.2)	2.6 (0.3) 0	2.3 (0.2)	2.4 (0.2) 0	2.1 (0.2)	1.5 (0.2) 0	2.0 (0.2)	1.5 (0.2) 0
PTSD	5.7 (0.7)	4.8 (0.5) 0	4.3 (0.7)	4.2 (0.5) 0	4.2 (0.7)	4.9 (0.6) 0	4.0 (0.7)	2.1 (0.5) 1	4.0 (0.6)	2.4 (0.5) 1
IED	4.6 (0.5)	3.5 (0.6) 0	2.8 (0.5)	2.8 (0.5) 0	2.7 (0.6)	3.1 (0.7) 0	3.5 (0.6)	2.5 (0.7) 0	4.0 (0.4)	2.2 (0.5) 1
Ulcer										
MDD or dysthymia	6.3 (0.4)	3.2 (0.5) 1	5.1 (0.4)	2.9 (0.4) 1	4.8 (0.4)	2.7 (0.4) 1	4.2 (0.4)	1.4 (0.3) 1	4.2 (0.5)	1.5 (0.3) 1
Social phobia	5.7 (0.5)	3.5 (0.8) 1	2.4 (0.5)	2.7 (0.7) 0	4.2 (0.6)	2.5 (0.6) 1	5.3 (0.5)	1.6 (0.4) 1	4.9 (0.5)	1.8 (0.6) 1
Specific phobia	2.9 (0.4)	3.0 (0.6) 0	2.1 (0.3)	2.6 (0.6) 0	2.0 (0.3)	2.6 (0.6) 0	2.4 (0.4)	1.8 (0.5) 0	1.9 (0.3)	1.8 (0.5) 0
IED	5.2 (0.5)	5.5 (0.9) 0	3.5 (0.5)	4.1 (0.8) 0	3.6 (0.5)	4.2 (0.8) 0	2.9 (0.5)	2.8 (0.6) 0	3.3 (0.5)	2.5 (0.7) 0
Low/lower- middle										
Arthritis										
MDD or dysthymia	4.6 (0.3)	4.8 (0.4) 0	4.3 (0.3)	4.6 (0.4) 0	3.9 (0.3)	3.9 (0.3) 0	3.5 (0.3)	2.6 (0.5) 0	3.7 (0.3)	2.7 (0.6) 0
Specific phobia	2.7 (0.2)	2.7 (0.5) 0	2.4 (0.2)	2.2 (0.4) 0	2.3 (0.2)	2.5 (0.5) 0	2.0 (0.2)	1.6 (0.4) 0	2.0 (0.2)	1.5 (0.3) 0
IED	3.4 (0.6)	4.8 (0.8) 0	3.0 (0.5)	4.6 (0.8) 0	3.0 (0.5)	4.6 (0.8) 0			2.8 (0.5)	3.1 (0.5) 0
Chronic back/neck pain										
MDD or dysthymia	5.5 (0.2)	4.9 (0.3) 1	4.5 (0.3)	4.6 (0.3) 0	4.1 (0.3)	4.2 (0.3) 0	3.7 (0.3)	1.7 (0.2) 1	3.8 (0.3)	1.6 (0.2) 1
GAD	4.8 (0.6)	5.2 (0.5) 0	4.3 (0.6)	4.9 (0.5) 0	3.0 (0.4)	3.1 (0.5) 0	2.7 (0.5)	2.4 (0.4) 0	4.0 (0.6)	2.4 (0.4) 1
Specific phobia	3.3 (0.4)	3.5 (0.5) 0	2.9 (0.4)	3.1 (0.5) 0	2.5 (0.4)	3.3 (0.6) 0	1.6 (0.6)	1.3 (0.3) 0	2.2 (0.3)	2.6 (0.5) 0
IED	3.1 (0.6)	3.7 (0.6) 0	2.4 (0.6)	2.8 (0.6) 0	3.3 (0.7)	4.9 (0.8) 0	3.4 (0.5)	3.3 (0.9) 0	1.9 (0.6)	1.2 (0.3) 0
Other chronic pain										
MDD or dysthymia	5.1 (0.4)	5.8 (0.6) 0	4.1 (0.4)	5.4 (0.6) 0	4.2 (0.4)				3.2 (0.3)	2.8 (0.4) 0
Headaches										
MDD or dysthymia	5.8 (0.2)	5.7 (0.4) 0	4.8 (0.3)	5.5 (0.4) 0	3.9 (0.3)	5.2 (0.5) 0	3.5 (0.3)	4.4 (0.6) 0	4.1 (0.4)	4.3 (0.5) 0
Social phobia	5.2 (0.6)	5.7 (0.5) 0	2.5 (0.8)	4.7 (0.6) 0	2.9 (0.8)	4.9 (0.6) 0	2.4 (0.3)	4.4 (0.6) 0	3.6 (0.6)	2.9 (0.8) 0
Specific phobia	3.0 (0.3)	4.0 (0.5) 0	2.2 (0.3)	3.7 (0.5) 0	2.4 (0.4)	3.8 (0.4) 0	2.9 (0.6)	2.9 (0.6) 0	2.2 (0.3)	2.8 (0.6) 0
IED	4.4 (0.6)	5.9 (0.6) 0	3.1 (0.6)	4.8 (0.5) 0	2.8 (0.4)	4.3 (0.6) 0	4.5 (0.7)	4.5 (0.7) 0	3.5 (0.6)	4.8 (0.7) 0
Heart disease										
MDD or dysthymia	5.7 (0.5)	5.1 (0.6) 0	4.2 (0.5)	5.1 (0.5) 0					4.3 (0.5)	3.1 (0.8) 0

Appendix Table 13.12 (cont.)

Country income level	Physical disorders	Mental disorders	Global Mental Mean	(SE)	Global Physical Mean	(SE)	Sig*	Home Mental Mean	(SE)	Home Physical Mean	(SE)	Sig*	Work Mental Mean	(SE)	Work Physical Mean	(SE)	Sig*	Social Mental Mean	(SE)	Social Physical Mean	(SE)	Sig*	Close relationships Mental Mean	(SE)	Close relationships Physical Mean	(SE)	Sig*
	Hypertension	MDD or dysthymia	5.4	(0.5)	6.5	(0.4)	0	4.3	(0.4)	6.4	(0.5)	0	4.4	(0.5)	5.9	(0.5)	0	3.8	(0.8)	3.6	(0.4)	0	3.5	(0.5)	3.5	(0.4)	0
		Specific phobia	3.5	(0.5)	4.1	(0.7)	0	2.6	(0.4)	3.4	(0.5)	0	3.0	(0.5)	3.8	(0.6)	0	3.0	(0.4)	3.3	(0.7)	0	3.0	(0.4)	3.2	(0.6)	0
	Ulcer	MDD or dysthymia	5.1	(0.6)	3.4	(0.5)	1	4.1	(0.4)	2.9	(0.5)	0	3.4	(0.5)	3.0	(0.5)	0	3.1	(0.7)	1.1	(0.4)	1	3.2	(0.8)	1.6	(0.4)	0
		Specific phobia	2.7	(0.6)	3.2	(0.8)	0	2.0	(0.3)	2.7	(0.7)	0	2.0	(0.3)	2.9	(0.7)	0	2.4	(0.6)	1.5	(0.5)	0	2.2	(0.5)	1.8	(0.6)	0
Upper-middle	Arthritis	MDD or dysthymia	6.4	(0.4)	4.9	(0.5)	1	5.2	(0.4)	4.7	(0.5)	0	5.1	(0.5)	4.5	(0.5)	0	4.6	(0.6)	2.9	(0.4)	1	4.8	(0.6)	2.6	(0.4)	1
		Specific phobia	4.4	(0.6)	5.9	(0.4)	0	3.8	(0.6)	5.6	(0.5)	0	3.1	(0.5)	5.5	(0.5)	0	2.7	(0.5)	3.2	(0.7)	0	3.1	(0.6)	3.1	(0.7)	0
	Chronic back/ neck pain	MDD or dysthymia	6.5	(0.3)	6.4	(0.3)	0	5.1	(0.3)	5.5	(0.3)	0	4.8	(0.4)	5.4	(0.3)	0	4.9	(0.4)	4.0	(0.4)	0	4.6	(0.4)	3.5	(0.3)	1
		GAD	5.4	(0.4)	6.0	(0.7)	0	4.0	(0.4)	5.2	(0.5)	0	4.6	(0.4)	5.7	(0.6)	0	4.2	(0.4)	3.5	(0.6)	0	3.9	(0.4)	2.8	(0.5)	0
		Social phobia	5.5	(0.4)	6.6	(0.4)	0	2.3	(0.5)	5.7	(0.5)	0	3.8	(0.5)	5.9	(0.5)	0	4.4	(0.4)	4.2	(0.6)	0	4.4	(0.4)	3.3	(0.5)	0
		Specific phobia	3.1	(0.4)	5.9	(0.3)	0	2.1	(0.4)	5.4	(0.3)	0	2.0	(0.3)	5.3	(0.4)	0	1.6	(0.2)	2.6	(0.3)	0	1.3	(0.2)	2.7	(0.4)	0
		IED	4.6	(0.6)	5.1	(0.6)	0	3.1	(0.4)	4.0	(0.5)	0	3.0	(0.5)	4.7	(0.5)	0	2.4	(0.4)	3.6	(0.6)	0	3.2	(0.6)	2.8	(0.5)	0
	Other chronic pain	MDD or dysthymia	7.2	(0.4)	6.3	(0.5)	0	5.5	(0.4)	5.8	(0.6)	0	5.6	(0.5)	5.6	(0.6)	0	6.1	(0.4)	4.3	(0.5)	1	6.0	(0.4)	4.1	(0.5)	1
		Social phobia	5.6	(0.6)	7.0	(0.5)	0	3.6	(0.6)	6.4	(0.6)	0	4.8	(0.5)	5.8	(0.6)	0	4.0	(0.6)	4.0	(0.9)	0	4.3	(0.6)	3.5	(0.9)	0
		Specific phobia	4.0	(0.4)	6.0	(0.6)	0	3.2	(0.4)	4.7	(0.5)	0	3.0	(0.5)	4.7	(0.5)	0	2.4	(0.5)	2.5	(0.6)	0	2.4	(0.5)	2.5	(0.6)	0
	Headaches	MDD or dysthymia	6.6	(0.2)	6.2	(0.3)	0	4.9	(0.3)	5.3	(0.3)	0	5.3	(0.3)	5.3	(0.3)	0	5.4	(0.2)	4.7	(0.3)	0	5.2	(0.2)	4.4	(0.3)	0
		GAD	5.6	(0.5)	6.0	(0.4)	0	3.5	(0.4)	5.1	(0.5)	0	4.4	(0.5)	5.2	(0.5)	0	4.0	(0.4)	5.2	(0.5)	0	4.1	(0.4)	4.5	(0.5)	0
		Panic	5.4	(0.8)	4.8	(1.3)	0											4.8	(0.8)	4.4	(1.1)	0	4.6	(0.8)	3.8	(1.0)	0
		Social phobia	5.4	(0.4)	5.7	(0.5)	0	2.2	(0.3)	4.6	(0.5)	0	3.0	(0.4)	5.2	(0.5)	0	4.7	(0.4)	4.0	(0.4)	0	4.2	(0.4)	3.9	(0.4)	0
		Specific phobia	3.4	(0.3)	5.5	(0.4)	0	2.6	(0.3)	4.8	(0.4)	0	2.7	(0.3)	5.1	(0.4)	0	1.9	(0.2)	4.2	(0.4)	0	1.9	(0.2)	4.2	(0.4)	0
		IED	4.4	(0.5)	5.0	(0.8)	0	2.6	(0.4)	4.0	(0.8)	0	2.8	(0.6)	4.7	(1.0)	0	3.8	(0.5)	3.2	(0.5)	0	3.3	(0.5)	3.7	(0.5)	0
	Heart disease	MDD or dysthymia	6.9	(0.6)	4.8	(0.7)	1	5.0	(0.7)	4.2	(0.7)	0	5.7	(0.7)	4.5	(0.8)	0	5.2	(0.7)	2.1	(0.6)	1	5.6	(0.7)	2.6	(0.6)	1

Table (rotated 90° on the page). Each disorder row reports five comparison blocks; within each block two estimates `value (SE)` are given followed by a 0/1 significance indicator. Cells shown as "." are missing in the source.

Condition	Disorder	B1 est 1	B1 est 2	B1 sig	B2 est 1	B2 est 2	B2 sig	B3 est 1	B3 est 2	B3 sig	B4 est 1	B4 est 2	B4 sig	B5 est 1	B5 est 2	B5 sig
Hypertension	MDD or dysthymia	6.7 (0.4)	5.1 (0.5)	1	5.6 (0.4)	4.4 (0.5)	0	5.5 (0.4)	4.8 (0.5)	0	5.4 (0.4)	4.0 (0.6)	1	5.6 (0.3)	3.8 (0.5)	1
	GAD	5.5 (0.6)	3.5 (0.6)	1	4.6 (0.5)	3.3 (0.6)	0	4.5 (0.6)	3.1 (0.6)	0	4.2 (0.6)	2.6 (0.7)	0	4.4 (0.6)	2.3 (0.6)	1
	Specific phobia	3.4 (0.4)	3.6 (0.5)	0	3.1 (0.5)	3.3 (0.5)	0	2.5 (0.4)	3.2 (0.5)	0	2.2 (0.4)	2.2 (0.5)	0	2.2 (0.4)	2.1 (0.4)	0
Arthritis (High)	MDD or dysthymia	7.2 (0.2)	5.0 (0.3)	1	5.5 (0.3)	4.2 (0.3)	1	5.6 (0.3)	4.1 (0.4)	1	5.9 (0.2)	2.4 (0.3)	1	5.1 (0.3)	2.0 (0.3)	1
	Bipolar	8.1 (0.3)	5.4 (0.6)	1	6.5 (0.4)	4.1 (0.7)	1	6.7 (0.6)	4.0 (0.9)	1	6.7 (0.4)	3.5 (0.6)	1	7.0 (0.4)	2.8 (0.6)	1
	GAD	6.5 (0.3)	5.2 (0.3)	1	4.3 (0.4)	4.1 (0.4)	1	4.9 (0.4)	4.1 (0.4)	1	5.4 (0.3)	2.9 (0.4)	1	4.9 (0.3)	2.1 (0.4)	1
	PTSD	6.4 (0.5)	5.8 (0.6)	0	4.0 (0.5)	4.5 (0.6)	0	4.6 (0.6)	4.2 (0.8)	1	5.3 (0.5)	3.5 (0.6)	1	4.9 (0.5)	3.1 (0.6)	1
	Panic	6.6 (0.5)	6.4 (0.6)	0	4.6 (0.5)	4.9 (0.7)	0	5.3 (0.6)	5.1 (0.7)	0	5.0 (0.6)	4.5 (0.7)	0	4.5 (0.5)	3.4 (0.7)	0
	Social phobia	5.4 (0.3)	4.7 (0.4)	0	2.2 (0.3)	3.6 (0.3)	0	3.4 (0.3)	3.8 (0.4)	1	5.0 (0.3)	2.2 (0.4)	1	4.2 (0.3)	1.9 (0.4)	1
	Specific phobia	3.4 (0.2)	4.3 (0.3)	0	2.0 (0.2)	3.8 (0.3)	0	2.1 (0.2)	3.1 (0.3)	0	1.9 (0.2)	1.5 (0.2)	0	1.6 (0.2)	1.1 (0.2)	0
	IED	4.8 (0.5)	4.7 (0.6)	0	3.7 (0.6)	4.2 (0.6)	0	3.6 (0.5)	3.1 (0.3)	0	2.1 (0.3)	1.0 (0.3)	0	1.9 (0.3)	1.0 (0.2)	0
Asthma (High)	MDD or dysthymia	6.5 (0.2)	2.4 (0.5)	1	4.7 (0.3)	1.8 (0.5)	1	4.2 (0.6)	4.2 (0.6)	1	2.5 (0.6)	2.1 (0.5)	0	3.6 (0.6)	1.9 (0.5)	1
	Bipolar	6.9 (0.5)	2.5 (1.0)	1	4.9 (0.6)	2.3 (1.0)	1	4.7 (0.3)	1.5 (0.4)	1	4.9 (0.3)	1.0 (0.3)	1	4.1 (0.3)	0.5 (0.1)	1
	GAD	6.3 (0.4)	2.7 (0.9)	1	4.4 (0.4)	2.4 (0.9)	1	5.1 (0.5)	0.6 (0.2)	1	5.0 (0.7)	0.4 (0.2)	1	4.9 (0.6)	0.3 (0.2)	1
	Panic	6.0 (0.7)	4.2 (1.1)	0	3.4 (0.6)	4.0 (1.1)	0	3.9 (0.5)	0.9 (0.3)	1	4.7 (0.4)	0.4 (0.2)	1	4.4 (0.4)	0.2 (0.1)	1
	Social phobia	5.0 (0.3)	2.5 (0.6)	1	1.7 (0.3)	2.1 (0.7)	1	3.1 (0.7)	1.3 (0.4)	0	4.8 (0.6)	2.1 (1.3)	0	4.9 (0.8)	1.9 (1.3)	1
	Specific phobia	2.8 (0.2)	2.4 (0.5)	0	1.5 (0.2)	1.9 (0.5)	0	3.1 (0.3)	1.0 (0.3)	1	4.3 (0.4)	0.8 (0.3)	1	3.5 (0.3)	0.6 (0.2)	1
	IED	4.7 (0.5)	4.7 (0.6)	0	4.3 (0.5)	3.1 (0.3)	0	2.4 (0.6)	0.9 (0.2)	1	1.8 (0.2)	1.0 (0.3)	0	1.3 (0.2)	0.7 (0.2)	1
Cancer (High)	Specific phobia	3.4 (0.6)	2.8 (0.7)	0	2.2 (0.5)	2.4 (0.7)	0	2.3 (0.6)	2.2 (0.6)	0	2.6 (0.6)	1.2 (0.4)	0	2.3 (0.5)	0.8 (0.2)	1
Chronic back/neck pain (High)	MDD or dysthymia	7.2 (0.2)	6.1 (0.2)	1	5.5 (0.2)	5.4 (0.2)	1	5.3 (0.2)	5.4 (0.2)	0	5.7 (0.2)	3.4 (0.2)	1	5.1 (0.2)	2.7 (0.2)	1
	Bipolar	7.8 (0.4)	6.9 (0.5)	0	6.3 (0.5)	6.2 (0.6)	0	6.1 (0.5)	5.5 (0.5)	0	6.4 (0.5)	4.0 (0.5)	1	6.2 (0.4)	3.9 (0.7)	1
	GAD	6.4 (0.3)	6.8 (0.2)	0	4.4 (0.3)	6.0 (0.3)	0	4.7 (0.3)	5.8 (0.3)	0	5.0 (0.3)	4.0 (0.3)	1	4.5 (0.3)	3.3 (0.3)	1
	Panic	5.3 (0.4)	6.3 (0.4)	0	3.6 (0.4)	5.8 (0.5)	0	4.3 (0.4)	5.1 (0.5)	0	3.4 (0.4)	3.4 (0.5)	0	3.2 (0.4)	2.7 (0.5)	0
	Social phobia	4.9 (0.2)	5.8 (0.3)	0	2.4 (0.2)	5.0 (0.3)	0	3.2 (0.2)	4.8 (0.3)	0	2.9 (0.2)	2.9 (0.3)	1	3.7 (0.2)	2.3 (0.2)	1
	Specific phobia	3.1 (0.2)	5.7 (0.3)	0	2.0 (0.2)	4.9 (0.3)	0	1.9 (0.2)	4.8 (0.3)	0	2.7 (0.2)	2.7 (0.3)	0	1.8 (0.2)	1.6 (0.2)	0
	PTSD	6.7 (0.5)	6.9 (0.6)	0	4.3 (0.5)	5.8 (0.6)	0	4.9 (0.6)	6.1 (0.7)	0	5.4 (0.6)	4.9 (0.8)	0	4.4 (0.5)	3.7 (0.5)	1
	IED	5.2 (0.6)	6.1 (0.6)	0	3.1 (0.5)	4.8 (0.6)	0	3.3 (0.6)	5.3 (0.6)	0	3.6 (0.6)	3.0 (0.5)	0	4.0 (0.7)	2.4 (0.5)	1
Other chronic pain (High)	MDD or dysthymia	7.1 (0.4)	6.3 (0.4)	0	5.6 (0.4)	5.6 (0.4)	0	5.3 (0.4)	5.7 (0.4)	0	5.7 (0.4)	3.7 (0.5)	1	5.6 (0.4)	3.3 (0.5)	1
	Bipolar	7.6 (0.7)	6.9 (1.1)	0	5.9 (0.6)	6.1 (1.1)	0	. (.)	6.1 (0.6)	0	. (.)	. (.)	.	6.4 (0.7)	5.3 (1.0)	0
	GAD	7.6 (0.3)	6.9 (0.4)	0	5.6 (0.4)	5.9 (0.4)	0	6.1 (0.6)	6.0 (0.5)	0	5.8 (0.4)	4.3 (0.4)	0	5.6 (0.4)	3.9 (0.5)	1

Appendix Table 13.12 (cont.)

Country income level	Physical disorders	Mental disorders	Global			Home			Work			Social			Close relationships		
			Mental	Physical		Mental	Physical		Mental	Physical		Mental	Physical		Mental	Physical	
			Mean (SE)	Mean (SE)	Sig*	Mean (SE)	Mean (SE)	Sig*	Mean (SE)	Mean (SE)	Sig*	Mean (SE)	Mean (SE)	Sig*	Mean (SE)	Mean (SE)	Sig*
		PTSD	7.0 (0.6)	6.0 (0.8)	0	.	.	.	.	6.3 (0.5)	0	5.1 (0.5)	5.0 (0.7)	0	4.2 (0.5)	4.3 (0.7)	0
		Social phobia	5.9 (0.5)	7.1 (0.5)	0	3.1 (0.5)	5.8 (0.5)	0	3.6 (0.5)	5.4 (0.8)	0	2.4 (0.3)	3.5 (0.7)	0	1.3 (0.3)	2.9 (0.6)	0
		Specific phobia	3.8 (0.4)	6.0 (0.7)	0	2.1 (0.4)	5.3 (0.7)	0	2.5 (0.5)	.	.	.	.	.	.	.	.
	Diabetes	MDD or dysthymia	7.3 (0.5)	2.6 (0.8)	1	5.8 (0.5)	1.9 (0.6)	1	5.6 (0.7)	2.3 (0.9)	1	5.8 (0.5)	0.7 (0.3)	1	5.6 (0.5)	0.8 (0.3)	1
		Specific phobia	2.5 (0.5)	6.1 (1.0)	0	1.4 (0.3)	5.4 (1.1)	0	1.9 (0.4)	4.6 (1.5)	0	1.6 (0.5)	2.0 (1.2)	0	1.3 (0.4)	1.9 (1.0)	0
	Headaches	MDD or dysthymia	7.6 (0.2)	6.7 (0.2)	1	5.7 (0.2)	5.7 (0.2)	0	5.8 (0.2)	5.6 (0.3)	0	6.0 (0.2)	5.0 (0.3)	1	5.6 (0.2)	4.4 (0.3)	1
		Bipolar	7.9 (0.3)	6.2 (0.4)	1	6.1 (0.4)	4.7 (0.4)	1	5.9 (0.4)	5.6 (0.4)	0	6.2 (0.4)	3.5 (0.6)	1	5.8 (0.4)	3.5 (0.5)	1
		GAD	6.8 (0.3)	6.6 (0.3)	0	4.3 (0.3)	5.6 (0.4)	0	4.5 (0.3)	5.3 (0.4)	0	5.4 (0.4)	4.5 (0.4)	0	5.1 (0.3)	4.1 (0.4)	0
		IED	4.9 (0.5)	6.6 (0.5)	0	2.7 (0.5)	5.0 (0.4)	0	2.5 (0.5)	5.1 (0.5)	0	4.2 (0.5)	4.7 (0.6)	0	4.1 (0.5)	4.8 (0.5)	0
		PTSD	6.5 (0.4)	7.4 (0.3)	0	3.7 (0.3)	6.2 (0.4)	0	3.9 (0.4)	6.3 (0.4)	0	5.4 (0.4)	5.4 (0.4)	0	5.2 (0.4)	3.9 (0.4)	1
		Panic	5.5 (0.5)	6.7 (0.5)	0	3.3 (0.4)	5.5 (0.6)	0	3.7 (0.3)	5.7 (0.6)	0	4.5 (0.5)	5.4 (0.6)	0	4.2 (0.5)	4.4 (0.6)	0
		Social phobia	5.6 (0.3)	6.6 (0.3)	0	2.2 (0.2)	5.3 (0.3)	0	3.2 (0.3)	5.6 (0.3)	0	5.1 (0.3)	5.1 (0.4)	0	4.3 (0.3)	3.9 (0.4)	0
		Specific phobia	3.1 (0.2)	6.6 (0.3)	0	2.0 (0.2)	5.8 (0.3)	0	1.9 (0.2)	5.6 (0.3)	0	2.0 (0.2)	5.1 (0.3)	0	1.7 (0.2)	3.9 (0.3)	0
		ADHD	6.1 (0.6)	7.0 (0.4)	0	4.7 (0.6)	5.9 (0.5)	0	4.0 (0.8)	6.5 (0.5)	0	4.1 (0.7)	5.3 (0.8)	0	4.0 (0.6)	4.4 (0.7)	0
	Heart disease	MDD or dysthymia	7.1 (0.5)	5.7 (0.9)	0	5.5 (0.5)	4.7 (0.8)	0	5.9 (0.6)	5.6 (1.0)	0	5.4 (0.6)	2.4 (0.7)	1	4.8 (0.8)	2.0 (0.6)	1
		Specific phobia	2.5 (0.5)	4.6 (0.8)	0	1.6 (0.4)	3.4 (0.8)	0	1.4 (0.4)	4.1 (0.8)	0	1.4 (0.5)	2.2 (0.8)	0	1.1 (0.4)	1.0 (0.3)	0
	Hypertension	MDD or dysthymia	6.6 (0.3)	2.5 (0.4)	1	4.9 (0.5)	2.1 (0.4)	1	4.5 (0.3)	2.0 (0.4)	1	5.1 (0.3)	1.3 (0.3)	1	4.8 (0.4)	1.3 (0.3)	1
		GAD	5.7 (0.5)	3.0 (0.9)	1	4.3 (0.5)	2.6 (0.7)	0	5.0 (0.6)	3.1 (0.9)	0	4.3 (0.6)	1.8 (0.8)	1	3.9 (0.6)	1.7 (0.8)	1
		PTSD	6.7 (0.6)	3.9 (1.0)	1	5.1 (0.8)	3.1 (0.9)	0	.	.	.	5.1 (0.6)	1.2 (0.5)	1	4.5 (0.6)	1.3 (0.7)	1
		Panic	6.1 (0.7)	2.3 (0.7)	1	4.2 (0.8)	1.7 (0.7)	1	3.7 (0.7)	2.1 (0.8)	0	4.4 (0.7)	0.4 (0.2)	1	3.2 (0.6)	0.5 (0.2)	1
		Social phobia	5.8 (0.3)	2.0 (0.4)	1	2.7 (0.4)	1.7 (0.5)	0	3.5 (0.4)	1.4 (0.4)	1	4.9 (0.3)	0.9 (0.2)	1	3.8 (0.4)	0.9 (0.3)	1
		Specific phobia	3.3 (0.3)	2.1 (0.3)	1	1.7 (0.2)	1.9 (0.3)	0	2.0 (0.3)	1.6 (0.3)	0	1.9 (0.2)	0.8 (0.2)	1	1.8 (0.3)	0.7 (0.2)	1

[a] Only cells with 30 or more respondents with a given pair of disorders and a valid disability score are included.

* Significance at the 0.05 level of difference between mental and physical within-person SDS means, two-sided test. 1 = yes; 0 = no.

Appendix Table 14.1 Best model selection according to AIC and BIC. The WMH surveys.

Variables included in the models	Cognition	Mobility	Self-care	Getting along	Role functioning	Family burden	Stigma	Discrimination
AIC: Aikaike's information criterion								
Disorders only	2307757	6588769	2951357	1915936	14153035	8488943	8426149	4979962
Number of disorders only	2343271	6631574	2984689	1959479	14141810	8438438	8360675	4984584
Disorders + number	2258278	6528093	2934776	1876493	13994554	8342059	8287826	4917482
Disorders + number*disorder	2217596	6485826	2917338	1849685	13923079	8279563	8195016	4870078
With disorder's importance score	2211649	6469735	2911669	1846738	13918598	8286993	8199664	4870972
BIC: Bayesian information criterion								
Disorders only	2308215	6589227	2951815	1916393	14153493	8489401	8426607	4980420
Number of disorders only	2343613	6631915	2985030	1959821	14142152	8438779	8361016	4984925
Disorders + number	2258781	6528596	2935279	1876996	13995056	8342562	8288329	4917985
Disorders + number*disorder	2218233	6486464	2917976	1850322	13923716	8280201	8195654	4870716
With disorder's importance score	2212287	6470373	2912307	1847376	13919235	8287631	8200301	4871610

Appendix Table 14.2 Individual-level effects of mental and physical disorders on WHODAS scores by country income level. The WMH surveys.

Country income level / Disorders	Cognition		Mobility		Self-care		Getting along		Role functioning		Family burden		Stigma		Discrimination		Combined	
	Est[a]	(SE)	Est[a]	(SE)	Est[a]	(SE)	Est[a]	(SE)	Est[a]	(SE)	Est[a]	(SE)	Est[a]	(SE)	Est[a]	(SE)	Est[a]	(SE)
Low/lower-middle																		
Alcohol abuse	0.4	(0.3)	0.5	(0.6)	0.5	(0.4)	0.8	(0.4)	4.0	(1.7)	3.1	(1.2)	1.9	(1.3)	2.0	(1.3)	1.7	(0.6)
Bipolar	3.1	(0.9)	1.0	(0.6)	2.6	(8.8)	0.7	(0.7)	13.5	(3.4)	3.7	(2.4)	5.5	(2.4)	4.9	(3.6)	4.7	(1.3)
Drug abuse	2.6	(2.3)	2.5	(2.9)	-0.8	(0.4)	4.8	(5.7)	10.4	(4.1)	10.5	(5.3)	9.5	(3.0)	8.9	(6.7)	6.0	(2.0)
Generalized anxiety	1.5	(1.0)	2.5	(1.7)	2.4	(1.4)	3.1	(1.5)	6.5	(2.5)	6.9	(2.3)	7.8	(1.9)	2.2	(1.8)	4.3	(1.2)
Major depressive disorder	1.0	(0.4)	2.3	(0.7)	2.4	(0.5)	1.2	(0.4)	4.9	(1.1)	2.7	(0.8)	4.7	(0.9)	2.2	(0.6)	2.8	(0.5)
Panic and/or agoraphobia	1.4	(0.8)	1.3	(1.1)	0.4	(1.0)	1.2	(0.8)	5.9	(2.7)	2.1	(1.7)	4.3	(2.1)	0.8	(1.3)	2.2	(1.0)
Post-traumatic stress	2.9	(1.8)	6.9	(2.5)	4.7	(4.9)	0.7	(1.1)	9.4	(3.4)	9.2	(2.7)	5	(3.5)	5.2	(2.4)	5.6	(1.6)
Social phobia	1.9	(1.0)	0.5	(0.8)	0.3	(3.5)	0.4	(0.7)	1.8	(1.7)	2.5	(1.5)	2	(1.6)	3.2	(1.4)	1.6	(0.8)
Specific phobia	0.7	(0.3)	-0.1	(0.4)	0.1	(0.4)	0.1	(0.3)	0.5	(0.8)	1.5	(0.9)	1.7	(0.9)	0.9	(0.7)	0.7	(0.4)
Arthritis	0.3	(0.3)	1.5	(0.7)	-0.6	(0.6)	-0.3	(0.4)	2.3	(1.0)	0.9	(0.8)	0.7	(0.9)	-0.8	(0.7)	0.7	(0.5)
Cancer	0.1	(0.7)	5.9	(2.7)	4.7	(2.4)	0.8	(0.6)	9.9	(4.4)	4.7	(3.0)	4.8	(3.4)	2.7	(2.0)	4.2	(1.9)
Cardiovascular	0.7	(0.4)	0.8	(0.8)	0.2	(0.6)	0.0	(0.2)	3.1	(1.2)	2.1	(0.8)	2.4	(1.0)	1.1	(0.6)	1.4	(0.5)
Chronic pain	0.3	(0.2)	1.4	(0.6)	0.3	(0.4)	0.1	(0.2)	2.6	(0.8)	0.7	(0.6)	1.8	(0.9)	0.6	(0.5)	1.0	(0.3)
Diabetes	1.1	(0.5)	0.2	(1.0)	0.6	(0.9)	0.3	(0.5)	3.1	(1.6)	2.6	(1.4)	2.9	(1.4)	0.9	(1.1)	1.6	(0.6)
Digestive	-0.2	(0.3)	-0.6	(0.4)	-0.3	(0.4)	0.1	(0.2)	0.8	(1.2)	0.6	(0.8)	0.2	(0.8)	-0.1	(0.7)	0.0	(0.4)
Headache/migraine	1.4	(0.3)	0.6	(0.6)	1.1	(0.6)	0.2	(0.3)	4.1	(0.9)	3.4	(0.7)	2.7	(0.9)	2.0	(0.6)	2.1	(0.4)
Insomnia	0.0	(0.5)	1.7	(0.8)	0.3	(0.5)	0.6	(0.5)	8.9	(1.9)	3.6	(1.2)	6.1	(1.2)	2.8	(0.9)	3.2	(0.7)
Neurological	2.0	(1.0)	3.5	(2.5)	3.6	(2.0)	0.3	(0.5)	11.1	(4.0)	12.5	(2.2)	13.7	(2.4)	8.9	(2.2)	7.1	(1.5)
Respiratory	0.0	(0.2)	1.2	(0.5)	0.2	(0.4)	0.3	(0.2)	3.0	(0.9)	1.4	(0.6)	1.3	(0.7)	1.1	(0.5)	1.1	(0.4)
All mental	1.3	(0.2)	2.1	(0.4)	1.8	(0.3)	1.2	(0.2)	6.0	(0.7)	3.9	(0.4)	4.8	(0.5)	2.6	(0.3)	3.1	(0.2)
All physical	1.0	(0.1)	2.4	(0.3)	0.8	(0.2)	0.3	(0.1)	7.6	(0.4)	4.0	(0.3)	5.2	(0.4)	2.0	(0.3)	3.1	(0.2)
All disorders	1.1	(0.1)	2.8	(0.2)	1.1	(0.1)	0.7	(0.1)	9.2	(0.4)	4.7	(0.2)	6.1	(0.3)	2.6	(0.2)	3.8	(0.1)
Upper-middle																		
Alcohol abuse	0.5	(0.6)	-0.5	(0.8)	0.1	(0.6)	0.1	(0.6)	4.9	(2.1)	3.0	(1.6)	4.9	(2.0)	3.1	(1.5)	2.1	(1.0)
Bipolar	5.3	(1.5)	1.1	(1.1)	0.9	(1.4)	3.9	(1.3)	8.5	(3.1)	14.2	(3.0)	11.5	(3.5)	3.8	(2.5)	6.6	(1.7)
Drug abuse	0.2	(1.1)	0.7	(2.2)	0.0	(0.4)	1.2	(2.3)	0.9	(3.5)	0.7	(4.0)	1.6	(6.4)	-1.0	(2.4)	0.6	(2.0)
Generalized anxiety	1.9	(1.1)	2.3	(1.5)	0.3	(0.8)	1.6	(1.1)	6.2	(2.8)	3.5	(2.0)	3.7	(3.0)	1.7	(2.0)	2.6	(1.2)
Major depressive disorder	3.8	(0.7)	3.5	(0.7)	0.9	(0.3)	2.0	(0.4)	12.5	(1.4)	8.7	(1.0)	8.3	(1.2)	5.5	(0.9)	5.9	(0.5)
Panic and/or agoraphobia	3.6	(0.9)	4.0	(1.2)	1.3	(0.6)	1.9	(1.3)	13.0	(2.9)	13.1	(2.6)	12.9	(2.4)	5.1	(2.0)	7.5	(1.3)
Post-traumatic stress	1.0	(1.4)	4.0	(2.0)	-0.3	(0.8)	0.8	(1.0)	6.1	(3.8)	6.3	(2.7)	8.7	(3.3)	4.4	(2.9)	4.1	(1.9)
Social phobia	0.0	(0.9)	1.4	(0.9)	0.6	(0.6)	3.6	(1.1)	7.4	(2.0)	4.2	(1.9)	4.9	(2.2)	3.6	(1.5)	3.5	(1.1)
Specific phobia	0.5	(0.5)	0.4	(1.1)	0.6	(0.5)	0.2	(0.5)	3.6	(1.6)	0.3	(1.5)	1.4	(1.8)	1.0	(1.4)	1.0	(0.9)

Arthritis	−0.6 (0.3)	0.8 (0.7)	−0.4 (0.4)	−0.5 (0.4)	1.7 (1.2)	1.2 (0.8)	3.0 (1.0)	0.9 (0.5)
Cancer	0.4 (1.4)	4.0 (3.3)	−0.6 (1.1)	−1.6 (0.9)	3.2 (4.8)	1.1 (3.1)	0.9 (3.6)	0.8 (1.9)
Cardiovascular	−0.1 (0.4)	0.3 (0.8)	−0.1 (0.4)	−0.5 (0.4)	2.5 (1.2)	2.2 (0.7)	1.3 (1.1)	1.0 (0.5)
Chronic pain	0.9 (0.3)	3.3 (0.5)	0.8 (0.3)	0.8 (0.2)	6.2 (1.1)	2.9 (0.9)	3.8 (1.0)	2.7 (0.5)
Diabetes	−0.2 (0.7)	1.2 (1.4)	0.3 (0.6)	0.6 (0.5)	3.8 (2.0)	−0.2 (1.3)	1.2 (1.6)	0.8 (1.0)
Digestive	−1.0 (0.8)	−1.5 (0.9)	−0.3 (0.4)	−0.1 (0.5)	−1.0 (1.7)	0.6 (1.5)	1.0 (1.6)	−0.2 (1.2)
Headache/migraine	1.2 (0.5)	1.1 (0.6)	0.8 (0.3)	0.7 (0.4)	4.3 (1.1)	2.6 (1.1)	4.4 (1.2)	2.2 (0.6)
Insomnia	2.8 (0.8)	1.0 (1.0)	0.4 (0.5)	0.3 (0.5)	5.2 (1.5)	5.1 (1.5)	5.7 (1.4)	3.3 (0.8)
Neurological	2.6 (1.3)	7.6 (2.6)	2.2 (1.8)	1.7 (0.9)	11.7 (4.2)	7.1 (2.6)	3.5 (3.9)	4.8 (1.7)
Respiratory	−0.4 (0.3)	−0.7 (0.5)	−0.1 (0.3)	0.1 (0.3)	−0.7 (1.2)	0.2 (0.7)	0.6 (1.0)	−0.1 (0.4)
All mental	2.5 (0.3)	2.7 (0.4)	0.8 (0.2)	1.5 (0.2)	9.8 (0.9)	7.2 (0.6)	8.0 (0.8)	5.0 (0.4)
All physical	1.1 (0.2)	3.3 (0.3)	0.7 (0.2)	0.6 (0.1)	6.8 (0.7)	4.4 (0.4)	6.4 (0.5)	3.4 (0.3)
All disorders	1.6 (0.1)	3.9 (0.2)	1.0 (0.1)	1.0 (0.1)	9.0 (0.4)	6.0 (0.3)	8.3 (0.3)	4.6 (0.2)
High								
Alcohol abuse	0.3 (0.3)	−1.0 (0.4)	−0.3 (0.2)	0.3 (0.4)	2.9 (1.2)	0.7 (0.8)	1.8 (0.8)	0.7 (0.6)
Bipolar	3.2 (0.7)	2.5 (0.9)	1.4 (0.6)	2.4 (0.7)	9.0 (1.6)	5.6 (1.4)	5.2 (1.1)	4.4 (1.0)
Drug abuse	1.0 (0.5)	0.3 (0.7)	0.2 (0.3)	1.5 (0.9)	5.3 (2.3)	3.0 (1.6)	1.1 (1.4)	1.7 (1.1)
Generalized anxiety	1.6 (0.5)	1.1 (0.8)	0.2 (0.3)	1.4 (0.4)	5.2 (1.4)	3.6 (1.0)	2.5 (0.9)	2.2 (0.6)
Major depressive disorder	2.1 (0.3)	1.3 (0.4)	0.2 (0.2)	1.4 (0.2)	7.5 (0.7)	3.4 (0.5)	3.9 (0.5)	2.9 (0.3)
Panic and/or agoraphobia	2.9 (0.5)	2.0 (0.8)	0.9 (0.5)	2.3 (0.5)	6.9 (1.2)	3.6 (1.0)	5.3 (0.9)	3.3 (0.6)
Post-traumatic stress	3.3 (0.6)	3.8 (0.8)	1.9 (0.6)	2.1 (0.5)	8.9 (1.3)	4.9 (1.1)	4.2 (0.9)	4.0 (0.6)
Social phobia	2.5 (0.4)	1.1 (0.5)	−0.1 (0.3)	1.8 (0.3)	4.7 (0.9)	5.0 (0.8)	4.2 (0.7)	2.7 (0.4)
Specific phobia	0.7 (0.2)	1.7 (0.5)	0.5 (0.3)	0.6 (0.3)	4.7 (1.0)	3.0 (0.7)	2.2 (0.6)	1.9 (0.4)
Arthritis	0.4 (0.2)	3.3 (0.5)	0.9 (0.3)	0.3 (0.2)	3.8 (0.7)	1.2 (0.5)	2.1 (0.4)	1.6 (0.2)
Cancer	0.5 (0.3)	1.1 (0.8)	0.5 (0.6)	0.6 (0.3)	4.8 (1.2)	1.7 (0.7)	0.8 (0.5)	1.4 (0.4)
Cardiovascular	0.3 (0.2)	3.1 (0.5)	0.9 (0.3)	0.3 (0.2)	4.6 (0.8)	2.0 (0.4)	1.7 (0.4)	1.8 (0.3)
Chronic pain	0.9 (0.2)	5.7 (0.4)	1.4 (0.5)	0.9 (0.1)	10.4 (0.7)	4.0 (0.4)	3.6 (0.4)	3.7 (0.2)
Diabetes	0.4 (0.3)	2.1 (0.8)	1.6 (0.5)	0.3 (0.2)	4.3 (1.1)	1.2 (0.6)	1.6 (0.6)	1.6 (0.4)
Digestive	0.8 (0.5)	5.0 (0.9)	1.0 (0.6)	1.5 (0.5)	9.4 (1.4)	4.2 (1.0)	4.8 (1.0)	3.7 (0.6)
Headache/migraine	1.2 (0.2)	0.6 (0.4)	0.6 (0.3)	0.4 (0.2)	3.3 (0.7)	2.7 (0.4)	1.5 (0.4)	1.5 (0.2)
Insomnia	1.4 (0.3)	4.0 (0.6)	1.4 (0.5)	1.3 (0.3)	6.4 (1.0)	4.2 (0.7)	3.7 (0.5)	3.2 (0.3)
Neurological	2.8 (0.7)	5.6 (1.8)	3.5 (1.1)	2.2 (0.7)	7.9 (2.0)	3.6 (1.8)	4.9 (1.7)	4.3 (1.2)
Respiratory	0.3 (0.1)	0.5 (0.3)	0.0 (0.2)	0.1 (0.1)	1.2 (0.4)	−0.2 (0.3)	0.3 (0.2)	0.3 (0.2)
All mental	2.5 (0.1)	2.1 (0.2)	0.8 (0.1)	1.9 (0.1)	9.0 (0.4)	5.2 (0.3)	4.8 (0.2)	3.7 (0.2)
All physical	1.1 (0.1)	5.4 (0.2)	1.3 (0.1)	0.8 (0.1)	9.5 (0.3)	4.0 (0.2)	3.5 (0.2)	3.5 (0.1)
All disorders	1.6 (0.1)	5.2 (0.2)	1.4 (0.1)	1.2 (0.1)	11.2 (0.3)	5.0 (0.2)	4.4 (0.1)	4.2 (0.1)

[a] Individual-level estimate.

Appendix Table 14.3 Population attributable risk proportions (PARPs) of different WHODAS dimensions due to disorders by country income level. The WMH surveys.

Country income level / Disorders	Cognition		Mobility		Self-care		Getting along		Role functioning		Family burden		Stigma		Discrimination		Combined	
	PARP (%)	(SE)	PARP (%)	(SE)	PARP (%)	(SE)	PARP (%)	(SE)	PARP (%)	(SE)	PARP (%)	(SE)	PARP (%)	(SE)	PARP (%)	(SE)	PARP (%)	(SE)
Low/lower-middle																		
Alcohol abuse	1.3	(1.0)	0.5	(0.7)	1.5	(1.2)	4.2	(2.1)	1.2	(0.5)	2.1	(0.8)	1.0	(0.7)	2.3	(1.5)	1.4	(0.5)
Bipolar	2.7	(0.8)	0.3	(0.2)	1.9	(6.3)	0.8	(0.9)	1.0	(0.3)	0.6	(0.4)	0.7	(0.3)	1.4	(1.0)	1.0	(0.3)
Drug abuse	1.0	(0.9)	0.3	(0.4)	-0.3	(0.1)	2.6	(2.9)	0.3	(0.1)	0.8	(0.4)	0.5	(0.2)	1.1	(0.8)	0.5	(0.2)
Generalized anxiety	3.0	(2.1)	1.8	(1.2)	4.3	(2.6)	9.2	(4.4)	1.2	(0.5)	2.8	(0.9)	2.5	(0.6)	1.5	(1.3)	2.1	(0.6)
Major depressive disorder	12.4	(4.2)	9.6	(2.9)	25.2	(5.0)	21.2	(5.7)	5.2	(1.2)	6.6	(2.0)	8.8	(1.7)	8.9	(2.6)	8.2	(1.4)
Panic and/or agoraphobia	3.6	(2.2)	1.2	(1.0)	0.8	(2.2)	4.5	(3.3)	1.4	(0.6)	1.1	(0.9)	1.7	(0.9)	0.8	(1.2)	1.4	(0.6)
Post-traumatic stress	4.5	(2.6)	3.5	(1.3)	6.2	(6.3)	1.6	(2.4)	1.3	(0.5)	2.8	(0.8)	1.2	(0.8)	2.7	(1.2)	2.0	(0.6)
Social phobia	4.3	(2.0)	0.4	(0.6)	0.7	(6.4)	1.1	(2.0)	0.4	(0.3)	1.1	(0.6)	0.7	(0.5)	2.4	(1.0)	0.8	(0.4)
Specific phobia	5.7	(2.7)	-0.2	(0.9)	0.8	(2.5)	1.4	(3.5)	0.3	(0.6)	2.4	(1.4)	2.1	(1.1)	2.3	(1.7)	1.3	(0.7)
Arthritis	5.8	(6.4)	10.8	(4.8)	-10.6	(0.1)	-8.0	(1.7)	4.2	(1.9)	3.7	(3.2)	2.2	(2.8)	-5.8	(4.8)	3.2	(2.3)
Cancer	0.1	(0.5)	1.4	(0.7)	2.9	(1.5)	0.8	(0.6)	0.6	(0.3)	0.7	(0.4)	0.5	(0.4)	0.7	(0.5)	0.7	(0.3)
Cardiovascular	12.4	(6.8)	4.7	(6.6)	2.6	(9.2)	0.0	(6.4)	4.9	(1.9)	7.7	(2.9)	6.7	(2.8)	6.9	(3.7)	6.2	(2.0)
Chronic pain	11.3	(7.6)	15.9	(7.6)	10.1	(2.9)	5.2	(9.2)	8.0	(2.5)	5.0	(4.3)	9.7	(4.6)	7.0	(5.8)	8.2	(2.6)
Diabetes	4.2	(1.7)	0.2	(1.2)	1.8	(2.8)	1.6	(2.7)	1.0	(0.5)	1.9	(1.0)	1.7	(0.8)	1.1	(1.3)	1.4	(0.5)
Digestive	-1.2	(2.2)	-1.5	(1.0)	-1.9	(2.3)	1.3	(2.2)	0.5	(0.7)	0.8	(1.2)	0.2	(0.8)	-0.2	(1.8)	0.1	(0.7)
Headache/migraine	31.6	(6.0)	4.5	(4.6)	21.7	(2.4)	6.5	(9.3)	8.3	(1.9)	15.4	(3.1)	9.4	(3.0)	15.1	(4.6)	11.3	(2.0)
Insomnia	0.0	(3.9)	4.5	(2.0)	1.9	(3.5)	6.3	(5.5)	6.0	(1.3)	5.5	(1.8)	7.2	(1.4)	7.4	(2.3)	5.9	(1.2)
Neurological	2.9	(1.4)	1.7	(1.2)	4.5	(2.5)	0.6	(1.0)	1.4	(0.5)	3.6	(0.6)	3.0	(0.5)	4.3	(1.0)	2.4	(0.5)
Respiratory	0.7	(3.9)	6.8	(2.7)	2.6	(5.7)	7.3	(5.7)	4.5	(1.3)	4.8	(2.2)	3.5	(1.8)	6.5	(2.9)	4.6	(1.4)
All mental	33.1	(4.6)	18.6	(3.2)	39	(5.3)	44.1	(5.5)	13.5	(1.5)	20.2	(2.1)	18.9	(2.1)	22.6	(2.8)	18.9	(1.5)
All physical	67.5	(5.3)	54.5	(5.4)	45	(3.2)	28.6	(9.4)	44.7	(2.4)	53.7	(3.3)	52.7	(3.3)	45.9	(5.2)	49.4	(2.4)
All disorders	84.8	(2.8)	69.8	(3.7)	71.4	(6.8)	74.8	(5.3)	60.7	(2.0)	70.6	(3.2)	70	(2.5)	66.8	(4.5)	67.1	(1.9)
Upper-middle																		
Alcohol abuse	1.1	(1.3)	-0.4	(1.3)	0.3	(1.8)	0.3	(2.1)	1.4	(0.6)	1.6	(0.9)	2.0	(0.8)	2.8	(1.4)	1.4	(0.7)
Bipolar	6.2	(1.7)	0.5	(1.0)	1.4	(2.1)	7.3	(2.2)	1.3	(0.5)	4.1	(0.9)	2.5	(0.8)	1.8	(1.2)	2.4	(0.6)
Drug abuse	0.1	(0.5)	0.1	(0.5)	0.0	(0.3)	0.9	(1.6)	0.1	(0.2)	0.1	(0.4)	0.1	(0.5)	-0.2	(0.4)	0.1	(0.3)
Generalized anxiety	3.2	(1.8)	1.6	(1.0)	0.7	(1.8)	4.2	(2.8)	1.4	(0.6)	1.5	(0.9)	1.2	(1.0)	1.2	(1.4)	1.4	(0.6)
Major depressive disorder	32.9	(4.4)	11.7	(2.1)	9.7	(3.4)	26.7	(4.5)	13.8	(1.5)	18.2	(2.0)	13.0	(1.9)	19.8	(2.9)	15.5	(1.4)
Panic and/or agoraphobia	8.6	(2.4)	3.7	(1.1)	4.1	(1.9)	7.2	(4.9)	4.0	(0.9)	7.6	(1.5)	5.6	(1.0)	5.0	(1.9)	5.4	(0.9)
Post-traumatic stress	1.5	(2.0)	2.3	(1.2)	-0.5	(1.6)	1.8	(2.3)	1.2	(0.7)	2.3	(1.0)	2.3	(0.9)	2.7	(1.8)	1.8	(0.9)
Social phobia	0.0	(2.6)	1.5	(1.0)	2.1	(2.2)	15.8	(4.8)	2.6	(0.7)	2.8	(1.3)	2.5	(1.1)	4.2	(1.7)	2.9	(0.9)
Specific phobia	4.2	(3.9)	1.3	(3.6)	6.0	(5.3)	2.9	(7.0)	3.8	(1.7)	0.7	(3.0)	2.1	(2.7)	3.3	(4.8)	2.5	(2.2)
Arthritis	-9.0	(4.5)	4.4	(4.1)	-6.9	(7.5)	-12.4	(7.6)	3.2	(2.2)	4.1	(2.6)	7.7	(2.6)	5.9	(4.5)	3.8	(2.1)
Cancer	0.3	(1.1)	1.3	(1.1)	-0.6	(1.1)	-2.1	(1.1)	0.3	(0.5)	0.2	(0.6)	0.1	(0.5)	-1.1	(0.7)	0.2	(0.5)
Cardiovascular	-2.7	(7.3)	2.5	(5.8)	-2.8	(0.0)	-14.0	(2.2)	6.3	(3.1)	10.5	(3.5)	4.4	(3.9)	9.5	(4.7)	5.8	(2.8)
Chronic pain	19.6	(4.9)	26.9	(4.0)	22.9	(7.5)	26.2	(7.6)	16.7	(2.8)	14.6	(4.2)	14.4	(3.9)	13	(5.9)	17.2	(2.9)

Diabetes	-0.7 (2.9)	2.1 (2.3)	1.5 (3.5)	4.2 (3.7)	2.2 (1.1)	-0.2 (1.4)	0.9 (1.9)	1.1 (1.2)
Digestive	-3.7 (2.9)	-2.2 (1.3)	-1.4 (2.1)	-0.9 (2.8)	-0.5 (0.8)	0.5 (1.4)	0.7 (1.8)	-0.2 (0.9)
Headache/migraine	18.2 (7.2)	6.3 (3.3)	15.2 (5.2)	17.5 (8.4)	8.1 (2.1)	9.3 (2.1)	11.9 (3.9)	10.1 (2.9)
Insomnia	18.8 (4.9)	2.6 (2.6)	3.7 (4.6)	3.6 (4.9)	4.5 (1.3)	8.5 (1.3)	7.0 (2.4)	6.8 (1.5)
Neurological	3.4 (1.7)	3.8 (1.3)	3.7 (2.9)	3.4 (1.7)	1.9 (0.7)	2.2 (0.7)	0.8 (0.8)	1.9 (0.7)
Respiratory	-3.8 (2.5)	-2.7 (1.9)	-1.2 (3.6)	1.6 (5.1)	-0.9 (1.5)	0.4 (1.5)	1.1 (1.7)	-0.2 (1.3)
All mental	51.0 (5.0)	21.2 (3.2)	21.7 (4.6)	49.0 (4.8)	25.6 (2.3)	35.6 (3.0)	29.4 (3.7)	30.6 (2.3)
All physical	51.7 (7.2)	62.7 (5.0)	46.3 (9.2)	44.9 (8.8)	42.1 (4.1)	52.2 (4.1)	55.8 (5.4)	50.0 (3.4)
All disorders	84.0 (2.8)	81.0 (2.9)	70.3 (7.7)	83.2 (4.8)	62.3 (2.3)	77.9 (2.1)	80.6 (2.8)	74.3 (1.8)

High

Alcohol abuse	0.7 (0.7)	-0.6 (0.2)	-0.6 (0.4)	0.7 (1.1)	0.4 (0.3)	0.4 (0.5)	1.2 (1.0)	0.5 (0.3)
Bipolar	4.8 (1.1)	1.0 (0.4)	2.2 (0.9)	4.9 (1.4)	1.5 (0.3)	2.4 (0.5)	4.6 (1.3)	2.1 (0.4)
Drug abuse	0.8 (0.5)	0.1 (0.2)	0.2 (0.3)	1.8 (1.0)	0.5 (0.2)	0.7 (0.4)	1.1 (0.8)	0.5 (0.2)
Generalized anxiety	3.6 (1.0)	0.6 (0.5)	0.5 (0.7)	4.4 (1.3)	1.3 (0.3)	2.3 (0.6)	1.6 (1.2)	1.6 (0.4)
Major depressive disorder	16.4 (2.0)	2.9 (1.0)	1.6 (1.0)	15.8 (2.4)	6.6 (0.6)	7.8 (1.2)	12.5 (1.4)	7.5 (0.7)
Panic and/or agoraphobia	7.9 (1.3)	1.5 (0.6)	2.5 (0.6)	8.6 (1.9)	2.0 (0.4)	2.8 (0.8)	2.6 (0.8)	2.9 (0.5)
Post-traumatic stress	9.0 (1.5)	2.8 (0.6)	5.2 (0.6)	8.1 (1.7)	2.7 (0.4)	3.9 (0.8)	4.5 (0.8)	3.6 (1.6)
Social phobia	10.9 (1.5)	1.3 (0.6)	-0.4 (1.4)	10.7 (1.8)	2.2 (0.4)	6.2 (1.0)	8.1 (1.1)	3.8 (2.1)
Specific phobia	4.9 (1.8)	3.3 (1.0)	3.6 (2.2)	6.4 (2.6)	3.8 (0.8)	6.5 (1.4)	7.9 (1.3)	4.5 (2.9)
Arthritis	5.6 (2.3)	12.5 (1.9)	11.8 (4.5)	5.3 (3.1)	5.8 (1.1)	4.9 (1.8)	7.8 (1.7)	7.4 (3.4)
Cancer	1.5 (0.9)	0.9 (0.6)	1.5 (1.7)	2.5 (1.2)	1.5 (0.4)	1.4 (0.6)	0.5 (0.5)	1.3 (1.0)
Cardiovascular	4.8 (2.5)	13.1 (2.1)	13.6 (4.9)	6.5 (3.3)	7.7 (1.3)	8.7 (1.9)	9.8 (2.0)	8.8 (3.6)
Chronic pain	17.0 (3.0)	29.8 (2.0)	27.7 (4.3)	23.3 (3.6)	21.7 (1.4)	22.2 (2.0)	21.2 (2.2)	23.3 (4.0)
Diabetes	1.7 (1.0)	2.3 (0.9)	6.5 (2.2)	1.8 (1.3)	1.9 (0.5)	1.4 (0.7)	2.8 (0.8)	2.1 (1.2)
Digestive	1.7 (1.1)	3.1 (0.6)	2.3 (1.5)	4.8 (1.5)	2.3 (0.3)	2.8 (0.8)	2.3 (0.8)	2.8 (1.3)
Headache/migraine	12.8 (2.3)	1.8 (1.2)	6.6 (2.8)	6.3 (2.7)	3.9 (0.8)	8.4 (1.3)	8.8 (1.5)	5.2 (2.8)
Insomnia	7.6 (1.7)	5.9 (0.9)	7.4 (1.9)	9.4 (2.3)	3.8 (0.6)	6.6 (1.0)	10.4 (1.0)	5.6 (2.1)
Neurological	3.2 (0.8)	1.8 (0.6)	4.1 (1.3)	3.5 (1.1)	1.0 (0.2)	1.2 (0.6)	3.6 (0.7)	1.6 (1.5)
Respiratory	4.9 (2.5)	2.7 (1.3)	-0.6 (2.9)	2.5 (2.7)	2.3 (0.9)	-0.9 (1.4)	0.3 (1.5)	1.6 (2.7)
All mental	51.4 (1.9)	11.7 (1.3)	16.0 (2.5)	52.8 (2.4)	20.4 (0.9)	30.8 (1.4)	38.0 (1.5)	25.2 (2.6)
All physical	49.9 (3.5)	69.4 (2.4)	60.3 (5.9)	51.5 (3.7)	48.7 (1.6)	53.9 (2.1)	57.8 (2.2)	54.5 (3.6)
All disorders	85.6 (1.3)	75.5 (2.3)	74.2 (5.0)	85.6 (1.6)	64.6 (1.4)	75.9 (1.7)	81.0 (1.6)	72.3 (2.1)

Appendix Table 15.1 Mean squared error (MSE) and mean absolute prediction error (MAPE) for VAS scores by country income level. The WMH surveys.

| One-part models | Country income level | | | | | | | |
| | All countries | | Low/lower-middle | | Upper-middle | | High | |
	MSE	MAPE	MSE	MAPE	MSE	MAPE	MSE	MAPE
OLS	289.7	12.4	277.2	12.2	354.1	13.3	264.6	11.9
GLM constant variance, link = log	292	12.4	279.6	12.3	354.5	13.3	267.6	11.9
GLM constant variance, link = square root	290.8	12.4	278.3	12.3	354.2	13.3	266.1	11.9
GLM variance proportional to mean, link = log	292.2	12.4	279.8	12.3	354.6	13.3	267.9	12
GLM variance proportional to mean squared, link = log	292.8	12.4	280.4	12.3	355.1	13.3	268.8	12
GLM variance proportional to mean, link = square root	291	12.4	278.5	12.3	354.3	13.3	266.3	11.9
GLM variance proportional to mean squared, link = square root[a]	771.5	22	584.2	19.3	962.1	24.8	1,038.9	26.1

[a] All countries: WARNING: The relative Hessian convergence criterion of 0.1384980578 is greater than the limit of 0.0001. The convergence is questionable.
Upper-middle: WARNING: The relative Hessian convergence criterion of 0.1292119351 is greater than the limit of 0.0001. The convergence is questionable.
High: WARNING: The relative Hessian convergence criterion of 0.1219400053 is greater than the limit of 0.0001. The convergence is questionable.

Appendix Table 15.2 Model comparisons for the multivariate associations of conditions on VAS scores (Aikaike information criterion; AIC) by country income level. The WMH surveys.

| Model | Country income level | | | |
| | All countries | Low/ lower-middle | Upper-middle | High |
	AIC	AIC	AIC	AIC
Model 1[a]	455365.4	142984.3	95780.9	215949.3
Model 2[b]	455835.3	143095.8	95682.9	216343.6
Model 3[c]	455293.7	142961.5	95680.7	215935
Model 4[d]	455258.7	142955.2	95643.6	215857.6

[a] Model 1: Additive model that included a separate predictor for each disorder without interactions.
[b] Model 2: Included a series of predictors for number of conditions (e.g., one predictor for having exactly one condition, another for exactly two, etc.) without information about type of disorder.
[c] Model 3: Included 19 predictors for type of disorder and predictor dummies for number of conditions, starting with exactly 2 conditions.
[d] Model 4: Included 19 predictors for type and predictor dummies for number of conditions, starting with exactly 2 conditions and interactions of type of conditions by the number of conditions.

Appendix Table 15.3 Individual-level condition-specific estimates based on bivariate and the best-fitting multivariate model by country income level. The WMH surveys.

Disorders	All countries			Low/lower-middle			Upper-middle			High		
	Bivariate	Multivariate	Multivariate/Bivariate	Bivariate	Multivariate	Multivariate/Bivariate	Bivariate	Multivariate	Multivariate/Bivariate	Bivariate	Multivariate	Multivariate/Bivariate
Alcohol abuse	-7.3	-3.1	0.42	-7.3	-3.7	0.51	-9.9	-5.4	0.55	-6.1	-1.7	0.28
Bipolar	-16.5	-8.6	0.52	-17.5	-11.3	0.65	-15.7	-8.3	0.53	-15.7	-7.5	0.48
Drug abuse	-11.3	-4.2	0.37	-23	-13.1	0.57	-6.1	-0.4	0.06	-9.6	-3.2	0.33
Generalized anxiety	-13.6	-5.0	0.37	-13.8	-4.5	0.33	-14.0	-5.4	0.39	-12.9	-4.9	0.38
Major depressive disorder	-13.6	-7.8	0.58	-13.3	-7.6	0.57	-14.4	-8.5	0.59	-13.1	-7.8	0.59
Panic and/or agoraphobia	-16.2	-6.8	0.42	-14.0	-5.5	0.39	-18.1	-8.8	0.49	-15.8	-6.6	0.42
Post-traumatic stress	-15.1	-5.6	0.37	-15.3	-5.6	0.36	-14.7	-6.0	0.41	-14.4	-5.0	0.35
Social phobia	-12.1	-3.6	0.30	-10.1	-3.0	0.29	-14.3	-4.8	0.34	-11.3	-3.0	0.27
Specific phobia	-8.1	-2.5	0.31	-5.7	-1.2	0.20	-9.0	-2.7	0.30	-8.8	-3.1	0.35
Arthritis	-9.4	-4.8	0.51	-10.3	-5.2	0.51	-8.7	-4.4	0.50	-9.0	-4.6	0.52
Cancer	-3.6	-2.1	0.58	-7.6	-8.1	1.07	-6.1	-5.2	0.86	-3.4	-1.5	0.44
Cardiovascular	-8.2	-4.9	0.60	-7.6	-4.1	0.53	-9.8	-5.9	0.60	-7.7	-4.9	0.64
Chronic pain	-10.7	-6.4	0.60	-10.2	-5.6	0.55	-11.1	-6.2	0.56	-10.6	-6.6	0.63
Diabetes	-7.9	-5.3	0.67	-7.7	-5.4	0.71	-8.5	-5.4	0.64	-7.5	-5.1	0.68
Digestive	-9.5	-4.1	0.43	-6.3	-2.4	0.38	-8.7	-2.1	0.24	-12.7	-6.3	0.50
Headache/migraine	-10.2	-4.8	0.47	-10.5	-5.4	0.52	-10.7	-5.2	0.49	-9.3	-4.2	0.45
Insomnia	-13.1	-5.9	0.45	-14.8	-7.3	0.49	-12.2	-4.4	0.36	-12.4	-5.7	0.46
Neurological	-14.5	-9.4	0.65	-12.3	-8.8	0.71	-14.0	-7.0	0.50	-15.1	-10.5	0.70
Respiratory	-4.6	-1.6	0.34	-5.4	-2.2	0.42	-7.0	-3.1	0.44	-3.5	-0.8	0.22
Statistics												
Median			0.45			0.51			0.49			0.45
Interquartile range (IQR)			0.37–0.58			0.39–0.57			0.38–0.56			0.35–0.56

Appendix Table 16.1 Effects (direct and indirect via WHODAS) of conditions on perceived health VAS. Low/lower-middle-income countries. The WMH surveys.

| | Total effects of conditions on VAS | | Direct effects of conditions | | Indirect effects via WHODAS scales | | Percentage of indirect effects over total effects | | Indirect effects via each WHODAS dimension[a] | | | | | | | | | |
| | | | | | | | | | Cognition | | Mobility | | Role functioning | | Family burden | | Stigma | |
	Coeff	(SE)	Coeff	(SE)	Coeff	(SE)	%	(SE)	Coeff	(SE)	Coeff	(SE)	Coeff	(SE)	Coeff	(SE)	Coeff	(SE)
Alcohol abuse	-3.2*	(1.4)	-3.1*	(1.3)	-0.1	(0.4)	3.2	(12.6)	.02	(0.04)	0.15	(0.08)	-0.14	(0.19)	-0.12	(0.15)	-0.06	(0.12)
Bipolar	-10.8*	(4.0)	-7.5*	(2.6)	-3.3	(2.1)	30.6*	(12.2)	-0.43	(0.34)	-0.08	(0.26)	-1.66*	(0.82)	-0.52	(0.37)	-0.36	(0.51)
Drug abuse	-11.9*	(4.6)	-7.4	(5.1)	-4.6*	(2.1)	38.3	(23.4)	-0.57	(0.39)	-0.02	(0.33)	-1.14	(0.63)	-1.94	(1.05)	-1.12	(0.64)
Generalized anxiety	-4.9*	(2.2)	0.4	(1.0)	-5.3*	(1.3)	107.9*	(37.3)	-0.37	(0.26)	-0.61	(0.35)	-1.54*	(0.43)	-1.47*	(0.54)	-1.04*	(0.33)
Major depressive disorder	-7.8*	(0.9)	-4.8*	(0.8)	-2.9*	(0.5)	37.9*	(5.6)	-0.16	(0.10)	-0.44*	(0.18)	-0.92*	(0.18)	-0.56*	(0.15)	-0.70*	(0.18)
Panic and/or agoraphobia	-5.6*	(2.3)	-2.3	(1.7)	-3.3*	(1.1)	58.8*	(18.0)	-0.28	(0.23)	-0.25	(0.18)	-1.22*	(0.48)	-0.68*	(0.33)	-0.83*	(0.29)
Post-traumatic stress	-5.9*	(2.7)	1.3	(2.7)	-7.2*	(1.1)	122.6*	(56.0)	-0.58*	(0.22)	-1.29*	(0.38)	-2.25*	(0.56)	-1.77*	(0.46)	-1.08*	(0.41)
Social phobia	-2.6	(1.7)	-2.0	(1.2)	-0.6	(0.9)	21.6	(24.8)	-0.27	(0.22)	0.07	(0.13)	0.00	(0.29)	-0.21	(0.26)	-0.20	(0.17)
Specific phobia	-1.0	(1.1)	-1.1	(0.9)	0.1	(0.3)	-10.0	(44.3)	-0.07	(0.05)	0.16*	(0.07)	0.15	(0.12)	-0.19	(0.13)	-0.01	(0.1)
Arthritis	-6.2*	(0.8)	-4.3*	(0.7)	-1.9*	(0.3)	30.0*	(5.0)	-0.10*	(0.04)	-0.42*	(0.12)	-0.71*	(0.15)	-0.35*	(0.10)	-0.26*	(0.11)
Cancer	-8.8*	(4.1)	-5.3	(3.9)	-3.5*	(1.6)	39.4	(21.7)	0.04	(0.07)	-0.81	(0.51)	-1.42*	(0.61)	-0.45	(0.31)	-0.58	(0.4)
Cardiovascular	-4.9*	(0.8)	-3.0*	(0.7)	-2.0*	(0.3)	39.9*	(6.6)	-0.05	(0.05)	-0.39*	(0.11)	-0.71*	(0.12)	-0.36*	(0.10)	-0.43*	(0.12)
Chronic pain	-5.9*	(0.6)	-4.7*	(0.6)	-1.2*	(0.2)	20.5*	(2.9)	-0.03	(0.02)	-0.19*	(0.06)	-0.48*	(0.09)	-0.20*	(0.06)	-0.30*	(0.08)
Diabetes	-6.4*	(1.4)	-3.9*	(1.3)	-2.5*	(0.6)	38.7*	(9.7)	-0.21	(0.11)	-0.26	(0.14)	-0.86*	(0.24)	-0.70*	(0.25)	-0.38*	(0.15)
Digestive	-2.0*	(0.8)	-2.9*	(0.7)	0.8*	(0.3)	-40.8	(24.8)	.07	(0.05)	0.23*	(0.07)	0.24	(0.14)	0.11	(0.11)	0.14	(0.09)
Headache /migraine	-5.8*	(0.7)	-3.4*	(0.6)	-2.4*	(0.3)	41.5	(5.3)	-0.19*	(0.09)	-0.22*	(0.08)	-0.91*	(0.13)	-0.54*	(0.13)	-0.46*	(0.13)
Insomnia	-7.8*	(1.3)	-3.9*	(1.2)	-3.9*	(0.6)	50.4*	(8.5)	-0.16	(0.10)	-0.49*	(0.17)	-1.64*	(0.29)	-0.78*	(0.23)	-0.81*	(0.2)
Neurological	-8.9*	(2.3)	-4.0*	(1.8)	-5.0*	(1.3)	55.6*	(12.5)	-0.21	(0.17)	-0.58	(0.34)	-1.43*	(0.57)	-1.26*	(0.40)	-1.38*	(0.51)
Respiratory	-2.5*	(0.6)	-1.5*	(0.6)	-1.0*	(0.3)	40.2*	(11.4)	-0.02	(0.03)	-0.16*	(0.07)	-0.47*	(0.13)	-0.21*	(0.10)	-0.12	(0.07)

Direct effects of scales

Cognition: -0.14 (0.06)* Mobility: -0.14 (0.03)* Self-care: -0.06 (0.04) Getting along: -0.03 (0.05)
Role functioning: -0.13 (0.01)* Family burden: -0.15 (0.03)* Stigma: -0.1 (0.02)* Discrimination: 0.02 (0.03)

[a] Only dimensions with statistically significant direct effect are included. Self-care, Getting along, and Discrimination not statistically significant.
* Significant at the 0.05 level, two-sided test.

Appendix Table 16.2 Effects (direct and indirect via WHODAS) of conditions on perceived health VAS. Upper-middle-income countries. The WMH surveys.

| | Total effects of conditions on VAS | | Direct effects of conditions | | Indirect effects via WHODAS scales | | Percentage of indirect effects over total effects | | Indirect effects via each WHODAS dimension[a] | | | | | | | |
| | | | | | | | | | Mobility | | Role functioning | | Family burden | | Stigma | |
	Coeff	(SE)	Coeff	(SE)	Coeff	(SE)	%	(SE)	Coeff	(SE)	Coeff	(SE)	Coeff	(SE)	Coeff	(SE)
Alcohol abuse	−5.9*	(2.5)	−5.1*	(2.4)	−0.8	(0.5)	13.9	(9.6)	0.15	(0.11)	−0.26	(0.15)	−0.20	(0.14)	−0.45	(0.26)
Bipolar	−6.5*	(2.2)	−2.6	(2.1)	−3.9*	(1.0)	60.3*	(21.1)	0.02	(0.11)	−0.63*	(0.24)	−1.32*	(0.40)	−1.83*	(0.57)
Drug abuse	−0.3	(3.8)	0.2	(3.3)	−0.4	(0.9)	163.2	(2253.9)	−0.03	(0.26)	−0.02	(0.25)	−0.12	(0.21)	−0.26	(0.43)
Generalized anxiety	−5.6*	(2.3)	−3.8	(2.3)	−1.9*	(0.9)	33.2	(17.8)	−0.38	(0.20)	−0.56*	(0.26)	−0.30	(0.20)	−0.59	(0.43)
Major depressive disorder	−8.3*	(1.0)	−4.8*	(1.0)	−3.5*	(0.4)	42.0*	(6.4)	−0.48*	(1.13)	−0.92*	(0.22)	−0.73*	(0.21)	−1.21*	(0.27)
Panic and/or agoraphobia	−7.8*	(1.8)	−3.8*	(1.9)	−4.0*	(0.9)	51.5*	(14.5)	−0.31	(0.20)	−0.74*	(0.22)	−1.05*	(0.35)	−1.81*	(0.54)
Post-traumatic stress	−5.2*	(2.4)	−2.0	(2.1)	−3.2*	(1.1)	61.1*	(25.5)	−0.55	(0.34)	−0.56	(0.30)	−0.59*	(0.27)	−1.42*	(0.42)
Social phobia	−5.0*	(1.7)	−3.2*	(1.6)	−1.8*	(0.7)	36.8*	(15.4)	−0.15	(0.18)	−0.46*	(0.22)	−0.38*	(0.18)	−0.83*	(0.37)
Specific phobia	−2.7*	(0.9)	−1.9*	(0.8)	−0.8*	(0.4)	29.7*	(12.9)	−0.09	(0.11)	−0.21*	(0.10)	−0.16	(0.11)	−0.32*	(0.15)
Arthritis	−5.7*	(0.8)	−3.5*	(0.8)	−2.2*	(0.3)	37.9*	(6.2)	−0.42*	(0.10)	−0.32*	(0.08)	−0.36*	(0.10)	−1.01*	(0.18)
Cancer	−4.9	(2.9)	−2.7	(2.2)	−2.3*	(1.1)	45.7*	(18.0)	−0.73	(0.42)	−0.55	(0.36)	−0.44	(0.33)	−0.53	(0.47)
Cardiovascular	−7.3*	(0.7)	−5.2*	(0.8)	−2.0*	(0.2)	28.0*	(4.1)	−0.39*	(0.09)	−0.51*	(0.10)	−0.37*	(0.11)	−0.73*	(0.18)
Chronic pain	−6.9*	(0.8)	−5.0*	(0.7)	−1.9*	(0.3)	27.2*	(3.7)	−0.56*	(0.13)	−0.50*	(0.11)	−0.21*	(0.08)	−0.58*	(0.15)
Diabetes	−5.5*	(1.5)	−4.5*	(1.4)	−1.0*	(0.5)	18.7*	(7.3)	−0.38*	(0.18)	−0.38*	(0.14)	−0.07	(0.10)	−0.23	(0.20)
Digestive	−1.8	(1.2)	−1.2	(1.3)	−0.6	(0.5)	32.9	(32.7)	0.07	(0.13)	−0.12	(0.13)	−0.12	(0.14)	−0.41	(0.24)
Headache/migraine	−5.0*	(0.7)	−4.2*	(0.7)	−0.8*	(0.3)	16.7*	(4.9)	−0.05	(0.07)	−0.18*	(0.08)	−0.14*	(0.07)	−0.43*	(0.13)
Insomnia	−4.4*	(1.2)	−3.2*	(1.1)	−1.1*	(0.4)	25.9*	(9.2)	−0.02	(0.09)	−0.15	(0.09)	−0.36*	(0.13)	−0.49*	(0.22)
Neurological	−6.9*	(2.6)	−2.9	(2.4)	−4.0*	(1.0)	58.5*	(21.1)	−1.24*	(0.48)	−1.1*	(0.20)	−0.78*	(0.33)	−0.89	(0.47)
Respiratory	−3.1*	(1.0)	−3.3*	(0.9)	0.2	(0.2)	−7.2	(8.8)	0.12	(0.08)	0.10	(0.00)	0.01	(0.05)	0.00	(0.11)

Direct effects of scales   Cognition: −0.02 (0.07) Mobility: −0.16 (0.03)* Self-care: 0.01 (0.05) Getting along: 0.02 (0.07)
Role functioning: −0.08 (0.01)* Family burden: −0.1 (0.03)* Stigma: −0.16 (0.03)* Discrimination: −0.02 (0.03)

[a] Only dimensions with statistically significant direct effect are included. Cognition, Self-care, Getting along, and Discrimination not statistically significant.

* Significant at the 0.05 level, two-sided test.

Appendix Table 16.3 Effects (direct and indirect via WHODAS) of conditions on perceived health VAS. High-income countries. The WMH surveys.

	Total effects of conditions on VAS		Direct effects of conditions on VAS		Indirect effects via WHODAS scales		Percentage of indirect effects over total effects		Indirect effects via each WHODAS dimension[a]											
									Cognition		Mobility		Self-care		Role functioning		Family burden		Stigma	
	Coeff	(SE)	Coeff	(SE)	Coeff	(SE)	%	(SE)	Coeff	(SE)	Coeff	(SE)	Coeff	(SE)	Coeff	(SE)	Coeff	(SE)	Coeff	(SE)
Alcohol abuse	-1.5	(0.8)	-1.8*	(0.7)	0.3	(0.3)	-23.0	(31.9)	0.01	(0.04)	0.38*	(0.09)	0.05*	(0.03)	-0.13	(0.17)	0.04	(0.08)	-0.03	(0.09)
Bipolar	-7.6*	(1.5)	-3.6*	(1.2)	-4.0*	(1.0)	52.4*	(11.1)	-0.64*	(0.19)	-0.40	(0.26)	-0.11	(0.08)	-1.3*	(0.33)	-0.64*	(0.23)	-0.61*	(0.21)
Drug abuse	-2.6	(1.5)	-2.8	(1.3)	0.2	(0.6)	-8.9	(28.3)	0.00	(0.00)	0.30*	(0.11)	0.01	(0.00)	-0.11	(0.29)	-0.03	(0.15)	0.13	(0.14)
Generalized anxiety	-5.2*	(1.1)	-2.4*	(0.9)	-2.8*	(0.7)	54.1*	(11.1)	-0.35*	(0.11)	-0.37	(0.20)	-0.02	(0.03)	-0.93*	(0.27)	-0.56*	(0.16)	-0.46*	(0.15)
Major depressive disorder	-8.3*	(0.5)	-5.5*	(0.5)	-2.8*	(0.3)	34.0*	(3.4)	-0.38*	(0.09)	-0.19*	(0.09)	-0.02	(0.02)	-1.18*	(0.13)	-0.44*	(0.09)	-0.49*	(0.10)
Panic and/or agoraphobia	-6.1*	(1.0)	-2.9*	(0.9)	-3.2*	(0.6)	52.0*	(9.4)	-0.46*	(0.12)	-0.47*	(0.16)	-0.09	(0.06)	-1.11*	(0.22)	-0.41*	(0.13)	-0.53*	(0.15)
Post-traumatic stress	-4.9*	(1.0)	-1.0	(0.8)	-3.9*	(0.8)	80.4*	(14.7)	-0.59*	(0.17)	-0.60*	(0.21)	-0.09	(0.07)	-1.46*	(0.28)	-0.58*	(0.18)	-0.47*	(0.16)
Social phobia	-2.4*	(0.8)	-1.5	(0.8)	-1.0*	(0.4)	39.3*	(16.6)	-0.25*	(0.08)	0.06	(0.09)	0.05	(0.03)	-0.28*	(0.12)	-0.26*	(0.10)	-0.22*	(0.09)
Specific phobia	-2.8*	(0.6)	-1.8*	(0.6)	-0.9*	(0.4)	33.5*	(12.3)	0.00	(0.00)	-0.09	(0.11)	0.00	(0.02)	-0.46*	(0.16)	-0.20*	(0.08)	-0.15*	(0.07)
Arthritis	-4.9*	(0.5)	-2.8*	(0.4)	-2.1*	(0.2)	42.6*	(4.2)	-0.05*	(0.02)	-0.87*	(0.10)	-0.08*	(0.04)	-0.70*	(0.11)	-0.14*	(0.04)	-0.23*	(0.05)
Cancer	-1.9*	(0.9)	-0.2	(0.8)	-1.7*	(0.4)	90.6*	(38.9)	-0.11	(0.06)	-0.40	(0.16)	-0.03	(0.03)	-0.73*	(0.17)	-0.29*	(0.09)	-0.13	(0.07)
Cardiovascular	-5.5*	(0.4)	-3.2*	(0.4)	-2.3*	(0.2)	42.6*	(4.1)	-0.10*	(0.03)	-0.86*	(0.11)	-0.10	(0.06)	-0.70*	(0.10)	-0.28*	(0.07)	-0.25*	(0.05)
Chronic pain	-6.7*	(0.4)	-3.3*	(0.3)	-3.4*	(0.2)	50.5*	(3.0)	-0.12*	(0.03)	-0.97*	(0.11)	-0.08*	(0.03)	-1.41*	(0.12)	-0.38*	(0.07)	-0.36*	(0.07)
Diabetes	-5.7*	(0.8)	-3.4*	(0.7)	-2.3*	(0.4)	39.9*	(6.4)	-0.11*	(0.04)	-0.72*	(0.16)	-0.10*	(0.04)	-0.92*	(0.18)	-0.18*	(0.07)	-0.19*	(0.07)
Digestive	-7.0*	(1.1)	-3.0*	(1.0)	-3.9*	(0.5)	56.4*	(8.3)	-0.12*	(0.06)	-1.05*	(0.20)	-0.09	(0.05)	-1.47*	(0.23)	-0.52*	(0.14)	-0.57*	(0.14)
Headache/migraine	-4.1*	(0.5)	-2.6*	(0.4)	-1.5*	(0.2)	36.4*	(4.9)	-0.16*	(0.04)	-0.14	(0.07)	-0.03	(0.02)	-0.61*	(0.10)	-0.30*	(0.06)	-0.20*	(0.05)
Insomnia	-6.2*	(0.6)	-2.8*	(0.6)	-3.4*	(0.3)	54.9*	(5.5)	-0.25*	(0.06)	-0.85*	(0.13)	-0.11*	(0.05)	-1.13*	(0.15)	-0.52*	(0.11)	-0.40*	(0.10)
Neurological	-11.3*	(1.4)	-4.7*	(1.2)	-6.5*	(1.3)	58.1*	(9.1)	-0.59*	(0.17)	-2.02*	(0.48)	-0.39	(0.21)	-1.75*	(0.39)	-0.65*	(0.24)	-0.84*	(0.26)
Respiratory	-0.6	(0.4)	-0.5	(0.3)	-0.1	(0.1)	12.5	(21.2)	-0.03	(0.02)	-0.04	(0.05)	0.01	(0.01)	-0.08	(0.06)	0.03	(0.03)	0.02	(0.02)
Direct effects of scales																				

Cognition: -0.15 (0.03)* Mobility: -0.17 (0.02)* Self-care: -0.06 (0.03)* Getting along: -0.02 (0.03)
Role functioning: -0.13 (0.01)* Family burden: -0.1 (0.02)* Stigma: -0.1 (0.02)* Discrimination: -0.04 (0.02)

[a] Only dimensions with statistically significant direct effect are included. Getting along and discrimination not statistically significant.
* Significant at the 0.05 level, two-sided test.

Index